# Basic Science in Gastroenterology

## Structure of the Gut

*Edited by:* J M Polak, S R Bloom, N A Wright, M J Daly

Glaxo Group Research Limited

Royal Postgraduate Medical School

GLAXO GROUP RESEARCH LIMITED
Ware, Herts, UK.

First published 1982

*Acknowledgements*
This volume has been prepared from published supplements to the Scandinavian Journal of Gastroenterology and the cooperation of Universitetsforlaget in facilitating the preparation of this volume is gratefully acknowledged.

Cloth bound ISBN 0 9500593 2 3
Limp bound ISBN 0 9500593 3 1

Printed in England by Page Bros (Norwich) Ltd

# Contents

## Section 1. Electronmicroscopy of the Gastrointestinal Tract

## Section 2. Autonomic Nerves of the Gut

# Section 3.   Adaptation

# Preface

The Royal Postgraduate Medical School has long had an interest in the basic science of various scientific disciplines. It was perhaps inevitable that a series of publications on basic science in gastroenterology should occur. It has therefore been fortunate that Glaxo Group Research Limited had the same interest and was willing to support such a venture. This project has proved to be a fruitful example of cooperation between Academia and Industry. The Editors are firmly of the opinion that the time is long past when university and industry can remain aloof and isolated. Multidisciplinary cooperation is now the order of the day for successful progress.

*J. M. Polak, S. R. Bloom, N. A. Wright, M. J. Daly*

*Section 1*

Electronmicroscopy of the Gastrointestinal Tract

# Ultrastructural Identification of Neurotransmitters

G. BURNSTOCK
Dept. of Anatomy & Embryology, and Centre for Neuroscience, University College London,
Gower Street, London WC1E 6BT, UK

It is apparent that the correlations made between intra-axonal vesicle types and the transmitters in cholinergic, adrenergic and non-adrenergic, non-cholinergic nerves in the early 1970's are too simplistic. The current proposals for 16 or more putative transmitters in the enteric nervous system and the additional possibility of co-existence of two or more transmitters within single nerve terminals, clearly complicate the issue. We must await preparative procedures that will lead to high quality electron-micrographs of nerve profiles following the application of specific cytochemical reactions for putative transmitters and associated enzymes before the problem will be resolved.

*Key-words:* Electronmicroscopy, neurotransmitters, gut, vesicles, autonomic.

*G. Burnstock, Dept. of Anatomy & Embryology and Centre for Neuroscience, University College London, Gower Street, London WC1E 6BT, UK*

## I. INTRODUCTION

The classical picture of the innervation of the gut is one of intramural cholinergic excitatory neurones controlled by preganglionic cholinergic vagal and sacral parasympathetic fibres, opposed by postganglionic sympathetic adrenergic inhibitory fibres (Fig. 1A).

Two findings in the early 1960's made it necessary to revise this picture (Fig. 1B). Firstly, the application of the fluorescence histochemical method for localising catecholamines showed that the terminal varicosities of the majority of adrenergic fibres were localised in Auerbach's and Meissner's plexuses and only supplied the smooth muscle of limited areas of the circular muscle coat (11). The second discovery was the demonstration of powerful nonadrenergic, noncholinergic inhibitory nerves supplying the smooth muscle of the gastrointestinal tract (4). These nerves are concerned with the propulsion of material through the alimentary canal, and are involved in reflex opening of sphincters, 'receptive relaxation' of the stomach and 'descending inhibition' during peristalsis, whereas the main role of adrenergic nerves is to modulate these activities mostly at the ganglion level (10).

In the early 1970's the ultrastructural identification of these three nerve components seemed clear and easily distinguishable from each other and from sensory nerve components (14). Cholinergic nerves contained a predominance of small agranular vesicles (45–60 nm in diameter) and a few large granular vesicles (Fig. 2A); adrenergic nerves contained a predominance of small granular vesicles (45–60 nm) together with some large granular vesicles (Fig. 2B), both vesicle types being 'loaded' and later destroyed by 6-hydroxy-dopamine (6-OHDA), while non-adrenergic, non-cholinergic nerves contained a predominance of vesicles termed either 'large opaque vesicles' (Fig. 2E) by Burnstock and his colleagues (55) or 'p-type' vesicles by Baumgarten's group (1). Sensory nerve terminals were characterised by many small vesicles (Fig. 2G).

Five criteria are generally regarded as necessary for establishing a substance as a neurotransmitter, namely: 1) synthesis and storage of transmitter in nerve terminals; 2) release of transmitter during nerve stimulation; 3) postjunctional responses to exogenous transmitter that mimic responses to nerve stimulation; 4) enzymes that inactivate the transmitter and/or an uptake system for the transmitter or its breakdown products; 5) drugs that produce parallel blocking or potentiating effects on the responses by both exogenous transmitter and nerve stimulation. In experiments designed to identify the transmitter in intramural nonad-

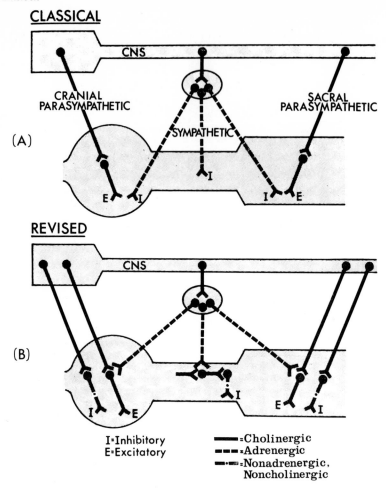

Fig. 1. Diagrammatic representation of the innervation of the gut, showing the classical picture and a revised picture. Modified from Burnstock (5).

Table I. Transmitters proposed in the autonomic nervous system

| | |
|---|---|
| Acetylcholine | ACh |
| Noradrenaline | NA |
| Adenosine Triphosphate | ATP |
| 5-Hydroxytryptamine | 5-HT |
| γ-Aminobutyric Acid | GABA |
| Dopamine | DA |
| Peptides: | |
| Enkephalin | Enk |
| Vasoactive Intestinal Polypeptide | VIP |
| Substance P | Sub P |
| Bombesin | Bom B |
| Somatostatin | ST |
| Neurotensin | NT |
| Luteinizing Hormone Releasing Hormone | LHRH |
| Cholecystokinin/Gastrin | CCK/G |
| Pancreatic Polypeptide | PP |
| (Bradykinin) | BK |
| Angiotensin | AII |
| Adrenocorticotrophic Hormone | ACTH |

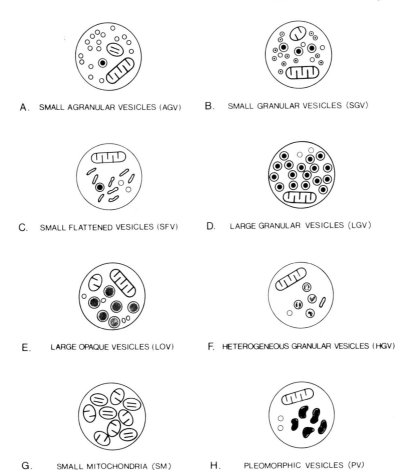

A. SMALL AGRANULAR VESICLES (AGV)    B. SMALL GRANULAR VESICLES (SGV)

C. SMALL FLATTENED VESICLES (SFV)    D. LARGE GRANULAR VESICLES (LGV)

E. LARGE OPAQUE VESICLES (LOV)    F. HETEROGENEOUS GRANULAR VESICLES (HGV)

G. SMALL MITOCHONDRIA (SM)    H. PLEOMORPHIC VESICLES (PV)

Fig. 2. Diagrammatic representation of the ultrastructure of the main nerve profiles in the gastrointestinal tract. The name given to each profile is based on the characteristic structure of the predominant vesicle type within that profile. Mitochondria are drawn in every profile.

renergic, noncholinergic inhibitory nerves supplying the gastrointestinal smooth muscle, a purine nucleotide, probably ATP, appeared to satisfy these criteria best, so these nerves were termed 'purinergic' (5). In more recent years with the application of immunohistochemistry and autoradiographic methods together with pharmacological studies, over 16 putative neurotransmitters have been postulated in enteric nerves (see Table I).

Six to nine ultrastucturally distinguishable nerve profile types in the gastrointestinal tract have now been claimed (18, 24, 27) and the task we face is to see if any relation exists between these ultrastuctural profiles and the different putative transmitters. The solution to this problem depends on the development of highly specific cytochemical methods that give sufficient resolution at the electron microscopic level. The question is compounded by the possibility that more than one transmitter substance may co-exist in some nerve fibres (6, 8, 13, 37), by the different appearance of vesicles in tissues prepared with different fixatives and the lack of homogeneity of intra-axonal content along the length of individual nerve fibres.

## II. ULTRASTRUCTURAL CHARACTER-ISTICS OF DIFFERENT NERVE PROFILES IN THE ENTERIC PLEXUSES

The enteric nervous system extends throughout the length of the gastrointestinal tract and consists of two ganglionated plexuses, the myenteric (or Auerbach's) plexus which is situated between the two external muscle coats and the submucous (or Meissner's) plexus which lies in the submucosa. Nerve fibres pass between the two plexuses as well as to and from the mucosa and serosa; fibres also reach them from the extrinsic sympathetic and parasympathetic nerve trunks (27).

In general, the ganglia of the myenteric plexus are larger than those of the submucous plexus, consisting of up to about 50 neurones which are packed tightly together with glial cells and a dense neuropil. However, as for the central nervous system but not sympathetic or parasympathetic ganglia, there is no connective tissue, basal lamina or blood vessel within them. 'Interstitial cells' form a more or less continuous sheath around the ganglia and large interconnecting strands. The neurones contained in the enteric ganglia are partly derived from special neural crest tissue and partly from that associated with the development of the parasympathetic system (45, 48). Some of the intermural neurones, particularly those in the submucous plexus, appear to be sensory, but many other afferent fibres in the gut are of extrinsic origin.

Nerve cell bodies in the myenteric plexus of the guinea-pig were tentatively classified by Cook & Burnstock (18) into nine different types according to their size, distribution of organelles, and location and relation to satellite cells but, since no progress has been made to date in relating these cell body ultrastructures to transmitter types, they will not be discussed in this article. What will now be described are the various types of axon profile that have been observed within the enteric plexuses, musculature and mucosa of the gastrointestinal tract of various mammalian species (1, 15, 18, 24, 26, 42).

### A. *Small agranular vesicles* (AGV)

Nerve profiles containing predominantly small agranular vesicles (45–60 nm in diameter) form over 50% of the total number of nerves present (Fig. 2A). A few (<5%) large granular vesicles (80–120 nm diameter) are usually also present.

### B. *Small granular vesicles* (SGV)

These profiles contain a predominance of small granular vesicles (45–70 nm diameter) (Fig. 2B). The core varies from a small central or eccentrically placed dot to a dark core occupying most of the vesicle, but the appearance varies considerably with different fixation procedures. Some large granular vesicles (<10%), as well as a few AGV and small flattened vesicles, are often also present.

### C. *Small flattened vesicles* (SFV)

These nerve profiles are characterised by a predominance of flattened vesicles (30–40 × 60–80 nm) together with a variable mixture of AGV and large granular vesicles (Fig. 2C).

### D. *Large granular vesicles* (LGV).

Many of these profiles contain only LGV (80–120 nm diameter), but some also contain a few AGV (Fig. 2D). The LGV generally have a dense granular core with a clear halo between the core and the vesicle membrane.

### E. *Large opaque vesicle* (LOV).

Profiles containing LOV can be clearly distinguished from those containing LGV (Fig. 2E). The vesicle is larger (80–180 nm), the core is usually less electron dense and the halo is indistinct. Some AGV are often also present.

### F. *Heterogenous granular vesicles* (HGV).

These profiles are characterised by granular vesicles (70–140 nm diameter) with cores that usually display an uneven granulated structure and a halo is rarely distinguishable (Fig. 2F). Sometimes the limiting vesicle membranes appear incomplete. Some AGV and SFV are often present.

### G. *Small mitochondria* (SM).

Axon profiles containing tightly packed clusters of small mitochondria have been described but appear to be relatively rare in the gut (Fig. 2G).

These profiles sometimes contain some small round profiles and may then be difficult to distinguish from profiles containing predominantly AGV.

## H. *Pleomorphic vesicles* (PV).

Profiles containing granular vesicles with irregular shape and sizes (70 to 300 nm) are present in some regions of the gut (Fig. 2H). The core is dense and finely granular and always surrounded by a narrow halo. A few AGV are sometimes present.

## I. *Other nerve profiles*

Several other types of nerve profiles have been described in the gut, but they are rare and it seems likely that they represent nerves either in the process of development or degeneration. These include profiles containing many lysosomes and dense bodies (18), profiles containing elongated tubular structures (18, 42), profiles with dense cytoplasm (24), and profiles packed with glycogen granules (18).

## III. LOCALISATION OF DIFFERENT NEUROTRANSMITTERS

The application at the electron microscope level of specific histochemical methods for localising different transmitters or associated synthesising or degrading enzymes is at a preliminary stage, but the results offer some possibilities for relating the types of profile described in Section II to the various transmitters claimed to be present in the gut.

## A. *Cholinergic nerves*

There is abundant pharmacological evidence for the presence of intramural cholinergic excitatory neurones in the gut (43). Profiles containing a predominance of AGV resemble the structure of established cholinergic nerve terminals of motor nerves in skeletal muscle and those in sympathetic ganglia or adrenal medulla. Many neurones in the myenteric and submucous plexuses stain intensely for acetylcholinesterase (32, 60), but unfortunately, a positive reaction for this enzyme is not invariably indicative of a chol-

inergic neuron (54) and there is a wide variation in intensity of staining within ganglia and between species. Furthermore, it has been shown recently that acetylcholinesterase not only degrades acetylcholine, but also substance P (17). Although a histochemical method for localising choline acetyltransferase has been applied with some success to cholinergic motor nerves (41) the activity of this enzyme in autonomic cholinergic nerves appears to be too low to allow histochemical localisation (8). Another complication is that it has been claimed that some 5-hydroxytryptamine-containing neurones (50) and some enkephalin-containing neurones (2) in the central nervous system also contain a predominance of AGV.

## B. *Noradrenergic nerves*

Postganglionic sympathetic noradrenergic nerves have been shown, using the Falck/Hillarp fluorescence histochemical method, to ramify extensively amongst nerve cell bodies in both myenteric and submucous plexuses as well as supply the circular muscle coat on some regions of the gut, particularly the sphincters (11). Some also supply arterioles and the mucosa. They produce inhibitory modulation of excitatory responses of the gut largely at the ganglion level, but can also affect smooth muscle when stimulated at high frequencies.

There is some controversy about the ultrastructural appearance of noradrenergic neurones in the gut. Profiles containing SFV (42, 46) and those containing LGV (1, 18) have been claimed to contain noradrenaline, as well as those characteristic of adrenergic nerves in other organs that contain a predominance of SGV. One reason for the confusion is that 'false transmitters' like 5-hydroxydopamine and 6-hydroxydopamine that 'load' adrenergic terminals, and 6-hydroxydopamine that later destroys adrenergic nerves in other organs (11), consistently fails to do this to SGV-type nerve profiles in the gut (23, 24, 31), and it has been suggested that these profiles might contain a different transmitter (intramural adrenergic neurones have been found only in the proximal colon of the guinea-pig). There is also a poor correspondence between the distribution

of autoradiographically-localised ³H-noradrena-
line and profiles containing SGV (27).

In contrast, SFV stain particularly well with the
chromaffin reaction (42) which has been claimed
to be specific for catecholamines (61). Adrenergic
fibres in the anococcygeus which contain SFV
have also been described (30). A few neurones
in the stomach show immunoreactivity for
dopamine-β-hydroxylase (57), but these have not
been identified yet at the electron microscope
level.

## C. *Purinergic neurones*

Since ATP was the only serious contender for
non-adrenergic, non-cholinergic nerves in the gut
until the mid-1970's, it was natural to relate profiles containing LOV to these nerves (5), but
direct evidence for this correlation is lacking.
However, preliminary autoradiographic studies
in gut preparations incubated in low concentrations of ³H-adenosine for short periods of less
than a minute show silver grains related to profiles
with LOV (Dennison and Burnstock, unpublished results). There is also evidence to suggest
that cells and nerves that are known to contain
high levels of ATP show fluorescence with quin-
acrine and contain LOV (19, 49).

The uranaffin reaction which has been claimed
to stain specifically for ATP associated with LOV
in platelets (53) stains a population of non-adrenergic neurones in the gut containing a mixture
of AGV and LGV (63) but it is not clear yet
whether uranaffin is specifically staining purinergic nerves or picking up non-specific phos-
phatases. It has also been suggested recently that
non-adrenergic (purinergic) inhibitory nerves
supplying gut muscle are a sub-category of 'p-
type' nerve endings containing vesicles 90–120 nm
in diameter (15).

## D.    5-*Hydroxytryptamine    (5-HT)-containing*
*nerves*

There is good evidence for the presence in the
gut of intramural 5-HT-containing neurones (or
amine-handling neurones as they are sometimes
called) (24, 28, 64). Neurones showing tryptophan hydroxylase-like immunoreactivity have
been    demonstrated    in    the    gut    (29).

Radioactive-labelled 5-HT has been shown to be
taken up by some enteric neurones by autoradiography (21). The labelled axons contained LGV,
(65–100 nm in diameter), although some AGV
were also present.

## E. *Peptide-containing nerves*

A variety of peptides have now been localised
in enteric nerves with immunocytochemical methods (37). Few studies have been carried out on
the immunoelectronmicroscopy of these nerves
and the results are not yet clear. Larsson (44)
claimed that VIP-containing nerves contain large
vesicles (70–160 nm in diameter), but it was not
clear whether these were LGV, HGV or LOV.
Axon profiles containing both large and small
vesicles were claimed to show immunostaining
for enkephalin in sympathetic ganglia (33). Most
recently, Polak and her colleagues (52) have
demonstrated LGV in substance-P-containing
nerves. Hopefully, this approach will be extended
to other peptides shortly.

## F. *Gamma-aminobutyric acid (GABA)-contain-*
*ing nerves*

Neurones that synthesise and take up GABA
have been shown in about 3–5% of the cells in
the myenteric plexus with autoradiographic methods, but none have been demonstrated in the
submucous plexus (40). No studies have been
carried out to date on the fine structure of nerve
varicosities that are related to silver grains following incubation in ³H-GABA. It is interesting,
however, that in the mammalian CNS, GABA
has been associated with SFV (39, 62).

## IV. CO-EXISTENCE OF TRANSMITTERS

The universality of the concept that one nerve
fibre contains only one transmitter, that has come
to be known as Dale's Principle, has been questioned in recent years (6, 7, 16, 37). Thus it seems
likely that nerve fibres containing more than one
transmitter in variable proportions will contain
mixtures of vesicle types (see for example Fig. 3).

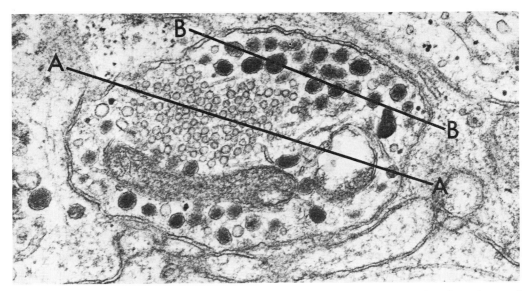

Fig. 3. A nerve profile from guinea-pig ileum illustrating a possible morphological expression of co-existence of transmitters in one nerve fibre (from Cook & Burnstock (18) with permission of the publishers).

A. *Acetylcholine with noradrenaline.*

In the adult animal, there are both structural and pharmacological indications that the distinction between adrenergic and cholinergic neurones in some organs of some species is not as rigid as previously supposed (3, 7). For example, nerves that are characterised as adrenergic because of a predominance of small granular vesicles may stain heavily for acetylcholinesterase. Conversely, sympathectomy with guanethidine destroys adrenergic neurones, but also reveals a weak amine uptake mechanism in adult cholinergic sympathetic neurones. Some sympathetic nerves in lower vertebrates appear to exhibit a combination of pharmacological and morphological characteristics of adrenergic and cholinergic nerves, both of which are abolished by 6-hydroxydopamine.

There is compelling evidence that under certain conditions *in vitro* a single sympathetic neurone may at different times release noradrenaline and acetylcholine (ACh) or a mixture of these two transmitter substances (25). It seems likely that this represents a true reflection of events that occur *in vivo* during perinatal development (34). Under the influence of conditioning factors, most of the cells appear to differentiate into either cholinergic or adrenergic neurones. The cells differentiating into cholinergic neurones gradually lose their ability to synthesise tyrosine hydroxylase, their ability to take up catecholamines is reduced, and they become unresponsive to NGF, while those differentiating into adrenergic neurones lose their ability to synthesise choline acetyltransferase. However, it is possible that some sympathetic neurones, supplying some organs in some animals, retain the ability to produce and release both ACh and noradrenaline (7).

B. *ATP with noradrenaline or acetylcholine*

ATP is found stored together with noradrenaline or ACh in autonomic nerve terminals, probably in vesicles. It is released together with catecholamines from adrenal medullary vesicles in perfused adrenal glands and it seems likely that ATP is released together with noradrenaline from some adrenergic nerves (9, 12, 22).

ATP is found together with ACh in synaptic vesicles of cholinergic nerves supplying the electric organ of *Torpedo* (20, 38). It has been shown that ATP is released together with ACh from phrenic nerves in the rat diaphragm (58, 59).

## C. Polypeptides with other transmitters

Certain peripheral endocrine cells, particularly those located in the gastrointestinal tract, contain both a biogenic amine, such as 5-HT or histamine, and a peptide hormone, such as substance P, somatostatin, or neurotensin; these cell systems are part of the so-called APUD ('Amine content or Precursor Uptake Decarboxylation') system (51).

Pearse (51) has postulated that this situation may also exist in neurones. In the peripheral nervous system, somatostatin-like immunoreactivity has been observed in about 60–70% of all principal adrenergic ganglion cells of the inferior mesenteric ganglion and of the coeliac superior mesenteric ganglion complex (35), suggesting the co-existence of noradrenaline and somatostatin, or a structurally related peptide, in the same peripheral neurone. In the superior cervical ganglion of the rat, enkephalin-like immunoreactivity has been observed in a rather small proportion of ganglion cells, at least some of which contain noradrenaline (56). Lundberg and co-workers (47) have discovered a further example: by combining immunocytochemistry and AChE staining, it was shown that the AChE-rich cells of the cat sympathetic ganglia contain a VIP-like peptide. Examples have also been observed in the C.N.S. In the lower brain stem, substance P-like immunoreactivity has been observed in 5-HT-containing neurones (16, 36).

## REFERENCES

1. Baumgarten, H. G., Holstein, A. F. & Owman, C. H. *Z. Zellforsch.* 1970, *106*, 376–397
2. Beauvillain, J. C., Tramu, G. & Croix D. *Neuroscience* 1980, *5*, 1705–1716
3. Burn, J. H. & Rand, M. J. *Ann. Rev. Pharmacol.* 1965, *5*, 163–182
4. Burnstock, G. *Pharmacol. Rev.* 1969, *21*, 247–324
5. Burnstock, G. *Pharmacol. Rev.* 1972, *24*, 509–581
6. Burnstock, G. *Neuroscience* 1976, *1*, 239–248
7. Burnstock, G. *Prog. Neurobiol.* 1978, *11*, 205–222
8. Burnstock, G. *Prog. Brain Res.* 1979, *49*, 3–21
9. Burnstock, G. *J. Physiol.* (Lond.) 1981, *313*, 1–35.
10. Burnstock, G & Costa, M. *Gastroenterol.* 1973, *64*, 141–144
11. Burnstock, G. & Costa, M. in *Adrenergic Neurons: Their Organisation, Function and Development in the Peripheral Nervous System,* Chapman and Hall, London, 1975
12. Burnstock, G., Crowe, R. & Wong, H. *Br. J. Pharmac,* 1979, *65*, 377–388
13. Burnstock, G., Hökfelt, T., Gershon, M. D., Iversen, L. L., Kosterlitz, H. W. & Szurszewski, J. H. in *Neuroscience Res. Prog. Bull. 17*, No. 3 MIT Press, Cambridge, Mass., 1979
14. Burnstock, G. & Iwayama, T. pp. 389–404 in Eränkö, O. (ed.) *Progress in Brain Research 34, Histochemistry of Nervous Transmission,* Elsevier, Amsterdam, 1971
15. Campbell, G. & Gibbins, I. L. pp. 103–144 in Kalsner, S. (ed.). *Trends in Autonomic Pharmacology,* Vol. 1. Urban and Schwarzenberg, Baltimore and Munich, 1979
16. Chan-Palay, V., Jonsson, G. & Palay, S. L. *Proc. nat. Acad. Sci. USA.* 1978, *75*, 1582–1586
17. Chubb, I. W., Hodgson, A. J. & White, G. H. *Neuroscience* 1980, *5*, 2065–2072
18. Cook, R. D. & Burnstock, G. *J. Neurocytol.* 1976, *5*, 171–194
19. Crowe, R. & Burnstock, G. *J. Aut. Nerv. Syst.* 1981 (In press)
20. Dowdall, M. J., Boyne, A. F. & Whittaker, V. P. *Biochem. J.* 1974, *140*, 1–12
21. Dreyfus, C. F., Sherman, D. L. & Gershon, M. D. *Brain Res.* 1977, *128*, 109–123
22. Fedan, J. S., Hogaboom, G. K., O'Donnell, J. P., Colby, J. & Westfall, D. P. *Eur, J. Pharmacol.* 1981, *69*, 41–53
23. Fehér, E., Csányi, K. & Vajda, J. *Acta. morphol. Acad. Sci. Hung.* 1974, *22*, 147–159
24. Furness, J. B. & Costa, M. *Neuroscience* 1980, *5*, 1–20
25. Furschpan, E. J., MacLeish, P. R., O'Lague, P. H. & Potter, D. D. *Proc. nat. Acad. Sci. U.S.A.* 1976, *73*, 4225–4229
26. Gabella, G. *J. Anat.* 1972, *111*, 69–97
27. Gabella, G. *Int. Rev. Cytol.* 1979, *59*, 129–193
28. Gershon, M. D. In Burnstock, G. *et al.* ref 13.
29. Gershon, M. D., Dreyfus, C. F., Pickel, V. M., Joh, T. H. & Reis, D. J. *Proc. nat. Acad. Sci. USA* 1977, *74*, 3086–3089
30. Gibbins, I. L. & Haller, C. J. *Cell Tissue Res.* 1979, *200*, 257–272
31. Gordon-Weeks, P. R. & Hobbs, M. J. *Neuroscience Letters* 1979, *12*, 81–86
32. Gunn, M. *J. Anat.* 1968, *102*, 223–239
33. Hervonen, A., Pelto-Huikko, M., Helén, P. & Alho, H. *Histochemistry* 1980, *70*, 1–6
34. Hill, C. E. & Hendry, I. A. *Neuroscience* 1977, *2*, 741–749
35. Hökfelt, T., Elfvin, L-G., Elde, R., Schultzberg, M., Goldstein, M. & Luft, R. *Proc. nat. Acad. Sci. USA.* 1977, *74*, 3587–3591
36. Hökfelt, T., Ljüngdahl, A., Steinbusch, H., Verhofstad, A., Nilsson, G., Brodin, E., Pernow, B. & Goldstein, M. *Neuroscience* 1978, *3*, 517–538
37. Hökfelt, T., Johansson, O., Ljüngdahl, A., Lundberg, J. M. & Schultzberg, M. *Nature (Lond.)* 1980, *284*, 515–521
38. Israël, M., Lesbats, B., Marsal, J. & Meunier, F. M. *C. R. Acad, Sci. Paris.* 1975, *280*, 905–908
39. Iversen, L. L. & Bloom, F. E. *Brain Res.* 1972, *41*, 131–143

40. Jessen, K. R., Mirsky, R., Dennison, M. & Burnstock, G. *Nature (Lond.)* 1979, *281*, 71–74
41. Kása, P., Mann, S. P. & Hebb, C. p. 298, Vol. 15 *Handbuch der Experimentellen Pharmakologie (Ergänzungswerk),* Springer-Verlag, Berlin, Heidelberg, 1970
42. Komuro, T., Baluk, P. & Burnstock, G. (1981). Neuroscience. In press.
43. Kosterlitz, H. W. & Lees, G. M. *Pharmac. Rev.* 1964, *16*, 301–339
44. Larsson, L-I. *Histochemistry* 1977, *54*, 173–176
45. Le Douarin, N. M. & Teillet, M. A. *J. Embryol. exp. Morph.* 1973, *30*, 31–48
46. Llewellyn-Smith, I. J., Wilson, A. J., Furness, J. B., Costa, M. & Rush, R. A. *Neurosci. Abstr.* 1980, *6*, 274
47. Lundberg, J. M., Hökfelt, T., Schultzberg, M., Uvnas-Wallenstein, K., Kohler, C. & Said, S. I. *Neuroscience* 1979, *4*, 1539–1559
48. Newgreen, D. F., Jahnke, I., Allan, I. J. & Gibbins, L. *Cell Tissue Res.* 1980, *208*, 1–19
49. Olson, L., Alund, M. & Norberg, K. *Cell Tissue Res.* 1976, *171*, 407–423
50. Palay, S. L. & Chan-Palay, V. *Cold Spring Harbor Symp. Quant. Biol.* 1975, *40*, 1–16
51. Pearse, A. G. *J. Histochem. Cytochem.* 1969, *17*, 303–313
52. Polak, J. M., Buchan, A. M. J., Probert, L., Tapia, F., De Mey, J. & Bloom, S. R. *Scand. J. Gastroent.* This supplement.
53. Richards, J. G. & Da Prada, M. *J. Histochem. Cytochem.* 1977, *25*, 1322–1336
54. Robinson, P. M. *J. Cell Biol.* 1969, *41*, 462–476
55. Robinson, P. M., McLean, J. R. and Burnstock, G. *J. Pharmacol. exp. Ther.* 1971, *179*, 149–160
56. Schultzberg, M. Hökfelt, T., Terenius, L., Elfvin, L.-G., Lundberg, J. M., Brandt, J., Elde, R. P. & Goldstein, M. *Neuroscience* 1979, *4*, 249–270
57. Schultzberg, M., Hökfelt, T., Nilsson, G., Terenius, L., Rehfeld, J. F., Brown, M., Elde, R., Goldstein, M. & Said, S. *Neuroscience* 1980, *5*, 689–744
58. Silinsky, E. M. *J. Physiol. (Lond.)* 1975, *247*, 145–162
59. Silinsky, E. M. & Hubbard, J. I. *Nature (Lond.)* 1973, *243*, 404–405
60. Taxi, J. *Ann. Sci. nat. Zool.* 1965, *7*, 413–674
61. Tranzer, J. P. & Richards, J. G. *J. Histochem. Cytochem.* 1976, *24*, 1178–1193
62. Uchizono, K. *Arch. Histol. Jap.* 1968, *29*, 399–424
63. Wilson, A. J., Furness, J. B. & Costa, M. *Neuroscience Letters* 1979, *14*, 303–308
64. Wood, J. D. & Mayer, C. J. *J. Neurophysiol.* 1979, *42*, 582–593

# Regulatory Peptides in Endocrine Cells and Autonomic Nerves

## Electron Immunocytochemistry

J. M. POLAK, A. M. J. BUCHAN, L. PROBERT, F. TAPIA, J. DE MEY* & S. R. BLOOM
Histochemistry Unit (Dept. of Histopathology) and Dept. of Medicine, Hammersmith Hospital,
London W12 0HS and *Dept. of Life Sciences, Laboratory of Oncology,
Janssen Pharmaceutical Research Laboratories, 2340 Beerse, Belgium

Advances in immunocytochemistry, particularly at the electron microscope level, have enabled us to establish further details of the ultrastructural appearance of endocrine cells and autonomic nerves of the gastrointestinal tract.

Its contribution can be summarised as follows:
a) Validation of previously recognised endocrine cell types.
b) Recognition of sub-groups within endocrine cells and autonomic nerve cell types previously included within one single type (e.g. $D_1$ cells and p-type autonomic nerves).
c) Discrimination of molecular forms now known to be stored in morphologically distinguishable secretory granules or parts thereof (e.g. pro-glucagon and glucagon in A cells and gut and antral gastrin-producing cells).

Advances in the techniques and the accurate quantification of the end products will enable us to recognise changes in gastrointestinal tract diseases in man.

*Key-words:* Autonomic nerves; electron microscopy; endocrine cells; gut; regulatory peptides

*J. M. Polak, Histochemistry Unit, Dept. of Histopathology, Hammersmith Hospital, London W12 0HS*

Since the discovery of secretin in 1902 (2), more than 25 regulatory peptides have been shown to be present in the gastrointestinal tract, localised to endocrine cells and/or autonomic nerves (14). It is known that most of these regulatory peptides are stored in distinct types of endocrine and neural cells which is in agreement with earlier ultrastructural observations that the gastrointestinal tract contains a wide variety of cell types (22). The different cells are distinguished by the presence of electron-dense secretory granules varying in their shape, their size and the form of their limiting membrane (see Solcia et al., this issue). Until recently, the functional classification of the various endocrine cell types was based mainly in the parallel distribution of a predominating cell type and a particular regulatory peptide (see Solcia et al., this issue).

As a result of advances in immunocytochemical methods it has now been possible, in many instances, (e.g. antral G cells) to validate earlier classifications. In addition, sub-groups of cells previously considered to be of one type (e.g. $D_1$ cells) have been recognised as, indeed, have sub-groups of autonomic, peptide-containing (p-type) nerves (23, 24). The refined methods have even been able to reveal the localisation of various molecular forms (pro-hormones—hormone) in different areas of the secretory granules (e.g. pro-glucagon and glucagon in the A cells of the pancreatic islets) (19).

## ELECTRON IMMUNOCYTOCHEMICAL METHODS

The introduction of peroxidase labelling of antibodies for immunocytochemistry (25) and the realisation that the end-product of the reaction could be made electron-dense by osmium tetroxide has led to the development of several other electron immunocytochemical methods (26). The most popular techniques at present are the peroxidase anti-peroxidase (PAP) method and a variety of gold-labelling procedures including protein A gold (20), gold-labelled immunoglobulin (10) and the directly labelled antigen procedure (11) (GLAD Gold Labelled Antigen Detection method) (Fig. 1).

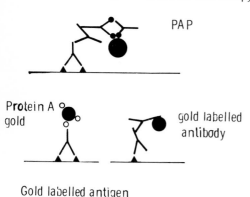

Immunostaining for Electron microscopy

PAP

Protein A gold

gold labelled antibody

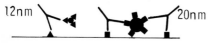

Gold labelled antigen

12nm          20nm

Fig. 1. Diagrammatic representation of the immunostaining methods commonly used in electron microscopy. The top diagram shows the end product of the peroxidase anti-peroxidase method. The middle diagram shows, on the left protein A-conjugated colloidal gold and on the right, colloidal gold-labelled immunoglobulin. The final diagram shows the antigen linked to colloidal gold and also demonstrates the use of two different sizes of gold particles.

We shall now discuss the contributions made by electron immunocytochemistry to a number of problems of particular interest to gastroenterologists.

A) *Validation of earlier ultrastructural classifications*

Electron immunocytochemical procedures have been instrumental in confirming many earlier suggestions that distinct cell types were responsible for the production of particular gut peptides. Examples include the gastrin-producing G cell of the antral mucosa, the secretin-producing S cell and the CCK-producing I cell of the small intestine.

B) *Subclassification of the $D_1$ cells (small granuled) and L cells (large granuled)*

Small granuled cells were first described in 1965 (21) and were termed $D_1$ in 1972 (6). These cells were present in all areas of the gut (stomach, small and large intestine and pancreas). A separate population of large granuled cells (L) was found mainly in the ileum and large intestine.

No particular peptide product was identified within the $D_1$ cells but Solcia and co-workers suggested that the L cells were responsible for the production of gut glucagon (enteroglucagon) (27).

i) *$D_1$ cell subclassification*

The first indication that the $D_1$ cells were a more heterogenous group than was originally suspected came in 1979 (15). At this time comparative light microscopical immunocytochemistry and electron microscopical morphology (serial semithin/thin method) revealed the presence of gastrin-like immunoreactivity (gastrin of intestinal origin) in a subpopulation of $D_1$ cells thereafter termed IG (intestinal gastrin) cells (4). This discovery was soon followed by the localisation of motilin-like immunoreactivity to another subpopulation of $D_1$ cells (15, 16), separate from that responsible for the production of intestinal gastrin, and now internationally recognised as the Mo cells (23, 24) (Figs. 2 and 3).

ii) *L cell subclassification*

In 1977 we, as well as others, reported the electron immunocytochemical localisation of a newly discovered 'brain and gut' regulatory peptide, neurotensin. Neurotensin was found to be produced by a subpopulation of large granuled (L) cells of the ileal mucosa (Figs. 4 and 5), thus establishing the subclassification of the L cells of the lower gut, originally considered to be a single cell type containing gut glucagon (13).

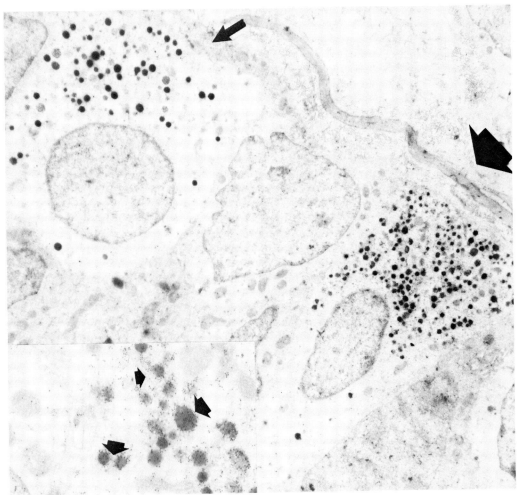

Fig. 2. 80 nm section of human duodenum showing a gastrin-containing cell (large arrow) labelled by 12 nm colloidal gold and an unlabelled endocrine cell (small arrow). × 10,000
The insert shows the labelled secretory granules. Note the concentration of gold particles over the granules (arrows) with unlabelled mitochondria and cytoplasm. × 30,000

## C) *Electron immunocytochemistry of variant forms of peptide molecules*

It is now well recognised that most, if not all, gut regulatory peptides are present in both the tissue and the circulation in a variety of molecular forms of differing sizes (8) (Fig. 6). Usually these differing molecular forms suggest the existence of precursors or pro-hormones, capable of giving rise, by biosynthetic processes to increasingly bioactive smaller fragments (see Fig. 6 for illustrative examples). The fact that antibodies can be raised to specific regions of a peptide molecule

has permitted the immunocytochemical identification of the site of production of different molecular forms of a single peptide. Two examples illustrate this point.

i) The localisation of antral gastrin and of intestinal gastrin to two types of endocrine cells containing distinctly different secretory granules has recently been achieved by the use of region specific antibodies to gastrin 17 and gastrin 34. The antral G cells, known to store mainly the smaller molecular form of gastrin, G17, are characterised by mostly large (average size 340 ±

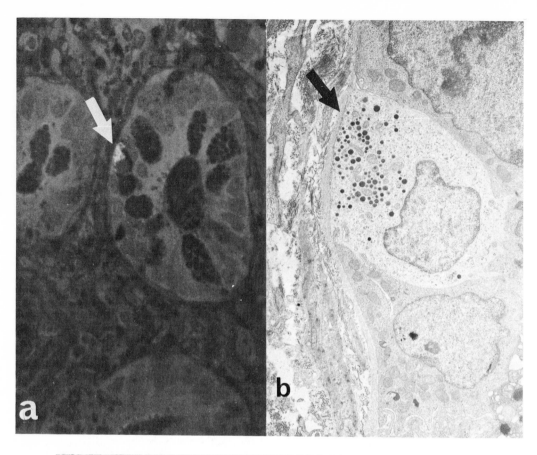

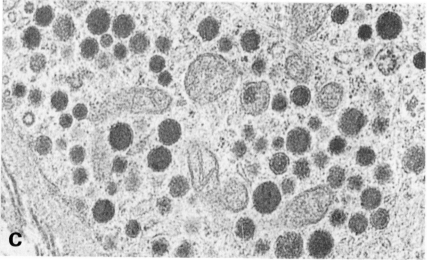

Fig. 3. a) Semithin (500 nm) section of duodenum showing a motilin-containing cell (arrow) detected using a C-terminal directed antiserum by the indirect immunofluorescent method.   × 500
b) The same cell identified in a serial thin (60 nm) section (arrow).   × 5,000
c) At higher magnification details of the characteristic secretory granules are visible.   × 30,000

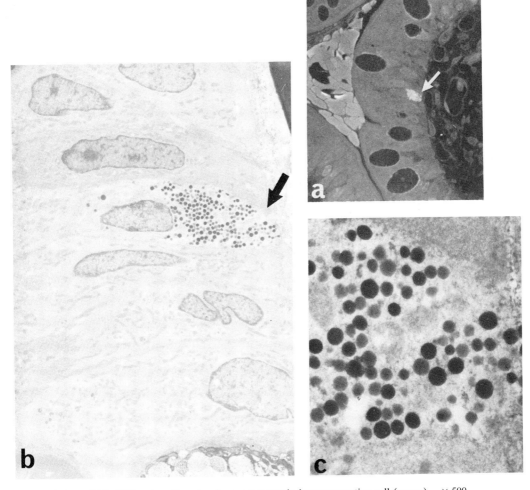

Fig. 4. a) A semithin (500 nm) section showing a neurotensin-immunoreactive cell (arrow).    × 500
b) A serial thin (60 nm) section of the same area, with the immunostained cell indicated by the arrow.    × 5,000
c) Higher magnification of the cell, revealing details of the secretory granules (compare with Fig. 5c).    × 30,000

54 nm) electron-lucent secretory granules, whereas intestinal gastrin cells, known (at least in man) to store predominantly the larger molecular form of gastrin, G34, are characterised by small (average size 175 ± 21 nm) round, electron-dense secretory granules (4). These granules are quite distinct from those of the I cells in the same area which secrete a chemically related peptide, CCK, but have larger (300 ± 28 nm) secretory granules (3). Thus it would appear that the predominance of a particular molecular form (gastrin 17 or gastrin 34) deter-

mines the structure of the secretory granules (Fig. 7). This phenomenon is also noticeable in tumours. The cells of the rare gastrinomas found to produce predominantly gastrin 17, contain mainly the antral gastrin type of secretory granules, whereas the granules of tumors which produce gastrin 34 as the main molecular form are mostly small and electron-dense resembling those of the 'intestinal gastrin cells' (Fig. 8).

ii) Glicentin or 'glucagon of intestinal origin', is a newly discovered regulatory peptide (12). It has now been found to be chemically identical

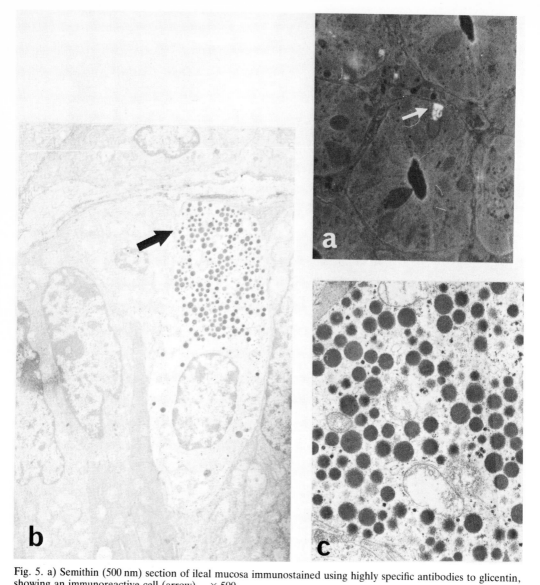

Fig. 5. a) Semithin (500 nm) section of ileal mucosa immunostained using highly specific antibodies to glicentin, showing an immunoreactive cell (arrow).  × 500

b) Electron micrograph of a serial thin (60 nm) section showing the same cell (arrow).  × 5,000

c) Details of the secretory granules present in the glicentin-immunoreactive cell (compare to Fig. 4c).  × 30,000

## MOLECULAR FORMS OF GASTRIN AND GLUCAGON

*Gastrin*

G34   QLGPQGPHSLVADPSKKQGPWLEEEEEAYGWMDF

G17                    QGPWLEEEEEAYGWMDF

*Glucagon*

Glicentin    RRAQKFVQWLMNTKRNKNNIA—

              HSQGTFTSDYDKYLDSRRAQDFVQWLMNTKRNKNNIA

Glucagon   HSQGTFTSDYSKYLDSRRAQDFVQWLMNT

Fig. 6. Gastrin 34 and Gastrin 17 share the whole of their common C-terminal sequence whereas glicentin has both an N-terminal and a C-terminal extension to the glucagon molecule. The whole of the glicentin sequence cannot be given as it has yet to be completely sequenced.

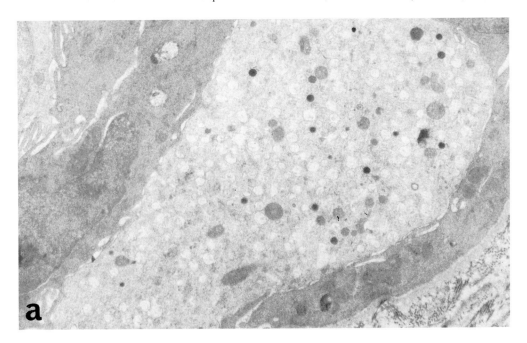

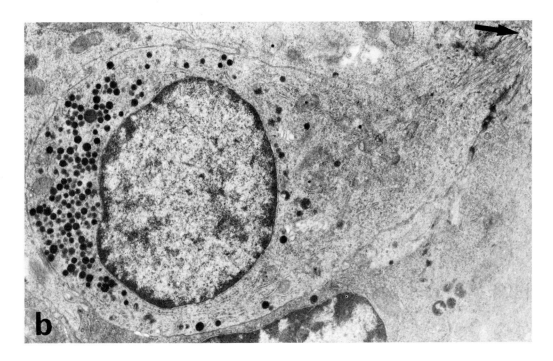

Fig. 7. (a) Antral G cell, Note the numerous electron-lucent vesicles.    × 12,000
(b) Intestinal gastrin $D_1$ type cell. Note connection with the lumen (arrow).    × 12,000

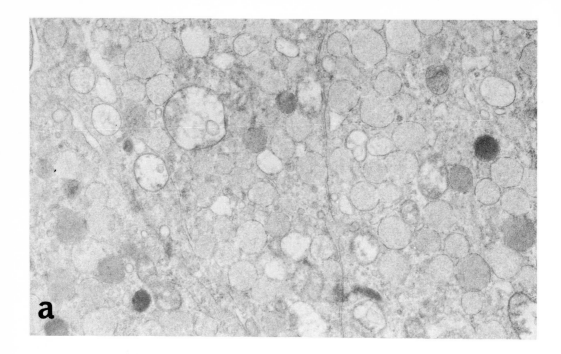

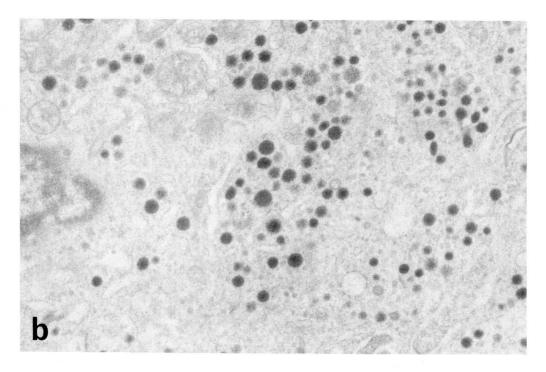

Fig. 8. (a) Secretory granules in a tumour producing predominantly gastrin 17.   × 30,000
(b) Secretory granules in a tumour producing predominantly gastrin 34.   × 30,000

GASTRINOMAS

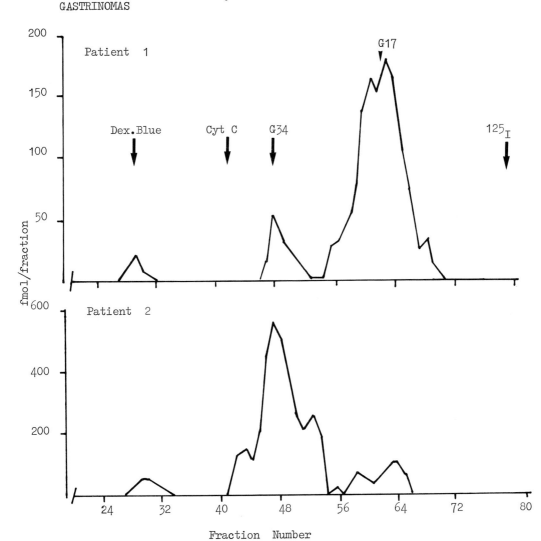

Fig. 9. Gel chromatography of tissue extracts from two gastrinomas. Patient 1. 10% gastrin 34 and 90% gastrin 17 (see Fig. 8a). Patient 2. 90% gastrin 34 and 10% gastrin 17 (see Fig. 8b). Column calibration
Dex. Blue = Dextran Blue
Cyt. c = Cytochrome c
$125_I$ = Iodine 125.

with pro-glucagon, the precursor hormone of pancreatic glucagon. Using electron immunocytochemistry with the immunogold method and antibodies to glicentin (pro-glucagon) and glucagon, these two different molecular forms of the peptide have been localised to different areas of the pancreatic A cell granule (19). Glicentin is present in the outer (halo) portion of the secretory granules and glucagon, in the core (Fig. 10). This may indicate that some of the post-transitional

enzymatic processes involved in converting the pro-hormone (glicentin) into the smaller more active form (pancreatic glucagon) have taken place prior to granule packaging.

The core of the glucagon granule had previously been distinguishable from the outer halo by its distinct reactivity to the Grimelius silver impregnation but the underlying difference in peptide content of the two areas was not understood (9).

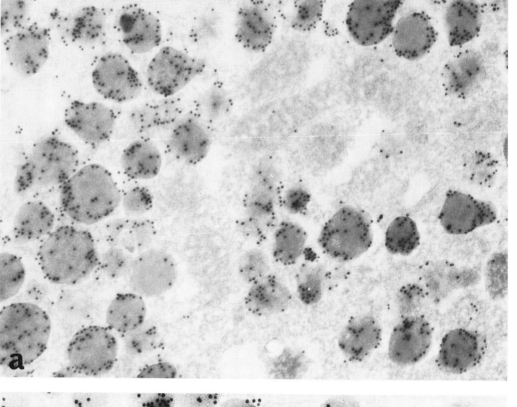

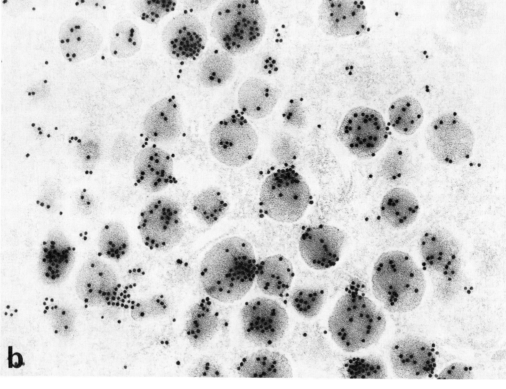

D) *Functional classification of p (peptidergic)-type autonomic neurosecretory granules*

In 1970 Baumgarten and his co-workers described autonomic nerves of a new class in the gastrointestinal tract (1). The nerves were characterised by the presence of ultrastructurally distinct neurosecretory granules, which were larger and more electron-dense than the vesicles associated with the classical neurotransmitters, acetycholine and noradrenalin.

Baumgarten termed these granules p-type because of their resemblance to the peptidergic neurosecretory granules of the posterior pituitary which contained the peptides vasopressin and oxytocin. At the time of their description Baumgarten had little suspicion of the imminent discovery of a massive peptidergic component of the autonomic nervous system which occurred from 1976 onwards.

Baumgarten's description was followed by the ultrastructural observations of Cook and Burnstock of significant differences between the newly recognised p-type nerves (7). At least 3 types were then recognised. Our recent observations using immunocytochemistry at the electron microscopial level fully support Burnstock's claim of a marked heterogeneity among the non-adrenergic, non-cholinergic (p-type) components of the autonomic nervous system. For example, substance P is an eleven amino acid peptide which is known to be a powerful regulator of gastrointestinal functions. Using the immunogold 'on grid' staining procedure we have been able to localise substance P to a sub-population of p-type nerves in the guinea pig colon (17). These substance P-containing nerves are characterised by the presence of round neurosecretory granules of medium electron density with a distinct halo between the core and the limiting membrane, which were classified by Cook and Burnstock as Type 5b (Fig. 11).

Preliminary observations seem to indicate that vasoactive intestinal polypeptide (VIP), a twenty-eight amino acid brain and gut peptide, is present in a different sub-population of p-type nerves (18). These are characterised by a preponderance of small, agranular vesicles intermingled with large, dense round granules (Type 5c of Cook and Burnstock), that are specifically labelled by VIP antibodies using the peroxidase anti-peroxidase procedure carried out on vibrotome sections before embedding.

Systematic analysis of ultrathin sections immunostained for substance P and VIP shows a significant proportion of distinct p-type nerves which remain unstained by either substance P or VIP antibodies (18). These findings are in keeping with the widely accepted view that there are many peptides, other than VIP and substance P, in the p-type nerves of the gut, e.g. enkephalin, TRH, CCK, bombesin, neurotensin and somatostatin.

## CONCLUSIONS

Early ultrastructural studies using conventional methods revealed the existence in the gut of numerous endocrine cell types characterised by the presence of distinct secretory granules, suggesting the production of a wide variety of active peptides. Thus, electron microscopists stimulated the successful search for peptide hormones and their chemical characterisation. To date more than 25 regulatory peptides have been identified. Immunocytochemistry has become the 'obligatory' tool for investigating their cellular localisation. Advances in the technique, in particular its successful use at the electron microscopial level have led to the more functional classification of the endocrine cells of the gut. Increasing emphasis is placed on establishing the type of peptide produced rather than relying solely on the size and shape of the intracellular secretory granules.

Electron immunocytochemistry has, in addition, contributed to the recognition of new endocrine cell types previously included as part of a poorly understood group of cells (e.g. intestinal gastrin and motilin cells were previously grouped together under the general term of $D_1$ cell).

Although in its infancy, the classification of the

---

Fig. 10. A-cell granules from human pancreas immunostained using gold-labelled antibodies.
(a) Gut glucagon (glicentin). The immunoreactivity is localised to the halo of the granules.   × 60,000
(b) Pancreatic glucagon. The immunoreactivity is localised to the core of the granules.   × 60,000

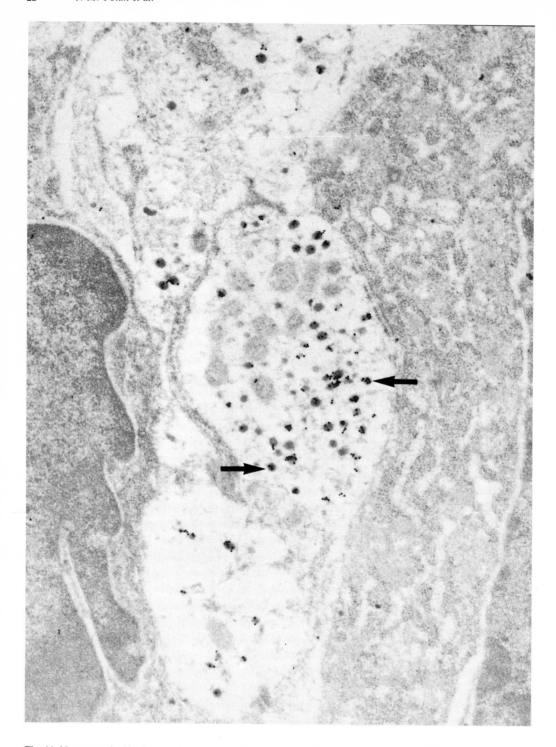

Fig. 11. Nerve terminal in the myenteric plexus of the guinea pig colon, showing substance P-like immunoreactivity. Antibodies were labelled with colloidal gold particles of 20 nm diameter. Note the concentration of the gold label over the granular secretory vesicles.    × 35,000

autonomic nerves of the gut, especially of the p-type, into distinct groups is beginning to be a possibility. Substance P-, in particular, and VIP-containing terminals can now be distinguished from the rest of the p-type (peptidergic) nerves which have yet to be identified. The future looks exceedingly promising. The availability of highly specific 'monoclonal' antibodies seems a near reality and with it the opportunity for different groups of scientists to compare their findings. The use of antibodies labelled with colloidal gold particles of different sizes will allow the accurate demonstration of separate antigens (peptides in cells and/or nerves) in a single tissue section.

Quantification of immunocytochemical staining at the ultrastructural level is advancing at a rapid pace. We shall soon be able to obtain precise information on the amount of hormone release from a cell as well as the amount stored. The years to come promise exciting new vistas.

## REFERENCES

1. Baumgarten, H. G., Holstein, A. F. & Owman, C. H. *Z. Zellforsch* 1970, *106*, 376–379
2. Bayliss, W. M. & Starling, E. H. *J. Physiol.* 1902, *28*, 325–353
3. Buchan, A. M. J., Polak, J. M., Solcia, E., Capella, C., Hudson, D. & Pearse, A. G. E. *Gut* 1978, *19*, 403–407
4. Buchan, A. M. J., Polak, J. M., Solcia, E. & Pearse, A. G. E. *Nature* 1979, *277*, 138–140
5. Buchan, A. M. J., Bryant, M. G., Timson, C. M., Polak, J. M. & Bloom, S. R. *Gut* 1979, *20*, A454
6. Capella, C., Solcia, E., Vassallo, G. p. 282 in Taylor, S. (ed.), *Endocrinology* 1971. Heinemann, London, 1972
7. Cook, R. D. & Burnstock, G. *J. Neurocytol.* 1976, *5*, 171–194
8. Dockray, G. J. pp. 43–48 in Bloom, S. R. & Polak, J. M. (eds.), *Gut Hormones.* 2nd ed. Churchill Livingstone, Edinburgh, 1981
9. Grimelius, L., Polak, J. M., Solcia, E. & Pearse, A. G. E. pp. 365–368 in Bloom, S. R. (ed.), *Gut Hormones.* Churchill Livingstone, Edinburgh, 1978
10. Gu, J., De Mey, J., Moeremans, M. & Polak, J. M. *Regulatory Peptides* 1981, 1, 365–374
11. Larsson, L-I. *Nature,* 1979, *282*, 743–746
12. Moody, A. J. & Thim, L. pp. 312–319 in Bloom, S. R. & Polak, J. M. (eds.), *Gut Hormones,* 2nd ed. Churchill Livingstone, Edinburgh, 1981
13. Polak, J. M., Sullivan, S. N., Bloom, S. R., Buchan, A. M. J., Facer, P., Brown, M. R. & Pearse, A. G. E. *Nature* 1977, *270*, 183–184
14. Polak, J. M. & Bloom, S. R. *Clinics in Endoc. Metab.* 1979, *8*, 313–330
15. Polak, J. M. & Buchan, A. M. J. *Gastroenterol.* 1979, *76*, 1065–1066
16. Polak, J. M. & Buchan, A. M. J. in Grossman, M. I., Brazier, M. A. B. & Lechago, J. (eds.), *Cellular basis of chemical messengers in the digestive system.* Academic Press, New York, 1981 (in press)
17. Polak, J. M. & Probert, L. *Gastroenterol.* 1981, **80**, 1253
18. Polak, J. M. & Probert, L. unpublished observations
19. Ravazzola, M. & Orci, L. *Nature* 1980, *284*, 66–67
20. Roth, J., Bendayan, M. & Orci L. *J. Histochem. Cytochem.* 1978, *26*, 1074–1081
21. Solcia, E. & Sampietro, R. *Z. Zellforsch* 1965, *68*, 689–698
22. Solcia, E., Vassallo, G. & Capella, C. pp. 3–29 in Creutzfeldt, W. (ed.), *Origin, Chemistry, Physiology and Pathophysiology of the Gastrointestinal Hormones.* Schattauer-Verlag, Stuttgart, 1970
23. Solcia, E., Polak, J. M., Pearse, A. G. E., Forssmann, W. G., Larsson, L-I., Sundler, F., Lechago, J., Grimelius, L., Fujita T., Creutzfeldt, W., Gepts, W., Falkmer, S., Lefranc, G., Heitz, Ph., Hage, E., Buchan, A. M. J., Bloom, S. R. & Grossman, M. I. pp. 40–48 in Bloom, S. R. (ed.) *Gut Hormones.* Churchill Livingstone, Edinburgh, 1978
24. Solcia, E., Polak, J. M., Larsson, L-I., Hakanson, R., Lechago, J., Fujita, T., Rubin, W., Grube, D., Falkmer, S., Grieder, M. H., Creutzfeldt, W. & Grossman, M. I. in Grossman, M. I., Brazier, M. A. B. & Lechago, J. *Cellular basis of chemical messengers in the digestive system.* Academic Press, New York, 1981 in press
25. Sternberger, L. *Immunocytochemistry.* (2nd ed.). Prentice Hall, N.J. 1979
26. Van Noorden, S. & Polak, J. M. pp. 80–89 in Bloom, S. R. & Polak, J. M. (eds.), *Gut Hormones.* 2nd ed. Churchill Livingstone, Edinburgh, 1981
27. Vassallo, G., Solcia, E. & Capella, C. *Z. Zellforsch* 1969, *98*, 333–356

# The Diffuse Endocrine-Paracrine System of the Gut in Health and Disease: Ultrastructural Features

E. SOLCIA, C. CAPELLA, R. BUFFA, L. USELLINI, R. FIOCCA,
B. FRIGERIO, P. TENTI & F. SESSA
Institute of Pathological Anatomy and Histopathology, and Histochemistry and Ultrastructure Centre,
University of Pavia—Via Forlanini 16, 27100 Pavia, Italy

At least 16 types of endocrine-paracrine cells have been identified ultrastructurally in the gastrointestinal mucosa. The production of hormones and local messengers such as 5-hydroxytryptamine, gastrin, cholecystokinin, somatostatin, secretin, gastric inhibitory peptide (GIP), enteroglucagon (glicentin, GLI), motilin, neurotensin, substance P and the enkephalins, by these cells, has been established.

Progress has also been made in cytological studies of gut and pancreatic endocrine tumours. Argentaffin EC cell carcinoids, gastrinomas (of several ultrastructurally different varieties of gastrin cells), L-cell tumours and D-cell tumours are among those cytologically and functionally defined in the gut. Functionally undefined tumours include the so-called non-argentaffin carcinoids arising in various parts of the gut, some of which have been characterised cytologically as gastric ECL cell tumours and gastroduodenal P-D$_1$-cell tumours. Gastrinomas, vipomas and rare argentaffin carcinoids are among gut-related pancreatic endocrine tumours. Non-functional paragangliomas, usually with some neuromatous component, occur in the duodenal wall. Extrapancreatic vipomas display ultrastructural features of ganglioneuroblastomas with peptidergic granules.

*E. Solcia, Institute of Pathological Anatomy and Histopathology, University of Pavia—Via Forlanini 16, 27100 Pavia, Italy*

The endocrine-paracrine cells scattered in the gastrointestinal mucosa are now regarded as a diffuse modulatory system of digestive motor and secretory functions. They appear to be sensitive to chemical and mechanical stimuli acting from the lumen, to which they respond by releasing a series of extracellular mediators (34). Such mediators are mostly the same as those released by nerve endings disseminated in the gastrointestinal wall, including substance P, somatostatin, enkephalin, gastrin-cholecystokinin C-terminal sequences, bombesin and catecholamines (18). Other mediators detected in the endocrine-paracrine cells whose presence in gut nerves have been suggested, although not fully proven yet, are gastrin, neurotensin, pancreatic polypeptide (PP), motilin and 5-hydroxytryptamine (5-HT). Among neural mediators possibly displaying some counterpart in gut endocrine-paracrine cells are vasoactive intestinal peptide (VIP), gamma-aminobutyric acid (GABA) and acetylcholine.

It seems clear that in the gut the endocrine-paracrine cells and nerves function as two integrated regulatory systems, (acting through the same extracellular mediators on targets largely in common). They differ mainly in the mechanism by which their mediators are released at the receptor site.

## A. *General cytology and physiology of endocrine-paracrine cells*

Endocrine-paracrine cells are specialised cells scattered in the epithelium lining the gastric glands, intestinal crypts and villi. They are characterised by secretory granules, which, as a rule, are concentrated in the basal part of the cytoplasm, whilst the Golgi complex is supranuclear (Fig. 1). In the pyloric and intestinal mucosa most of such cells reach the lumen in a narrow, specialised area showing tufts of microvilli and a centriole (Fig. 2). It is likely that this area acts as a receptor surface facing the luminal contents (38).

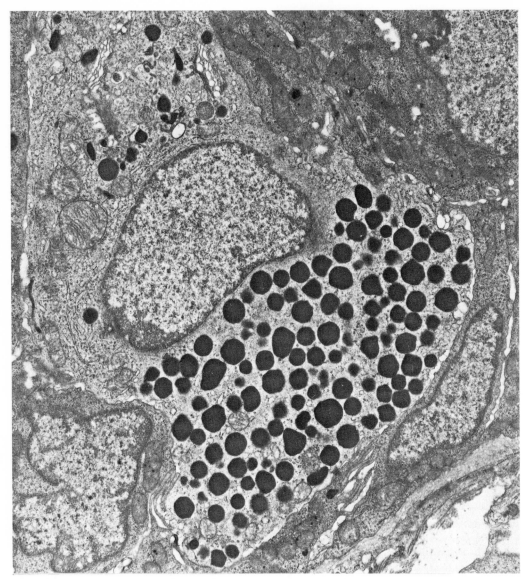

Fig. 1. Endocrine-paracrine cell of VL type in the human jejunum showing secretory granules grouped at the base of the cell, with progranules in the supranuclear Golgi zone. Note thin intraepithelial intercellular spaces surrounding endocrine and non-endocrine cells.   × 9,800

Such pattern suggests some functional polarity of the cell. In the fundic mucosa endocrine-paracrine cells lack luminal contacts and show less evident polarity (36).

Secretory granules are released at the basal surface of the cell or along the lower part of its lateral surface (21), where intervening cells may form interstitial spaces and canaliculi (Fig. 1). In the upper (juxtaluminal) part of the epithelium these spaces are closed by junctional complexes with neighbouring cells (Fig. 2). Granule release at the luminal surface has never been observed.

The endocrine-like cells may exert a local modulatory activity (paracrine) on neighbouring exocrine and endocrine cells of gut epithelia. This may occur either by direct cell to cell contact,

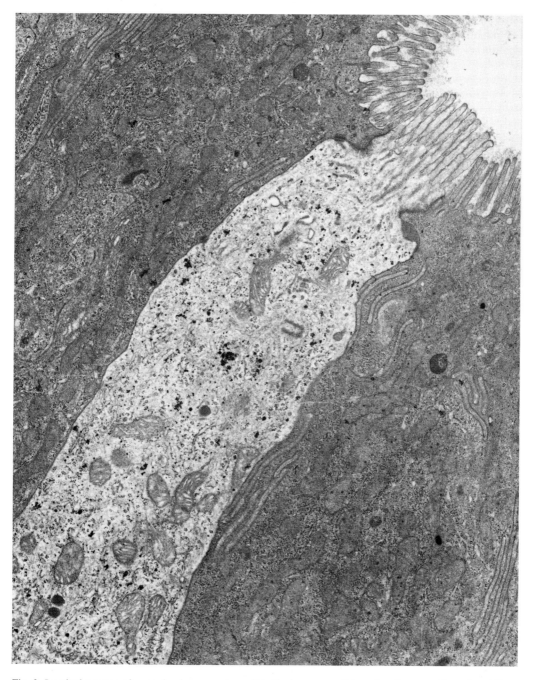

Fig. 2. Luminal process of an endocrine-paracrine cell in the human small intestine; its protruding microvilli are thicker than those of the surrounding enterocytes, whilst showing less surface coat. Note smooth cisternae filled with electron opaque amorphous material in the juxtaluminal cytoplasm, a centrosome and a well developed junctional complex in the apical part of the lateral membranes.  × 14,000

sometimes through long cytoplasmic processes, or by the diffusion of secretory products throughout the intercellular intraepithelial spaces. Secretory products may also cross the basal membrane of the glands and villi and diffuse in the lamina propria, where they may either exert a paracrine action on nerve endings, blood vessels and smooth muscles or enter the circulation (through fenestrated capillaries) and display truly *endocrine* activities on distant targets.

## Identification and classification of endocrine-paracrine cells

First attempts to classify the endocrine-paracrine cells of the gut were based mainly on ultrastructural findings, with special reference to the size, shape, density, fine structure and reactivity of secretory granules (40). Parallel immunohistochemical studies and hormone assays on tissue

extracts helped in the functional identification of some cell types (5). More recently, the semithin/ultrathin section technique has been used for the simultaneous characterisation of the hormone content and ultrastructural pattern of the same cell (8, 9). Ultrastructural cytochemistry (Fig. 3) and immunocytochemistry (Fig. 4) are now being extensively applied. The revised Lausanne classification of gastro-enteropancreatic endocrine cells (Table I) is based on these refined technical developments (37). The final identification of specific motilin (Mo) cells (Fig. 5) and the recognition of gastrin cell variants (IG and TG cells) are among the more recent achievements (7, 10, 24).

Together with the main secretory products reported in Table I, a number of peptides or related sequences have been found in subpopulations of endocrine cells, as for instance substance P (30) or enkephalin (3) in some argentaffin EC cells, N-terminal ACTH-$\alpha$-MSH

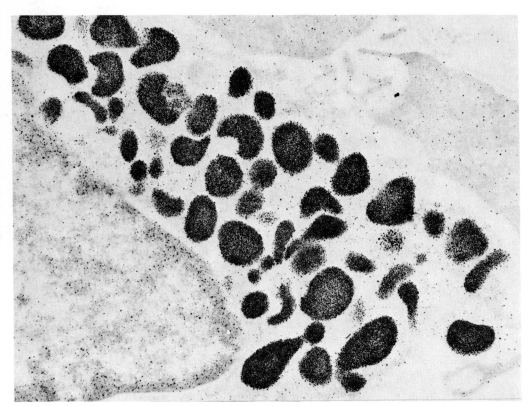

Fig. 3. Pleomorph granules of an EC cell in the human small intestine showing intense deposition of reduced silver grains, due to their 5-hydroxytryptamine content. Masson's argentaffin reaction,  × 28,000

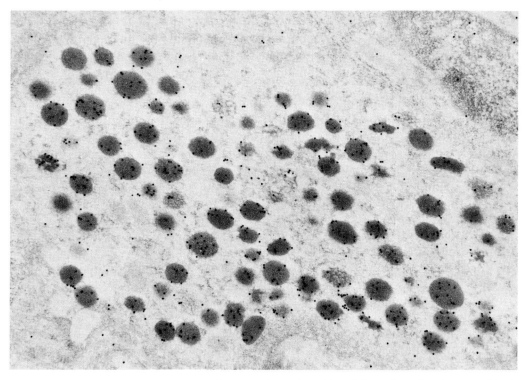

Fig. 4. Granules of an L-cell in the human large bowel reacting with anti-C-terminal glicentin serum (kindly provided by Prof. N. Yanaihara, Shizuoka, Japan) revealed by the protein A-gold technique: note the deposition of gold particles on secretory granules. Similar results were obtained with R-64 anti-glicentin serum (from Dr. A. J. Moody, Novo Research Institute, Copenhagen, Denmark), non-C-terminal antiglucagon serum n.4842 (Dr. V. L. W. Go, Mayo Foundation, Rochester, U.S.A.), anti-BPP serum n.146/6 (Dr. R. E. Chance, Lilly Research Institute, Indianapolis, USA) and anti-C-terminal PP serum n.221 (Prof. K. D. Buchanan, Queen's University, Belfast, U.K.) while no reactivity was obtained with anti-C-terminal glucagon serum n.K5563 (Dr. L. Heading, Novo Research Institute, Copenhagen) and anti-HPP serum n.248/4 (Dr. Chance).  × 28,000

sequence in some gastrin cells (22) and C-terminal PP sequence in most L-cells (16).

Besides the cell types reported in Table I, cells with irregularly shaped, moderately dense granules of variable, usually large, size (variable large granule or VL cells) have been observed (Fig. 1). Some of these cells may correspond to type III gastrin-immunoreactive cells of Larsson and Jørgensen (25) and might display ACTH-α-MSH-like immunoreactivity (23).

*Tumours*

In the past, only two types of gut endocrine tumours were diagnosed by pathologists, the argentaffin and the non-argentaffin carcinoids. Then, some twenty years ago duodenal gastri-

nomas were added and for many years no further progress was made. As shown in Table I, as many as 14 or 15 endocrine cell types may occur in the gut, suggesting that the situation of gut endocrine tumours is probably more complicated than generally recognised. Although for technical reasons the majority of such tumours still escape appropriate histochemical and ultrastructural study, progress has been made in the last few years in detecting new tumour entities. The present status of studies concerning the identification and classification of gut endocrine tumours is outlined in Table II. It must be stressed that many tumours show more than one endocrine cell type (35, 41); these are to be classified according to the prevalent cell type. When major cell populations

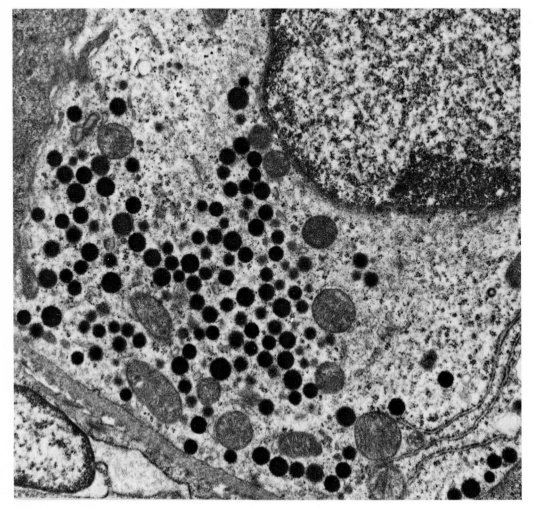

Fig. 5. Motilin cell of the human duodenum showing small, round, fairly dense granules and perinuclear filaments.   × 17,600

coexist or when a minor cell population accounts for the hyperfunctional syndrome, a diagnosis of mixed endocrine tumour should be made and the coexisting cells should be specified. The widely used term 'carcinoid', apart from the case of EC cell tumours (argentaffin carcinoids), should be applied only to endocrine tumours whose cells are either unknown or functionally undetermined (non-argentaffin carcinoids). The latter tumours are better subdivided according to the site of origin or, when known, the cell type(s) involved. Immunohistochemical tests and electron microscopy are recommended for the study of group

A tumours related with functionally defined cells; a proportion of these tumours (especially among gastrin and EC tumours) will develop hyperfunctional syndromes. Only electron microscopy is available for the exact cellular characterisation of group B and C tumours, usually lacking hyperfunctional syndromes.

On cytological grounds pancreatic endocrine tumours should be distinguished into a) *islet cell tumours* (A, B, D and PP cell tumours) reproducing the morphology of the cell types occurring in adult islets, independently from their actual origin, from differentiated islet cells or from duc-

Table I. Human Gastroenteropancreatic endocrine cells

| Cell | Main Product | PANCREAS | STOMACH | | INTESTINE | | |
| --- | --- | --- | --- | --- | --- | --- | --- |
| | | | | | Small | | |
| | | | Oxyntic | Antral | Upper | Lower | Large |
| P | Peptides? | a | + | + | + | | |
| D$_1$ | Peptides? | f | + | f | f | f | f |
| EC | 5-HT, Peptides | r,b | + | + | + | + | + |
| D | Somatostatin | + | + | + | + | f | f |
| B | Insulin | + | | | | | |
| PP (F) | Pancreatic polypeptide | + | | | | | |
| A | Glucagon | + | a,b | | | | |
| X | Unknown | | + | | | | |
| ECL | Unknown (b:histamine) | | + | | | | |
| G | Gastrin | | | + | f | | |
| IG | Gastrin | | | b | + | r | |
| TG | C-terminal gastrin/CCK | | | b | + | b | |
| I | CCK | | | | + | f | |
| S | Secretin | | | | + | f | |
| K | GIP | | | | + | f | |
| Mo | Motilin | | | | + | f | |
| N | Neurotensin | | | | r | + | r |
| L | GLI | | | | f | + | + |

a = foetus or newborn; b = animals; f = few; r = rare; GLI = Glucagon-like immunoreactivity

tular stem cells; b) *diffuse endocrine system* (DES) and *ectopic tumours*, reproducing the morphology of cells lacking in adult human islets—although occasionally present in the juxtaduodenal pancreas (EC cells) or in rat foetal pancreas (gastrin cells)—but well represented in extrapancreatic tissues, with special reference to the gastrointestinal mucosa; and c) *rare poorly differentiated*

Table II. Endocrine tumours of the gut

A. Functionally defined tumours:
  —Gastrin cell tumour (gastrinoma)
  —D-cell tumour (somatostatinoma)
  —L-cell tumour (enteroglucagonoma)
  —EC cell tumour (argentaffin carcinoid)
    1. 5-HT with Substance P
    2. 5-HT without Substance P
  —Ectopic tumours (ACTH, HCG, insulin, etc.)

B. Functionally undefined tumours
  (Non-argentaffin carcinoids):
    1. ECL cell carcinoid
    2. P-D$_1$ cell carcinoid
    3. Paraganglioma
    4. Others

C. Poorly differentiated endocrine carcinoma
  (Argyrophil carcinoma; endocrine microcitoma)

*endocrine carcinomas*. Tumours with more than one cell type occur very often. Benign growths prevail among group a) tumours, low grade malignancies among group b) tumours and high grade malignancies among group c) tumours (33).

So far, among gut endocrine tumours and gut-related endocrine tumours of the pancreas, the following entities have been characterised on cytologic and/or clinicopathologic grounds:

1) *Argentaffin EC cell carcinoids* producing 5-HT, kallikreins and sometimes also the active peptide substance P. Although they may arise in any part of the gastrointestinal tract, pancreas, biliary tree and oesophagus, their sites of higher incidence are the appendix and the lower small intestine. An overwhelming population of well differentiated argentaffin EC cells has been found in most of these tumours (35, 36).

2) *L-cell tumours and non-argentaffin colorectal carcinoids*. The majority of the rectal endocrine tumours we have investigated so far showed various proportions of cells reacting with anti-glicentin sera and anti-pancreatic polypeptide C-terminal sera. In some of these cases L-cells have been identified at the electromicroscopial level

(16). It seems interesting that in some pancreatic glucagonoma cells we found in the tumour cells both diagnostic target-cells, α-granules and poorly diagnostic, homogeneous granules (proglucagon granules?) resembling those of L-cells, now reputed to be the ancestor cell of glucagon A-cells (34). Substance P, enkephalin, β-endorphin, somatostatin or neurotensin cells have been found in a few of our rectal carcinoids and in occasional tumours previously reported in the literature (2).

3) *Gastric cell tumours (Gastrinomas).* 13% of gastrin-producing tumours are found in the duodenum (20), about 1% in the stomach, upper jejunum and biliary tree collectively, and 85% in the pancreas. This distribution of tumours is in sharp contrast to the distribution of human gastrin cells, which are mostly concentrated in the gastric mucosa of the pylorus, with much fewer cells in the upper small bowel and no gastrin cells in the pancreas (10, 27, 36).

The immunohistochemical demonstration of gastrin in tumour cells is essential for a correct diagnosis of this kind of tumour and its distinction from other endocrine tumours of the upper small intestine or pancreas. In our cases pyloric-type G-cells with partly vesicular granules, TG type cells with round, solid, sometimes haloed granules, cells with smaller, solid granules resembling those of the so-called 'intestinal gastrin' (IG) cells, or cells with various admixtures of G, TG and IG granules were present in the pancreatic and intestinal gastrinomas (Fig. 6) have been investigated ultrastructurally (32, 39). The IG cells, which appear early in embryogenesis (29) and whose granules somewhat resemble Golgi-associated progranules of G-cells, should store higher proportions of larger molecular forms (gastrin 34 or big gastrin, component 1, etc.), as found in extracts of tumour tissue and intestinal mucosa (4, 15). In some tumours, large, dense, irregular granules appear in gastrin cells, together with G- or IG-type granules (12, 32); such granules might be related with the production of ACTH-like peptides, known to occur in both normal G-cells and gastrinomas (14, 22).

4) *Somatostatin D-cell tumour.* Only one pure somatostatin D-cell tumour seems to have been observed so far in the gut (17), although D-cells have been detected in several gut tumours, especially in those also showing gastrin cells (1, 32). Unlike somatostatinoma in the pancreas, no somatostatinomas syndrome has been reported so far in association with intestinal tumours; instead, a gastrinoma syndrome has been found in a patient whose jejunal tumour showed somatostatin cells largely prevalent over gastrin cells (32).

In a pancreatic somatostinoma associated with diarrhoea and cholelytiasis we found a prevalent population of well differentiated D-cells, together with few PP cells and some functionally undefined cells (33).

5) *Argyrophil gastric carcinoids.* A consistent proportion of gastric endocrine tumours have been found to arise in a background of chronic atrophic gastritis (35, 41). Multifocal endocrine cell hyperplasia, either intraepithelial or extra-epithelial, often chain-forming and micronodular, occurs very often in this disease, with or without associated pernicious anaemia. Although most of these very frequent hyperplastic foci remain as harmless lesions of no clinicopathologic relevance, in a few cases histologic patterns suggesting direct development of endocrine tumours from such hyperplastic growths have been observed (35). ECL, EC, P-, $D_1$- and X-cells have been found quite frequently in gastric carcinoids, either arising in chronic atrophic gastritis or in normal mucosa (6, 28, 35, 41). The *ECL cell argyrophil carcinoid* (Fig. 7) seems to represent a definite pathologic entity and to occur more frequently than other types of gastric endocrine tumours (11). Intestinal-type endocrine tumours, showing various kinds of intestinal endocrine cells, have been found to arise from extensively intestinalised gastric mucosa (35). As a rule, no hyperfunctional syndrome is observed in association with gastric carcinoids, apart from a few reports of 'carcinoid' syndrome, sometimes coupled with histamine secretion. It seems pertinent to recall here that histamine-producing argyrophil ECL cell carcinoids arise very frequently in the gastric mucosa of the South African rodent *Mastomys natalensis* (13) and that murine ECL cells produce large amounts of histamine (19).

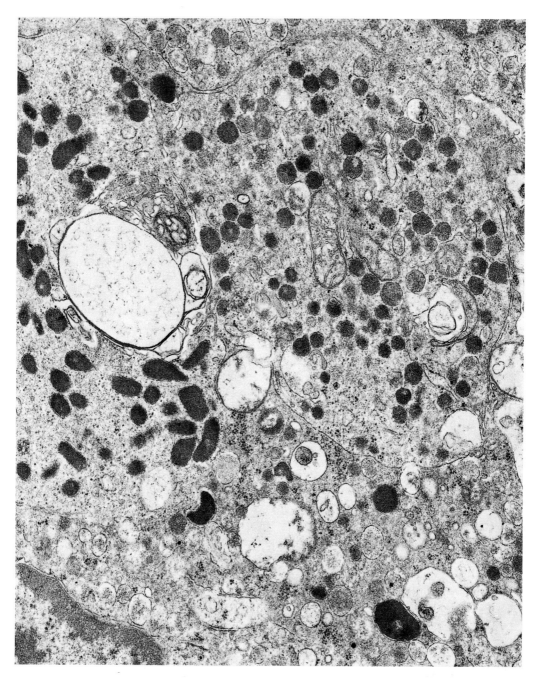

Fig. 6. Endocrine tumour of the upper jejunum associated with severe hypergastrinaemia and the Zollinger–Ellison syndrome. Note part of an EC cell (left side), a cell with plenty of TG granules plus some G granules (mixed TG/G cell; centre-right part of the micrograph) and two G-cells (lower and upper part). × 21,000

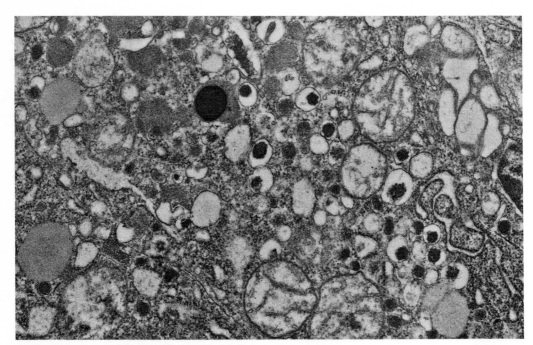

Fig. 7. Gastric argyrophil carcinoid showing ECL granules.    × 28,000

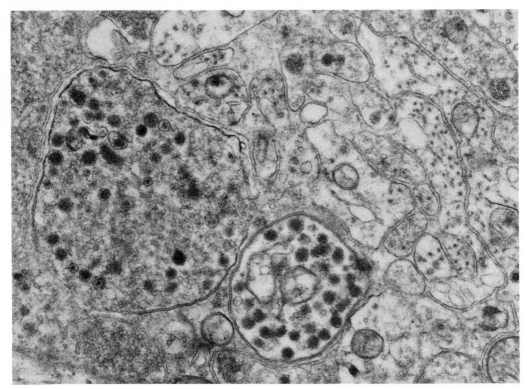

Fig. 8. VIP-producing adrenal ganglioneuroma with watery diarrhoea syndrome: nerve fibres and nerve endings with small 'synaptic' vesicles and dense 'peptidergic' granules.    × 28,000

6) *Vipomas*—Most, but not all, pancreatic tumours associated with severe *secretory diarrhoea* (diarrheogenic, Verner-Morrison's or WDHA tumours) have been found to produce excessive amounts of vasoactive intestinal peptide (VIP), which is reputed to be the most likely mediator of the syndrome. Extrapancreatic neurogenic tumours (Fig. 8) have also been found to produce VIP as well as secretory diarrhoea (5, 31). This is not surprising since VIP has been localised in a number of central and peripheral nerve cells and fibres. However, all the diarrheogenic VIP-producing tumours (*vipomas*) of the pancreas we have investigated so far proved to be epithelial endocrine tumours lacking any neural component. Most of them were malignant and poorly differentiated, with only a minority of tumour cells reacting with anti-VIP sera.

So far, despite extensive investigation, a specific epithelial endocrine VIP cell has not been identified in the pancreas or in the gastrointestinal mucosa (26). Thus, at present the production of VIP by epithelial pancreatic tumours seems to be accounted for by a deviation in the differentiation process of tumour stem cells.

7) *Paragangliomas and neurogenic tumours*— Paragangliomas with more or less developed gangliocytic and/or neuromatous components are known to arise in the intestinal wall, with special reference to the duodenum. Although granules resembling peptide-storing secretory granules of nerve cells have been found in such tumours, no pertinent hyperfunctional syndrome has been reported so far. In particular, it seems surprising that, despite the very large number of VIP-producing neurons found everywhere in the digestive tract, no one neurogenic vipoma has been documented so far in this area.

## ACKNOWLEDGEMENTS

This work was supported in part by research grants from Italian Consiglio Nazionale delle Ricerche (CT 80.00585.04) and Ministero della Pubblica Istruzione.

## REFERENCES

1. Alumets, J., Ekelund, G., Håkanson, R., Ljunberg, O., Ljungqvist, U., Sundler, F. & Tibblin, S. *Virchows Arch. A Path. Anat. Histol.* 1978, *378*, 17–22
2. Alumets, J., Fålkmer, S., Grimelius, L., Håkanson, R., Ljunberg, O., Sundler, F. & Wilander, E. *Acta Path. Microbiol. Scand. Sect. A* 1980, *88*, 103–109
3. Alumets, J., Håkanson, R., Sundler, F. & Chang, K.-J. *Histochemistry* 1978, *56*, 187–196
4. Berson, S. A. & Yalow, R. S. *Gastroenterology* 1971, *60*, 215–222
5. Bloom, S. R., Polak, J. M. & Pearse, A. G. E. *Lancet* 1973, *2*, 14–16
6. Bordi, C., Senatore, S. & Missale, G. *Amer. J. Dig. Dis.* 1976, *21*, 667–671
7. Buchan, A. M. J., Polak, J. M., Capella, C. & Solcia, E. *Histochemistry* (In preparation)
8. Buchan, A. M. J., Polak, J. M., Solcia, E., Capella, C., Hudson, D. & Pearse, A. G. E. *Gut* 1978, *19*, 403–407
9. Buchan, A. M. J., Polak, J. M., Solcia, E., Capella, C. & Pearse, A. G. E. *Histochemistry* 1978, *56*, 37–44
10. Buchan, A. M. J., Polak, J. M., Solcia, E. & Pearse, A. G. E. *Nature* 1979, *277*, 138–140.
11. Capella, C., Polak, J. M., Frigerio, B. & Solcia, E. *Ultrastructural Path.* 1980, *1*, 411–418
12. Capella, C., Solcia, E., Frigerio, B., Buffa, R., Usellini, L. & Fontana, P. *Virchows Arch. A Path. Anat. Histol.* 1977, *373*, 327–352
13. Capella, C., Solcia, E. & Snell K. C. *J. Nat. Cancer Inst.* 1973, *50*, 1471–1485
14. Creutzfeldt, W. in Wellman, K. F. & Volk B. W. (eds.) *The Diabetic Pancreas.* Plenum Publ. Co. New York, 1977
15. Creutzfeldt, W., Arnold, R., Creutzfeldt, C. & Track, N. S. *Human Path.* 1975, *6*, 47–76
16. Fiocca, R., Capella, C., Buffa, R., Fontana, P., Solcia, E., Hage, E., Chance, R. E. & Moody, A. J. *Amer. J. Path.* 1980, *100*, 81–92
17. Fujita, T. Communicated at the Santa Monica Meeting on GEP endocrine cells classification. January 1980
18. Furness, J. B. & Costa, M. *Neuroscience* 1980, *5*, 1–20
19. Håkanson, R., Larsson, L.-I., Liedberg, G. & Sundler, F. pp. 243–263 in Coupland, R. E. & Fujita, T. (eds.) *Chromaffin, Enterochromaffin and Related Cells.* Elsevier, Amsterdam, 1976
20. Hofmann, J. W., Fox, P. S. & Milwaukee, S. D. W. *Arch. Surg.* 1973, *107*, 334–338
21. Kobayashi, S. & Sasagawa, T. pp. 255–271 in Fujita, T. (ed.) *Endocrine Gut and Pancreas.* Elsevier, Amsterdam 1976
22. Larsson, L.-I. *Histochemistry,* 1978, *56*, 245–251
23. Larsson, L.-I. *Regulatory Peptides, Suppl. 1,* 1980, 65
24. Larsson, L.-I., Capella, C., Jørgensen, L. M. & Solcia, E. in Lechago, J., Grossman, M. I. & Walsh, J. H. (eds.). *Cellular Basis of Chemical Messengers in the Digestive System.* Academic Press, New York, 1981
25. Larsson, L.-I. & Jørgensen, L. M. *Cell. Tiss. Res.* 1978, *194*, 79–102
26. Larsson, L.-I., Polak, J. M., Buffa, R., Sundler,

F. & Solcia, E. *J. Histochem. Cytochem.* 1979, *27,* 936–938

27. Larsson, L.-I., Rehfeld, J. F. & Goltermann, N. *Scand. J. Gastroent.* 1977, *12,* 869–872
28. Larsson, L.-I., Rehfeld, J. F., Stockbrügger, R., Blohme, G., Schöön, I.-M., Lundqvist, G., Kindblom, L. G., Säve-Söderberg, J., Grimelius, L. & Olbe, L. *Amer. J. Path.* 1978, *93,* 53–68
29. Larsson, L.-I., Rehfeld, J. F., Sundler, F. & Hakanson, R. *Nature* 1976, *262,* 609–610.
30. Pearse, A. G. E. & Polak, J. M. *Histochemistry* 1975, *41,* 373–375
31. Said, S. I. & Faloona, G. R. *New Engl. J. Med.* 1975, *293,* 155–160
32. Solcia, E., Capella, C., Buffa, R., Frigerio, B. & Fiocca R. pp. 119–133 in Fenoglio C. M. (ed.) *Progress in Surgical Pathology* (vol. 1). Masson Publishing, USA, New York 1980
33. Solcia, E., Capella, C., Buffa, R., Frigerio, B., Sessa, F. & Tenti, P. in *Diagnosis and Treatment of Upper Gastro-Intestinal Tumors.* Excerpta Medica, Amsterdam, 1981
34. Solcia, E., Capella, C., Buffa, R., Usellini, L., Fiocca, R. & Sessa, F. In Johnson, L., Christensen, J., Grossman, M., Jacobson, E. D., Schultz, S. G. (eds.) *Physiology of the digestive tract.* Raven Press, New York, 1981 (In press)
35. Solcia, E., Capella, C., Buffa, R., Usellini, L., Frigerio, B. & Fontana, P. *Pathobiology Annual* 1979, *9,* 163–203
36. Solcia, E., Capella, C., Vassallo, G. & Buffa, R. *Internat. Rev. Cytol.* 1975, *42,* 223–286
37. Solcia, E., Polak, J. M., Larsson, L.-I., Buchan, A. M. J. & Capella, C. pp. 96–100 in Bloom, S. R., Polak, J. M. (eds.) *Gut Hormones,* 2nd ed. Churchill Livingstone, Edinburgh 1981
38. Solcia, E., Vassallo, G. & Sampietro, R. *Z. Zellforsch.* 1967, *81,* 474–486
39. Vassallo, G., Solcia, E., Bussolati, G., Polak, J. M., & Pearse, A. G. E. *Virchows Arch. B Zellpath.* 1972, *11,* 66–79
40. Vassallo, G., Solcia, E. & Capella, C. *Z. Zellforsch.* 1969, *98,* 333–356
41. Wilander, E., Grimelius, L., Lundqvist, G. & Skoog, V. *Amer. J. Path.* 1979, *96,* 519–530

# The quantification of Zinc in the Mucosal Cells of Human Small Intestine using X-ray Microanalysis

J. GWYN JONES & MARGARET E. ELMES
Dept. of Pathology, University Hospital of Wales, Cardiff

The intracellular zinc concentration of human small intestinal mucosal cells was estimated using X-ray microanalysis. Jejunum and ileum from 11 patients resected during surgery was fixed in 2.5% glutaraldehyde and acetone and the estimations performed with an AEI EMMA 4. The zinc content of undifferentiated stem cells, enterocytes, goblet cells and Paneth cells was determined and all the cell types were found to contain significant amounts of zinc.

The highest levels were found in the stem cells and enterocytes with a maximum in the ileal enterocytes in Crohn's disease. In non-inflammatory conditions the ileal enterocytes had a higher zinc content than the jejunal enterocytes. Stem cells had comparable levels in all tissues analysed.

Goblet cells showed a wide variation in zinc levels that may be due to their secretory status.

Paneth cells had the lowest zinc levels. The whole Paneth cell zinc and granule zinc were of the same order in all tissues sampled. The cytoplasmic zinc was higher than the granule zinc in all samples of ileum analysed, but there was no significant difference in the jejunum.

The limitations of the technique are considered and observations made on the role of zinc in intestinal mucosa.

*Key-words:* Electron probe microanalysis; intestinal mucosa; zinc

*Dr. Margaret E. Elmes, Dept. of Pathology, University Hospital of Wales, Heath Park, Cardiff*

Zinc is one of the essential trace elements and is necessary for the activity of many enzymes involved in major metabolic pathways both as a constituent of metalloenzymes such as carbonic anhydrase, various peptidases and dehydrogenases and also as a co-factor in thymidine kinase activity and nucleic acid synthesis. Analysis of the tissue content of zinc has been largely confined to the major tissues such as liver, bone, muscle, skin and blood until interest in the absorption of zinc by the gut arose. Analysis of total mucosal zinc in 24-hour-fasted normal rats using neutron activation analysis showed levels in the duodenum, jejunum and ileum of 18.5; 14.8; and 26.6 µg/g wet weight (2). These are of the same order as muscle and brain levels and only exceeded by liver and prostate. In man levels of 97 and 99 µg/g dry weight were found in the jejunal mucosa of 2 normal children (4).

Histochemically detectable zinc was found in rat Paneth cells by Okamoto (10) using dithizone and Millar, Vincent & Mawson (9) found that $^{65}Zn$ injected into zinc deficient rats was concentrated in Paneth cells in the ileum. Mager, McNary & Lionetti (8) using a dithizone complex-forming solution demonstrated zinc in the intestinal epithelium of both small and large intestine of rabbits given intravenous zinc acetate 24 hrs. prior to death. However, no dithizone-reactive zinc was found in human Paneth cells (3) and the current work was done to determine the total intracellular zinc content of human intestinal mucosal cells and to see if the Paneth cells, in view of their histochemical reactivity in animals, contained significantly higher zinc levels than the non-reactive cells.

## MATERIALS AND METHODS

Samples of histologically normal jejunum and ileum were obtained at operation from patients undergoing partial gastrectomy or intestinal resection. Details of the patients are given in Table I. The specimens were placed in transparent polythene specimen bags in the operating theatre, transported as quickly as possible to the laboratory and placed in fixative with the minimum of delay. Fixation was at room temperature and the procedure was as follows:

2 hrs. in 2.5% glutaraldehyde made up in 0.1 M phosphate buffer pH 7.4.
100% Acetone 75 minutes
100% Acetone 15 minutes
1:1 Acetone/Epon mixture 2 hrs.
Pure Epon overnight

The samples were then subdivided into smaller pieces suitable for electron microscopy and polymerised in Epon at 60°C for 24 hrs. Six blocks of tissue were prepared for each patient.

Ultrathin sections were cut from five separate resin blocks of each patient using an LKB Ultramicrotome III. The sections were floated on distilled water, collected on aluminium grids and carbon-coated. The carbon coating was necessary to prevent the sections from breaking up in the analytical electron microscope which was used without an objective aperture during the analysis.

The sections were analysed in an AEI EMMA 4 transmission electron microscope fitted with a KEVEX solid state detector linked to a TEKTRONIX multi-channel analyser. Each analysis was performed at an accelerating voltage of 80 kV, a beam current of 0.1 µA and a counting time of 40 seconds.

The following cells were analysed:

Enterocytes on the lower part of the villus between the crypt/villus junction and the mid-zone of the villus.
Goblet cells in a similar region.
Paneth cells and undifferentiated stem cells at the base of the crypt.

Whole cell zinc concentrations were measured in enterocytes, goblet cells, Paneth cells and stem cells and the aim was to analyse each cell type per section in each of the 5 sections per patient, using a beam with a diameter sufficient to include as much of the cell as possible. For stem cells, enterocytes and Paneth cells, this generally included most of the cytoplasm (including granules in Paneth cells) and part of the nucleus (Figs. 1 and 2). The cytoplasm of goblet cells however is packed with secretory product and therefore the whole cell analysis was, to a large extent, a measure of the secretory product zinc level (Fig. 3).

To determine mean granule and cytoplasmic zinc concentrations in Paneth cells the 5 sections per patient were used and in one Paneth cell per section 5 granules and 5 points in the cytoplasm adjacent to these granules were analysed.

The analysis of cells in different sections of each patient was performed to compensate for any variability between resin blocks. In practice it was not always possible to obtain whole cell zinc concentrations of two cells of each type in

Table I. Details of Patients analysed

| Patient | Sex | Age | Diagnosis | Region Sampled |
|---|---|---|---|---|
| 1 | F | 83 | Gastric Ulcer | Jejunum |
| 2 | F | 56 | Carcinoma Stomach | Jejunum |
| 3 | M | 74 | Carcinoma Stomach | Jejunum |
| 4 | M | 56 | Carcinoma Stomach | Jejunum |
| 5 | F | 79 | Carcinoma Caecum | Ileum |
| 6 | M | 54 | Angiodysplasia | Ileum |
| 7 | F | 69 | Carcinoma Caecum | Ileum |
| 8 | F | 31 | Crohn's Disease | Ileum |
| 9 | M | 34 | Crohn's Disease | Ileum |
| 10 | M | 20 | Crohn's Disease | Ileum |
| 11 | F | 28 | Crohn's Disease | Ileum |

Table II. Total numbers of cells used to estimate the mean whole cell zinc concentrations

| Patient | Paneth | Goblet | Stem | Enterocyte |
|---|---|---|---|---|
| 1 | 6 | 8 | 6 | 8 |
| 2 | 6 | 4 | 8 | 5 |
| 3 | 8 | 7 | 7 | 9 |
| 4 | 8 | 9 | 6 | 9 |
| 5 | 9 | 12 | 8 | 10 |
| 6 | 12 | 15 | 9 | 9 |
| 7 | 8 | 10 | 6 | 10 |
| 8 | 9 | 10 | 10 | 9 |
| 9 | 5 | 8 | 3 | 9 |
| 10 | 4 | 8 | 3 | 8 |
| 11 | 6 | 7 | 4 | 8 |

every section and the actual figures are given in Table II.

In each analysis the zinc concentration was measured by integrating energy regions 8.30 to 8.46 KeV (Zn background) and 8.56 to 8.72 KeV (Zn peak, $K_\alpha$) in the energy spectrum produced by the multi-channel analyser. In addition, the white radiation (WR) produced by the resin of the section was measured by integrating energy region 4.85 to 7.45 KeV which had no elemental peaks and subtracting any white radiation due to the aluminium of the grid. The WR of the resin was used as a measure of resin thickness and a Zn/WR resin ratio was calculated for each analysis using the following formula:

$$\frac{(\text{Zn peak } K\alpha\text{-Zn background})}{\text{WR resin}}$$

The actual zinc concentration (in parts per million) was obtained from a calibration curve of levels of zinc standard resin sections (provided by Dr. J. A. Chandler of the Tenovus Institute, Cardiff) which had been analysed under the same conditions. The performance of the instrument was checked at regular intervals during an analysis session using the zinc standards.

The precision of the technique was estimated by testing the whole cell zinc data using the following statistical methods:

i) Performing a one-way analysis of variance testing the between section variability within cell types in every patient.

ii) Calculating the pooled coefficient of variation for each cell type in every patient.

The mean whole cell concentrations of the different cell types were calculated for each patient. The patients were grouped in the following categories:

Group 1 (patients 1, 2, 3 and 4). Jejunum from patients with gastric ulcers or gastric carcinoma—i.e. non-inflammatory disease.

Group 2 (patients 5, 6 and 7). Ileum from patients with non-inflammatory disease of the ileum and caecum.

Group 3 (patients 8, 9, 10 and 11). Ileum adjacent to areas resected for Crohn's disease.

A two-way analysis of variance was performed for each cell group taking into account variation arising between patients and cell types. A significant 'F' test in the analysis of variance was further tested for significant differences using a multiple range test. The mean whole cell concentrations of the different cell types in each group was calculated by pooling the data of all the patients within a group and differences between groups were tested using an analysis of variance.

The mean Paneth cell granule and cytoplasmic zinc data were also subdivided as above into three patient groups and differences between granule and cytoplasmic levels within groups were tested using the paired t-test.

RESULTS

Figs. 1, 2 and 3 show the appearance of the cells analysed, viewed unstained and identified by position and characteristic morphology.

Fig. 4 shows the contamination marks which indicate the precise site and extent of the area analysed.

*Assessment of technique*

The precision of the technique was assessed by analysing the variability between cells of the same type in each patient, for example: the whole goblet cell zinc concentrations measured in the jejunum of Patient 1 are given in Table III. The standard deviations between duplicate readings within sections range from 283 to 4950 ppm and the variability appeared to be independent of the means. The means range from 1800 to 21,500 ppm

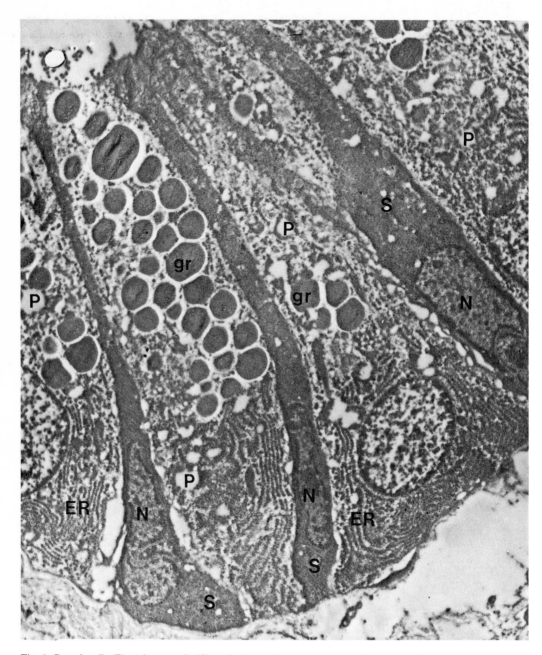

Fig. 1. Paneth cells (P) and stem cells (S) at the base of a crypt. In spite of poor definition due to the mode of fixation the characteristic Paneth cell granules (gr) and rough endoplasmic reticulum (E.R.) are seen. Stem cells are identified by their position between Paneth cells and by their nuclei (N).
Patient 2. Jejunum, unstained.   × 8,700.

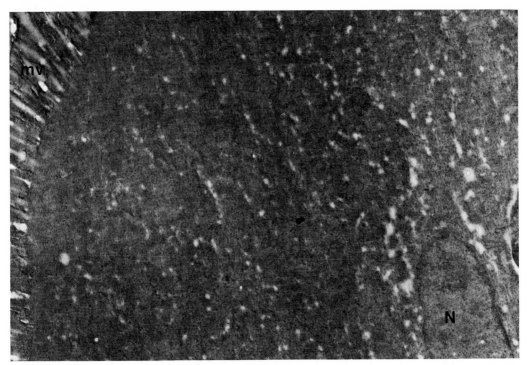

Fig. 2. Villar enterocytes identified by their microvillous border (mv) and nuclei (N). The cytoplasm is too electron dense for identification of organelles.     Patient 1. Jejunum, unstained.   × 12,700.

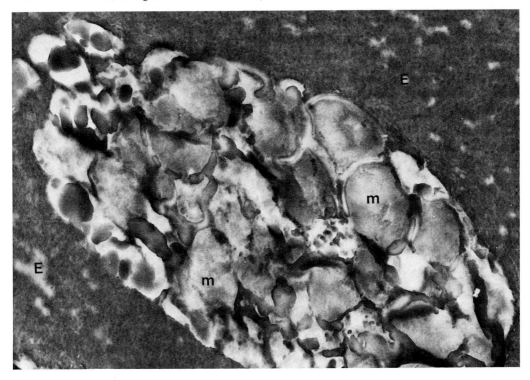

Fig. 3. Goblet cell at the base of a villus identified by the characteristic mucigen granules (m). Parts of two enterocytes (E) are also shown.     Patient 1. Jejunum, unstained.   × 19,600.

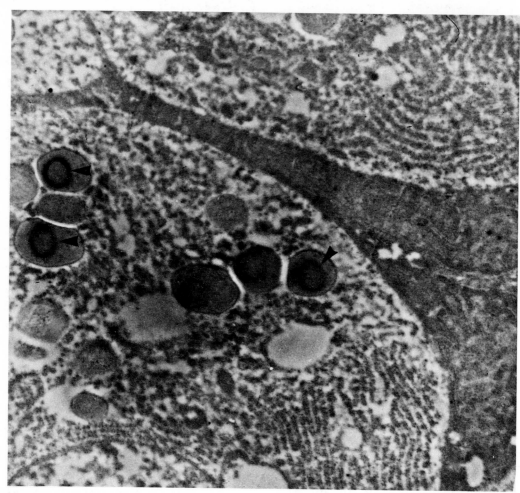

Fig. 4. Contamination marks (arrowheads) produced during x-ray microprobe analysis of a Paneth cell showing that the electron beam can be focused well within the granules. Patient 1. Jejunum, unstained.   × 12,500.

Table III. Goblet cell whole cell zinc concentrations (ppm) in four ultrathin sections of Patient 1 (jejunum)

|  | Sections | | | | |
|  | 1 | 2 | 3 | 4 | Totals |
|---|---|---|---|---|---|
| 1st reading* | 4,200 | 1,600 | 7,000 | 25,000 | 37,800 |
| 2nd reading* | 11,000 | 2,000 | 8,800 | 18,000 | 39,800 |
| Totals | 15,200 | 3,600 | 15,800 | 43,000 | 77,600 |
| Means | 7,600 | 1,800 | 7,900 | 21,500 | 9,700 |
| S.D. | 4,808 | 283 | 1,273 | 4,950 | 3,500 |
| C.V. % | 63 | 16 | 16 | 23 | 36 |
|  |  |  |  |  | (pooled) |

*Two cells analysed in each section.

Table IV. Analysis of variance of data given in Table III

| Source | Degrees of Freedom | Sums of squares | Mean squares | F ratio |
|--------|--------------------|-----------------|--------------|---------|
| Total | 7 | 46,837 | 6,691 | |
| Between sections | 3 | 41,905 | 13,968 | 11.33* |
| Error | 4 | 4,932 | 1,233 | |

Data transformed to units of $1 \times 10^{-2}$ to avoid use of large numbers.
*P < 0.05

and an analysis of variance (Table IV) gave an F ratio of 11.3 (p < 0.05). The pooled coefficient of variation from Tables III and IV is 36%. Although the analysis shows the variability within sections is very large the significant F ratio shows that the between cell variability in Patient 1 is mainly due to differences between goblet cells of different sections rather than between cells of the same section.

Similar analyses were performed to examine the variability between sections for the other cell types in Patient 1 and the different cell types in the other patients. A summary of the results is given in Table V. The variation between sections was least in the Paneth cells (except in Patient 11 with Crohn's disease), low in stem cells and greatest in goblet cells and enterocytes. The pooled coefficient of variation of the whole cell zinc concentrations for each patient ranged from 13% to 67% (mean 41%) for Paneth cells; 28% to 56% (mean 36%) for goblet cells; 21% to 72% (mean 44%) for stem cells and 12% to 58% (mean 32%) for enterocytes.

## Whole Cell Zinc Concentrations

The mean whole cell zinc concentrations of the four mucosal cell types for the three groups of patients are given in Tables VI, VII and VIII. In the jejunum a two-way analysis of variance (Table VI) showed significant differences between patients and between cell types (F ratios; patients = 39.36, df 3/9; cell types = 8.78, df 3/9; p < 0.01 in both cases). A multiple range test

Table V. Results of the analyses of variance of whole cell zinc concentration between sections

| | Patient | Paneth | Goblet | Stem | Enterocyte |
|--|---------|--------|--------|------|------------|
| Group 1 (Jejunum) | 1 | — | * | N.S. | N.S. |
| | 2 | — | — | N.S. | — |
| | 3 | N.S. | N.S. | N.S. | N.S. |
| | 4 | N.S. | * | — | ** |
| Group 2 (Ileum) | 5 | N.S. | * | N.S. | N.S. |
| | 6 | N.S. | ** | * | ** |
| | 7 | N.S. | * | — | ** |
| Group 3 (Ileum) | 8 | — | — | * | N.S. |
| | 9 | — | N.S. | — | ** |
| | 10 | — | ** | — | * |
| | 11 | ** | — | — | N.S. |

N.S. = not significant; * = P < 0.05; ** = P < 0.01; — = unsuitable data for analysis.

Table VI. Mean whole cell zinc concentrations (ppm) in Patient Group 1 (jejunum)

| Patient | Paneth | Goblet | Stem | Enterocyte | Patient mean |
|---------|--------|--------|------|------------|--------------|
| 1 | 4,700 | 9,700 | 10,100 | 9,300 | 8,500 |
| 2 | 10,000 | 15,300 | 19,700 | 16,400 | 15,400 |
| 3 | 4,200 | 5,300 | 8,000 | 8,200 | 6,400 |
| 4 | 2,400 | 4,700 | 4,100 | 5,300 | 4,100 |
| Group mean | 5,300 | 8,800 | 11,000 | 9,800 | |

Table VII. Mean whole cell zinc concentrations (ppm) in Patient Group 2 (ileum)

| Patient | Paneth | Goblet | Stem | Enterocyte | Patient mean |
|---|---|---|---|---|---|
| 5 | 6,600 | 9,900 | 11,800 | 13,200 | 10,400 |
| 6 | 3,400 | 6,500 | 8,700 | 11,000 | 7,400 |
| 7 | 9,400 | 6,800 | 9,100 | 13,200 | 9,600 |
| Group mean | 7,000 | 7,700 | 9,900 | 12,500 | |

Table VIII. Mean whole cell concentrations (ppm) in Patient Group 3 (ileum)

| Patient | Paneth | Goblet | Stem | Enterocyte | Patient mean |
|---|---|---|---|---|---|
| 8 | 14,600 | 14,400 | 17,500 | 23,000 | 17,400 |
| 9 | 2,000 | 7,000 | 3,900 | 8,900 | 5,500 |
| 10 | 5,200 | 9,500 | 9,100 | 13,300 | 9,300 |
| 11 | 5,400 | 12,600 | 6,900 | 18,000 | 10,700 |
| Group mean | 6,800 | 10,900 | 9,400 | 15,800 | |

revealed a significant difference between Paneth cells, which had the lowest zinc concentration and the other three mucosal cell types as a group. Stem cells, enterocytes and goblet cells did not differ significantly (see Fig. 5). The between patient variability was mainly due to the extremely high mucosal cell zinc concentrations in Patient 2 (gastric carcinoma) with some contribution from Patient 1 who had a significantly higher concentration than Patient 4.

An analysis of variance of the ileal cells from patients without Crohn's disease (Table VII)

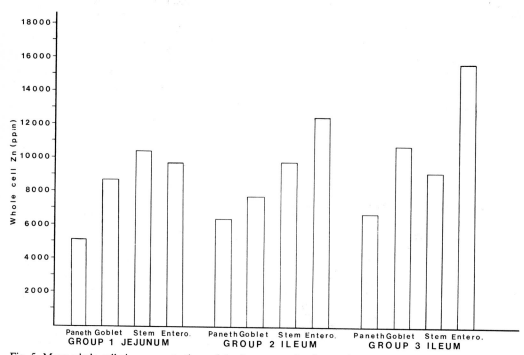

Fig. 5. Mean whole cell zinc concentrations of the four mucosal cell types in the three patient groups.

showed significant differences between cell types (P < 0.05) and no significant difference between patients (F ratios, cell types = 8.35, df 3/6; patients = 3.86, df 2/6). The highest mean zinc concentrations were found in the enterocytes and again with the exception of Patient 7, Paneth cells had the lowest zinc levels. A multiple range test showed a significant difference between entero- cytes on the one hand and goblet and Paneth cells on the other (see Fig. 5).

higher than in the jejunum of similar patients. In patients with Crohn's disease the mean zinc con- centrations in both goblet cells and enterocytes were much higher in the ileum than in either jejunum or ileum when compared to patients without Crohn's disease.

### Paneth Cell Zinc Concentrations

The values for granules and cytoplasm in each patient are shown in Table IX.

Table IX. Mean Paneth cell granule and cytoplasm zinc concentration (ppm)

| | Group 1 | | | Group 2 | | | Group 3 | |
|---|---|---|---|---|---|---|---|---|
| Patient | Granules | Cyto. | Patient | Granules | Cyto. | Patient | Granules | Cyto. |
| 1 | 8,200 | 5,400 | 5 | 6,800 | 7,800 | 8 | 12,400 | 15,600 |
| 2 | 8,600 | 8,900 | 6 | 3,800 | 6,400 | 9 | 1,400 | 2,900 |
| 3 | 2,400 | 3,100 | 7 | 2,900 | 5,600 | 10 | 3,100 | 4,200 |
| 4 | 3,300 | 1,900 | | | | 11 | 1,800 | 4,300 |
| Group mean | 5,600 | 4,800 | Group mean | 4,500 | 6,600 | Group mean | 4,700 | 6,800 |
| S.E. | 800 | 800 | S.E. | 1,200 | 600 | S.E. | 2,600 | 3,000 |

An analysis of variance of the values for the ileum in patients with Crohn's disease (Table VIII) showed a highly significant difference between patients and between cell types (F ratios; cell types = 14.03, df 3/9; patients = 24.16, df 3/9; P < 0.01 in both cases). A multiple range test showed that the variations between cell types were mainly due to the higher mean zinc con- centrations in enterocytes compared with the other mucosal cell types. The variability between patients was due to the very high mucosal cell zinc concentrations in Patient 8 and also the high levels in Patient 11 compared with Patient 9.

When the mean whole cell zinc concentrations of the cell types in each group (calculated by pooling the data of the patients within a group) were analysed, statistically significant differences could not be demonstrated in the whole cell zinc concentration in each cell type between the groups. However, the Paneth cell zinc concen- tration was slightly higher in both ileal groups compared with the jejunal group (Fig. 5), and the mean enterocyte zinc concentration in ileum from patients without Crohn's disease was appreciably

In the jejunum of patients in Group 1 the mean granule zinc concentration was higher than the cytoplasmic concentration (Fig. 6). However, in the ileum of patient groups 2 and 3 the converse was true – the cytoplasmic zinc concentration was higher than the granule zinc concentration and there was no significant difference between the two groups (Fig. 6).

In patients without Crohn's disease this differ- ence between granules and cytoplasm was stat- istically significant (paired t-test p < 0.05) but due to the wide variability in values in patients with Crohn's disease a statistical difference could not be demonstrated.

## DISCUSSION

The zinc levels measured in this study of intra- cellular zinc are 60–100 times those found in the whole tissue analyses reported previously (4). The variation in zinc content between sections is a measure both of the zinc retention within the tissue after processing and biological variation between cells in one patient's tissues. To obtain

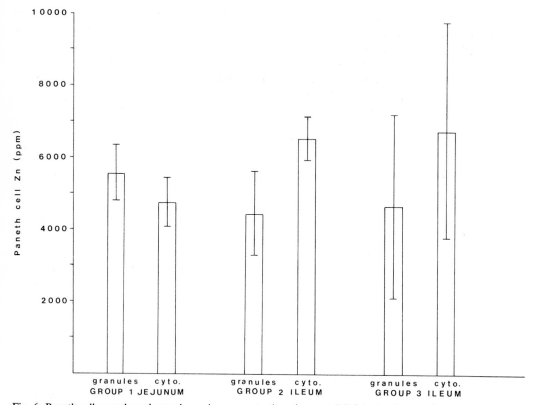

Fig. 6. Paneth cell granule and cytoplasm zinc concentrations (mean ± S.E.) in the three patient groups.

good estimations of the mean mucosal cell zinc concentrations within a sample of intestinal tissue it is clearly important to analyse a large number of sections from as many blocks and as many levels within a block as possible.

We have been able, in spite of this problem, to demonstrate significant variations between cell types and between patients.

To our surprise Paneth cells did not have the high zinc levels we were anticipating from the previous histochemical studies and in fact had generally lower mean zinc levels than the other three cell types analysed, the enterocytes having the highest levels especially in the ileum. Another unexpected finding was the high level of zinc in the goblet cells and enterocytes of non-diseased areas of mucosa from patients with Crohn's disease; and one patient with carcinoma of the stomach (Patient 2) had very high zinc levels in all four types of cell examined.

If we consider the non-secretory cells first, that is the enterocytes and the undifferentiated stem cells, then we find that in both jejunum and ileum and in patients without Crohn's disease the highest zinc levels are found in these cells. As the stem cells are metabolically active and zinc is essential for normal cell division this is not a surprising observation. The levels for jejunum and ileum are of the same order and there is no marked increase in Crohn's disease.

The enterocytes show a significant increase in zinc level in the ileum when compared with the jejunum and a marked increase in Crohn's disease. Animal experiments (1) indicate that the ileum has the greatest capacity for zinc absorption. We would postulate that there may be high levels of free zinc and metallothionein; a metal-binding protein with a significant role in zinc absorption (11) in the enterocytes examined. Numerous essential metalloenzymes contain zinc but as the technique of X-ray microanalysis will not detect zinc in concentrations below 100 ppm (Chandler, J. A., personal communication) and as most enzymes are large molecules (M.W. ranging from approximately, 10,000 to 900,000), the integral zinc (A.W. 65) may not be measurable. Thus the detectable zinc is more likely to be free zinc or a part of a small molecule. Zinc both forms an integral part of the metallothionein molecule and binds to it. The molecular weight of metallothionein is between 6,000 and 7,000 (5) and so even if only one atom of zinc is present it should be well within the detectable capabilities of the technique. Zinc deficiency has been reported in Crohn's disease with impaired zinc absorption (12) and this could be due to excess metallothionein binding zinc and preventing normal transport of zinc into the blood stream.

If we now consider the goblet cells these were found to have much higher zinc levels than we were anticipating. Although the zinc level in these cells in the ileum was slightly lower than that in the jejunum it was not statistically significant in patients without Crohn's disease. However, patients with Crohn's disease had a slightly higher goblet cell zinc in the ileum than patients without Crohn's disease but due to the small sample we were unable to confirm this statistically.

In this study the whole goblet cell zinc concentration is a measure of the zinc content of both the secretory mucigen granules and also the mucus mass (see Fig. 3). We have found in unpublished work on human and rat goblet cells that the mucigen granules had a much higher zinc concentration than the mucus mass awaiting secretion in the cell. As the relative proportions of granule mass and mucus mass vary from cell to cell this may contribute to the wide variations in results obtained. We suggest that zinc is essential for normal secretory processes with a role in maintaining secretory granule stability. We have observed unusual jejunal goblet cells in zinc deficiency due to acrodermatitis enteropathica in addition to the abnormal Paneth cell granules already described (7).

In the majority of Paneth cells examined the whole cell zinc concentration was lower than that found in goblet cells. The whole Paneth cell zinc

concentrations found in the ileum of patient Groups 2 and 3 were slightly higher than those found in the jejunum of Group 1 and this is due to the increase in cytoplasmic zinc (Fig. 6).

The granule zinc concentration was much less variable between groups than the whole goblet cell zinc concentration (a measure of the mucigen granule mucus mass concentration) and this may relate to the different modes of secretion. Paneth cells usually show discrete electron dense granules which are serially extruded in the merocrine mode of secretion and can be seen as granules in the crypt lumen. In contrast the discrete mucigen granules of goblet cells coalesce into a mucus mass which is extruded as a whole. Thus the Paneth cell granules seen and analysed in electron microscopy are more likely to be of consistent composition than the goblet cell secretory product which may be at any stage of the secretory process.

The one case of gastric carcinoma with very high jejunal zinc levels needs to be investigated further. Previous zinc medication and accidental contamination were eliminated and it was not possible to obtain a history of environmental exposure. These very high levels were not found in the other two cases of gastric carcinoma.

This was a preliminary survey and we made no attempt to assess the zinc status of patients by measuring plasma zinc or nucleated tissue zinc (6) and all patients were fasted prior to resection.

## ACKNOWLEDGEMENTS

J. G. Jones was supported by the Welsh Scheme for the Development of Health and Social Research.

Our thanks are due to Dr. J. A. Chandler of the Tenovus Institute for Cancer Research, Cardiff for access to the AEI EMMA 4 and general assistance and advice and to Dr. T. Khosla, Department of Medical Statistics, Welsh National School of Medicine for advice on statistical analysis.

## REFERENCES

1. Antonson, D. L., Barak, A. J. & Vanderhoof, J. A. *J. Nutr.* 1979, *109,* 142–147

2. Elmes, M. E. *Studies on the Role of the Paneth Cell in Zinc Metabolism in the Rat.* Ph.D. Thesis, Faculty of Medicine, Queen's University of Belfast, 1974, p. 62

3. Elmes, M. E. & Gwyn Jones, J. *Histochem. J.* 1981. *13,* 335–336

4. Hambidge, K. M., Neldner, K. H., Walravens, P. A., Weston, W. L., Silverman, A., Sabol, J. S. & Brown, R. M. *Zinc and Acrodermatitis Enteropathica.* In *Zinc and Copper in Clinical Medicine,* Spectrum Publications Inc., Holliswood, N.Y. 1978. pp. 81–98

5. Kagi, J. H. R., Himmelhoch, S. R., Whanger, P. D., Bethune, J. L. & Vallee, B. L. *J. Biol. Chem.* 1974, *249,* 3537–3542

6. Keeling, P. W. N. Jones, R. B., Hilton, P. J. & Thompson, R. P. H. *Gut,* 1980, *21,* 561–564

7. Lombeck, I., Bassewitz, D. B. von., Becker, K., Tinschmann, P. & Kastner, H. *Pediat. Res.* 1974, *8,* 82–88

8. Mager, M., McNary, W. F. & Lionetti, F. *J. Histochem. and Cytochem.* 1953, *1,* 493–504

9. Millar, M. J., Vincent, N. R. & Mawson, C. A. *J. Histochem. Cytochem.* 1961, *9,* 111–116

10. Okamoto, K. *Hyogo, J. Med. Sci.,* 1951, *1,* 77–88

11. Starcher, B. C., Glauber, J. G. & Madaras, J. G. 1980 *J. Nutr. 110,* 1391–1397

12. Sturniolo, G. C., Molokhia, M. M., Shields, R. & Turnberg, L. A. *Gut,* 1980, *21,* 387–391

# Ultrastructural Features of Allergic Manifestations in the Small Intestine of Children

MARGOT SHINER

Intestinal Studies Group, Clinical Research Centre, Harrow HA1 3UJ, UK

A comparison has been made between the fine structural damage of the small intestinal mucosa of children caused by the entry of 2 types of allergens:– milk proteins in cow's milk protein intolerance and gluten proteins in coeliac disease. These were discussed in the light of possible local hypersensitivity reactions.

*Key-words:* Coeliac disease; cow's milk protein intolerance; local hypersensitivity mechanisms; ultrastructure

*Dr. M. Shiner, FRCP FRCPath DCH, Intestinal Studies Group, Division of Clinical Sciences, Clinical Research Centre, Harrow HA1 3UJ, UK*

Food intolerances in children under the age of 2 years are mainly confined to those associated with the ingestion of either cow's milk or wheat. It is customary to refer to the symptoms they evoke as primary, due to an allergic response within the small intestine, or secondary, associated with a preceding intestinal condition such as gastro-enteritis. Since the secondary type often produces only transient intolerance to both foods and causes mucosal damage through different etiol-ogical mechanisms it will not be dealt with any further.

Primary allergic manifestations in the small intestinal mucosa due to cow's milk protein intolerance (CMPI) or coeliac disease (CD) have many features in common: they may occur together, allergy may not be confined to a single protein in cow's milk or gluten, symptoms usually start several weeks after first ingestion of the allergen and they may both lead to secondary carbohydrate intolerance, particularly lactose. The differences between CMPI and CD are, how-ever, more striking: CMPI is usually self-limiting whereas CD may be lifelong, CMPI is more fre-quently associated with infant and family atopy than CD and CMPI usually produces mild to moderately severe mucosal damage whereas CD causes a subtotal or villous atrophy which remains the diagnostic hallmark of the disease.

If the mucosal damage in CMPI and CD is etiologically related to their respective allergens and the immune reactions that follow their inges-tion, then the histological and ultrastructural appearances of the jejunal mucosa in untreated patients and in those treated and challenged with food to which they are intolerant should be stud-ied in the light of a local expression of possible hypersensitivity reactions.

*Cow's milk protein intolerance (CMPI)*

The histology of the small intestinal mucosa in untreated CMPI varies from normal to severe partial villous atrophy (3, 15) though a moder-ately severe partial villous atrophy with crypt hypertrophy is most common. Enterocyte height may be reduced and theliolymphocytes increased. Inflammatory cell infiltration of the lamina pro-pria is usually increased, especially plasma cells, eosinophils and mast cells.

Ultrastructurally, the enterocytes appear of mature type and their only abnormality is mod-erate shortening and branching of microvilli and increase in lysosomal number in the apical cyto-plasm (Fig. 1). Plasma cells in the lamina propria appear increased and moderately active (Fig. 2). Mast cells are either granulated or partly degran-ulated (Fig. 3). Variable increase in fibrocytes and macrophage activity may be seen. The eos-inophils show the typical well defined granules (Fig. 4). Mucosal immunofluorescence studies

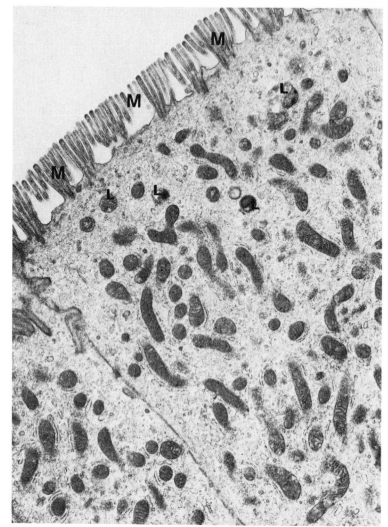

Fig. 1. Apical portion of enterocyte from the small intestineal mucosa of untreated cow's milk protein intolerance (CMPI). The microvilli (M) appear short and branched. The cytoplasmic organelles are typical of mature absorbing type of columnar epithelium. Lysosomes (L) are increased.    × 5,200

showed an increase in IgE plasma cells in 1 of 12, IgA in 4 of 5 and IgM in 1 of 5 patients (unpublished data).

Mucosal biopsies, obtained from children after cow's milk exclusion for several weeks, show histologically normal mucosae or a mild partial villous atrophy (2, 12) with normal enterocytes on fine structural examination (Fig. 5). Time sequence studies after a single oral challenge with cow's milk may show histological damage as early as 11 hours (12) with oedema and polymorphonuclear infiltration. More severe mucosal damage is seen at 24 hours but appears to subside at 48 hours (unpublished observation). Ultrastructurally, this damage affects the enterocytes leading to shortening of the cell, irregularity of the microvilli, increase in lysosomal number and mitochondrial damage (Fig. 6). In other areas

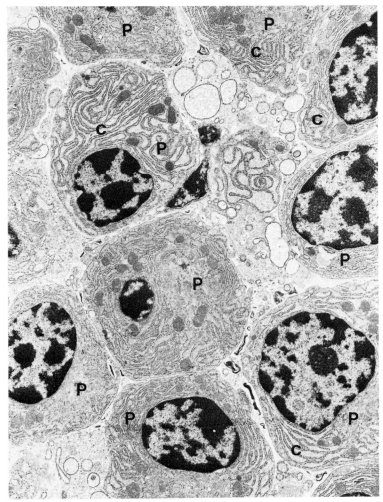

Fig. 2. Plasma cells (P) in the lamina propria in untreated CMPI. No other inflammatory cell type is visible, indicating increased infiltration of plasma cells whose cisternae (C) demonstrate all degrees of dilatation. × 3,500

intense polymorphonuclear infiltration between the enterocytes (Fig. 7) and in the lamina propria was observed (Fig. 8). Mast cells appear in an advanced state of degranulation (Fig. 9). Increased numbers of eosinophils may be seen with variable degranulated vacuoles (Fig. 10). Plasma cells appear moderately active and there may be some hypertrophy of the endothelium of small blood vessels and increase in fibrous tissue and collagen, none of these changes being marked when compared to pre-challenge ultrastructural appearances. Mucosal immunofluorescence showed increase in IgE plasma cells in 5 out of 6 patients, in IgA plasma cells in 3 of 6 and in IgM plasma cells in 2 of 6.

*Coeliac Disease (CD)*

The subtotal villous atrophy of the jejunal mucosa in children with untreated CD can usually but not always be differentiated from the histologically severest form of villous atrophy in untreated CMPI. Enterocyte height in CD is

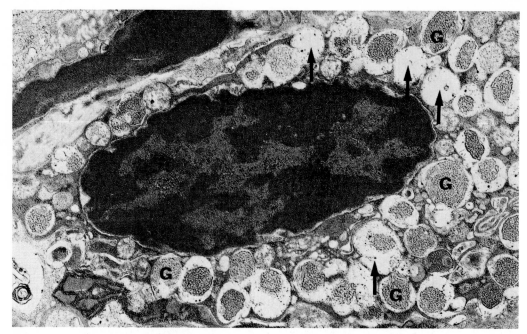

Fig. 3. A mast cell in untreated CMPI seen in the lamina propria containing typical granules (G) enclosed in smooth membranes of the endoplasmic reticulum. About ⅓ of the vacoules are empty (arrow) indicating degranulation.   × 8,300

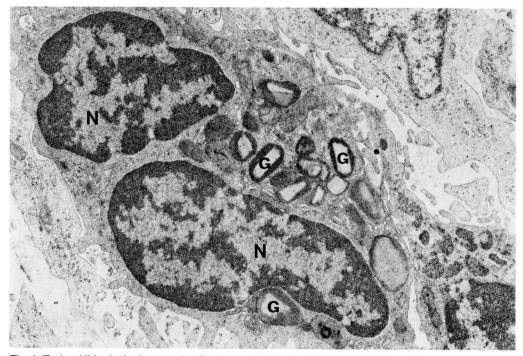

Fig. 4. Eosinophil in the lamina propria of untreated CMPI, showing two nuclei (N) and characteristic granules (G) with light crystalline central structures surrounded by dense homogenous material enclosed in smooth-membraned vacuoles.   × 5,800

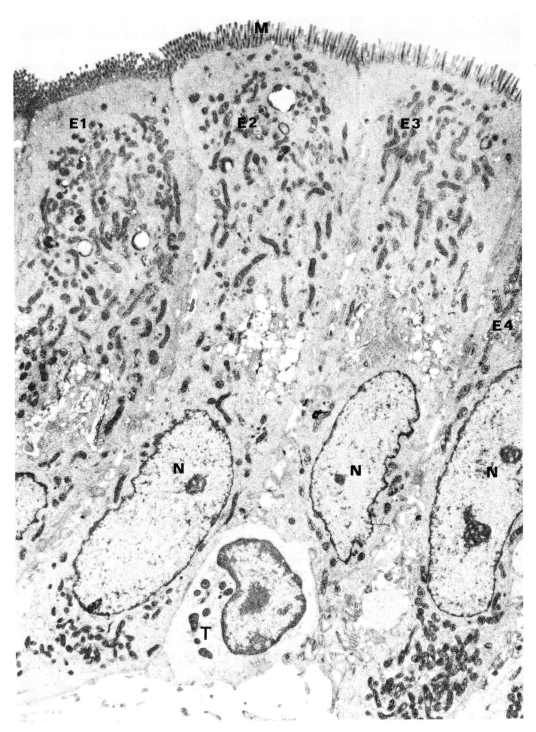

Fig. 5. Four enterocytes (E1–4) from the mucosa in CMPI after exclusion of cow's milk. Entirely normal appearance. T = theliolymphocyte.   × 2,200

markedly diminished and theliolymphocytes often twice as numerous as in CMPI. Other mucosal abnormalities include crypt hypertrophy with increase in mitosis, and an increase in inflammatory cells, predominantly mature plasma cells to be cleared normally (all jejunal biopsies were taken after a 12 hour fast). Numerous immature enterocytes may reach the luminal surface (Fig. 13) characterized by an excess of cytoplasmic ribosomes and polysomes. Lysosomes are

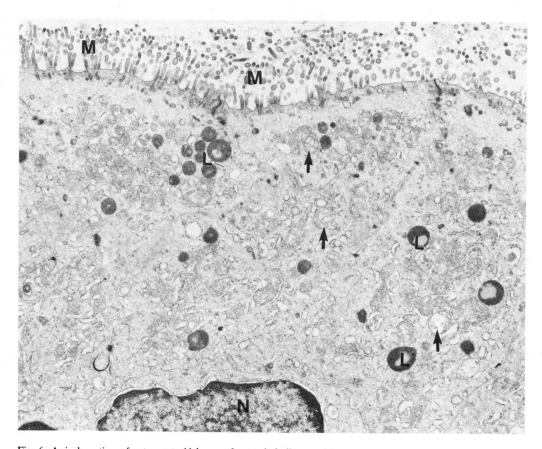

Fig. 6. Apical portion of enterocyte 11 hours after oral challenge with cow's milk. Same patient as Fig. 5. Note short amount of cytoplasm apical to the nucleus (N), the increase in lysosomes (L) and the irregularity and swelling of the microvilli (M). The mitochondria (arrows) appear swollen, with greater electron translucency and breaking up of the cristae.   × 2,900

but also lymphocytes, eosinophils and even polymorphs.

The fine structural appearances of the enterocyte layer in untreated coeliac disease is severely abnormal (Fig. 11). The microvilli show similar but more severe branching and shortening (Fig. 12). The more mature enterocytes (Fig. 11) may be filled with retained material (? fat), enclosed in membrane bound vacuoles, which has failed increased, mitochondria are swollen and the Golgi complex shows dilated vesicles (Figs. 13 and 11). Theliolymphocytes are very numerous in the enterocyte layer (Fig. 11). In the lamina propria isolated polymorphs may be seen (Fig. 14) but the predominant cells are plasma cells with dilated cisternae. Most of the mast cells are either partly or wholly degranulated (Fig. 15).

Similar pre- and post-challenge biopsy studies

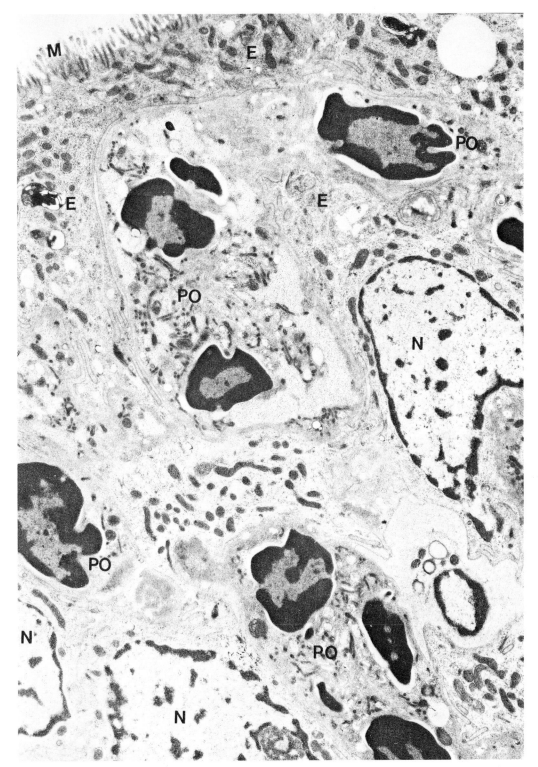

Fig. 7. Polymorphonuclear (PO) infiltration between enterocytes (E) 20 hours after cow's milk challenge in CMPI. The enterocyte nucleus (N) is easily distinguished from the smaller and densely staining nuclei of the 4 polymorphs. × 4,400

to those described for CMPI were carried out in children with CD. The jejunal mucosa reverted to normal on a gluten-free diet and was compared ultrastructurally in each child with those taken tation of plasma cells (Fig. 18), degranulated mast cells and moderate increase in eosinophils and polymorphs. In the early hours after gluten challenge the lamina propria appeared oedematous,

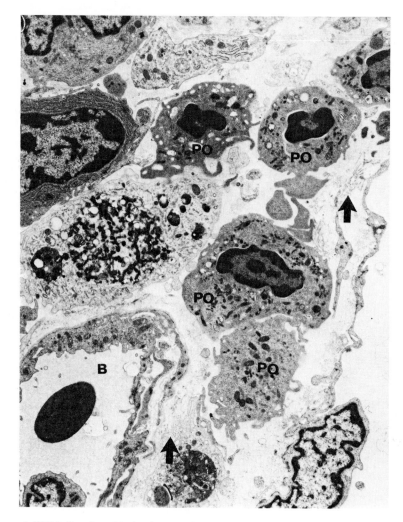

Fig. 8. Polymorph (PO) infiltration of the lamina propria in the same mucosa as Fig. 7. In this area the inflammatory cells are widely separated suggesting oedema although some fibrous tissue proliferation (arrow) is also evident. A blood vessel (B) is seen in the lower left hand corner.   × 3,000

sequentially up to 4 days (14). Throughout this period the enterocytes remained normal but the lamina propria showed distinct ultrastructural changes consisting of thickening of the basal laminae of enterocytes and blood vessels (Fig. 16), endothelial hypertrophy (Fig. 17), cisternal dila- but fibrous tissue increase and collagen fibres appeared after 20 hours (11). Immunofluorescence studies in 6 children with untreated coeliac disease showed an average IgA plasma cell count of 132.1 (normal range 26–65 cells per mucosal unit (5)) whereas the average IgA count in 4

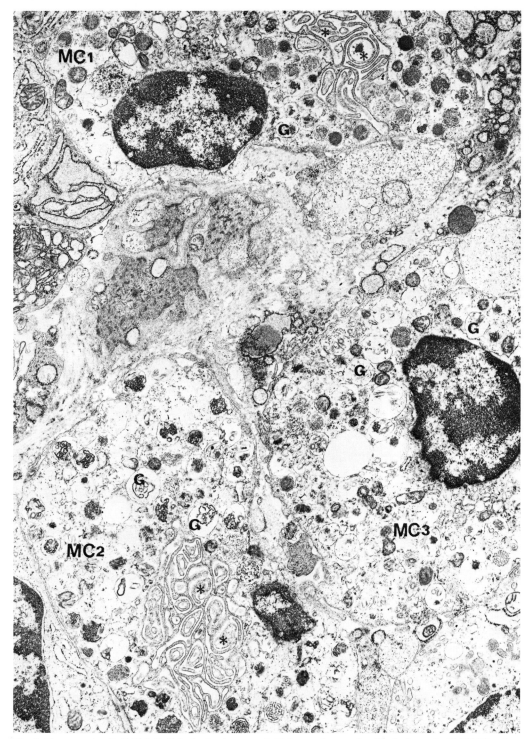

Fig. 9. Three mast cells (MC 1, 2, 3) in the lamina propria 11 hours after cow's milk challenge in CMPI. The close proximity of these cells to each other suggests an increase in number. The mast cell granules (G) are small and shrivelled and many empty vacuoles are seen. Cells MC 1 and 2 show an elaborate tubular system in their cytoplasm (asterisk), the so-called labyrinthine system through which the granular material is discharged. × 2,800

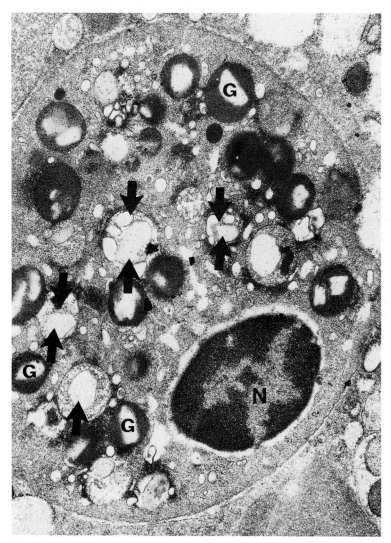

Fig. 10. Eosinophil showing typical nucleus (N) and cytoplasm granules (G), some of which are granulated (arrow). Compare with Fig. 4.   × 6,300

patients with CMPI was 89.6 cells. Similar values for IgM plasma cell counts were 37.1 in CD and 18.2 in CMPI (normal range 4–19 per mucosal unit). A numerical increase in IgE plasma cells was seen in all 4 children with CD tested, pronounced in 3 of the 4 (unpublished).

## DISCUSSION

There are undoubted similarities between the histological, ultrastructural and immunological appearances within the jejunal mucosa of untreated CMPI and CD which might suggest a common mode of damage caused by the respective allergens, differing only in degree. However, food challenges and repeat biopsies within hours of the ingested allergen have revealed certain differences in morphological events which are best shown by electron microscopy. Early (20 hours +) damage to the enterocytes in CMPI contrasts with delayed damage in CD. Jos et al. (1) reported histological damage in CD mainly

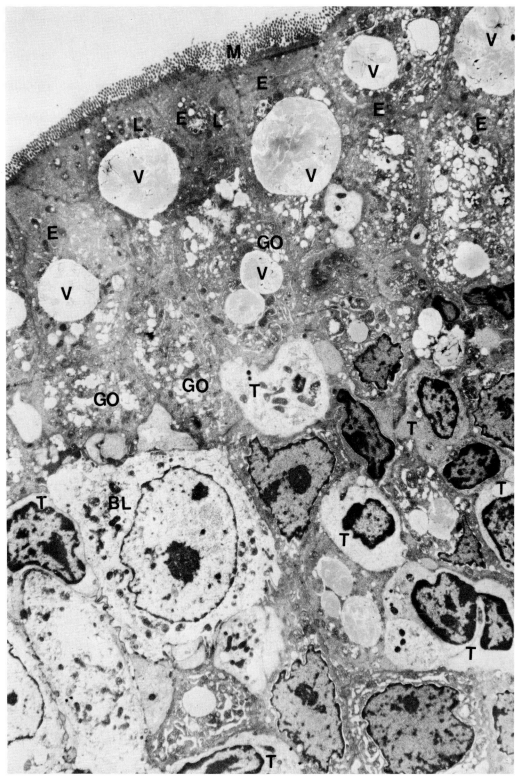

Fig. 11. Low magnification of several enterocytes (E) in untreated coeliac disease. The cells contain large vacuoles (V) filled with a homogenous material, probably fat. The Golgi vesicules (Go) are dilated and lysosomes (L) are numerous. Theliolymphocytes (T) invade the enterocyte layer. Note cell (BL) (? blast cell) apparently intra-epithelial, with large, pale nucleus containing 2 nucleoli.   × 1,800

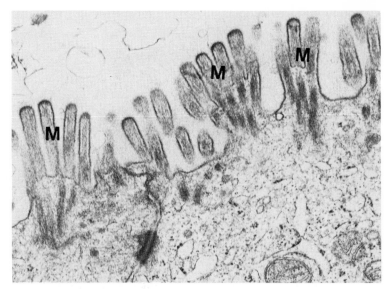

Fig. 12. Microvilli (M) of 2 enterocytes in untreated coeliac disease showing shortening and branching.   × 11,400

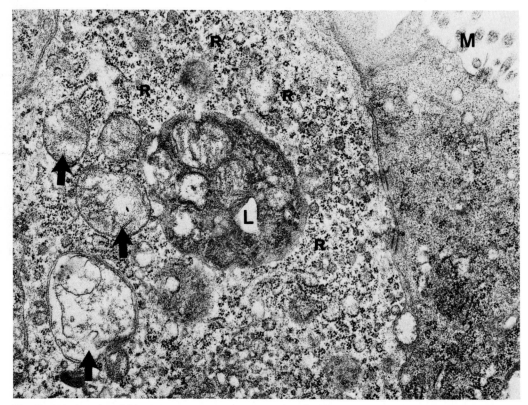

Fig. 13. Apical portion of 2 immature enterocytes in untreated coeliac disease, showing large numbers of ribosomes (R) and polysomes, a large lysosome (L) displaying autophagy and swollen mitochondria (arrow) in which the cristae are disrupted. M = microvilli.   × 9,200

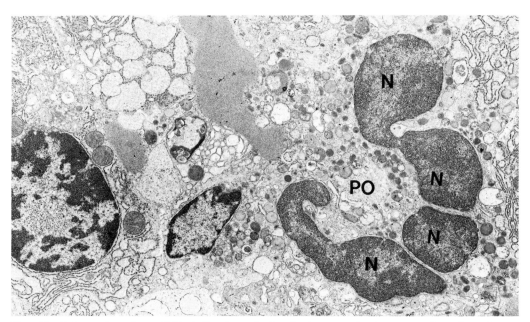

Fig. 14. Polymorphonuclear (PO) infiltration of the lamina propria in untreated coeliac disease.
N = nuclei.   × 4,500

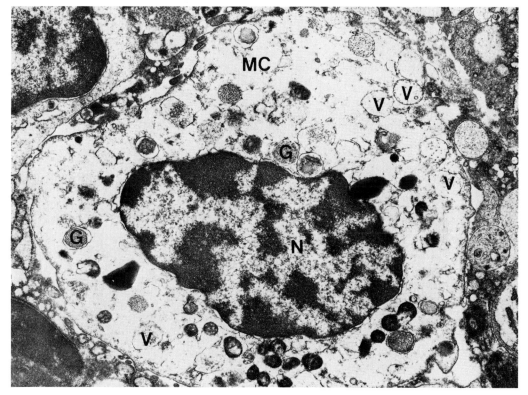

Fig. 15. Almost totally degranulated mast cell (MC) in the lamina propria in untreated coeliac disease.
V = vacuole. Compare with Fig. 3.   × 7,900

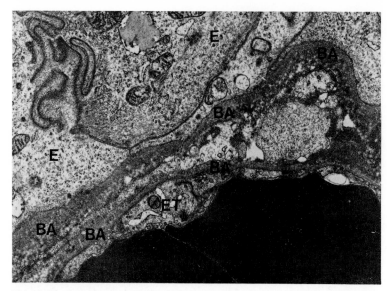

Fig. 16. The basal laminae (BA) of enterocytes (E) and blood vessels endothelium (ET) showing thickening and increased electron density. From the jejunal mucosa of treated coeliac disease after gluten challenge. RBC = red blood corpuscle.   × 3,100

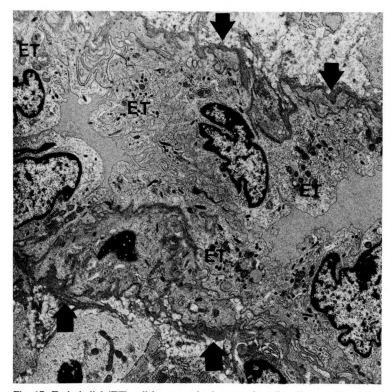

Fig. 17. Endothelial (ET) cell hypertrophy in treated coeliac disease after gluten challenge. Compare with Fig. 8. The basal lamina (arrow) is thickened around the swollen endothelium.   × 3,300

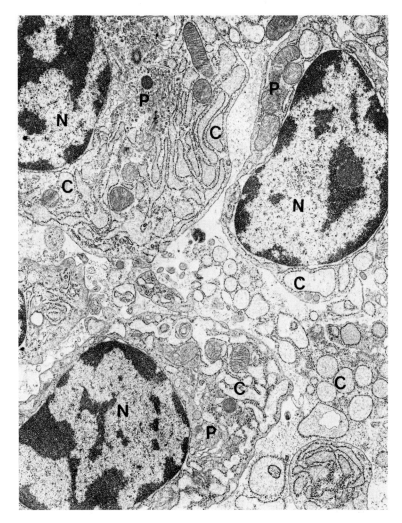

Fig. 18. Three plasma cells (P) in treated coeliac disease after gluten challenge with typical nuclear chromatin pattern and grossly dilated cytoplasmic cysternae (C). Some cisternae appear outside the limits of the cells. Compare with Fig. 2. × 7,100

after 5 days. Mast cell degranulation and polymorphonuclear infiltration is more marked in CMPI, whereas thickening of the basal laminae of epithelium and endothelium, endothelial hypertrophy, increase in fibrous tissue and collagen, and cisternal dilatation of plasma cells is greater in CD. In terms of possible hypersensitivity reactions initiated locally by the entry of allergen into the mucosa there is evidence of a reaginic type hypersensitivity (Type I) in the early

hours in both CMPI and CD. Whereas our own and others' immunofluorescence studies have not shown increases in IgE plasma cells in untreated CMPI (8) we demonstrated an increase in IgE cells within 6–23 hours after challenge (12, 13). Rosekrans *et al*. (9) found no increase at 48 hours after milk challenge. Similarly IgE cells were increased in untreated CD and also after challenge (2, 16). There was also ultrastructural and immunological evidence for a Type III hypersensitivity reaction (Arthus): in CMPI increase in polymorphs and in IgG and C3 complement in the basal laminae and connective tissue 6 and 23 hours post-challenge (12, 13) and in CD (10) thickening of the basal laminae, increase in polymorphs and IgA plasma cells with deposition of immune complexes in the basal laminae. If cytotoxicity were the result of this type of humoral-mediated hypersensitivity alone it would not explain the observed time difference between CMPI and CD in enterocyte damage. It might be postulated that in CMPI Type II hypersensitivity reactions cause direct enterocyte damage via antibody- (and complement?) dependent mechanisms and K-cells. In CMPI we have recently demonstrated the presence of plasma cells of IgA and IgE class within the jejunal mucosa producing specific antibodies to two milk proteins, β-lactoglobulin and bovine serum albumin (7) and complement is also activated after milk challenge (6). There is, therefore, at least evidence for both requirements of Type II hypersensitivity but so far no immunological evidence of K-cell activity. The delayed damage to enterocytes in CD on the other hand might be mediated via a delayed type hypersensitivity reaction (Type IV) and may involve T-lymphocytes and lymphokines which, in response to gluten challenge, may cause damage to the crypt epithelium, increased mitosis and faulty maturation of enterocytes. This may be accompanied by increased theliolymphocytes. Such a mechanism, leading to villous atrophy, has been shown experimentally to be due to a graft versus host reaction (4). It is clear that further immunological data on the precise mechanism of local hypersensitivity reactions are required to explain the observed fine structural changes after allergen challenge.

## ACKNOWLEDGEMENT

I am grateful to Mr. Ray Sapsford for technical assistance.

Figs. 1, 2, 6–9, 11–15 reproduced with permission from: Shiner, M. 'Normal and disease related ultrastructure of the small intestinal mucosa'. In publication, Springer-Verlag, London. Medical ed: M. Jackson.

## REFERENCES

1. Jos, J., Rey, J. & Frézal, J. *Arch. franç.Pédiat.* 1969, *26*, 849–859
2. Kingston, D., Pearson, J. & Shiner, M. pp. 394–405, in Pepys, J. & Edwards, A. M. (eds.), *The Mast Cell*, Pitman Medical, Bath, England, 1979
3. Kuitunen, P., Visakorpi, J. K., Savilahti, E. & Pelkonen, P. *Arch. dis. Childh.* 1975, *50*, 351–356
4. MacDonald, T. T. & Ferguson, A. *Gut* 1976, *17*, 81–91
5. Maffei, H. V. L., Kingston, D., Hill, I. D. & Shiner, M. *Pediat. Res.* 1979, *13*, 733–736
6. Matthews, T. S. & Soothill, J. F. *Lancet* 1970, *ii*, 893–895
7. Pearson, J., Kingston, D. & Shiner, M. 1981. In press
8. Perkkiö, M. *Allergy* 1980 *35*, 573–580
9. Rosekrans, P. C. M., Meijer, C. J. L. M., Cornelisse, C. J., Wal, A. M. & Lindeman, J. *J. clin. Pathol.* 1980, *33*, 125–130
10. Shiner, M. & Ballard, J. *Lancet* 1972, i, 1202–1205
11. Shiner, M. pp. 33–54, in Cooke, W. T. & Asquith, P. (eds.), *Clinics in Gastroenterology, Coeliac Disease*, Saunders Co. Ltd., London vol. 3 no.1, 1974
12. Shiner, M., Ballard, J. & Smith, M. E. *Lancet* 1975, i, 136–140
13. Shiner, M., Ballard, J., Brook, C. G. D. & Herman, S. *Lancet* 1975, ii, 1060–1063
14. Shmerling, D. H. & Shiner, M. pp. 64–75, in Booth, C. C. & Dowling, R. H. (eds.), *Coeliac Disease*, Churchill Livingstone, Edinburgh and London, 1970
15. Walker-Smith, J. p. 148, in Walker-Smith, J. (ed.) *Diseases of the Small Intestine in Childhood*. 2nd ed. Pitman Press, Bath, 1979
16. Walker-Smith, J. p. 224, in Walker-Smith, J. (ed.), *Diseases of the Small Intestine in Childhood*. 2nd ed. Pitman Press, Bath 1979

# Small Intestinal Mucosa in Childhood in Health and Disease

ALAN D. PHILLIPS
Electron Microscopist, Queen Elizabeth Hospital for Children,
Hackney Road, London, E2 8PS, UK

A great increase in the knowledge of human small intestinal mucosal pathology has resulted from the use of the peroral small intestinal biopsy technique.

This paper highlights some different applications of electron microscopy to such biopsy samples in order to obtain diagnostic criteria and to further the understanding of enteric processes in childhood in health and disease. The importance of control data in childhood is emphasized and differences are described between adult and childhood mucosa.

The possibilities of quantitative studies at the ultrastructural level and the link between structure and function are demonstrated by studies on microvillous appearance in relation to disaccharidase enzyme levels; the potential for experimental work is shown in studies using tracer molecules to investigate antigen permeability of the small intestine; and finally descriptive observation is highlighted in a section concerned with parasitic, bacterial and viral infections of the small intestine in childhood.

*A. D. Phillips, Queen Elizabeth Hospital for Children, Hackney Road, London, E2 8PS, UK*

The use of the peroral small intestine biopsy technique is now commonplace in medical centres investigating gastrointestinal disorder. Its introduction by Dr. Margot Shiner (56) in the U.K. and by Crosby & Kugler (14) in the U.S.A. has led to a great increase in the knowledge of small intestinal mucosal pathology. The vast majority of studies have been at the light microscopical level and in several disease states diagnostic pathology has been established, for example in coeliac disease (35) and in the cow's milk sensitive enteropathy of childhood (67) with the use of dietary challenges. The application of electron microscopy to such biopsy samples in order to further the understanding of enteric processes and to establish diagnostic criteria, has by no means been fully exploited. In this paper I wish to present some basic studies of small intestinal mucosa in childhood at the ultrastructural level in health and disease.

## Practical considerations

All the samples were from children undergoing peroral small intestinal biopsies at Queen Elizabeth hospital for Children, London, using a double port paediatric biopsy capsule (28). The children were fasted overnight and the biopsy was taken between 9.30 and 11.00 a.m. the following morning. All biopsies were taken from the 3rd or 4th part of the duodenum, the duodeno-jejunal flexure or the 1st part of the jejunum. After removal from the capsule each specimen was placed luminal side upwards on black filter paper, immersed in cold saline and viewed under a dissecting microscope. Routinely, a sample for electron microscopy was taken and fixed in 3% glutaraldehyde in 0.1 M phosphate (or cacodylate) buffer at pH 7.3. Additional samples, if required for other purposes, were taken at this stage. Conventional processing was used for routine transmission or scanning electron microscopy (44).

The small bowel biopsy capsule relies on suction pressure to draw mucosa into the port holes and to release a knife blade within the capsule to cut off the specimens. It is conceivable that artefacts may arise during this procedure, however, little work has been carried out to investigate such possibilities.

In a preliminary study we found that surgically removed samples of mouse small intestine placed in chambers and subjected to momentary suction pressures in the region of minus 8 to minus 14 psi exhibit few artefacts and certainly no more than surgically removed samples placed immediately into a fixative (52).

However, artefacts are most likely to arise when suction pressure is applied directly to the intact mucosa and include haemorrhage, epithelial stripping and trauma. These areas can easily be avoided either before taking the sample for EM, when the biopsy is viewed under the dissecting microscope, or subsequently when the sample is examined in the light microscope as a $\frac{1}{2}$–1 μm thick toluidine blue stained section prior to taking thin sections.

The biospy technique provides a small specimen of the small intestine, (often likened to a postage-stamp sized sample from a tennis court,) and only a part of this is taken for EM. Thus only a very small sample of the intestine is studied, an inevitability when using EM, but a necessary consideration when interpreting results. Because of the small sample size, it is important to orientate the specimen so that the maximum amount of information is obtained. It is assumed that all enterocytes pass through the same process of differentiation, maturation, ageing and exfoliation. Therefore, if the mucosa is sectioned along the axis on which these changes occur, information can be obtained at all stages of their life cycle, i.e. the mucosa is sectioned on a line parallel to the villi, from crypt base to villous tip. Similarly, the lamina propria will be sectioned at all levels in the mucosa. This approach has enabled us to describe changes in enterocyte ultrastructure occurring as they mature and age (44) which might otherwise have not been appreciated.

*"Normal" small intestinal mucosa in childhood*

At the present time the accepted ultrastuctural appearance of normal small intestinal mucosa is based, to a large extent, on the examination of biopsy specimens obtained from adults. Indeed, children without any past or present gastrointestinal complaints are not biopsied due to ethical considerations. However, there are several childhood diseases not found in adults (e.g. toddler's diarrhoea (66), the post-enteritis syndrome (18) and cow's milk protein intolerance (20)), susceptibility to gastroenteritis is greater in children, especially malnourished children and those under two years of age, and it is important to study the early stages of diseases that can occur throughout life (e.g. coeliac disease, Crohn's disease). Thus, it is of paramount importance to obtain information concerning the appearance of the gut in childhood, that is at a time when the above phenomena occur. Indeed, differences between adult and childhood intestinal mucosa are becoming apparent. Wright, Watson, Morley, Appleton & Marks (69) comparing epithelial cell kinetics in adults and children found that epithelial cell transit time in the crypts was 40% less in children and that the corrected mitotic index was 20% greater. Also post mortem studies on children dying from non-gastroenterological causes (64) demonstrated by gross examination that the villi in the duodenum and jejunum of children presented less surface-area than in adults. Recently, in an electron microscopical study of the appearance of the enterocyte in relation to its position on the villus in healthy children (44), we found differences from earlier observations made on adult small intestinal mucosa. It was noticeable that enterocytes had certain characteristics, depending on their villous position. These are described below, including some observations on crypt enteroblasts. These healthy children had no gastrointestinal symptoms at the time of biopsy and their mucosae were histologically normal, although they had had gastrointestinal symptoms previously.

*Crypt enteroblasts:*

Flask-shaped cells with basally located nuclei and little sub-nuclear cytoplasm. The apical cytoplasm contained few organelles but a noticeable number of free- and poly-ribosomes and some multivesicular lysosomes. Microvilli were present but not well organised and there was evidence of apocrine secretion (Fig. 1). Proceeding towards the villus the organelles, apart from free- and poly-ribosomes, increased in number and complexity, and lateral inter-digitations between the cells further developed, as did the brush border.

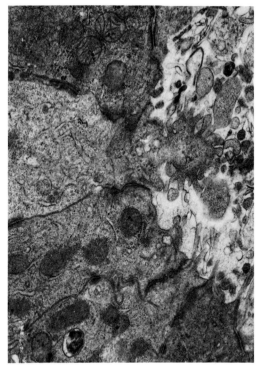

Fig. 1. Apical region of crypt enteroblasts. ×16,500

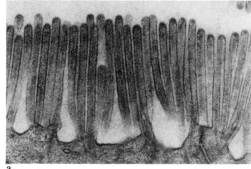

a

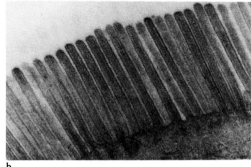

b

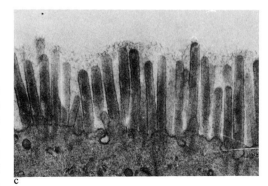

c

Fig. 2. The appearance of microvilli in a) low villous, b) mid villous and c) upper villous regions. ×26,000.

*Low-villous enterocytes:*

In this region two populations of enterocytes were evident. The most numerous cells were those with organelles of normal appearance, although there was some tufting of the microvilli (Fig. 2a). The other cells appeared to be suffering some osmotic imbalance or to be in the process of extrusion. That is, there was a variable appearance in which the various organelles were equally affected, including some or all of the following —dilation and/or vesiculation of rough endoplasmic reticulum (ER), mitochondrial swelling, microvillous decay, increased free- and polyribosomes and extrusion of cytoplasm (Fig. 3). These cells were usually adjacent to normal enterocytes and thus, it is unlikely that they represent an artefact of tissue collection or preparation (17). Cells in this region showing swollen mitochondria and/or dilated rER alone were similar to the 'undifferentiated' cells described by Shiner (57).

*Mid-villous enterocytes*

Enterocytes in the mid-region presented tall, thin close-packed microvilli (Fig. 2b). Organelle organisation was most marked in these cells, that is the various organelles only occurred, or were concentrated in, certain parts of the enterocyte, presumably a functional arrangement. If one proceeds from the apical to the basal cell region this organisation becomes apparent—the microvilli,

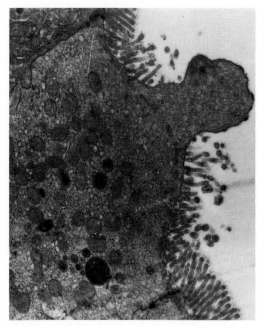

Fig. 3. An extruding cell in the low villous region.   ×11,500.

with their associated glycocalyx are an obvious specialization of the apical membrane and their filamentous cores run into the cell at right angles to other filaments which stretch across the cell from desmosomes on the lateral cell membrane to form the terminal web. Immediately below the terminal web is found smooth endoplasmic reticulum, multivesicular bodies and the paired centrioles (Fig. 4). Some secondary lysosomes may also be found in this region. Below this is an area rich in mitochondria, and rough ER extending to the nucleus. A prominent Golgi complex is found just above the nucleus, and below the nucleus the basal cytoplasm contains mitochondria, some rough ER and a noticeable quantity of free- and poly-ribosomes. Pinocytosis was evident in all cellular membranes but was most prominent in between the bases of the microvilli (Fig. 4).

*Upper-villous enterocytes*

In the upper part of the villus some changes in

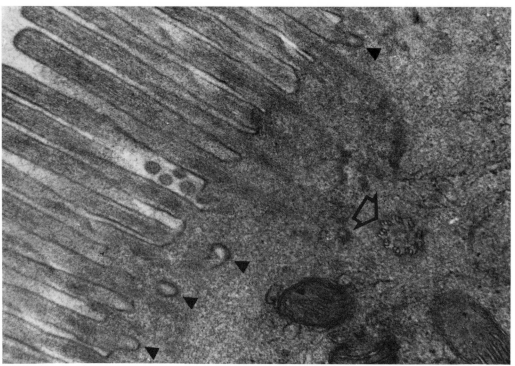

Fig. 4. Brush border region of enterocyte. Note centriole (open arrow) and pinocytotic vesicles (small arrows).   ×61,250.

organelle appearance became apparent. Microvilli, especially towards the villous tip, were shorter, uneven in height and often irregularly arranged (Fig. 2c). Three types of mitochondrial dissolution were observed in cells also containing normal mitochondria: swollen and burst mitochondria (Fig. 5a), pyknotic mitochondria, some of which appeared as 'signet-rings' (Fig. 5b), and mitochondria undergoing lysosomal digestion in autophagic vacuoles, as described by Biempica, Toccalino & O'Donnel (5) and Brunser, Castillo & Araya (9). These changes were present in all samples but were not widespread as the appear-

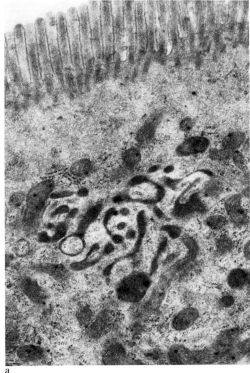

a

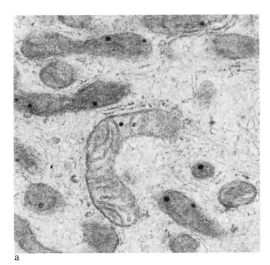

a

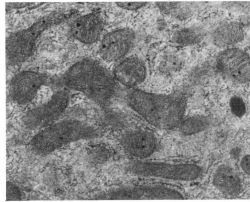

b

Fig. 6. a) Bizarre bodies in upper villous enterocyte. ×28,500. b) Branched mitochondrion. ×28,000.

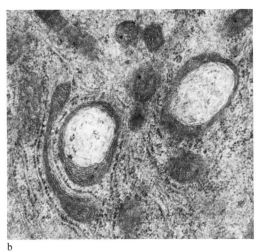

b

Fig. 5. a) Swollen mictochondrion. ×32,000. b) Pyknotic and signet-ring mitochondria. ×34,000.

ance of the majority of the mitochondria was normal.

Dense residual bodies, some having bizarre shapes (Fig. 6a) were seen in the apical region of some upper-villous enterocytes. The outlines of these bizarre bodies were similar to those of branched mitochondria (Fig. 6b). It is often assumed that mitochondria are simple sausage-shaped organelles and that there are numerous individual mitochondria present in cells. Figure 6(b) and other observations we have made on serial thin sections, and studies made on thick ($\frac{1}{2}$ μm) sections at 100 kV accelerating voltage suggest that this is not so. Many of the mitochondria present in enterocytes and intraepithelial lymphocytes are not simple sausage shapes but are quite branched and extend some distance through the cell (52). Similar observations have been made in mouse lymphocytes (50) and single cell algae (19). This effectively reduces the number of individual mitochondria present and imparts some rigidity to the cellular organisation, unless of course the joints between mitochondria are not stable and there is a constant interchange of mitochondrial connections. However, as described earlier there is a marked degree of intracellular organisation in the enterocytes and so it seems likely that the mitochondria are more complex in three dimensions than it would appear from two dimensional observation. It also seems likely that the bizarre bodies in the upper villous region represent such mitochondria undergoing pyknosis and lysosomal degeneration. (Fig. 6a).

Autophagic vacuoles (or cytolysosomes) were consistently found near the tips of the villi, where one would expect to find the oldest enterocytes, but in only one or two cells per section.

Extruding cells, where the various organelles were equally, but variably affected, as described earlier for a minority of low villous enterocytes, were observed near the villous tip (Fig. 7).

These organelle changes, seen in the upper parts of the villi are indicative of cytological damage. This could be the result of an adverse luminal effect due to the exposed position of these cells or be symptomatic of a natural ageing phenomenon occurring prior to extrusion. It is also possible, and perhaps more likely, that there is a combination of the two processes—older cells being less capable of resisting the noxious influence of substances in the gut lumen, so that both external and internal factors influence the morphology of the cells.

It is usually assumed that extrusion occurs in

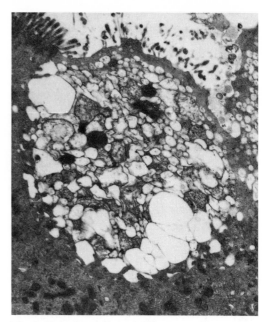

Fig. 7. Extruding cell.   ×9,200.

extrusion zones found near the villous tips. However, our observations suggest that extrusion is not limited to the villous tip region in healthy children, but can occur at other points particularly in the low villous region. Potten & Allen (49) observed extrusion occurring over the whole villus in an ultrastuctural study of cell loss in mouse small intestine, supporting our findings, although we found little evidence of extrusion occurring in the mid-villous region. We applied scanning electron microscopy (SEM) to extend the observations made by transmission electron microscopy (TEM) and found two apparent populations of enterocytes. One population, where the glycocalyx overlying the microvilli was present obscuring the underlying microvilli, and the other population, where the glycocalyx was absent so that the microvilli were clearly visible. These latter cells were particularly evident near the villous tips (Fig. 8) and to a lesser extent towards the bases of the villi, coinciding with the distribution of extruding cells seen by T.E.M. I have assumed that these cells observed by S.E.M. are extruding cells, and indeed some of them showed evidence of cytoplasmic extrusion. However, definitive

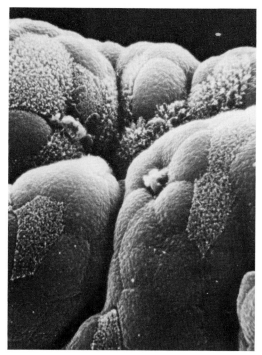

Fig. 8. SEM. Extrusion zone at villous tip.   ×2,000.

proof that they are one and the same is lacking. Iancu & Elian (22) stated that only exfoliating cells lack or have a disrupted glycocalyx and as it has been suggested (63) that the glycocalyx is a necessary part of the cell's defences against antigens and toxic molecules it seems logical to assume that when it is missing the enterocyte is no longer viable.

Thus, in small intestinal mucosa from healthy children we found the mid-region of the villus to be morphologically best adapted for digestion and absorption in contrast to the concept that cells at the tips of the villi are the most active (42). This concept was based on three pieces of evidence:

1) The microvilli have maximal surface area at the villous apices—we have found this not to be true for intestinal mucosa in childhood and will be discussed in more detail in the next section.

2) There is a reduction in ribonucleoprotein as the enterocyte travels up the villus—implying a decrease in free- and poly-ribosomes which are said to synthesize proteins for endogenous cellular needs (17). It may be that towards the villus tip

the amount of ribonucleoprotein present is insufficient to meet the cell's demands. The organelle damage we have observed (44) and the reduction in digestive enzymes reported by Nordström & Dalqvist (38) would support this (see next section).

3) The cells at the tips of the villi concentrate foodstuffs to a greater degree than the younger enterocytes below—this, however, may be a result of the maximal exposure to foodstuffs coupled with a relative inefficiency of transport out of the cell. Also, the occurrence of cellular extrusion near the villous tip argues against the presence of maximally active cells in the same region.

*Microvilli—Quantitative Studies*

Most EM studies are descriptive and thus rely on the subjective interpretation of observation. Where possible objective results are preferable as they provide information in a manner which is more easily verified by other workers and should reduce any bias the observer might hold. In order to confirm and extend the observation made on microvillous appearance over the villus (see previous section and Fig. 2) we quantified the microvillous surface area per square micron of cell surface (44). The microvilli are particularly important in the small intestine as they separate the enterocyte from the lumen of the gut, with its potentially cytotoxic constituents, house many digestive enzymes, which break down food products facilitating their absorption into the cell, and contain other enzymes responsible for maintaining the cells ionic balance (alkaline phosphatase, ATPase). Their finger-like shape is an obvious means of increasing the cell's luminal surface area both for digestion and absorption.

For purposes of quantification the appearance of a microvillus was approximated to a cylinder (surface area $2\pi rl$) with a flat cap (surface area $\pi r^2$). The number of microvilli (n) along a length of cell surface (d) was counted, allowing the number of microvilli per micron of cell surface to be calculated (n/d). This was squared to give the number of microvilli per square micron. The mean height (l) and the width (2r) of the microvilli were found and the mean surface area calculated. Multiplying this by the number of microvilli per square micron of cell surface gave the microvillous surface area per square micron of cell surface, i.e. $(n/d^2 \times (2\pi rl + \pi r^2)$.

By measuring microvillous surface area per square micron of cell surface the variable parameters of height, width and density of microvilli were all taken into consideration giving a more accurate measurement of differences in appearance than by measuring height alone. Also, errors of calibration were minimized as the result was expressed as a ratio of two areas from the same micrograph, not as a measurement per se.

The villus was split into three regions and the results from the children were meaned in each region. We found that the site of maximal microvillus surface area was the mid-villous region being statistically significantly greater than the tip region ($p < 0.005$) and the low region ($p = 0.025 - 0.01$) (Fig. 9).

These results conflict with observations made by Brown (8), who found that microvilli were tallest, most numerous, and hence presented the maximal surface area at the villous crests; those over the rest of the villus were shorter and less numerous. Support for our findings comes from a study by Merril, Sprinz & Tousimis (36) who found in prenatal, post-natal and adult guinea pig ileum that there was a reduction in height, number, and surface area of microvilli in the upper villous region, compared to the mid region. Also Brunser, Castillo & Araya (9) reported finding shorter microvilli in the cells at the villous tips of 3 control infants. Brown (8) gave no details of the ages of the patients in his study, however, Iancu & Elian (22) reported finding the same observations in microvillous appearance as Brown (8) in control patients with a mean age of 28 years (ranging from 5 years to 64 years). It is possible that adult mucosa has a different pattern of microvillous appearance to that in childhood, perhaps a reflection of the differences in cell turnover rate (69) and surface area (64) mentioned earlier.

The majority of small intestinal disaccharidase enzymes are found in the brush border of the enterocyte (12) and have been shown to be associated with the microvillous membrane (1, 26). It seems likely in view of this association that there

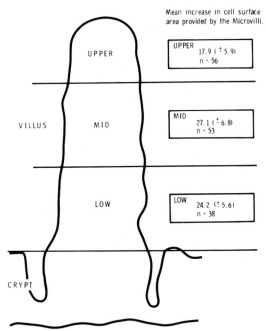

Fig. 9. The mean increase in surface area provided by the microvilli in each villous region (n = number of observations per region).

would be a relationship between microvillous surface area and the level of disaccharidase activity. In coeliac disease, for example, there is a reduction in microvillous height (57) and a reduction in mucosal disaccharidase activity (3, 34). It is thus of interest that Nordström & Dalqvist (38) investigating the quantitative distribution of some enzymes along the villus of human small intestine found that digestive enzymes, 'were almost exclusively present along the villi with the highest activities in the mid villi or apical halves of the villi'. Activities of sucrase, maltase, isomaltase, trehalase, and to some extent alkaline phosphatase, decreased in the upper parts of the duodenal villus. This distribution is similar to the pattern of microvillous surface area over the villus in childhood.

To further investigate this relationship we quantified the microvillous appearance in a group of seven children with secondary disaccharidase deficiency in contrast to five children with normal disaccharidase levels (45). The microvillous surface area was quantified as before, although the villus was split into five regions rather than three. Results from the control group confirmed our earlier report (44) of maximal surface area in the mid region of the villus in childhood and a reduction in surface area in the tip. A similar trend was seen in the children with secondary disaccharidase deficiency but at statistically significantly lower levels of microvillous surface area measurements (Fig. 10). Thus, when disaccharidase activities were reduced the microvillus surface area was also reduced. An example of the change in microvillous appearance is shown in Fig. 11.

The occurrence of a reduction in surface area rather than generalised microvillous disruption in these cases of disaccharidase deficiency suggested an alteration in microvillous membrane metabolism, perhaps as a result of a restriction in the supply of necessary metabolites, or a case of demand exceeding supply when turnover of microvillous membrane is high. In contrast to this, Klish et al. (29) found severe distortion and fragmentation of microvilli, as well as a reduction in surface area, in acute acquired monosaccharide intolerance.

Acquired monosaccharide tolerance is said to be a more complete manifestation of sugar intolerance than intolerance to just disaccharide, when occurring in the same clinical condition (2), and thus the extent of microvillous damage probably determines the extent of carbohydrate intolerance.

*Small Intestinal Permeability to Macromolecules*

The changes described so far are obviously important in relation to the small intestine's specialised functions of digestion and absorption. However, the gut also plays an especially important role in excluding potentially harmful substances present in the gut lumen, e.g. ingested antigens, bacterial toxins, proteolytic enzymes. In this respect, the single thick epithelial covering of the mucosa acts as a barrier preventing macromolecules from entering the internal milieu of the body. It is not a perfect barrier, however, as intact protein can cross the epithelium. Lippard, Schloss & Johnson (31) for example, demonstrated the presence of cow's milk antigen and cow's milk antibody in children's serum following milk drinking and it is now generally accepted that minute quantities of whole protein can enter the mucosa, producing no ill effects in the majority of people.

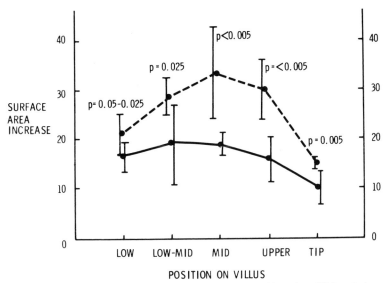

Fig. 10. The mean increase in cell surface area provided by microvilli in relation to position on the villus from 5 patients with normal disaccharidase activities (hatched line) and 7 patients with reduced disaccharidase activities (solid line). Vertical bar = ± 1 S.D.

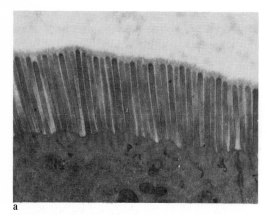

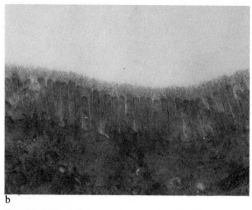

Fig. 11. Microvillous appearance in mid villous region in relation to disaccharidase activity. a) Normal disaccharidase (child on cow's milk free diet). b) Low disaccharidases (same child after clinical relapse following cow's milk feeding).

How macromolecules gain entry into the mucosa is under much study at the present time and two possible methods of entry are usually considered:

a) Diffusion—a passive, energy independent process whereby macromolecules enter through damaged or dying enterocytes or pass between epithelial cells through 'leaky' tight junctions.

b) Absorption—a process of active uptake of macromolecules by the enterocytes themselves in pinocytotic vesicles. The macromolecules somehow avoid breakdown by the lysosomes, positioned just below the brush border, to enter the lateral intracellular spaces by reverse pinocytosis.

The relative importance of either method is unknown and very few studies have been performed to confirm or deny their existence in human tissue, although several experimental animal studies have been carried out (10, 39). Such studies have a particular clinical relevance as antigenic molecules have been implicated in the pathogenesis of some gastrointestinal diseases. In the cow's milk protein induced enteropathy of childhood increased antigen entry into damaged mucosa during gastroenteritis has been suggested as the means by which susceptible individuals become sensitised to cow's milk protein (20). Re-exposure to milk protein, when the mucosa has healed but the individual is hypersensitive, results in mucosal damage. Thus antigen entry into normal as well as abnormal mucosa merits investigation.

We have recently been studying the anatomical pathways of macromolecular uptake in small intestinal biopsy samples using light- and electron-dense tracer molecules.

*Diffusion*

The rate of diffusion of molecules in solution can be deduced from Fick's law which states that the amount of dissolved substances crossing a plane of equal concentration in unit time is proportional to the concentration gradient.

$$N_{AD} = -D_{AB}\frac{dCA}{dZ}$$

where $N_{AD}$ is the rate of diffusion in moles per square centimetre per second, $D_{AB}$ is the diffusion coefficient, CA is the concentration of A in moles per cubic centimetre and Z is the distance in the direction of diffusion in centimetres.

If we consider the situation in the small intestine the distance of diffusion is effectively the thickness of the epithelium, around 30 µm in normal mucosa and less in abnormal mucosa. The concentration gradient will be extremely variable. However, if we take cow's milk proteins as an example, then there are around 3.3 g of protein per 100 ml made up largely of lactalbumin (0.3 mM) and casein (1.1 mM). Allowing for dilution and some digestion of the protein in digestive juices there could be micromolar concentrations of protein in the lumen of the proximal small intestine. The diffusion coefficients of proteins in the molecular weight range of 20 to 60,000 vary from eleven to six $\times$ $10^{-7}$ cm$^2$ per second (37).

In order to obtain some idea of what diffusion rates might be expected in the intestine, an imaginary protein can be taken in assumed conditions:

For example, a protein 'X' (M. Wt. 25,000) with an intestinal luminal concentration of 10 $\mu$M ($10 \times 10^{-9}$ moles per cm$^3$), a diffusion coefficient of $10 \times 10^{-7}$ cm$^2$ per second diffusing across a 25 $\mu$m thick epithelial layer would diffuse at a rate of:

$$\frac{-10}{10^7} \times \frac{10 \times 10^{-9}}{25 \times 10^{-4}} \text{ moles per cm}^2 \text{ per second}$$

(using Fick's Law).

$= 4 \times 10^{-12}$ moles (4 picomoles) per cm$^2$ per second.

This assumes that its effective concentration in the lamina propria is zero, as it will be carried away in the capillary system, and there is a linear concentration gradient across the epithelium. It is, of course, only an approximation as it ignores molecular shape and charge (if any) and assumes that the epithelium presents no barrier to macromolecular penetration. However, if pico-molar concentrations of protein can enter the mucosa it should be of immunological significance.

To investigate what pathways of entry by diffusion were present in the gut, in the absence of active processes, we exposed pieces of small intestinal biopsies to fixative solutions containing 0.5% ruthenium red or 10 $\mu$M horseradish peroxidase (23). The biopsy specimens were divided into two groups based on their histological appearance, i.e. 'normal' or 'abnormal'. The abnormal specimens came from children with a variety of gastrointestinal diseases, including coeliac disease, post-enteritis syndrome, giardiasis and cow's milk protein intolerance. Ruthenium red (RR) was applied as a test of cell integrity as it only enters damaged cells (33). It has a molecular weight around 1,000, a molecular diameter of approximately 1 nm and carries 6 positive charges per molecule. In 'normals', although in

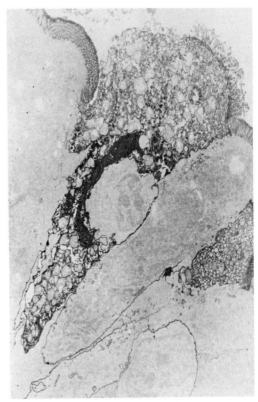

Fig. 12. Extruding cells penetrated by ruthenium red. Unstained section. $\times$4,000.

the most part excluded from the epithelium, ruthenium red entered some enterocytes at the tips and, to a lesser extent, at the base of the villi. Electron microscopy demonstrated that the cells penetrated were either damaged or extruding (Fig. 12). In the abnormal group more enterocytes, both singly and in small patches, were penetrated by ruthenium red. Intracellular staining occurred next to stained enterocytes in both groups and in the 'abnormals', where a number of neighbouring enterocytes were stained, ruthenium red also entered the basement membrane and lamina propria. The number of enterocytes entered by ruthenium red was counted, using light microscopy, and expressed as a percentage of the total number of enterocytes over the villus or, in the case of total villous atrophy, in the exposed surface epithelium. There was a significant increase ($p = 0.01 - 0.005$) in ruthenium red stained cells in the abnormal group (8.2% ± 3.6) in comparison to the normal group (3.7 ± 1.6).

The distribution of ruthenium red stained cells in normal mucosa coincides with the previous observations on the location of extruding cells (44) and the increased number of damaged enterocytes in abnormal mucosae agrees with other studies which have shown increased epithelial cell turnover rates in such situations (13, 16, 32, 47, 69). The penetration of ruthenium red into the lamina propria demonstrates that small molecular weight substances can cross the epithelial barrier through damaged enterocytes; however, the important question is whether these damaged cells are permeable to antigen-sized molecules.

Horseradish peroxidase (HRP) has a molecular weight of 40,000 (of a similar order to other food antigens), a molecular diameter of 5 nm, is a naturally occurring antigen protein, and has the ability to generate light- and electron-dense reaction product with no diffusion artefact when used in low concentrations (55, 58). It is then, an ideal macromolecule to use for studies on antigen permeability.

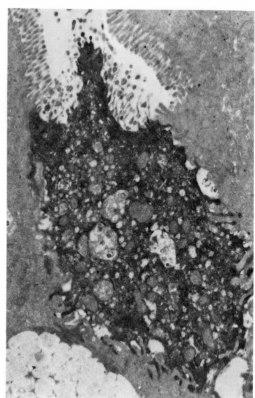

Fig. 14. Extruding cell penetrated by horseradish peroxidase. Unstained section.   ×9,000.

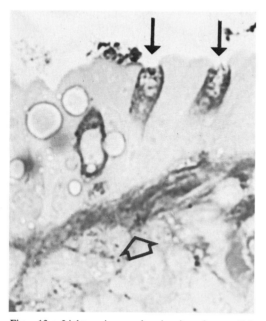

Fig. 13. Light micrograph showing horseradish peroxidase-penetrated enterocytes in abnormal mucosa (arrows) and peroxidase in the basement membrane region (open arrow). Unstained section.   ×1,000.

When histologically normal and abnormal groups of fixed biopsy samples were treated with horseradish peroxidase there was a general absence of exogenous reaction product in the normals (the method described by Cornell, Walker & Isselbacher (10) was used to develop the reaction product). Some enterocytes at the tips and bases of the villi were stained, as were a few goblet cells. Control incubations, omitting the exogenous horseradish peroxidase, were performed to reveal endogenous peroxidase activity. In abnormal mucosae increased numbers of enterocytes were diffusely penetrated by horseradish peroxidase; interepithelial staining and some penetration of HRP into the basement membrane was observed near stained enterocytes (Fig. 13), as found previously with ruthenium red. Quantifying the observations showed a significant increase (p < 0.005) in the number of HRP-penetrated cells in 'abnormals' (3.7% ± 0.8) compared to 'normals' (0.9% ± 0.8), and electron microscopy confirmed that HRP-stained cells were extruding or suffered gross organelle damage (Fig. 14). Reflecting their difference in molecular size, significantly less cells were penetrated by HRP than by RR in both normal and abnormal groups. This has also been observed by Köhler & Geyer (30) in a study of the guinea pig organ of Corti, using the same two tracers.

We were unable to find evidence of HRP within epithelial tight junctions, although reaction product was identified on either side of the junction. Interepithelial staining below the tight junction, by and large, occurred near stained enterocytes and it seems likely that diffusion of HRP from these cells into the intercellular spaces produced this phenomenon.

The entry of HRP into normal mucosa through extruding or non-viable enterocytes demonstrates a potential site of antigen entry and may account for some or all of the antigen entry in healthy children after an oral load. Entry through non-viable enterocytes avoids the lysosomal barrier found in viable enterocytes. The significant increase in HRP entry (a four fold increase) in abnormal mucosae indicates a greater proportion of enterocytes permeable to antigen through passive diffusion. Returning to the hypothetical situation described earlier, it is now clear that normal mucosa represents a 99% effective barrier to macromolecular diffusion so that any calculation of the rate of macromolecular entry must take this into account. In abnormal mucosa the efficiency of this barrier is significantly impaired. However, these observations were made on fixed tissue—the time taken for a damaged enterocyte to be exfoliated, i.e. the length of time to which it is permeable to macromolecules in vivo is unknown. Neither is it known if the process of extrusion takes a longer or shorter time in abnormal mucosae. Therefore, whilst we have shown that anatomical pathways for passive diffusion exist in small intestinal mucosa in childhood and that these pathways could theoretically account for immunologically significant macromolecular entry in normal, as well as in abnormal mucosa, their presence in living tissue needs to be established and investigated.

## Absorption and Diffusion

In order to investigate this point and study the role of active uptake of antigen we incubated biopsy specimens under conditions of organ culture (27) with 10 μM HRP (24). Again normal and abnormal mucosae were studied and the numbers of diffusely stained enterocytes were quantified as before.

In normal mucosae HRP was observed within pinocytotic vesicles in the apical region of enterocytes over the whole villus. It was also seen between enterocytes and in the basement membrane mainly at the bases of the villi. Occasionally HRP exocytosis was seen at enterocyte lateral membranes. However, staining was also evident within multivesicular bodies, indicating that the fate of some HRP was coalescence with lysosomal bodies within the enterocyte rather than passage out of the cell (Fig. 15). In abnormal mucosae there was a more varied pattern of HRP uptake in pinocytotic vesicles, that is less evidence of pinocytosis occurred in the more disrupted enterocytes, although normal or increased uptake of HRP was evident in more normal enterocytes.

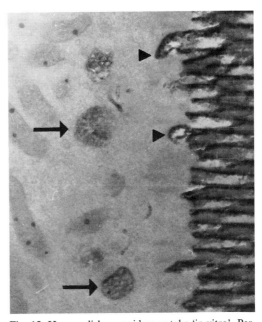

Fig. 15. Horseradish peroxidase uptake 'in vitro'. Peroxidase is seen in pinocytotic vesicles (short arrows) and in multivesicular bodies (long arrows). Unstained section. ×28,500.

Increased staining of the basement membrane was seen particularly in three cases of flat mucosae.

Diffuse staining of enterocytes, as described in the earlier study, was recognised and again significantly more enterocytes were stained by HRP in abnormal mucosae ($1.9\% \pm 1.98$, n = 7) in comparison to normal mucosae ($0.2\% \pm 0.14$, n = 7). The diffusely stained cells showed ultrastructural characteristics of damaged or extruding cells confirming the occurrence of macromolecular diffusion through damaged enterocytes in living tissue. In vivo studies in animals have also shown this phenomenon using HRP (10, 39) as well as demonstrating active uptake.

Thus two pathways of macromolecular entry into small intestinal mucosa have been identified. In normal mucosa passive diffusion and active absorption exist together and would account for the penetration of whole protein found in healthy children. In abnormal mucosa there is a significant increase in passive diffusion but no similar detectable increase in active absorption, suggesting that the passive diffusion of macromolecules through damaged enterocytes is the more important pathway in abnormal small intestinal mucosa.

## Gut Infections

The previous sections have been concerned with healthy small intestinal mucosa and its appearance in certain states, e.g. secondary disaccharidase deficiency and increased enterocyte turnover, which are common to several gastrointestinal diseases. However, there are certain conditions where more specific diagnoses can be made, for example when the mucosal appearance is distinguished by the presence of parasitic or infective agents.

## Giardia lamblia

Although *Giardia lamblia* is a common gastrointestinal parasite world-wide, it is not that frequently seen in our experience (approximately 2% of children undergoing gastrointestinal investigation have *Giardia* found on stool examination or small bowel biopsy). It is easily recognised in the scanning or transmission EM (Fig. 16)

although light microscopical analysis of stools or duodenal juice is the diagnostic method of choice.

A related parasite of rodents, *Giardia muris* has been suggested as an animal model of the

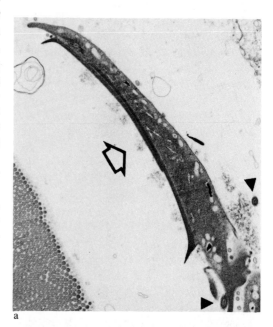

a

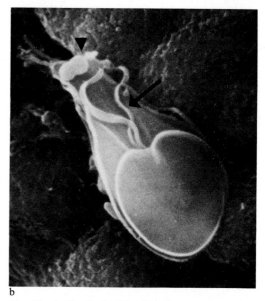

b

Fig. 16. a) *Giardia lamblia* (TEM). Note sucker disc (open arrow) and flagella (arrows). ×8,000. b) *G. lamblia* (SEM). Ventral surface displayed. Note spiral nature of sucker disc, flattened ventral flagella (arrow), and adherent diplococcus (short arrow). ×5,700.

human parasite (53), however, we have found certain differences between the two parasite species which suggest that *G. lamblia* is less pathogenic.

Using scanning electron microscopy we found that *G. lamblia* was not attached in great numbers to exposed mucosal areas but favoured the bases of villi and mucosal folds, presumably where there is some protection against physical dislocation. *Giardia* appeared 'adhesive disc' up as well as down and was often entwined with strands of mucus. There was no evidence of surface lesions as reported with infected mice (15). In the jejunum of the rat *G. muris* is reported to cover the villi (15) promoting the suggestion that *Giardia* forms a competitive barrier against absorption of foodstuffs. This theory would not be applicable to childhood infections in our experience. Indeed, in 9 recent cases *G. lamblia* appeared to have little overt effect on mucosal structure, some children had mild villous atrophy usually associated with reduced disaccharidase levels, especially lactase, and a minority had raised intraepithelial lymphocytes. All the 9 infected children were of low weight and short stature and although gastrointestinal symptoms improved following treatment, only one child showed a gain in weight and height.

One association not reported previously is the finding that isolated mucosal lymphoid follicles were more commonly seen in biopsies from children with *Giardia lamblia* infections. Over a five year period a total of 33% (263/796) of biopsies had lymphoid follicles present, whereas 60% (10/17) of the biopsies containing *G. lamblia* contained lymphoid follicles (25). There was no preferential localisation of *Giardia lamblia* to the epithelium overlying the follicles has been described for some organisms (41, 43). Owen, Allen & Stevens (40) have recently made the intriguing observation of *G. muris* trapping by macrophages in the epithelium overlying lymphoid follicles in normal and nude mice (Fig. 17). Most infected children mount an antibody response against *G. lamblia* and mucosal lymphoid follicles would be prime suspects for sites of antigen entry in man, although this has yet to be established.

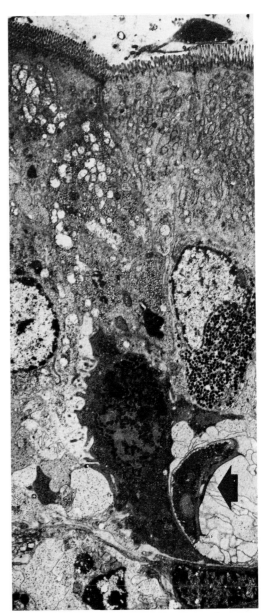

Fig. 17. Epithelium over lymphoid follicle of nude mouse. Note *G. muris* within a macrophage extension (arrow). 3,600. Reproduced from Owen et al (40) with kind permission of Dr R. Owen.

## Bacterial and Viral Infections

The children undergoing small bowel biopsy at Queen Elizabeth Hospital by and large do not have acute gastrointestinal problems but are being investigated for more long term complaints such as failure to thrive, food intolerances, and persistent diarrhoea. Also ethical considerations discourage small intestinal biopsy during acute episodes. As a result of this it is a rare event to find viruses or bacteria associated with the small intestine, although for this very reason when such associations arise they are especially intriguing.

I previously mentioned the increased incidence of IMLF in *Giardia* infections. In germ-free mice Peyer's patches (collections of lymphoid follicles) are present but do not develop germinal centres except when exposed to bacteria (48).

It is thus of interest that we have found preferential localisation of bacteria to the epithelium overlying an isolated mucosal lymphoid follicle in a histologically normal biopsy from a child who had had chronic diarrhoea for 7 months (43). Using SEM we identified many rod-like bacteria adhering to enterocytes overlying the follicle with evidence of increased cellular extrusion (Fig. 18)

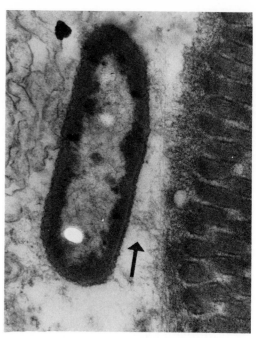

Fig. 19. Bacillus adhering to enterocyte surface. Note filamentous connections (arrow).    ×51,800

although not necessarily asscociated with adherent bacteria. Occasional bacteria were found adhering to villi away from the follicle but were not seen in sections taken from the rest of the biopsy for routine histological assessment. No evidence of invasion was found using TEM and no microvillous decay was observed in areas where bacterial adhesion occurred. Filamentous connections between the bacteria and microvilli were seen in some instances (Fig. 19). There was little evidence of ultrastructural alteration apart from a noticeable increase in cytolysosomes in nearly all villous enterocytes and the presence of variably sized fat droplets in some enterocytes.

Stool microbiology failed to demonstrate any pathogens during her 2 months admission apart from one rectal swab 7 days after the biopsy which grew *Salmonella agona*. A detailed microbiological examination of the biopsy and duodenal juice did not show the presence of any pathogens but there was local antibody production against an unidentified rod-like bacillus (4). Peyer's patches have been proposed as sites where antigen entry occurs (7, 62) and where priming of

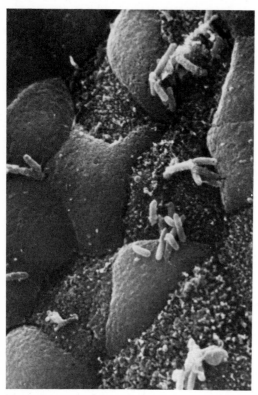

Fig. 18. Bacteria adhering to epithelium over a lymphoid follicle. Note extruding cells. SEM   ×5,000.

immunoblast cells takes place prior to migration to the lamina propria of the gut, where they secrete immunoglobulin (11). This in vivo adherence of bacteria to the epithelium overlying the lymphoid follicle suggests an involvement in the pathogenesis of the child's protracted diarrhoea. Indeed, the observations in this section on mucosal lymphoid follicles indicate that they may have important roles to play in gut infections and merit further detailed study.

*E. coli* may be grouped into enteropathogenic (EPEC), enterotoxigenic (ETEC), and invasive strains. EPEC can cause diarrhoea in man yet do not produce recognised toxins, whereas ETEC release recognised enterotoxins. An important factor in the pathogenicity of *E. coli* is the ability to adhere to the mucosal surface. The phenomenon of bacterial adherence without invasion or overt mucosal damage was illustrated above and has also been described for normal gut flora (see review (54)). Adhesion of *E. coli* with microvillous damage but no invasion or recognised toxin production has recently been recognised (61) and we have seen a similar case involving *E. coli* 0128 adhesion in a boy suffering a severe form of traveller's diarrhoea (21), although we were unable to determine toxin production.

The child's small intestinal biopsy showed a severe enteropathy with adhering gram-negative bacilli, and his duodenal juice grew *E. coli* 0128 and *Pseudomonas aeruginosa*. These organisms were detected in his stool for 6 and 8 weeks respectively. TEM showed many rod-like bacteria adhering to enterocyte surfaces on raised cup-like projections lacking microvilli (Fig. 20). No bacterial invasion was identified and enterocytes without bacteria adhesion possessed short microvilli. Neutrophil polymorphs were present in the epithelium. The terminal web near sites of adhesion was disorganised and increased free- and poly-ribosomes, dilated rough ER and swollen mitochondria were observed in enterocytes. Indirect immunofluorescence using 0128 agglutinating serum demonstrated *E. coli* 0128 adhering to the brush border and in mucus above the mucosa. There was no cross reaction with *Pseudomonas aeruginosa*. This appearance has been described as a cytotoxic enteritis (61) and may represent a novel method of causing diarrhoea in man. It has also been seen in *E. coli*. infections in adult rabbits (60).

*E. coli* 0128 is usually referred to as an EPEC, however, it is now recognised that it can produce stable toxin (51), underlining the importance of determining the toxin producing capacity of isolated strains.

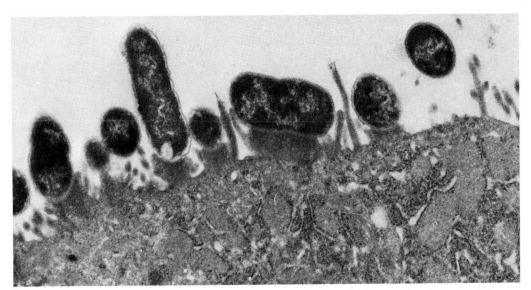

Fig. 20. Bacteria adhering to enterocyte surface on cup-like projections with loss of microvilli. ×16,500

*Viral Infections*

Direct visualisation of rotavirus particles within the small intestinal mucosa has only been reported on two occasions (6, 59) in children with acute gastroenteritis. Recently we have found rotavirus particles within the abnormal small intestinal mucosae of two children with cow's milk protein intolerance (46). The two cases provide an interesting comparison as the distribution of rotavirus was not identical and one child did not have any of the symptoms normally associated with rotavirus infection.

One child whose weight had been static for four months since commencing cow's milk feedings, had had diarrhoea for five days precipitating his hospital admission. His diarrhoea continued and he was biopsied on day 10 of his illness. Stools collected on days 10 and 14 of illness were examined by negative staining EM and contained rotavirus particles. On ultrastructural examination of his biopsy, rotavirus particles were found within expanded rough endoplasmic reticulum of villous enterocytes (Fig. 21) and within macrophages of the lamina propria. Two attempts to return him to a cow's milk feed failed. He was put on a cow's milk-free diet, and showed a rapid

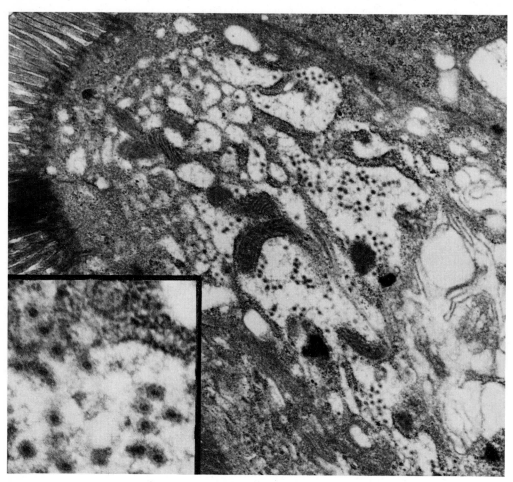

Fig. 21. Rotavirus within expanded rough ER of enterocyte.   ×22,000. Insert: detail showing rotavirus particles.   × 76,300

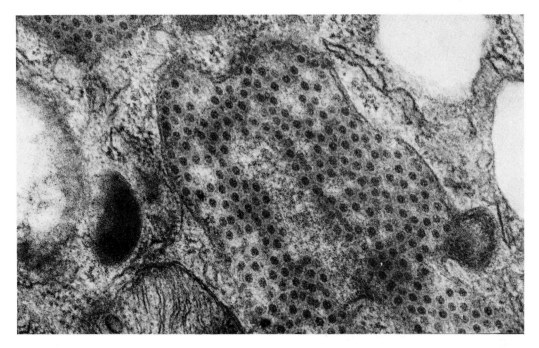

Fig. 22. Rotavirus particles in a membrane bound inclusion within a macrophage.   ×70,700

clinical improvement with weight gain. Normally acute rotavirus infections are mild self-limiting illnesses only lasting 5–8 days and the return to cow's milk is uneventful (65).

The other child had a history of failure to thrive for four months with no acute gastrointestinal symptoms. His biopsy was abnormal and showed crypt atrophy. Rotavirus particles were seen, as above, within macrophages in the lamina propria of the villi (Fig. 22) but not within expanded rough endoplasmic reticulum of enterocytes. Rotavirus was seen, however, within a few enterocyte autophagic vacuoles (Fig. 23). Macrophages were also seen within the epithelium. The absence of rotavirus from rough endoplasmic reticulum is interesting in view of the subclinical nature of the infection. It is feasible that macrophage phagocytosis and lysosomal containment has prevented the development of overt acute symptoms. When the child was placed on a cow's milk-free diet he rapidly gained weight.

To ensure that the particles seen in section were rotavirus, mucosal homogenates from both children were studied by negative staining EM and typical rotavirus particles were identified.

The presence of rotavirus in damaged mucosa at a time of cow's milk intolerance may indicate

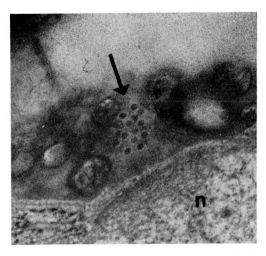

Fig. 23. Rotavirus particles (arrow) within autophagic vacuole. n = nucleus.   ×62,000

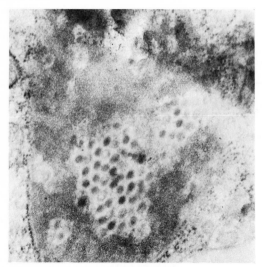

Fig. 24. Adenovirus particles within a nucleus. Histological sample reprocessed for T.E.M.   ×83,000

a viral role in the pathogenesis of this disease and demonstrates the need for further ultrastructural studies in similar cases to investigate the frequency of such findings.

Several morphologically distinct viruses, as well as rotavirus, have been found by EM examination of stools from children with gastroenteritis. These include calicivirus, astrovirus, adenovirus, coronavirus, and small viral particles. Adenovirus has been reported in the small intestinal mucosa of a child who died from gastroenteritis (68) and we have made a similar finding (Fig. 24) in a child suffering a sudden infant death. As far as I am aware, the other viruses have not been recognised within the small intestinal mucosa in man and such findings would obviously enhance their status as aetiological agents of gastrointestinal disease.

## ACKNOWLEDGEMENTS:

I would like to acknowledge my debt to Dr. John Walker-Smith and thank him for his helpful encouragement and advice. I must also thank Derek Jackson, Steve Rice, and colleagues in gastroenterology at Queen Elizabeth Hospital for Children for their assistance, and Judi Hills for typing the manuscript.

Figs. 2, 3, 5 & 9 are from Phillips et al. (44) and are reproduced with permission of the Editor of *Histopathology*.

Figs. 10 and 11 are from Phillips et al. (45) and are reproduced with permission of the Editor of *Gut*.

## REFERENCES

1. Alpers, D. H. & Seetharam, B. *New England Journal of Medicine* 1977, *296*, 1047–1050
2. Anderson, C. M. & Burke, V. pp. 199–217 in Anderson, C. M. & Burke, V. (eds.), *Paediatric Gastroenterology* Blackwell, Oxford, 1975
3. Anderson, C. M., Burke, V., Messer, M. & Kerry, K. R. *Lancet.* 1966 (*i*), 1322
4. Avigad, S., Manuel, P., Bampoe, V., Walker-Smith, J. A. & Shiner, M. *Lancet* 1978 (*i*), 1130–1132
5. Biempica, L., Toccalino, H. & O'Donnell, J. C. *Am. J. Pathol.* 1968, *52*, 795–823
6. Bishop, R. F., Davidson, G. P., Holmes, I. H. & Ruck, B. J. *Lancet.* 1973 (*ii*), 1281–1283
7. Bockman, D. E. & Cooper, M. D. *Am. J. Anat.* 1973, *136*, 455–478
8. Brown, A. L. Jr. *J. Cell Biol.* 1962, *12*, 623–627
9. Brunser, O., Castillo, C. & Araya, M. *Gastroenterology* 1976, *70*, 495–507
10. Cornell, R., Walker, W. A. & Isselbacher, K. J. *Lab. Invest.* 1971, *25*, 42–48
11. Craig, S. W. & Cebra, J. J. *J. Exp. Med.* 1971, *134*, 188–200
12. Crane, R. K. pp. 25–51 in Dickens, F., Randle, P. J. & Whelan, W. J. (eds.) *Carbohydrate Metabolism and its Disorders.* Academic Press, London, 1968
13. Croft, D. N., Loehry, C. A. & Creamer, B. *Lancet* 1969 (*ii*), 68–70
14. Crosby, W. H. & Kugler, H. W. *Am. J. Dig. Dis.* 1957, *2*, 236–241
15. Erlandsen, S. L. & Chase, D. G. *Am. J. Clin. Nutrition* 1974, *27*, 1277–1286
16. Ferguson, A. & Snodgrass, D. R. *Acta. Paed. Belgica.* 1978, *31*, 109
17. Ghadially, F. N. *Ultrastructural Pathology of the Cell.* Butterworths, London & Boston, 1975
18. Gribbin, M., Walker-Smith, J. A. & Wood, C. B. S. *Acta. Paed. Belgica.* 1976, *29*, 167–176
19. Grobe, B. & Arnold, C. G. *Protoplasma.* 1975, *86*, 291–294
20. Harrison, M., Kilby, A., Walker-Smith, J. A. & Wood, C. B. S. *Brit. Med. J.* 1976, *1*, 1501–1504
21. Hutchins, P., Hindocha, P., Phillips, A. & Walker-Smith, J. *Lancet,* 1979 (*ii*), 1373–1374
22. Iancu, T. & Elian, E. *Acta. Paed. Scandinavica.* 1976, *65*, 65–73
23. Jackson, D., Walker-Smith, J. A. & Phillips, A. D. *Acta. Paed. Belgica.* 1980, *33*, 133–134
24. Jackson, D., Walker-Smith, J. A. & Phillips, A. D. in preparation
25. Jackson, D., Walker-Smith, J. A & Phillips, A. D. Unpublished observations
26. Johnson, C. F. *Science* 1957, *155*, 1670–1672
27. Jos, J., Lenoir, G., de Ritis, G. & Rey, J. *Scand. J. Gastroent.* 1975, *10*, 121–128

28. Kilby, A. *Gut* 1976, *17*, 158–159
29. Klish, W. J., Udall, J. N., Rodriguez, J. T., Singer, D. B. & Nichols, B. L. *J. Paediatrics.* 1978, *92*, 566–571
30. Köhler, B. & Geyer, G. *Acta. Histochemica.* 1978, *63*, 261–264
31. Lippard, V. M., Schloss, O. M. & Johnson, P. A. *Am. J. Dis. Childhood* 1936, *51*, 562–574
32. Loehry, C. A., Croft, D. N., Singh, A. K. & Creamer, B. *Gut* 1969, *10*, 13–18
33. Luft, J. H. *Anat. Record.* 1971, *171*, 347–426
34. McNeish, A. S. & Sweet, E. M. *Arch. Dis. Childhood* 1968, *42*, 433–437
35. Meeuwisse, G. W. *Acta. Paed. Scandinavica* 1970, *59*, 461–463
36. Merril, T. G., Sprinz, H. & Tousimis, A. J. *J. Ultrastr. Res.* 1967, *19*, 304–326
37. Moore, W. J. *Physical Chemistry* (4th ed.). Longman, 1962
38. Nordström, C. & Dalqvist, A. *Scand. J. Gastroent.* 1973, *8*, 407–416
39. Owen, R. L. *Gastroenterology* 1977, *72*, 440–451
40. Owen, R. L., Allen, C. L. & Stevens, D. P. *Infection and Immunity* (In press)
41. Owen, R. L. & Nemanic, P. pp. 367–378 in Becker, R. P. & Johari, O. (eds.), *Scanning Electron Microscopy/1978 Vol II.* Illinois SEM, Inc. 1978
42. Padykula, H. A. *Fed. Proceedings* 1962, *21*, 873–879
43. Phillips, A. D., Rice, S., France, N. E. & Walker-Smith, J. A. *Lancet* 1978 (*i*), 454
44. Phillips, A.D., France, N.E. & Walker-Smith, J. A. *Histopathology* 1979, *3*, 117–130
45. Phillips, A. D., Avigad, S., Sacks, J., Rice, S., France, N. E. & Walker-Smith, J. A. *Gut* 1980, *21*, 44–48
46. Phillips, A. D., Rice, S., Variend, S. & Walker-Smith, J. A. In preparation
47. Pink, I. J., Croft, D. N. & Creamer, B. *Gut* 1970, *11*, 217–222
48. Pollard, M. & Sharon, N. *Infec. Immun.* 1970, *2*, 96
49. Potten, C. S., & Allen, T. D. *J. Ultrastr. Res.* 1977, *60*, 272–277
50. Rancourt, M. W., McKee, A. P. & Pollack, W. *J. Ultrastr. Res.* 1975, *51*, 418–424
51. Reis, M. H. L., Castro, A. F. P., Toledo, M. R. F. & Trabusi, L. R. *Infec. Immun.* 1979, *24*, 289–290
52. Rice, S. & Phillips, A. D. Unpublished observation
53. Roberts-Thomson, I. C., Stevens, D. P., Mahmoud, D. F. & Warren, K. S. *Gastroenterology* 1976, *71*, 57–61
54. Savage, D. pp 31–59 in Beachy, E. M. (ed.), *Bacterial Adherence.* Chapman & Hall, London & New York, 1980
55. Seligman, A. M., Shannon, W. A., Hoshino, Y. & Plapinger, R. E. *J. Histochem. Cytochem.* 1973, *21*, 756–758
56. Shiner, M. *Lancet.* 1956 (*i*), 85
57. Shiner, M. *Clinics in Gastroenterology.* 1974, *3*, 33–53
58. Strauss, W. *Methods & Achievments in Experimental Pathology* 1969, *4*, 54–91
59. Suzuki, H. & Konno, T. *Tohoku J. exp. Med.* 1975, *115*, 199–211
60. Takeuchi, A., Inman, L. R., O'Hanley, P. D., Cantley, J. R. & Lushbangh, W. B. *Infec. Immun.* 1978, *19*, 686–694
61. Ulshen, M. H. & Rollo, J. L. *N. England J. Med.* 1980, *302*, 99–101
62. Wacksmann, B. H. *J. Immunology* 1973, *111*, 878–884
63. Walker, W. A. *Pediatric Clinics of North America.* 1975, *22*, 731–746.
64. Walker-Smith, J. A. M.D. Thesis, University of Sydney. 1970
65. Walker-Smith, J. A. *Diseases of the Small Intestine in Childhood.* (2nd ed.) Pitman Medical, 1979
66 Walker-Smith, J. A. *Arch. Dis. Childhood* 1980, *55*, 329–330
67. Walker-Smith, J. A., Harrison, M., Kilby, A., Phillips, A. D. & France, N. E. *Arch. Dis. Childhood* 1978, *53*, 375–380
68. Whitelaw, A., Davies, H. & Parry, J. *Lancet,* 1977, (*i*) 361
69. Wright, N., Watson, A., Morley, A., Appleton, D. & Marks, J. *Gut* 1973, *14*, 701–710

# Studies of Intestinal Lymphoid Tissue

## The Cytology and Electron Microscopy of Gluten-Sensitive Enteropathy, with Particular Reference to its Immunopathology

M. N. MARSH

University Dept. of Medicine, Hope Hospital (University of Manchester School of Medicine), Eccles Old Road, Salford, Manchester, UK

Knowledge of the cytology, ultrastructure and histochemistry of the small intestinal mucosa has advanced considerably over the last 20 years, particularly in regard to the changes associated with coeliac disease. Many of the known structural and cytological changes in coeliac mucosa are probably non-specific, and not directly related to its pathogenesis. It seems important to move away from purely descriptive images of mucosal abnormality such as 'villous atrophy', and static measurements, such as crypt-villous ratios. Rather, the mucosa should be viewed as a dynamic, three-dimensional structure and evaluated in terms of total villous cell counts, crypt cell production rates, and so on. The organisation of the lamina propria is still poorly documented, and requires further exploration at the ultrastructural level. More thought should be given to the meaning of mucosal permeability and to its structural counterparts.

The immunocytopathology of the coeliac lesion is far from understood; it is questionable whether local humoral activity is central to the pathogenesis of the condition. More needs to be learned of the role of T cells, not only in local mucosal reactions, but also in terms of possible regulatory effects on crypt cell kinetics, villous shape and hence mucosal structure. Increased mitotic activity of epithelial lymphocytes in coeliac disease appears to correlate exclusively with gluten-sensitivity and the use of this presumed immunological marker in the histological diagnosis, and thus prediction, of gluten-sensitised individuals is proposed in this paper.

*Key-words:* Small intestine; coeliac disease; epithelial lymphocytes; mitotic index; cell-mediated immunity

*M. N. Marsh, Univ. Dept. of Medicine, Hope Hospital, Eccles Old Road, Salford, Manchester, UK*

## THE JEJUNAL LESION IN COELIAC DISEASE

### Introduction

The development (173) and widespread use of intestinal biopsy techniques, whereby specimens of jejunal mucosa are obtained from unanaesthetised human subjects, has revolutionised our understanding of many physiological functions and pathological abnormalities of the small bowel (161, 190, 191). Such advances, in particular, are exemplified by the numerous studies conducted into the physiopathology of gluten-sensitive enteropathy (GSE). It is with these investigations, and especially the associated immunological perturbations in this condition, that this paper is concerned.

### Non-specific Alterations in Gluten-sensitive enteropathy: Cytology & Ultrastructure (Figs. 1, 3)

Although first demonstrated in operative specimens (143), the broad outlines of the cytologic, and ultrastructural, features of the 'coeliac lesion' sprang from numerous detailed studies of specimens obtained by the peroral suction-biopsy technique (160, 162, 174, 175, 176). Much of this description was directed towards the grossly disorganised, irregular, and flattened epithelial cells, and their damaged microvilli (42) as compared with normal. At the time, however, these observations focussed attention on the epithelium as the prime (and perhaps, only) target of gluten-induced damage. Descriptions of the deranged intracellular ultrastructure of the enterocyte encouraged this view, which seemed

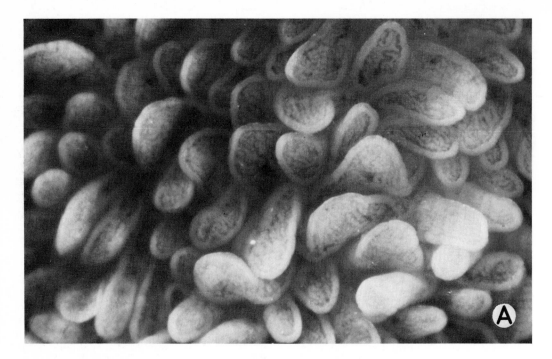

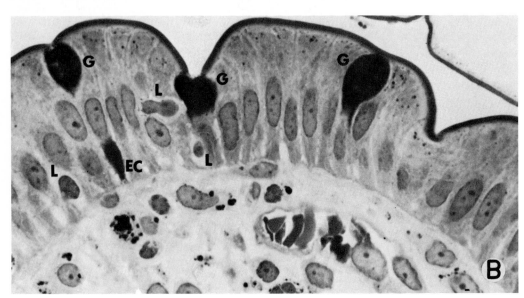

Fig. 1. These micrographs illustrate typical normal structural appearances of human jejunal mucosa as viewed (a) through the dissecting microscope and (b) in 1 μm Epon sections. Dissecting microscopy affords an important means of assessing villous shape: the epithelium is transparent beneath which the capillary network within each villus is clearly seen. Histologically, the regular arrangement of the epithelium, together with goblet cells, G, 'endocrine cell', EC, and inter-epithelial space lymphocytes, L, is apparent (Magnifications: (a) × 52 (b) approx. ×1,030).

entirely consistent with Frazer's (63) idea of a supposed congenital mucosal (or intracellular) peptidase deficiency, the absence of which resulted in exposure to intermediate "toxic" break-down products of the gluten molecule (16). Additional information from well-controlled histochemical studies (139, 157, 164, 179) provided further evidence for the central importance of the enterocyte, and of its diffused lysosomal enzymes (the intracellular 'suicide kit') (157), in the genesis of intestinal dysfunction.

In looking back over those exciting years, during which so much that was new and unexpected became known about the jejunal mucosa, it is clear that the key to elucidating the pathogenesis of coeliac disease was not contained within the epithelial cell. Even with the use of the most advanced centrifugal techniques (146, 147), there is little to suggest that the epithelial cell is primarily at fault. Furthermore, the critical observation that gluten is not apparently directly toxic to the epithelium of mucosa exposed in organ culture (53, 91) is proof enough of the central inadequacy of Frazer's 'digestive' aetiology. These, and other objections to a primary biochemical aetiology of coeliac disease, are discussed in greater detail elsewhere (118) and where the current position regarding the immunological basis of the condition is critically reviewed.

### Surface Structure of Mucosal Specimens (Figs. 2, 4, 5)

Two supposedly distinct lesions were originally described by Shiner & Doniach (176)—'subtotal villous atrophy' and 'partial villous atrophy'. In subsequent studies with the dissecting microscope (82, 83) the former lesion appeared uniformly flat and without villous projections, whereas the latter comprised twisted, whorl-like convolutions which, in section, were thought to be stunted villi. However, the low resolving power of the dissecting microscope limited progress in reconciling these seemingly different, and unrelated, appearances, but the advent of the scanning electron microscope permitted study of surface ultrastructure with far greater precision (113, 121, 122, 123, 185). This technique provided

the means of tracing how villi progressively develop from an initially flat, untreated mucosa (Marsh (113)). It is now clear that convolutions are, indeed, part of the continuously evolving 'terrain' of the mucosal surface, and that these various intermediate stages correlate with progressively changing rates of crypt cell proliferation (203). Thus the terms 'subtotal' and 'partial' villous atrophy are no longer apt descriptions, since they merely represent phases of a dynamic and progressively evolving surface contour varying from a normal villous pattern, to the other extreme where no villi are present at all.

### Crypt Cell Proliferation Kinetics

Apart from the obvious epithelial damage, the other major, striking abnormality of coeliac mucosa is the crypt hypertrophy associated with numerous mitotic figures. Shiner & Doniach (176) accepted that this represented increased proliferation consequent upon excessive loss of epithelial cells to the lumen, just as haemolysis causes compensatory hypertrophy of bone marrow. The opposing view (34, 36), i.e., 'maturation arrest' of crypt epithelium was supported by much other contemporary experimental evidence indicating that a variety of mitotic antagonists could produce 'flat' lesions superficially resembling the coeliac lesion (Table 1). Subsequent evidence, obtained from luminal DNA washings (37); examination of enzyme activities reflecting pyrimidine metabolism (21); organ culture of mucosa with $^3$H-TdR (192); and finally, stathmokinetic studies (197, 201, 202), convincingly proved that cell turnover is markedly increased in the untreated lesion, as a compensatory response to excessive desquamation of epithelial cells into the lumen. Such elegant studies have shown that (i) the maturation compartment is expanded within the crypt, (ii) cell cycle time is decreased and (iii) the proliferative compartment is somewhat enlarged. The resulting increase in length and circumferential girth of the crypts leads to a sixfold output of new cells per crypt, which is in keeping with biochemical data monitoring $^3$H-TdR uptake by cultured whole mucosa by Jones & Peters (90).

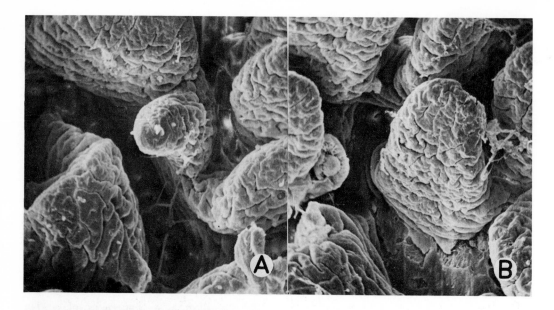

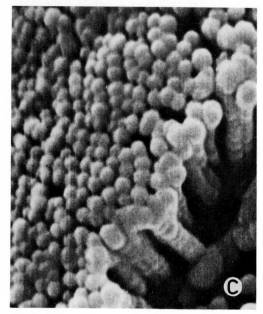

Fig. 2. These three panels illustrate scanning EM appearances of normal villi (a, b) and a spectacular display of the micro-villous 'brush border' of an isolated enterocyte (c). (Magnifications: (a) × 550 (b) × 550 (c) × 80,000). (From Marsh, 112, 113, 124).

*Basement Membrane and Subepithelial Region*

The intestinal basement membrane lies between epithelium and lamina propria. Following the introduction of the periodic acid-Schiff technique (99, 103, 105), basement membranes, in general, were found to be positive and hence rich in glycoprotein. More recent studies with the electron microscope reveal three distinct zones: (i) the *lamina lucida*, which lies immediately adjacent to the epithelium and is continuous with the extracellular coat (99): (ii) the *lamina densa*, which appears as a dense linear structure, and (iii) a third region comprising loose connective tissue intermingled with subepithelial fibroblasts (54, 55). The lamina densa is a continuous structure which is exposed after removal of epithelium by mechanical or enzymatic means (113, 123), and which appears to be the real basement membrane: it has been shown to be perforated when viewed directly by scanning EM (113), probably by cells, especially lymphocytes, and cellular processes of macrophages and epithelial cells.

In coeliac disease, the membrane is often thickened (43, 80, 85, 133, 166) sometimes with a dense band of collagen (198); whether the latter represents a particular variant of coeliac disease ('collagenous sprue') is hard to tell—it may be an unusual occurrence in certain individuals, rather like collagenous colitis (10). In addition, there is ultrastructural evidence of reduplication of the lamina densa (Fig. 6) a change that is also seen in other chronic pathological conditions, (8, 204, 208). These alterations have not however,

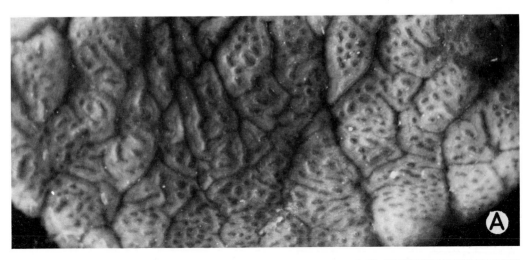

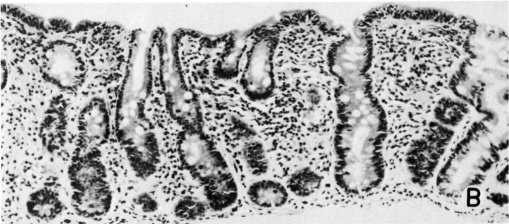

Fig. 3. These are corresponding views of untreated coeliac mucosa seen (a) through the dissecting microscope and (b) in histological section. The former illustrates the typical mosaic surface appearance, perforated by large crypt wells (see Fig. 4). Histological features include damaged epithelial cells: elongated and hypertrophied crypts and infiltrate into lamina propria of many plasma cells. (Magnifications: (a) × 78.5 (b) × 150).

Table I. Clinical and experimental causes of villous flattening of jejunal mucosa (13, 27, 145, 162)

| | Reference | | Reference |
|---|---|---|---|
| 1. Coeliac Disease | 160 | 14. Giardiasis | 101 |
| 2. Dermatitis Herpetiformis | 111 | 15. Cytomegalovirus | 193 |
| 3. Soy Bean Protein | 1 | 16. Coccidiosis | 102 |
| 4. Other Dietary Proteins | 4 | 17. Nippostrongylus infestation | 186 |
| 5. Tropical Sprue | 20, 184 | 18. Zollinger-Ellison Syndrome | 172 |
| 6. Acute Gastroenteritis | 28, 69 | 19. Systemic Mastocytosis | 15 |
| 7. Eosinophilic Gastroenteritis | 160 | 20. X-irradiation | 154 |
| 8. Inflammatory (collagen) | 187 | 21. Antimetabolites | 199 |
| 9. Malignancy | 34 | 22. Colchicine Administration | 22 |
| 10. Hypogammaglobulinaemia | 151 | 23. Triparanol Ingestion | 107 |
| 11. IgA Deficiency | 31 | 24. Acid Perfusion | 189 |
| 12. Alpha Chain Disease | 156 | 25. Mucosal Transplantation | 196 |
| 13. Intestinal Lymphoma | 48 | 26. Mucosal Exteriorisation | 182 |

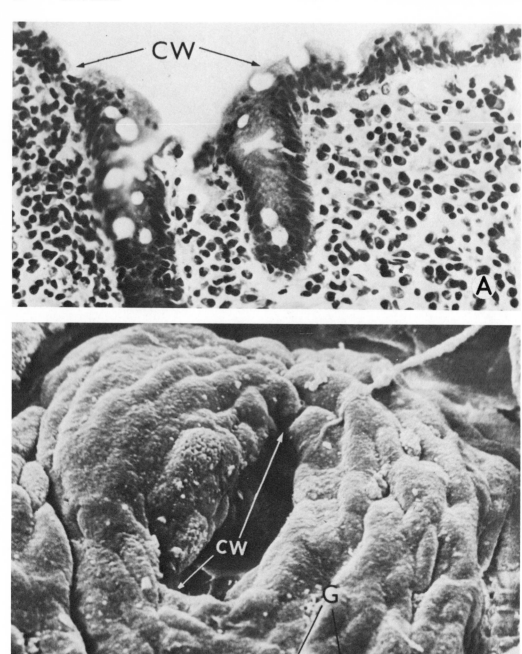

Fig. 4. The scanning EM appearance of a flat specimen, compared with a section of same mucosa are illustrated. The former shows in detail the appearance of a crypt well (CW), approximately 100–150 μm diameter, into which several individual crypt tubes open. The well is surrounded by a characteristic cuff of irregular enterocytes interspersed with goblet cells, G, and arranged concentrically around the well. Note that surface pits seen through the dissecting microscope (Fig. 3a) are not individual crypt openings, as is often incorrectly thought. (Magnifications: (a) × 350 (b) × 1,250).

attracted a great deal of attention from electron microscopists. Further it is not known whether this fibrogenesis results from immunological processes, or merely reflects non-specific injury to epithelial cells: this is certainly an area for future work.

In some earlier studies in colon (92, 142), attention was drawn to the subepithelial fibroblast sheath, as a replicating structure that ascended the colonic crypt in synchrony with the advancing column of epithelial cells. Furthermore, in areas of adenomatous polyps, the fibroblasts appeared altered and degenerate (93). Studies of normal jejunal mucosa show that this sheath is not continuous along the villi (125, 132); neither does it replicate in synchrony with the epithelium (126, 132). Although detailed studies have not been made, there do not appear to be any ultrastructural changes in subepithelial fibroblasts in coeliac mucosa (Fig. 6), analogous to those occurring adjacent to colonic polyps (93).

### Intestinal Permeability in Coeliac Disease

The damaged mucosa in coeliac disease may be associated with functional disorders including secretion of water, electrolytes (29, 62, 167) and proteins (40, 140). Furthermore, increased permeability is thought to account for immunisation to dietary proteins, and hence to high-titre antibodies to various dietary components (95). The lipid membrane of the intestine contains hydrophilic "pores" of theoretical diameter 4 Å (104, 178, 200). Other possible sites of increased permeability could be extrusion zones, altered or "leaky" tight junctions between adjacent epithelial cells; damage to basement membrane or even subepithelial capillaries.

One of the simplest methods of quantifying intestinal permeability employs determination of urinary ratios of ingested cellobiose and mannitol (23, 24, 25, 128). This ratio has proved to be highly discriminatory in distinguishing controls from coeliac patients, but not other inflammatory lesions (e.g., Crohn's disease) affecting the small intestine. Recent ultrastructural observations of freeze-fracture carbon replicas showed considerable disorganisation of tight junctions which, compared with other normally "leaky" epithelia,

provide a structural basis to account for these known alterations in mucosal permeability (108).

It is often assumed that circulating, high-titre food antibodies are a direct measure of increased mucosal permeability. A more critical appraisal should take account of hepatic extraction of such absorbed antigens by Kupffer cells during their first passage through the portal sinusoids. Absolute levels of antibody titre are dependent also on the degree of concurrent antigen-antibody formation (87) and thus are likely to be underestimated if this is not taken into account. Moreover, antibody synthesis may result (a) from migration and seeding of primed cells from Peyer's patches to the spleen—thus escaping antigen surveillance by the liver, or (b) from direct systemic immunisation should large amounts of antigen overwhelm local mucosal immune defences (14). One further point to be remembered is that, in general, exaggerated humoral responses to given antigens are characteristic of HLA A1, B8 individuals, including coeliacs (168) compared with other haplotypes (38, 61). This has been abundantly confirmed from antibody responses in B8 individuals with various other types of disease, e.g., anti-cholinesterase antibody in myasthenia gravis (131); anti-B islet cell antibodies in diabetics (134) and circulating precipitins in certain forms of external allergic alveolitis (129). Enhanced antibody responses to oral polio vaccine have been shown to occur in coeliac patients relative to controls (110). Furthermore, circulating non-gluten food antibodies are almost twice as common in coeliacs at least four months after starting a gluten-free diet compared with controls; and are only about 10–15% less prevalent among coeliacs after this period of dietary restriction (Etermann, 49). The presence of circulating food antibody should therefore not be taken as a good guide of mucosal permeability; responsiveness to the diet; or to the strictness of patients' dietary habit.

### THE GUT-ASSOCIATED LYMPHOID TISSUE (GALT)

The concept of GALT derives from several observations: (i) the high proportion of IgA in

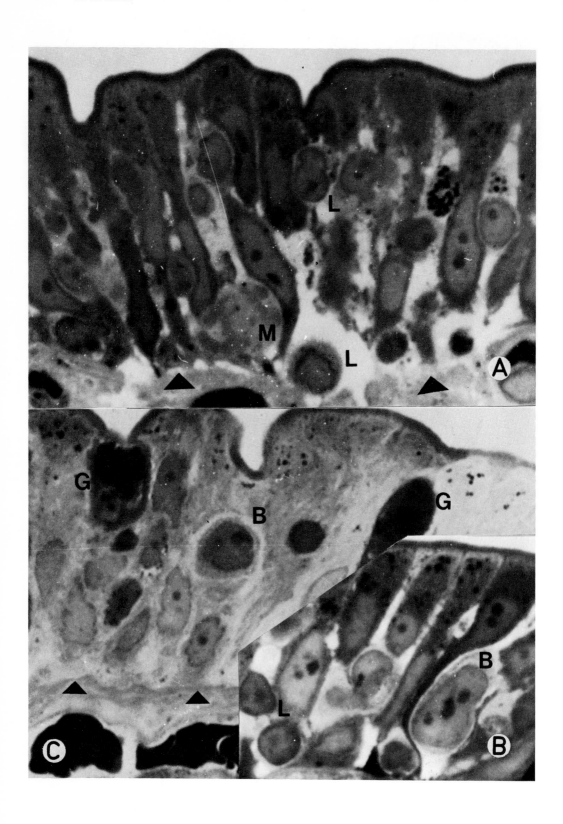

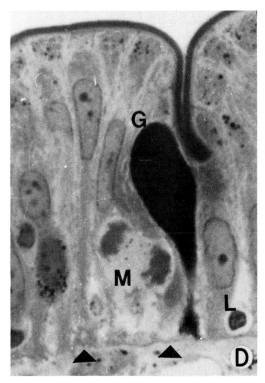

Fig. 5. (a, b, c): These are representative 1 μm Epon sections of untreated coeliac mucosa, illustrating the disruption of the epithelial cell layer by medium–sized lymphocytes, L, and including large immunoblasts, B. Note mitotic figure, M, of dividing epithelial lympho-cyte. (d): Mucosa from treated patient, showing nor-malized epithelium, smaller lymphocytes, L, and also dividing lymphocyte, M. Goblet cells, G; basement membrane, arrow heads. (Magnifications: (a) × 2,125 (b) × 1,500 (c) × 2,300 (d) × 1,670).

secretions, relative to serum (78, 188), (ii) the marked preponderance of mucosal IgA cells (30) and (iii) that coproantibody formation is inde-pendent of serum antibody production (9, 19, 39, 64) and brought about by a set of specifically-committed lymphoid cells which provide the first-line defence of mucosal surfaces (194, 195).

*Humoral Features*

Local polymeric Ig (i.e., IgA dimers or IgM pentamers, secretory component and J chain) is effective in neutralising bacteria and viruses, and of promoting fixation of antigen thus reducing absorption and aiding its proteolytic digestion,

probably within the glycocalyx (195). The local role of IgG is unknown, but the idea (14) that it provides back-up to IgA offers a rational basis for further work in evaluating its role in mucosal defence. Specific local antibody production has been demonstrated with many soluble and parti-culate antigens (19, 32, 39, 44, 47, 135, 136, 153, 207). Plasma cells are 'end cells' and represent the final effector phase of interactions initiated when antigen priming first occurred. Their turn-over is rapid (127) and are replaced by a stream of immunoblasts returning to lamina propria via thoracic duct lymph or mesenteric lymph nodes (7, 70, 74, 75); they are derived from Peyer's patches (33).

Peyer's patches are also important antigen-sensing devices, by virtue of their 'M' cells (138) whose ultrastructural appearances seem to allow direct access of antigen to organised lymphoid tissue subjacent to the dome epithelium; it is likely that sensitisation may occur elsewhere within the intestinal mucosa (77), however. Peyer's patches provide precursors of T, as opposed to B, lymphocytes (74, 130, 180) but their role in cell-mediated events, or in the pro-motion of humoral antibody synthesis within the mucosa, is poorly understood.

The return of immunoblasts (B & T) to lamina depends on many factors, such as inter-actions with high-walled endothelial vessels (177), blood flow and inflammation (137), presence of bacteria and other antigen (86, 135, 136, 150) although the latter cannot be solely regulatory (141).

Another physiological role of immunoblasts, and encompassed within the philosophy of GALT, is their return to other secretory surfaces, e.g. mammary gland. Hence milk, rich in secreted (copro)-antibody derived from blasts of intestinal origin, confers distinct advantages upon the suck-ling neonate; indeed, the lower prevalence of 'gastroenteritis' in breast-fed infants is testimony of the effectiveness of this recirculating potential of GALT-derived cells.

*Cellular Features*

GALT also comprises other diffusely scattered lymphocytes throughout the lamina propria and

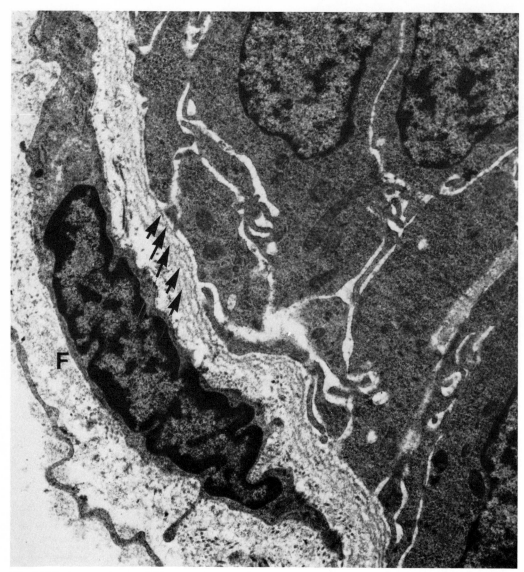

Fig. 6. This electron micrograph illustrates the subepithelial region of untreated coeliac epithelium. Note thickening and reduplication of basal laminae (Arrows), and adjacent cell body of sheath fibroblast, F. (Magnification × 15,000). (From Marsh, 113).

epithelium. In animals, epithelial lymphocytes take up tritiated thymidine (26, 67, 114), undergo mitosis and appear to migrate rapidly through the epithelium (68, 115, 159). Studies with surface markers (3) and monoclonal antibodies (171) show that the majority of epithelial lymphocytes are T suppressor/cytolytic cells, which are also selectively concentrated within the epithelium (3).

Some epithelial lymphocytes exhibit blast-trans-

formation (26, 114, 159). In a detailed study of such immunoblasts (114), they were shown to display ribosome-studded cytoplasm identical to cells stimulated polyclonally (46, 89). Such observations suggest that epithelial lymphocytes might be responding to antigen to which they had previously been sensitised, a belief strengthened by more recent studies of coeliac mucosa (116, 117).

Thus there are considerable cytological, ultrastructural and immunohistological data indicating that epithelial lymphocytes are immunocompetent cells. These ideas are contrary to the views of Ferguson (56) that such cells are dedifferentiated—recalling notions expressed earlier in this century that considered epithelial lymphocytes effect, and merely passing through the epithelium to be discarded into the lumen. Rather, it appears that this is an important subpopulation of cells which, because of their strategic position within the mucosa, provides a wide repertoire of effector functions likely to be of considerable importance in local host defences.

## IMMUNOLOGICAL FEATURES OF COELIAC DISEASE MUCOSA

If it is supposed that coeliac disease results from a local immunological reaction to gluten, then the cytologic appearances of the target tissue—the jejunal mucosa—should provide the most important clues as to the mechanisms underlying such processes. Historically, the year 1970 may be taken as the point when the immunological basis for coeliac disease began to assume prominence. This followed the realisation, as crystallised in Booth's classic exposition on the coeliac enterocyte (11, 12), that a digestive theory of gluten-sensitivity, as originally hinted at by Frazer (63), was becoming untenable as a working hypothesis.

### Cellular Basis of Humoral Reactivity to Gluten

Some of the earliest observations, made in parallel with other contemporary studies of GALT (Section II), showed that the lamina propria contains large numbers of IgA and IgM plasma cells (14, 45, 71, 73, 97, 165) located in the upper third of the mucosa, along with numerous macrophages. What is critical, and still largely unknown, is to what extent this marked accumulation of plasma cells is involved in *specific reactivity to gluten*. Data on such specificity are hard to come by, and rest solely on the demonstration that mucosa produces IgA anti-gliadin antibody in organ culture (52).

Conversely, studies with labelled anti-gliadin antibody (14) successfully identified anti-gluten activity within plasma cells of IgG isotype only. Very few cells were observed, although this is less surprising, and consistent with other experimental work with defined antigens where the number of specific antibody cells is always small. There is, however, a very significant rise in the density of IgG plasma cells within untreated coeliac mucosa (14); insufficient is known of IgG responses in the small intestine to conclude whether this represents direct local immunisation, or secondary influx of cells from extra-intestinal sources.

Circulating antibody predominantly appears to be of IgG type, although lesser amounts of IgM, and of IgA, are also detectable in coeliac sera (50, 181). Despite the paucity of data, the humoral response to gluten, both locally and systemically, is heightened. Neither is there any generalised impairment of local antibody production (6), and responses to oral polio vaccination (110) are enhanced in coeliacs compared with controls (q.v. Section I, 6).

### Mucosal Lymphocyte Abnormalities in Coeliac Disease

Lymphoid infiltration of the epithelium is supposedly one of the main 'hallmarks' of the coeliac lesion. This doctrine has become so ingrained in the literature that it has acquired "rubber-stamp" status, and is rarely lacking from most commentaries on this subject. Such a view, however, requires critical modification in the light of recent controlled, morphometric analyses which indicate that the actual number of lymphocytes within the epithelium is either normal (72), or slightly reduced (116). With particular reference to coeliac disease, therefore, it would seem that the apparent 'infiltration' is largely due to crowding of lymphocytes into a fairly small volume of epithelium resulting from loss of villi rather than to any real increase in lymphocyte numbers.

The flaw stems from adopting the universally-employed method of Ferguson and Murray (57) of relating lymphocytes to *a fixed volume of epi-*

Table II. Screening test and other 'markers' of gluten-sensitive enteropathy

| Test | %yield | Reference | Test | % yield | Reference |
|---|---|---|---|---|---|
| Folate deficiency: | 86 | 79 | Characteristic 'flat' mucosa: (see Table I) | | 160 |
| 'Figlu' excretion: | 90 | 79 | HLA Status: | | |
| Film suggesting splenic atrophy: | 10–15 | 79 | A1, B8 | 80 | 51 |
| | 65 | 18 | Dr(W)3 | 90 | 94 |
| Reticulin autoantibody: | | | Cellobiose/mannitol ratio (urinary) | 95 | 23, 24, 25 |
| children | 70 | 169, 205 | Elevated Mitotic Index in | | |
| adults | 35 | 170 | Epithelial Lymphocytes: (see Fig. 10) | ? 100 | 116, 117 |
| Xylose Malabsorption: | 55 | 25 | | | |

It should be remembered that although many of these tests give a good yield of positive coeliac diagnoses, they may also be positive for a variable number of non-coeliacs, thus blunting their discriminatory value in distinguishing gluten-sensitivity from other causes of malabsorption, even though the mucosa is 'flat'.

*thelium*; this approach is erroneous if major reductions in surface area, and hence epithelial volume, exist between mucosae, as indeed occurs between normal mucosa, untreated coeliac mucosa and partially-treated mucosa (119). Furthermore, since the numbers of epithelial lymphocytes, both in normal and disease specimens vary so considerably, their immediate clinical, and diagnostic relevance remains uncertain (119). Much care should therefore be exercised in accepting the pathogenetic and other implications drawn from such counts particularly where they supposedly relate to responses to a gluten-free diet (57, 66, 81), cell-mediated events within the epithelium (17), risks of neoplasia (60) and possible relationships to other dietary sensitivities (96, 149).

*Turnover of Epithelial Lymphocytes*

The use of $^3$H-TdR as a marker of cell proliferation has been considerably exploited in crypt cell activity of intestinal epithelium. Similar dynamic studies of epithelial lymphocyte kinetics have been less satisfactory because a) these cells do not form a closed population, b) division occurs within the inter-epithelial cell spaces, and c) rates of cell entry into, and out of, the epithelium (either via lumen or lamina propria) cannot be accurately measured (115). In the human, ethical considerations also restrict the use of nuclear label ($^3$H-TdR).

In order to circumvent the latter, an attempt to gain some idea of lymphocyte fluxes across the basement membrane was made by determining the ratio of lymphocytes within the epithelium to those actually in transit through the basal lamina (116). Compared with control mucosae, "flux ratios" for coeliac lymphocytes were markedly elevated, indicating increased lymphocyte traffic across the membrane and correlating directly with a large number of perforations observed by scanning EM in the exposed basement membrane of coeliac mucosae denuded of epithelium (113). What this raised lymphocyte 'flux' means in relation to pathogenesis, and to gluten-driven events within the epithelium, requires further analysis, however.

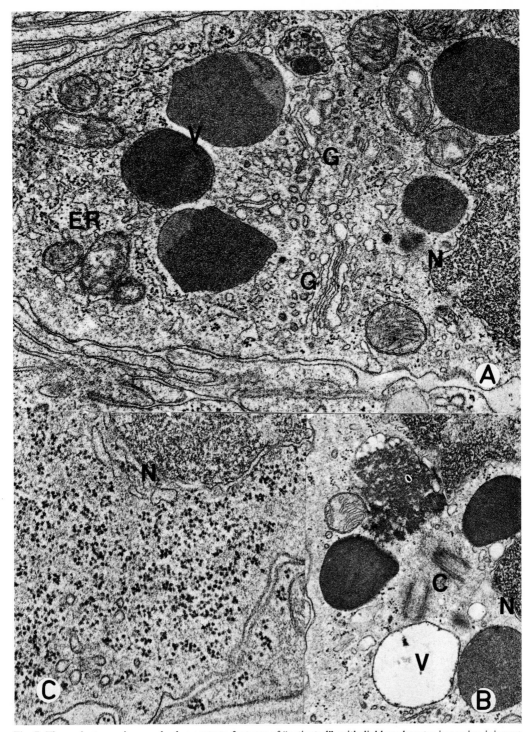

Fig. 7. These electron micrographs demonstrate features of "activated" epithelial lymphocytes in murine jejunum (From Marsh, 114). (a) shows supranuclear region containing dark, osmiophilic vacuoles, V (i.e. granules); extensive Golgi membrane formation, G, and rough endoplasmic reticulum, ER. (b): two centrioles, C, apposed perpendicularly, are characteristic of developing cell. Other large vacuoles, V, are evident. (c): Part of cytoplasm of epithelial immunoblast, showing extensive polyribosome formation. Nuclei, N. (Magnifications: (a) × 28,000 (b) × 25,200 (c) × 52,000).

*Evidence for Cell-Mediated Reactions in Coeliac Mucosa*

Little firm evidence exists that directly implicates cell-mediated immune local reactions to gluten. One study suggests that whole coeliac mucosa, cultured with gluten, secretes migration inhibition factor (MIF) (58)—a widely used test of cell-mediated immunity (76). However, problems in the interpretation of these data leaves some uncertainty as to whether the described effects could be due to gluten-sensitised lymphocytes and macrophages, or not.

Another study in *Nippostrongylus*-infested rats by Ferguson & Jarrett (59) showed that gross reductions in villous height could be caused by a T lymphocyte-dependent mechanism. This observation is certainly of great interest, pointing to a way whereby flattening could occur in coeliac mucosa. Clearly, more data on this effect are needed before the exact process of 'flattening' is understood.

Thirdly, in pursuing an earlier observation that blast-transformation of epithelial lymphocytes occurs in murine small intestine (Fig. 7) (114), untreated coeliac mucosa was analysed morphometrically to determine the size distribution and mitotic activity of these lymphocytes (116). A highly significant proportion of immunoblasts (8%) was found within the epithelium, compared with only 2% in controls (Fig. 8). Furthermore, construction of metaphase-accumulation curves (using colchicine as mitotic blocking agent, and multiple biopsies over a four-hour period) revealed a very high rate of proliferation in coeliac lymphocytes, whereas control lymphocytes showed little tendency to divide (Fig. 9). This relationship also held for other disease-controls with pseudo-coeliac lesions, e.g. lymphomas, immunodeficiencies, Crohn's disease and infections (117). Thus it was concluded that, irrespective of the degree of mucosal flattening, only high mitotic indices (Fig. 5) in epithelial lymphocytes correlate precisely with gluten-sensitivity. This feature, therefore, is a highly discriminatory cytological marker of gluten-sensitivity (117, 118, 120) and one that expresses likely *immunologic*

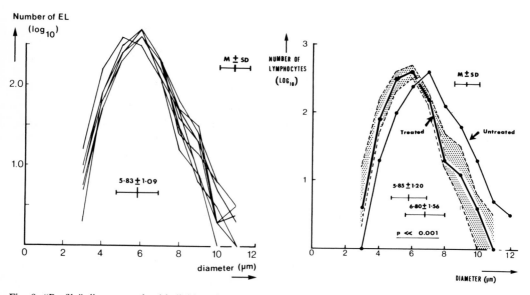

Fig. 8. "Profile" diameters of epithelial lymphocytes are shown here. On the left, distributions for samples of 1,000 lymphocytes from each of 10 control subjects: overall mean refers to total population of $10^4$ cells, of which 2% ⩾ 9 μm diameter. The right hand diagram features two distributions obtained from one coeliac patient before (arrow:untreated) and after (arrow:treated) gluten restriction. The former curve is shifted to the right, the proportion of blasts being 8%. The treated curve falls within control range. Means of both samples are highly significantly different (From Marsh, 116).

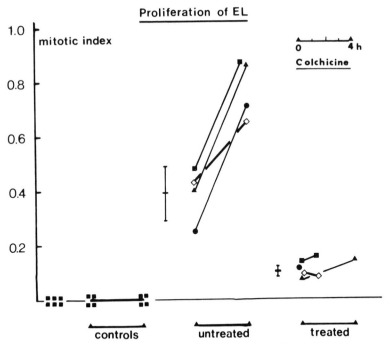

Fig. 9. This diagram illustrates the effect of a 4-hour period of colchicine administration on mitotic activity of epithelial lymphocytes. Basal mitotic indices in
untreated coeliacs are high and the steep rates of accumulation of metaphase arrests
during the period of colchicine blockade are striking in comparison with the control
group (From Marsh, 116).

specificity—as opposed to non-specific *morpho-logic* 'flattening' (Fig. 10) alone (See Table I).

Raised mitotic indices in epithelial lymphocytes have since been found in patients with the enter-opathy of dermatitis herpetiformis; in malignant histiocytosis of the intestine, this being a diffuse, multi-focal malignancy of intestinal macrophages associated specifically with gluten-sensitivity (88) and thirdly, in so-called non-responsive coeliac patients (117, 120) and who, by definition (11) fail to regrow villi after a long period of dietary gluten restriction (Fig. 10). Several important conclusions, therefore, are to be drawn from these recent observations:

(i) That a high mitotic index among epithelial lymphocytes in mucosa of untreated coeliac patients correlates very closely with a state of gluten-sensitivity. This is an easy and highly dis-criminatory morphologic marker than can be assessed quickly on any (routine) jejunal biopsy;

(ii) that similar features in pre-treatment biop-sies of so-called non-responding coeliacs indicates their underlying gluten-sensitivity, thus implying that failure of villous regrowth must be due to factors other than (c)overt gluten ingestion, or some other ill-defined dietary sensitivity;

(iii) that flat (pseudo-coeliac) lesions lacking high mitotic indices among epithelial lymphocytes cannot be deemed to be flat because of immune reactions to gluten;

(iv) that in such pseudo-coeliac lesions (lym-phoma, immunodeficiency, etc) lack of this marker provides a rational and positive reason for not prescribing a gluten-free diet;

(v) that the definition of coeliac disease, which currently requires a mucosal response to gluten withdrawal, is too restrictive since it can now be seen to be based on (a) a very non-specific mucosal lesion (Table I) and (b) because it excludes patients (ii, above) with apparent gluten-mediated enteropathy. In this regard, too

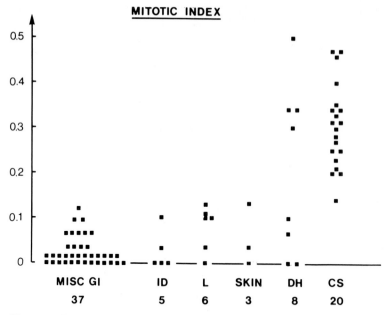

Fig. 10. This diagram illustrates basal mitotic indices in jejunal mucosa from miscellaneous gastrointestinal controls, GI; other selected disease controls including immunodeficiency, ID; intestinal lymphoma, L; dermatitis herpetiformis, DH; together with untreated coeliac sprue patients, CS. The high basal mitotic indices of epithelial lymphocytes in untreated coeliacs, and in those DH patients with enteropathy, are distinct from the remainder among which are several with 'flat', pseudo-coeliac mucosal lesions. The predictive value of this appearance in identifying gluten-sensitised patients is clear from these data (From Marsh, 117).

little attention has been paid to cellular responses to gluten restriction, (2, 65, 109, 144, 152, 183, 206) as these probably provide a quicker and more accurate guide to gluten-sensitivity, rather than overall mucosal recovery.

(vi) that only one biopsy is necessary to establish the diagnosis of gluten enteropathy. Further biopsies, either for assessing 'response' or determining true sensitivity with gluten re-challenge either in vivo (84), or in vitro (5, 41, 98), would be unnecessary in the majority of cases on these criteria.

(vii) that it provides to date the most highly specific test for gluten-sensitivity, compared with other 'markers' which over the years have been advocated (Table II), the majority of which are often associated with other conditions, thus causing some diagnostic confusion.

## ACKNOWLEDGEMENTS

This work has been supported by generous grants from the North Western Regional Health Authority; the Granada Foundation (Salford); the Smith, Kline & French Foundation, and the Medical Research Council of Great Britain.

Data in Figs. 2 and 7 are reproduced from *Gut* by permission of the Editor and Publisher and in Figs. 8 and 9 by permission of the Publisher of *Gastroenterology*, Volume 79; copyright 1980, by the American Gastroenterological Association.

## REFERENCES

1. Ament, M. & Rubin, C. E. *Gastroenterology* 1972, *62*, 227–234
2. Anderson, C. M. *Arch. dis. Childh.* 1960, *35*, 419–427

3. Arnaud-Battandier, F., Bundy, B., O'Neill, M. & Bienenstock, J. *J. Immunol.* 1979, *121*, 1059–1065

4. Baker, A. L. & Rosenberg, I. H. *Ann. Inter. Med.* 1978, *89*, 505–508

5. Bayless, T., Rubin, S., Topping, T., Yardley, J. & Hendrix, T. pp 76–89 in Booth, C. C. & Dowling, R. H. (eds.), *Coeliac Disease.* Churchill-Livingstone, Edinburgh, 1970

6. Beale, A., Parrish, W., Douglas, A. & Hobbs, J. *Lancet* 1971, *1*, 1198–1200

7. Bennell, M. & Husband, A. *Immunology* 1981, *42*, 469–474

8. Benscombe, S. A., West, R., Kerr, J. & Wilson, D. *Am. J. Med.* 1966, *40*, 67–77

9. Besredka, A. *Local Immunisation.* Williams & Wilkins, Baltimore, 1972

10. Bogomdetz, W., Adnet, J., Birembant, P., Feydy, P. & Dupont, P. *Gut* 1980, *21*, 164–168

11. Booth, C. C. *Br. Med. J.* 1970, *3*, 725–731

12. Booth, C. C. *Br. Med. J.* 1970, *4*, 14–17

13. Brandborg, L. *Am. J. Med.* 1979, *67*, 999–1006

14. Brandtzaeg, P. & Baklien, K. *Scand. J. Gastroenterol.* Suppl. *36*, 1976

15. Broitman, S., McCray, R., May, J., Deren, J., Ackroyd, F., Gottlieb, L., McDermott, W. & Zamchek, N. *Am. J. Med.* 1970, *48*, 382–389

16. Bronstein, H., Haeffner, L. & Kowlessar, O. D. *Clin. Chim. Acta.* 1966, *14*, 141–155

17. Bullen, A. & Losowsky, M. *Gut* 1978, *19*, 126–131

18. Bullen, A., Hall, R., Gowland, G., Rajah, S. & Losowsky, M. *Gut* 1981, *21*, 28–33

19. Burrows, W., Elliot, M. & Havens, I. *J. Infect. Dis.* 1947, *81*, 261–281

20. Butterworth, C. E. & Perez-Santiago, E. *Ann. Int. Med.* 1967, *42*, 319–326

21. Clark, M. L. & Senior, J. R. *Gastroenterology* 1969, *56*, 887–894

22. Clark, P. & Harland, W. *Br. J. exp. Path.* 1963 *44*, 520–523

23. Cobden, I., Dickinson, R. J. Rothwell, J. & Axon, A. T. R. *Br. Med. J.* 1978, *2*, 1060–1062

24. Cobden, I., Rothwell, J. & Axon, A. T. R. *Gut* 1979, *20*, 716–721

25. Cobden, I., Rothwell, J. & Axon, A. T. R. *Gut* 1980, *21*, 512–518

26. Collan, Y. *Scand. J. Gastroenterol.* Suppl. *18*, 1972

27. Collins, J. R. *Am. J. Clin. Path.* 1965, *44*, 36–44

28. Collins, J. R. & Isselbacher, K. *Gastroenterology* 1965, *49*, 425–432

29. Chadwick, V. S., Phillips, S. F. & Hoffman, A. F. *Gastroenterology* 1977, *73*, 247–251

30. Crabbe, P., Carbonara, A. & Heremans, J. F. *Lab. Invest.* 1965, *14*, 235–248

31. Crabbe, P. & Heremans, J. F. *Am. J. Med.* 1967, *42*, 319–326

32. Crabbe, P., Nash, D., Bazin, H., Eyssen, H. & Heremans, J. R. *J. exp. Med.* 1969, *130*, 723–738

33. Craig, S. & Cebra, J. *J. exp. Med.* 1971, *134*, 188–200

34. Creamer, B. *Gut* 1962, *3*, 295–300

35. Creamer, B. *Br. Med. J.* 1964, *2*, 1435–1436

36. Creamer, B. *Br. med. Bull.* 1967, *23*, 226–230

37. Croft, D. N., Loehry, C. & Creamer, B. *Lancet* 1968, *2*, 68–70

38. Dausset, J. & Contu, L. pp. 513–529 in Fougereau, M. & Dausset, J. (eds.), *Progress in Immunology, IV*, Academic Press, London, 1980

39. Davies, A. *Lancet* 1922, *2*, 1009–1012

40. Dawson, A. M. pp. 126–147 in Badenoch, J. & Brooke, B. N. (eds.), *Recent Advances in Gastroenterology* (1st ed.). Churchill, London, 1967

41. Dissanayake, A., Jerrome, D., Offord, R., Truelove, S. & Whitehead, R. *Gut* 1974, *15*, 931–946

42. Dobbins, W. O. *Am. J. Med. Sci.* 1969, *258*, 150–171

43. Doe, W., Evans, D., Hobbs, J. & Booth, C. C. *Gut* 1972, *13*, 112–123

44. Dolezel, J. & Bienenstock, J. *Cell Immunol.* 1971, *2*, 458–468

45. Douglas, A. P., Crabbe, P. & Hobbs, J. *Gastroenterology* 1970, *59*, 414–425

46. Douglas, S. D. *Transpl. Rev.* 1972, *11*, 39–59

47. Eddie, D., Schulkind, M. & Robbins, J. *J. Immunol.* 1971, *106*, 181–190

48. Eidelman, S., Parkins, A. & Rubin, C. E. *Medicine* 1966, *45*, 111–137

49. Eterman, K. P. Thesis, University of Amsterdam, 1977

50. Eterman, K. P., Hekkens, W., Pena, A., van Kan, P. & Feltkamp, T. *J. Immunol. Methods* 1977, *14*, 85–92

51. Falchuk, Z. M., Rogentine, G. & Strober, W. *J. Clin. Invest.* 1972, *51*, 1602–1605

52. Falchuk, Z. M. & Strober, W. *Gut* 1974, *15*, 947–952

53. Falchuk, Z. M., Gebhard, R., Sessons, C. & Strober, W. *J. Clin. Invest.* 1974, *53*, 487–500

54. Farquhar, M. G. & Palade, G. *J. Cell Biol.* 1963, *17*, 375–412

55. Fawcett, D. W. *Circulation*, 1962, *26*, 1105–1125

56. Ferguson, A. *Gut.* 1977, *18*, 921–937

57. Ferguson, A. & Murray, D. *Gut* 1971, *12*, 988–994

58. Ferguson, A., McClure, J., MacDonald, T. & Holden, R. *Lancet* 1975, *1*, 895–897

59. Ferguson, A. & Jarrett, E. *Gut* 1975, *16*, 114–117

60. Ferguson, R., Asquith, P. & Cooke, W. T. *Gut* 1974, *15*, 458–461

61. Festenstein, H. & Demant, P. *HLA & H-2 Basic Immunogenetics, biology and clinical relevance.* Arnold, London 1978

62. Fordtran, A., Rector, F. C., Lacklear, T. W. & Ewton, M. F. *J. Clin. Invest.* 1967, *46*, 287–298

63. Frazer, A. C. *Proc. Roy. Soc. Med.* 1956, *49*, 1009–1013

64. Freter, R. *J. Infect. Dis.* 1962, *111*, 37–48

65. Fry, L. *Lancet* 1968, *1*, 557–561

66. Fry, L., Seah, P., McMinn, R. *Br. Med. J.* 1972, *3*, 371–374

67. Glaister, J. R. *Int. Arch. Allergy Appl. Immunol.* 1973, *45*, 844–853

68. Glaister, J. R. *Int. Arch. Allergy Appl. Immunol.* 1973, *45*, 854–867

69. Gottlieb, S. & Brandborg, L. *Gastroenterology* 1966, *51*, 1037–1045

70. Gowans, J. L. & Knight, E. *Proc. Roy. Soc. B.* 1964, *159*, 257–282
71. Guix, M., Skinner, J. & Whitehead, R. *Gut* 1979, *20*, 504–508
72. Guix, M., Skinner, J. & Whitehead, R. *Gut* 1979, *20*, 275–278
73. Guix, M., Skinner, J. & Whitehead, R. *Scand. J. Gastroenterol.* 1979, *14*, 261–265
74. Guy-Grand, D., Griscelli, C. & Vassalli, P. *Eur. J. Immunol.* 1974, *4*, 435–443
75. Hall, J. G., Smith, M. E. & Parry, D. *Cell Tissue Kinet.* 1972, *5*, 269–281
76. Hamblin, A. S. & Maini R. N. p 243 in Thompson, R. A. (ed.), *Recent Advances in Clinical Immunology,* Churchill-Livingstone, Edinburgh, 1980
77. Hamilton, S. R., Keren, D., Yardley, J., Brown, G. *Immunology* 1981, *42*, 431–435
78. Heremans, J. F. pp 265–276 in Sela, M. (ed.), *The Antigens,* Academic Press, New York, 1974
79. Hoffbrand, A. V. pp 85–89, in Cooke, W. & Asquith, P. (eds.), *Coeliac Disease. Clinics in Gastroenterology,* Saunders, 1974
80. Holdstock, D. & Oleesky, S. *Postgrad. Med. J.* 1973, *49*, 664–667
81. Holmes, G., Asquith, P. & Stokes, P. *Gut* 1974, *15*, 278–283
82. Holmes, R., Hourihane, D. & Booth, C. C. *Lancet* 1961, *1*, 81–83
83. Holmes, R., Hourihane, D. & Booth, C. C. *Postgrad. J.* 1961, *37*, 717–724
84. Howdle, P., Corazza, G., Bullen, A. & Losowsky, M. *Gastroenterology* 1981, *80*, 442–450
85. Hourihane, D. *Proc. Roy. Soc. Med.* 1963, *56*, 1073–1077
86. Husband, A. & Gowans, J. *J. exp. Med.* 1978, *148*, 1146–1160
87. Inganas, M., Johansson, S. G. & Dannaeus, A. *Clin. Allergy* 1980, *10*, 293–302
88. Isaacson, P. & Wright, D. *Human Pathol.* 1978, *9*, 661–677
89. Janossy, G., Shohet, M., Greaves, M. F. & Dourmashkin, R. R. *Immunology* 1972, *24*, 211–227
90. Jones, P. E. & Peters, T. J. *Br. Med. J.* 1977, *1*, 1–4
91. Jos, J., Lenoir, G. de Ritis, G. & Rey, J. p. 91 in Hekkens, W. & Pena, A. S. (eds.), *Coeliac Disease,* Stenfert-Kroess, Leiden, 1974
92. Kaye, G. I., Lane, N. & Pascal, R. *Gastroenterology* 1968, *54*, 852–865
93. Kaye, G., Pascal, R. & Lane, N. *Gastroenterology* 1971, *60*, 515–536
94. Keuning, J., Pena, A., van Leuwen, A., van Hooff, J. & van Rood, J. *Lancet* 1976, *1*, 506–507
95. Kivel, R. M., Kearns, D. H. & Liebovitz, D. *New Engl. J. Med.* 1964, *271*, 769–772
96. Kumar, P., Ferguson, A. & Lancaster-Smith, M. *Scand. J. Gastroenterol.* 1976, *2*, 5–9
97. Lancaster-Smith, M., Kumar, P., Marks, R., Clark, M. & Dawson, A. *Gut* 1974, *15*, 371–376
98. Lancaster-Smith, M., Kumar, P. & Dawson, A. M. *Gut* 1975, *16*, 683–688
99. Leblond, C. P. *Am. J. Anat.* 1950, *86*, 1–25
100. Leinbach, G. & Rubin, C. E. *Gastroenterology* 1970, *59*, 874–889
101. Levinson, J. D. & Nastro, L. J. *Gastroenterology* 1978, *74*, 271–275
102. Liebman, W., Thaler, M., DeLorimer, A., Brandborg, L. & Goodman, J. *Gastroenterology* 1980, *78*, 579–584
103. Lillie, R. *J. Lab. Clin. Med.* 1947, *32*, 910–912
104. Lindemann, B. & Solomons, A. K. *J. Gen. Physiol.* 1962, *45*, 801–810
105. MacManus, J. F. *Stain Tech.* 1948, *23*, 99–108
106. McNeish, A. & Anderson, C. M. pp. 127–144, in Cooke, W. & Asquith, P. (eds.), *Coeliac Disease, Clinics in Gastroenterology,* Saunders, London, 1974
107. McPherson, J. & Summerskill, W. *Gastroenterology* 1963, *44*, 900–904
108. Madara, J. L. & Trier, J. S. *Lab. Invest.* 1980, *43*, 254–261
109. Magdanagopalan, N., Shiner, M. & Rowe, P. *Am. J. Med.* 1965, *38*, 42–53
110. Mahwhinney, H. & Love, A. *Clin. Exp. Immunol.* 1970, *21*, 399–406
111. Marks, J., Shuster, S. & Watson, A. J. *Lancet* 1966, *2*, 1280
112. Marsh, M. N. *Ann. Roy. Coll. Surg. Engl.* 1971, *48*, 356–368
113. Marsh, M. N. pp 81–135, in Badenoch, J. & Brooke, B. N. (eds.), *Recent Advances in Gastroenterology* (2nd ed.). Churchill-Livingstone, London, 1972
114. Marsh, M. N. *Gut* 1975, *16*, 665–674
115. Marsh, M. N. *Gut* 1975, *16*, 674–682
116. Marsh, M. N. *Gastroenterology* 1980, *79*, 481–492
117. Marsh, M. N. *Gastroenterology* 1980, *78*, 1218
118. Marsh, M. N. *Clin. Sci. molec. Med.* 1981, *61*, 1–7
119. Marsh, M. N. *Gastroenterology* 1981, *80*, 1086–1087
120. Marsh, M. N. 1981, *in manuscript*
121. Marsh, M. N., Swift, J. A. & Williams, E. D. *Br. Med. J.* 1968, *4*, 95–97
122. Marsh, M. N. & Swift, J. S. *Gut* 1969, *10*, 940–949
123. Marsh, M. N., Brown, A. C. & Swift, J. A. pp. 26–44, in Booth, C. C. & Dowling, R. H. (eds.), *Coeliac Disease,* Churchill-Livingstone, London, 1970
124. Marsh, M. N., Peters, T. J. & Brown, A. C. *Gut* 1971, *12*, 499–508
125. Marsh, M. N. & Trier, J. S. *Gastroenterology* 1975, *67*, 622–635
126. Marsh, M. N. & Trier, J. S. *Gastroenterology* 1975, *67*, 636–645
127. Mattioli, C. & Tomasi, T. B. *J. exp. Med.* 1973, *138*, 452–460
128. Menzies, I. S., Kaler, M. F., Pounder, R., Bull, J., Heyer, S., Wheeler, P. G. & Creamer, B. *Lancet* 1979, *2*, 1107–1109
129. Morris, M. J., Faux, J. A., Ting, A., Morris, P. J. & Lane, D. J. *Clin. Allergy* 1980, *10*, 173–179
130. Muller-Schoop, J. & Good, R. A. *J. Immunol.* 1975, *114*, 1757–1760
131. Naeim, F., Keesey, J., Herrmann, C., Lindstrom, J., Zeller, E. & Walford, R. *Tissue Antigens* 1978, *12*, 381–386

132. Neal, J. V. & Potter, C. S. *Gut* 1981, *22*, 19–24
133. Neale, G. *Br. Med. J.* 1968, *2*, 678–684
134. Nerup, J., Platz, P., Ryder, L., Thomsen, M. & Svejgaard, A. *Diabetes* 1978, *27*, 247–250
135. Ogra, P. L. & Karzon, D. T. *J. Immunol.* 1969, *102*, 1423–1430
136. Ogra, P. L., Coppola, P., MacGillivray, M. & Dzierba, J. L. *Proc. Soc. Exp. Med. Biol.* 1974, *145*, 811–816
137. Ottaway, C., Manson-Smith, D., Bruce, R. & Parrott, D. M. V. *Immunology* 1980, *41*, 963–971
138. Owen, R. L. & Jones, A. L. *Gastroenterology* 1974, *66*, 189–203
139. Padykula, H., Strauss, E., Ladman, A. & Gardner, F. *Gastroenterology* 1961, *40*, 735–765
140. Parkins, R. A. *Lancet* 1960, *2*, 1366–1368
141. Parrott, D. M. V. & Ferguson, A. *Immunology* 1974, *26*, 571–588
142. Pascal, R., Kaye, G. I. & Lane, N. *Gastroenterology* 1968, *54*, 835–851
143. Paulley, J. W. *Br. Med. J.* 1954, *2*, 1318–1321
144. Pena, A. S., Truelove, S. C. & Whitehead, R. *Quart. Jnl. Med.* 1972, *41*, 457–476
145. Perera, D., Weinstein, W. & Rubin, C. E. *Human. Pathol.* 1975, *6*, 157–217
146. Peters, T. J., Jones, P. & Wells, G. *Clin. Sci. molec. Med.* 1978, *55*, 285–292
147. Peters, T. J., Jones, P., Jenkins, W. & Wells, G. *Clin. Sci. Molec. Med.* 1978, *55*, 293–300
148. Petingale, K. *Gut* 1971, *12*, 291–296
149. Phillips, A., Rice, S. & France, N. *Gut* 1979, *20*, 509–512
150. Pierce, N. & Gowans, J. *J. exp. Med.* 1975, *142*, 1550–1563
151. Pitkaenen, R., Siurala, M. & Vuopio, P. *Acta med. Scand.* 1963, *173*, 549–555
152. Pollock, D., Nagle, R., Jeejeeboy, K. & Coghill, N. *Gut*, 1970, *11*, 567–575
153. Porter, P., Noakes, D. & Allen, W. *Immunology* 1970, *18*, 909–920
154. Quastler, H. & Hampton, J. C. *Radiat. Res.* 1962, *17*, 914–931
156. Rambaud, J., Bognel, C., Prost, A., Bernier, J., Le Qunitrec, Y., Lambling, A., Danon, F., Hurez, D. & Seligman, M. *Digestion* 1968, *1*, 321–336
157. Riecken, E., Stewart, J., Booth, C. & Pearse, A. *Gut* 1966, *7*, 317–332
158. Riecken, E. & Pearse, A. G. E. *Br. med. Bull.* 1967, *23*, 217–222
159. Ropke, C. & Everett, N. B. *Am. J. Anat.* 1976, *145*, 395–408
160. Rubin, C. E., Brandborg, L., Phelps, P. & Taylor, H. *Gastroenterology* 1960, *38*, 28–49
161. Rubin, C. E. & Dobbins, W. O. *Gastroenterology* 1965, *49*, 676–697
162. Rubin, C. E., Eidelman, S. & Weinstein, W. *Gastroenterology* 1970, *58*, 409
163. Rubin, W., Ross, L., Sleisenger, M. & Weser, E. *Lab. Invest.* 1966, *15*, 1720–1747
164. Samloff, I., Davis, J. & Shenck, E. *Gastroenterology* 1965, *48*, 155–172
165. Savilhati, E. *Gut* 1972, *13*, 958–964
166. Schein, J. *Gastroenterology* 1947, *8*, 438–460
167. Schmid, W. C., Phillips, S. F. & Summerskill, W. H. J. *J. Lab. Clin. Med.* 1969, *73*, 772–783

168. Scott, B., Rajah, S., Swinburne, M. & Losowsky, M. *Lancet* 1974, *2*, 374–377
169. Seah, P., Fry, L., Rossiter, M., Hoffbrand, A. & Holborow, E. *Lancet* 1971, *2*, 681–682
170. Seah, P., Fry, L., Hoffbrand, A. & Holborow, E. *Lancet* 1971, *1*, 834–846
171. Selby, W., Janossy, G., Goldstein, G. & Jewell, D. *Immunology* 1981, *in press*
172. Shimoda, S., Sandes, D. & Rubin, C. E. *Gastroenterology* 1968, *55*, 705–723
173. Shiner, M. *Lancet* 1956, *1*, 85
174. Shiner, M. *Br. Med. Bull.* 1967, *23*, 223–225
175. Shiner, M. pp 33–53, in Cooke, W. & Asquith, P. (eds.), *Coeliac Disease: Clinics in Gastroenterology*, Saunders, London, 1974
176. Shiner, M. & Doniach, I. *Gastroenterology* 1960, *38*, 419–440
177. Smith, M. E. & Ford, W. L. *Prog. Allergy* 1980, *26*, 203–232
178. Smyth, D. M. & Whittam, R. *Br. Med. Bull,* 1967, *23*, 231–235
179. Spiro, H., Filipe, M., Stewart, J. S. & Pearse, A. G. E. *Gut* 1964, *5*, 145–154
180. Sprent, J., Miller, J. F. A. *Cell Immunol.* 1972, *3*, 385–404
181. Stern, M., Fischer, K. & Gruttner, R. *In press*
182. Stevens, F. O. *Gastroenterology* 1964, *47*, 626–630
183. Stewart, J., Pollock, D., Hoffbrand, A., Mollin, D. & Booth, C. C. *Quart. Jnl. Med.* 1967, *36*, 425–444
184. Swanson, V. & Thomassen, R. W. *Am. J. Pathol.* 1965, *46*, 511–536
185. Swift, J. A. & Marsh, M. N. *Lancet* 1968, *2*, 915–916
186. Symons, L. & Fairburn, D. *Fed. Proc.* 1960, *21*, 913–918
187. Toivenen, S., Pitkanen, E. & Siurala, M. *Acta med. scand.* 1964, *175*, 91–95
188. Tomasi, T. B., Tall, E., Solomon, A. & Prendergast, R. *J. exp. Med.* 1965, *121*, 101–124
189. Townley, R., Cass, M., Finckh, E., Miton, G. & Anderson, C. M. *Gut* 1964, *47*, 626–630
190. Trier, J. S. pp 1125–1175 in Code, C. F. (ed.), *Handbook of Physiology,* Vol. 3, Section 6, *Amer. Physiol. Soc.* Washington, 1970
191. Trier, J. S. *New Engl. J. Med.* 1971, *285*, 1470–1473
192. Trier, J. S. & Browning, T. H. *New Engl. J. Med.* 1970, *283*, 1245–1250
193. Tytgat, G. N., Huibregtse, K., Schellekens, P. T. & Feltkamp-Vroom, T. H. *Gastroenterology* 1979, *76*, 1458–1465
194. Waldman, H. & Ganguly, R. *J. Infect. Dis.* 1974, *130*, 419–440
195. Walker, W. A. & Isselbacher, K. J. *New Engl. J. Med.* 1977, *297*, 767–773
196. Watson, A. J., Watson, J. & Walker, F. C. *Am. J. Path.* 1965, *46*, 553–556
197. Watson, A. J. & Wright, N. pp 11–31, in Cooke, W. & Asquith, P. (eds.), *Coeliac Disease. Clinics in Gastroenterology,* Saunders, London 1974
198. Weinstein, W., Saunders, D., Tytgat, G. & Rubin, C. E. *New Engl. J. Med.* 1970, *283*, 1297–1301
199. Williams, A. W. *Gut* 1961, *2*, 346–351

200. Wright, E. M. & Pietras, R. J. *J. membrane Biol.* 1974, *17*, 293–312
201. Wright, N., Watson, A. J., Morley, A., Appleton, D., Marks, J. & Douglas, A. P. *Gut* 1973, *14*, 603–606
202. Wright, N., Watson, A. J., Morley, A., Appleton, D., Marks, J. & Douglas, A. P. *Gut* 1973, *14*, 701–710
203. Wright, N., Appleton, D., Monks, J. & Watson, A. *J. Clin. Path.* 1979, *32*, 462–470
204. Vassalli, P., Simon, G. & Rouiller, C. *Am. J. Path.* 1963, *43*, 579-617
205. von Essen, R., Savilahti, E. & Pelkonen, P. *Lancet* 1972, *1*, 1157–1159
206. Yardley, J., Bayless, T., Norton, J. & Hendrix, T. *New Engl. J. Med.* 1962, *267*, 1173–1179
207. Yoshizawa, H., Itor, Y., Iwakiri, S., Tsuda, F., Makano, S., Miyakawa, Y. & Mayumi, M. *Gastroenterology* 1980, *78*, 114–118
208. Zacks, S., Pegues, J. & Elliott, F. *Metabolism* 1962, *11*, 381–393

# The Ultrastructure of some Gastrointestinal Lesions in Experimental Animals and Man

K. E. CARR, P. G. TONER, A. L. C. McLAY, & R. HAMLET
Dept. of Anatomy, University of Glasgow,
University Dept. of Pathology, Glasgow Royal Infirmary and Radiology Research Group,
Belvidere Hospital, Glasgow

This has been a brief and necessarily selective review, covering only a few of the numerous experimental and diagnostic uses of electron microscopy in the field of gastroenterology.

The roles of experimentalist and diagnostician have emerged in a kind of counterpoint. We have identified the contrasting themes of the controllable laboratory experiment and the uncontrollable experiment of disease; of the three-dimensional image of the surface scanning technique and the two-dimensional world of the thin section. There is harmony, also, in our common concern for morphology and our shared interest in any structural change. Altered morphology, whether in tissue architecture or cellular organisation, may offer a key to the better understanding of altered function.

In the future, both the experimental and the diagnostic electron microscopist will come to rely more on correlative procedures, such as the re-processing of specimens for a second look with a different technique. Functional dividends are promised to the morphologist by advances in detector technology and associated techniques such as analytical microscopy. It remains to be seen whether medical benefits will accrue, in terms of a more precise diagnosis or a more effective prognosis in individual cases of human gastrointestinal disease.

*Key-words:* Scanning electron microscopy, transmission electron microscopy, gastrointestinal tract, experimental radiation injury, diagnostic pathology

*K. E. Carr, Dept. of Anatomy, University of Glasgow, Scotland, U.K.*

It is a universally acknowledged truth that a cell in possession of a distinctive fine structure must be in want of a function. Starting from a baseline of anatomical and physiological normality, the gastrointestinal electron microscopist can both explore and exploit this relationship between structure and function. There are two broad frontiers of ultrastructural investigation, the experimental and the clinical.

Firstly, in the area of experimentation, there are almost infinite modifications of structure and function which can be produced in the laboratory using experimental animals. Here the investigator largely has control, through the design of experiments and the choice of specimens and methods, within the limits of technology. The results can thus be based upon adequate numbers and comprehensive specimen sampling. By definition, experiments of this kind should be reproducible.

In this paper, the experimental model at the centre of discussion is the structural response of the small intestinal mucosa to irradiation.

By contrast, the experiments of nature known as human disease are randomly designed and uncontrolled. Here the investigator has much less influence over specimens or methods, numbers or sampling. The electron microscopist must be satisfied, in many cases, with a protocol which would be regarded as unsatisfactory under experimental laboratory conditions. In this paper, the selected clinical cases deal with a number of diagnostic problems presented by human gastrointestinal tumours.

Through the juxtaposition of these selected experimental and clinical studies, certain fundamental differences of approach between the experimental and clinical electron microscopist will become apparent.

## EXPERIMENTAL AND CLINICAL METHODS

There are substantial differences in methodology between a typical 'experimental' study and a typical 'diagnostic' or 'clinical' investigation using the electron microscope. These differences are highlighted by studies of the effects of irradiation on the mucosa of the gut, using scanning and transmission electron microscopy.

Experimental studies involving laboratory rodents (3, 6, 9, 15, 16) allow detailed comparisons to be made between different doses and schedules of irradiation, between different forms of irradiation and between different time-points after given doses. The actual exposure of the gut can be accurately determined by the use of appropriate dosimetry techniques. The problem of individual variations may be caused by intercurrent animal house infection. Although often troublesome, this problem can be limited by the study of appropriate numbers of animals and of specimens at each experimental point.

By contrast, it is extremely difficult to study the mucosal effects of irradiation in the human gut. Ethical considerations restrict the taking of biopsies unless required for some appropriate clinical reason. In general, therefore, the specimens which do become available are those in which there is other disease, or in which only late effects of irradiation are apparent, such as vascular injury and ischaemia.

The actual radiation exposure suffered by the mucosa often cannot be accurately computed, since in the treatment of cancer, the radio-therapist aims at all times to avoid damage to surrounding tissues as far as possible. While the tumour dose may be accurately calculated, the actual level of mucosal exposure can often only be guessed. It is, therefore, almost impossible to assemble an adequately controlled series of human mucosal biopsies to provide accurate documentation of the effects of irradiation on the morphology of the gut. Such cases as may be gathered must be interpreted with the greatest of caution.

Ultrastructural studies of human biopsies are often seriously hampered by the limited availability of appropriate controls. There are obvious practical and ethical problems in obtaining adequate control material from normal healthy volunteers. Most controls used in clinical studies, therefore, come from patients undergoing clinical investigation for symptomatic disease, but in whom no organic cause is found. 'Normal' biopsies from such a selected population have their limitations. If matched roughly for age, they must be accepted as being at least adequate for the purpose. This is in contrast with the theoretically unlimited availability of appropriate controls for experimental laboratory studies.

Further limitations of the human biopsy become apparent on detailed consideration of specimen handling procedures. In the experimental animal, specimens of small or large intestine are most easily obtained as segmental resections carried out at the moment of death. A loop of bowel can be prepared by flushing through with fixative, tying off the distal end, inflating the loop with further fixative and finally tying off the proximal end and immersing the specimen in fixative. This procedure ensures uniform and even distension of the gut within physiological limits, thus optimising fixation and minimising tissue distortion. The large, flat, non-traumatised areas of the mucosa made available are of particular value in ultrastructural studies using the scanning electron microscope.

The typical human mucosal biopsy, on the other hand, is small and crushed, and is traumatised to a variable and uncontrolled degree by the avulsion procedure through which it was obtained. Uncontrolled contraction of the underlying muscularis mucosae causes curling of the mucosal sample, leading to unavoidable surface distortion. Artefacts introduced in this way seriously limit the study of most forms of human mucosal disease.

In general, it is in the experimental field that new technology is first deployed. Transmission electron microscopy was already widely used in the laboratory before it became accepted into regular diagnostic practice (17, 27). Scanning electron microscopy, recently popular in experimental work, has still to find a valid role in human medicine (4, 8, 11). It is, therefore, important for the diagnostic specialist to keep in touch with developments such as backscattered electron imaging and X-ray microanalysis, which may influence future diagnostic practice (1, 11).

Both experimental and clinical electron microscopists are becoming aware of the need to

for light microscopy and transmission electron microscopy (10).

Finally, whilst scanning electron microscopy is most commonly used to assess mucosal surface morphology, it is worth noting that special prep-

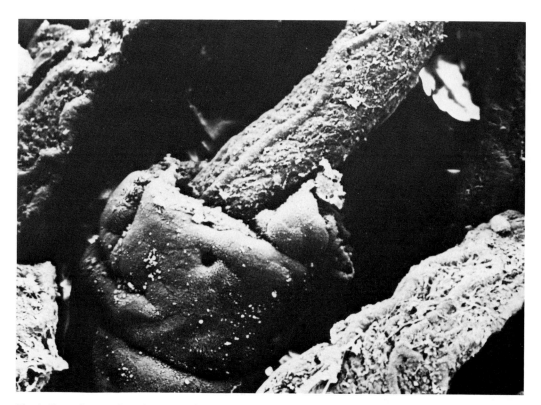

Fig. 1. Control mouse intestine exposed to ultrasonic disintegration for 5 minutes in saline. Half of the epithelial sheet covering the villus in the centre of the field has been removed, while the villus on the right has been completely stripped. Details of the subepithelial capillaries can be seen on both villi.

cross-reference the images of light microscopy, scanning microscopy and transmission microscopy into a total structural concept of tissue architecture. Where possible, particularly in experimental studies where the availability of tissue is not a problem, parallel samples are often sufficient. In the clinical context, however, the only available tissue may be a small sample which cannot be subdivided. Methods are now available, however, for dewaxing histological blocks for subsequent scanning and transmission electron microscopy (8). It is equally possible to reprocess scanning EM specimens through resin-embedding

aration methods can be employed which broaden the horizons of surface scanning. For example, the connective tissue framework of the mucosa can be exposed by ultrasonic disintegration or by controlled autolysis, allowing the study of stromal alterations (Figs. 1, 2, 3). Vascular patterns can be demonstrated by scanning microscopy using resin casts (13). Techniques such as these have proved useful in the experimental field.

REVIEW OF RESULTS

Although electron microscopy is traditionally associated with magnifications far beyond light

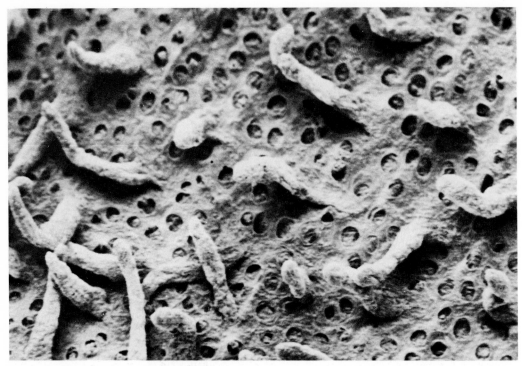

Fig. 2. S.E.M. of autolysed control gut. The connective tissue framework can be seen. Villous cores vary from erect to completely collapsed. Crypt mouths run in double rows in the intervillous basins between villi.

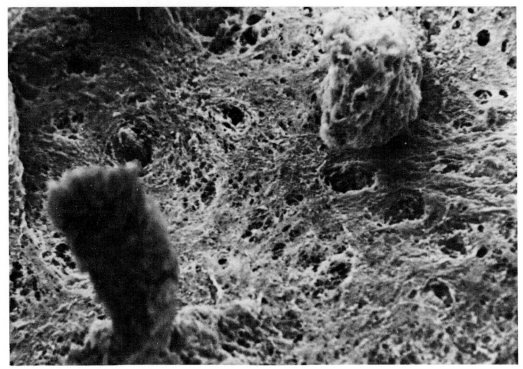

Fig. 3. S.E.M. of autolysed gut from irradiated mouse. A few villous cores can be seen projecting from the intervillous basin. A few crypt openings are also seen but most of them have been occluded by invasion of connective tissue.

microscopy, the recent growth of surface scanning electron microscopy has had the effect of re-awakening an interest in the lower ranges of mag-nification. Each range has its own contribution to make to our understanding of structural nor-mality or structural change. In the intestine, in particular, the overall surface morphology is a particularly sensitive indicator of response to environmental influences such as irradiation. In the study of tumours, however, while low mag-nification examination is essential to define the pattern, extent and behaviour of the disease as a whole, the analysis of cells at a much higher range of magnification is essential for the iden-tification of specific patterns of differentiation.

*Anatomical Normality*

There are various reviews of the morphology of the normal gastrointestinal tract as seen both by scanning and transmission electron microscopy (24, 25). Broadly speaking, scanning microscopy has shown itself best adapted to the recording of details of tissue organisation, such as regional mucosal specialisations. Transmission electron microscopy, on the other hand, provides a more sensitive record of cellular relationships within tissues, and of the ultrastructural details of the individual cells.

Distinctive regional specialisations of the mucosal surface include the wear-resistant squa-mous mucosa of the mouth and oesophagus; the mucus-secreting protective surface of the stomach, with its underlying glands; the elabor-ately expanded absorptive surfaces of the small bowel and the much flatter but still highly struc-tured contours of the large intestine. These natu-ral surfaces are ideal targets for the scanning microscopist with an interest in tissue architec-ture. The basic normal features have been exten-sively explored, although many uncertainties remain as to the significance of certain structural details which scanning microscopy has high-lighted. These include the distinctive creases which mark the surface of the intestinal villi and the variations in the prominence of the demar-cated territories around crypt orifices in the colon, known as crypt units.

Scanning microscopists are increasingly con-cerned with cellular details as well as tissue organisation. In the gut, for example, the varying patterns of intercellular boundaries and surface microvilli are of interest. In the oesophagus, the squamous cells have elaborate finger-print pat-terns of surface microridges, in contrast with the true microvilli seen in gastric and intestinal epi-thelial surfaces (Fig. 4). In specimens which have been accidently traumatised, causing disruption and shedding of parts of the surface epithelium, the lateral and basal aspects (Fig. 5) of the exposed epithelium can be studied. The com-plexity of epithelial cell lateral contours lining the intercellular spaces is particularly well seen. Intraepithelial lymphocytes can be recognised in the basal intercellular spaces (Fig. 5).

In general, however, in the examination of cytoplasmic detail, transmission electron micro-scopy is the dominant technique, revealing the relationships of epithelial cells to each other and to their underlying basal lamina. On occasion, apparently normal epithelial cells may show pro-jections of their basal cytoplasm through a narrow gap in the basal lamina, thus bringing epithelial and stromal elements into mutual contact. It has been speculated that herniations of this kind may mark the passage of migrating lymphocytes across the intestinal basal lamina. While much of the basic ultrastructure of the epithelium of the gut was established by early studies, it is only recently that the ultrastructural features of the M cells and the tuft cells have been properly documented. The recognition of these new cell types suggests new functional possibilities (21, 22).

*Tissue Changes, Experimental and Clinical*

In probing the relationships between structure and function, the electron microscopist will often begin by documenting the overall tissue response to experimental manipulation or disease. Tissue responses in the gastrointestinal tract often pro-duce subtle alterations of the mucosal surfaces by scanning electron microscopy, representing the integrated contribution of minor alterations of cells and stroma which might be individually unrecognisable. Surface morphology reflects not only epithelial, but also stromal and vascular reactions. Scanning microscopy is ideal for the

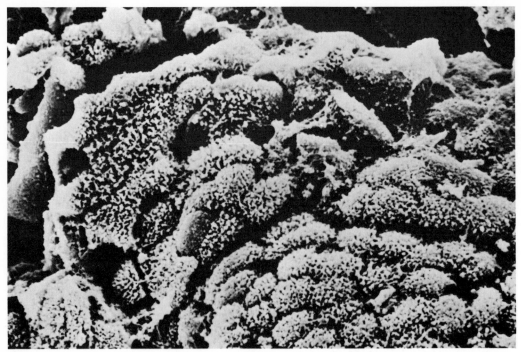

Fig. 4. S.E.M. of colonic mucosa from a case of Hirschsprung's disease. This biopsy was taken from the clinically identified junctional zone between the ganglionic and aganglionic segments. Both normal and abnormal patterns are seen here. The more normal region (bottom right) shows the conventional pattern of enterocytes each with apical microvilli. The abnormal region (top left) shows a shed enterocyte still with apical microvilli.

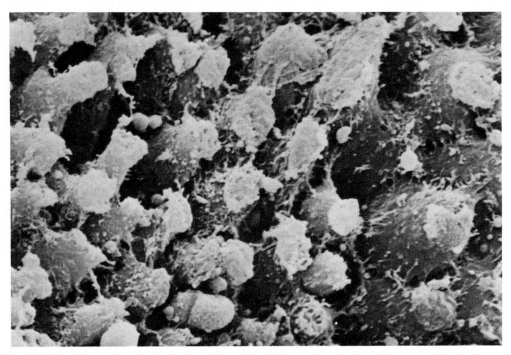

Fig. 5. S.E.M. of human intestinal epithelium. The epithelial sheet is detached from the core and the basal aspect of the cells can be seen. The spaces between the peg-like bases of the cells are clearly seen, with occasional lymphocytes lying in these clefts.

study of both localised and generalised changes in the mucosal surfaces of experimental animals.

Duodenal ulceration is a typical example of a localised intestinal response to damage. Gastric secretagogue administration (5) causes extensive local duodenal ulceration. Scanning microscopy tinal damage relies on the histological recognition and counting of microcolonies containing regenerating clones of epithelial cells, $3\frac{1}{2}$ days following radiation exposure. The results are expressed as the number of regenerating 'crypts' per circumference of the gut. This assay, which relies entirely

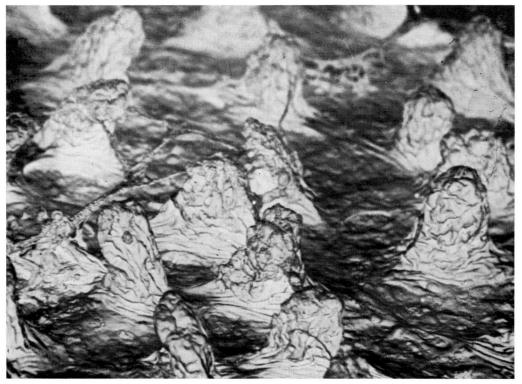

Fig. 6. S.E.M. of villi which have collapsed after irradiation. The villi have lost their erect, finger-like shape and are almost conical in shape.

shows swollen and abnormal villi at the edge of the ulcer crater, merging at a distance with a more normal pattern. The surface phenomena of re-epithelialisation can be studied in ulcers of different ages.

The mucosal alterations produced by irradiation provide a typical example of a generalised or diffuse intestinal response (Fig. 6). Various studies have observed the degradation of rodent intestinal mucosa following large doses of radiation (9) and the structural phenomena accompanying the process of repair (3, 15).

The conventional radiobiological assay of intes-

on the response of the epithelial cell population to injury, is unable to record damage below a threshold of around 900 rads of photon irradiation.

Scanning electron microscopy has proved a more sensitive indicator of low dose radiation injury than the crypt counting method (16). Presumably this reflects the broader scope of the surface structure 'assay', which can take note of modulations associated with multiple different aspects of tissue response.

The ability to identify integrated tissue responses in the gut is both a strength and a weakness of the technique of scanning electron microscopy. The crypt count assay of epithelial proliferative response has the advantage of a numerical result, lending itself to the graphic expression of changes within an experimental series. Surface morphology, on the other hand, with more fully below, under the heading of cellular changes.

For reasons discussed above, there are no satisfactory comparable studies of clinical radiation injury. While therapeutic irradiation has occasional well recognised gastrointestinal side-

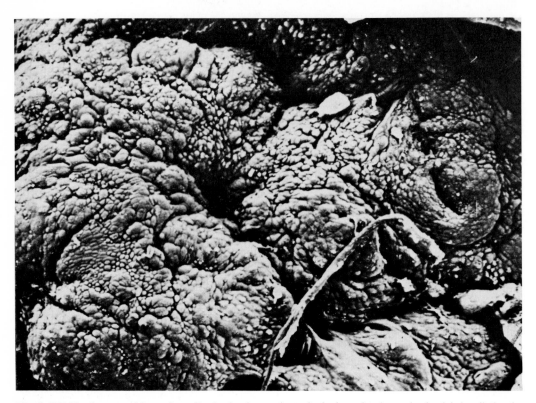

Fig. 7. S.E.M. of mucosal biopsy from distal colon in a patient who had previously received pelvic irradiation for malignancy. The surface has a cobblestone appearance, differing from the usual regular pattern of crypt units and furrows.

while sensitive both to epithelial and to stromal effects, and perhaps even to neuromuscular and functional changes, is more of a qualitative rather than a quantitive assay. Attempts have been made to identify individual factors in the mucosal response to fractionated radiation and to score these on a numerical scale in an attempt to progress towards a graphic representation of the results. A feature of some recent experiments has been the occurrence, under certain circumstances, of bizarre radiation-induced multinucleated epithelial giant cells (7). These are dealt

effects, the opportunity to study appropriate tissue samples rarely presents itself, especially in the phase of the acute response. Such changes as may be observed at a later stage may be related to incidental factors such as the presence of mild non-specific inflammatory disease or the existence of circulatory inadequacy due to vascular damage. Figure 7 shows an example of a mucosal biopsy of large intestine from a patient with a functional disturbance of the bowel some months following pelvic irradiation for cervical carcinoma. The obvious distortion of the surface pattern may be related to previous irradiation, although perhaps only in an indirect way.

One of the commonest clinical examples of an abnormal tissue response is seen in coeliac disease. Tissue sampling is less restricted in this condition, since patients with suspected intestinal malabsorption are routinely biopsied to establish the diagnosis and to assess the progress of treatment. Extensive ultrastructural information has therefore become available concerning the mucosal changes of coeliac disease. The typical surface features include the absence of villi and the presence of irregular heaped-up collars around the orifices of the crypts (20). These mucosal changes can be shown to regress slowly on the withdrawal of gluten from the diet. Unfortunately, there is no direct experimental counterpart of coeliac disease, the model of intestinal homograft rejection being perhaps the closest approach (14).

The effect of coeliac disease on cellular proliferation is the opposite to that seen in irradiation and cytotoxic therapy. In coeliac disease, cell turnover is enhanced with increased crypt cell proliferation. One might therefore expect the morphological expression of these different conditions to differ widely. Curiously, however, the distinctive collars of heaped-up cells around crypt mouths which are typical of severe coeliac disease can occasionally be recognised in the mouse intestine as part of a severe mucosal abnormality following certain schedules of heavy irradiation (6).

While there are many examples of human disease in which the tissue changes have been investigated by both transmission and scanning electron microscopy (17, 27), it is notable that in general the ultrastructural information has not been used by diagnostic pathologists for the purposes of routine service work. It appears that the recognition of tissue changes by electron microscopy has not displaced other simpler and less expensive established histological methods in the diagnostic laboratory.

*Cellular Changes, Experimental and Clinical*

Up to this point, in the discussion of tissue responses, the role of the scanning electron micro-scope has received considerable emphasis. This is hardly surprising, since the instrument is adapted for surveying large tissue samples, while retaining a significant high resolution capability. Even at the cellular level, while the transmission microscope is the traditional investigative tool, the increased resolution of the modern scanning microscope can now be of significant use.

Ultrastructural analysis has played an important part in the study of the cellular effects of radiation injury. A particular feature of recent experiments has been the abnormal frequency of protrusions or herniations of the epithelial cells of the intestinal villus through the underlying basal lamina into the lamina propria. When this happens, there is often close contact between epithelial cells and underlying macrophages and other inflammatory cell types (Fig. 8). Although similar herniations are occasionally seen in the normal intestinal mucosa, the extent of the change in the irradiated intestine is unusual. The possible functional consequences of this observation remain unexplored.

Frequently, it appears that the attachment of the villous epithelial cells to their underlying basal lamina is insecure, as shown by the presence of small areas of detachment along the cell base (Fig. 9). This abnormality can become much more extensive (Figs. 10, 11) resulting in the formation of what amount to blisters at the tips of villi, caused by the linear detachment of a number of adjacent cells. When these blisters collapse, as sometimes happens, on processing, they give rise to areas of indentation. The enterocytes themselves show evidence of functional impairment in the presence of abnormal amounts of cytoplasmic lipid, a feature also seen in the macrophages of the lamina propria.

During recent experiments on the time course of recovery from radiation injury, a distinctive cellular abnormality was identified at around five days. Warty outgrowths or blebs were noticed on many villi (Fig. 12). Re-embedding of the SEM specimens confirmed that these blebs represented multinucleated epithelial giant cells. Transmission electron microscopy showed the persistence of a distorted but recognisable microvillous border (Fig. 13) and the presence of epithelial adhe-

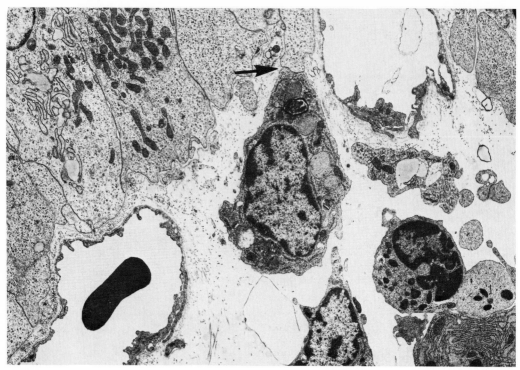

Fig. 8. T.E.M. of base of epithelial sheet in a villus after irradiation. The junction between the epithelium and stroma can be seen. In one position, there is close juxtaposition of a herniated enterocyte process with a connective tissue cell (arrow).

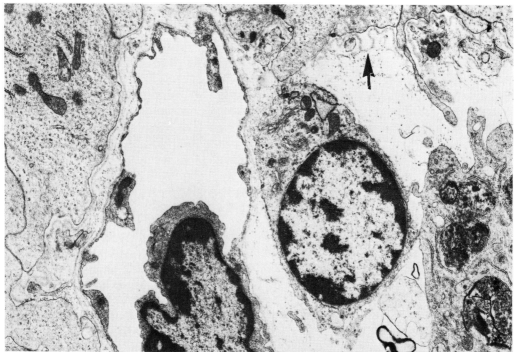

Fig. 9. T.E.M. of junction between epithelium and stroma in a small intestinal villus after irradiation. The basal lamina can be seen looping away (arrow) from the base of an enterocyte. Note the thin herniated epithelial cell process just to the right of the arrow.

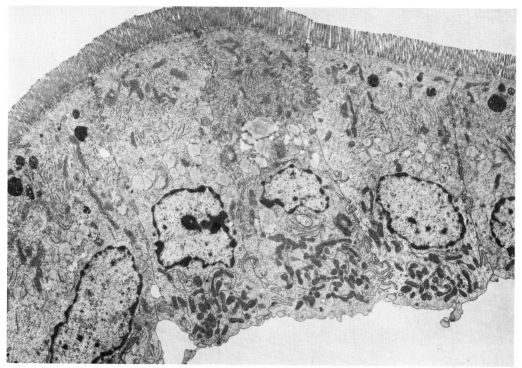

Fig. 10. T.E.M. of epithelial sheet, from irradiated intestinal villus. The epithelial sheet consists of enterocytes firmly bound to each other, but lacking basal lamina, or underlying connective tissue.

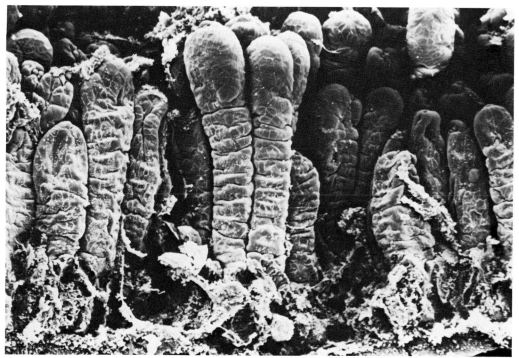

Fig. 11. S.E.M. of irradiated intestinal villi, showing abnormalities at the villous tips. These may be swollen, or collapsed, probably both reflecting abnormalities similar to that seen in Fig. 10.

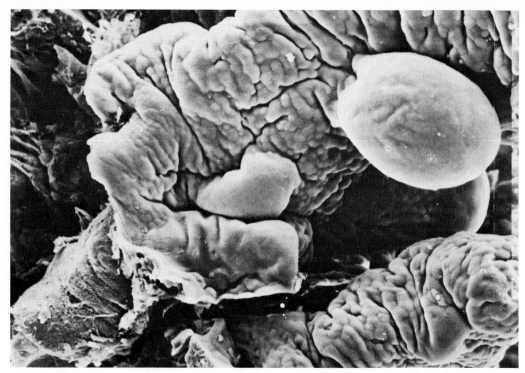

Fig. 12. S.E.M. of villus from irradiated mouse small intestine. Several giant cells can be seen. These lack enterocyte or goblet cell boundary patterns. The giant cell furthest up the villus from the base shows a greatly swollen profile.

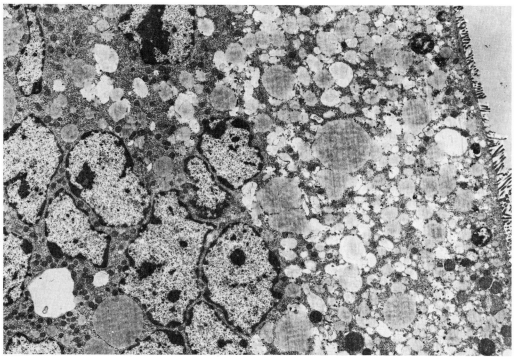

Fig. 13. T.E.M. of giant cell similar to those seen in Fig. 12. The apical cell membrane has sparse microvilli. There are several irregular nuclei and many lipid profiles.

sion specialisations between the giant cell and the adjacent enterocytes. The cytoplasm of these giant cells also contained many fat droplets (7). The nuclear chromatin patterns differed from those of the surrounding epithelial cells. The basal cytoplasm of the giant cell was sometimes herniated into the lamina propria. Intracytoplasmic

plasmic virus arrrays however, have been found in these cells.

In the clinical sphere, one might anticipate a harvest of valuable new diagnostic criteria from the ultrastructural examination of the cellular changes in human intestinal disease. On the contrary, however, with one exception, electron

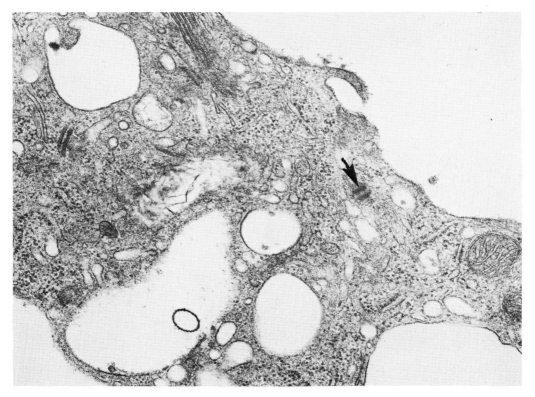

Fig. 14. T.E.M. of giant cell, showing membrane-bound cytoplasmic vacuoles and intracytoplasmic desmosome (arrow).

desmosomes (Fig. 14) occasionally seen within these cells may reflect a contribution of cell fusion to their formation, although incomplete cell division may be a more important factor. The presence of large cytoplasmic vacuoles (Fig. 14) and 'myelin figures' provides further nonspecific evidence of functional irregularity. It remains to be seen whether these giant cells are produced simply by the effects of irradiation, or by radiation combined with some other factor, such as viral infection. Neither intranuclear nor intracyto-

microscopy has not so far significantly influenced the practice of diagnostic pathology. The single exception, the field of tumour pathology, is discussed below, with detailed examples.

This is not to deny the value of electron microscopy in the scientific study of disease. For example, electron microscopy has been the key to the identification of various common gastrointestinal infections due to viruses, previously recognised as ill-defined clinical entities (23). This technique remains invaluable in further investigations in this field where faecal samples must be screened for the presence of viral particles (2).

Recent reviews (12, 26) document the various ultrastructural changes which have been recognised in common and uncommon diseases such

essential starting point, its resolution is often insufficient to allow the recognition of cellular patterns of differentiation. With current advances in cytotoxic pharmacology, cellular fine structure can be of greater diagnostic relevance than tissue

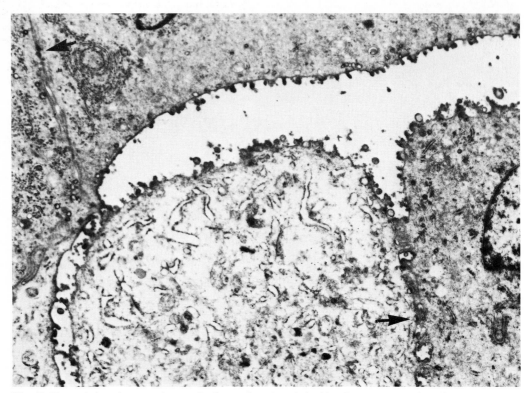

Fig. 15. Transmission electron micrograph of secondary deposit in skin of a mucus-secreting adenocarcinoma of colon. The open space between cells is lined by microvilli and the areas of intimate cell/cell contact are characterised by small but relatively well developed adhesion specialisations (arrows).

as coeliac disease, abetalipoproteinaemia, Whipple's disease, amyloidosis, blind loop syndrome, and storage diseases. In general, however, these ultrastructural observations do not amount to a significant diagnostic advance. The clinician and the histopathologist have other well-established ways of identifying these diseases. If electron microscopy is more complex, more time consuming or more expensive, it will not displace simpler methods already in use (18).

The situation is different in human oncology. In this special area of cellular pathology the electron microscopist can contribute most to diagnostic accuracy. While light microscopy is the

response. In such cases the transmission electron microscope has the greatest part to play, while the scanning microscope has no defined role (4, 8, 11).

Although tumour cells often show gross ultrastructural aberrations, they still tend to reflect their tissue origin, or histogenesis, through the structural patterns which they display. When electron microscopy can make a positive contribution to diagnosis, it is usually through the recognition of some normal ultrastructural marker rather than some unique cellular aberration. The questions at issue usually relate to the differential diagnosis of tumours of epithelial, muscular or connective tissue cell differentiation, which are the commonest varieties in the gut.

The typical epithelial tumour, such as a carcinoma, has markers such as junctional complexes, desmosomes and small spaces lined by microvilli,

their expected different special features, reflecting the appropriate differentiation patterns.

A simple introduction such as this inevitably involves a degree of oversimplification. For example, most gastrointestinal lymphomas, in our

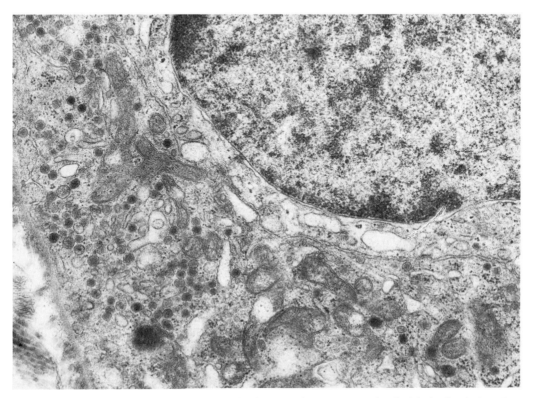

Fig. 16. Micrograph from lymph node metastasis of pancreatic tumour associated with duodenal ulceration. Numerous dense core, membrane bound granules are evident in a predominantly basal location.

corresponding to gland lumina (Fig. 15). The special epithelial category of neuroendocrine tumour has its own distinctive secretory granules (Fig. 16) which can persist when few or none of the histological markers of endocrine tumours are present. Smooth muscle tumours form a significant minority of gastrointestinal neoplasms. When typical, they are distinguished by the presence of myofilaments, cytoplasmic and subsurface dense bodies, extensive intervening basal lamina and patchy close cellular contact. Finally, lymphoid tumours are to some extent diagnosed by exclusion, although a typical lymphocytic tumour (Fig.17) and a typical plasma cell tumour have

experience, are far from typical in these simple terms. The following illustrative case histories of a group of gastrointestinal tumours will indicate the ways in which the ultrastructural pathologist can contribute to the differential diagnosis in such cases

*Case 1. Tumour of Stomach*

Histology shows a highly undifferentiated malignant tumour (Fig. 18). The probable diagnosis is undifferentiated carcinoma, but the possibility of lymphoma cannot be excluded. Electron microscopy (Fig. 19) confirms the presence of cytoplasmic tonofilaments and adhesion spe-

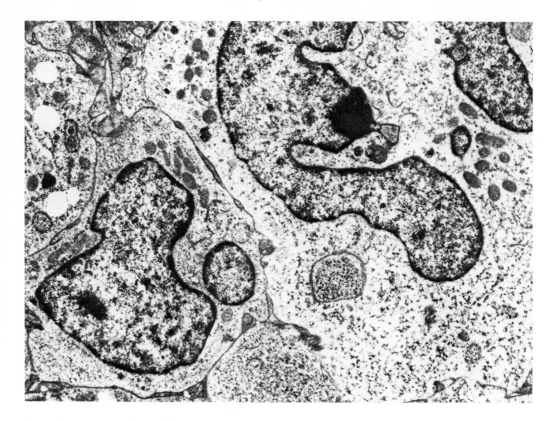

Fig. 17. T.E.M. of small intestinal lymphoma. The cells here are characterised by a relative paucity of organelles and by the lack of adhesion specialisations.

cialisations, consistent with an epithelial differentiation pattern. The diagnosis of carcinoma is thus reinforced.

### Case 2. Tumour of Stomach

Histology shows a poorly differentiated adenocarcinoma of stomach with no distinctive fea-

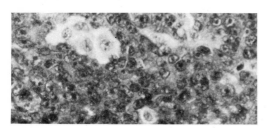

Fig. 18. Case 1. H & E section of gastric tumour. No specific differentiated features are seen.

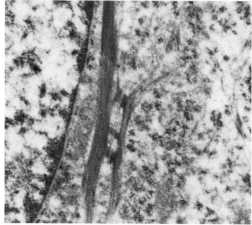

Fig. 19. Case 1. T.E.M. shows cytoplasmic tonofilaments and relatively well developed adhesion specialisations towards the centre of the illustration.

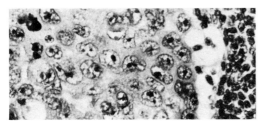

Fig. 20. Case 2. H & E section from lymph node metastasis of what appeared to be a rather poorly differentiated gastric carcinoma.

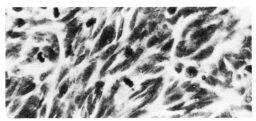

Fig. 22. Case 3. H & E preparation from tumour of small intestine. A spindle cell pattern is clearly evident.

tures (Fig. 20). Electron microscopy shows the presence of significant numbers of neuroendocrine granules in most cells (Fig. 21). This unexpected finding indicates endocrine differentiation.

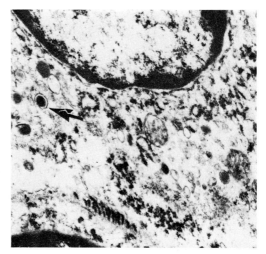

Fig. 23. Case 3. In this micrograph portions of two adjacent cells are seen. In one of these a typical neuroendocrine granule (arrow) is identified. There are no significant arrays of cytoplasmic microfilaments.

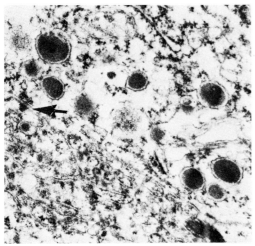

Fig. 21. Case 2. This electron micrograph shows a poorly developed adhesion specialisation (arrow) and several dense core, membrane bound neuroendocrine type granules.

### Case 4. Needle Biopsy of Liver

Secondary tumour in liver, clinical mass in stomach and pancreas. Histology shows infiltrating malignant tumour of widely variable pattern, with areas of spindle cell morphology and a suggestion of packeting (Fig. 24). The tissue was

### Case 3. Tumour of Small Intestine

Incidental finding at cholecystectomy. Histology shows a spindle cell malignant tumour of uncertain type (Fig. 22), provisionally diagnosed as leiomyosarcoma. Electron microscopy shows epithelial differentiation, with scanty neuroendocrine granules (Fig. 23) in keeping with a diagnosis of spindle cell carcinoid tumour. There are no features suggestive of muscle differentiation.

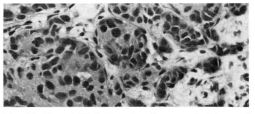

Fig. 24. Case 4. H & E section from needle biopsy of liver. Elements of an infiltrating tumour of relatively small cell type are evident. There is some evidence of packeting.

not available for electron microscopy. Remnants of the paraffin block were reprocessed and embedded in resin for thin sections. Electron microscopy shows abundant neuroendocrine granules, suggesting a diagnosis of malignant islet cell tumour (Fig. 25).

type, with abundant neuroendocrine granules, principally basal in location (Fig. 27). These granules appear between numerous large foamy lipid droplets which dominate the histological appearances. Electron microscopy allows a diagnosis of an unusual variant of islet cell tumour.

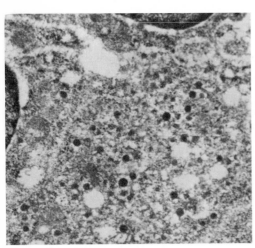

Fig. 25. Case 4. The corresponding electron micrograph shows numerous neuroendocrine type granules. Since this material is reprocessed from paraffin the membrane definition is poor.

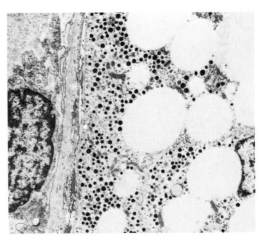

Fig. 27. Case 5. The cell on the right of this electron micrograph is characterised by basally located neuroendocrine granules interspersed with large, lipid droplets which gave the cell its foamy appearance on light microscopy.

## Case 5. Cyst of Pancreas

A cystic lesion in tail of pancreas removed as an incidental finding during gastrectomy for carcinoma of stomach. The gastric carcinoma was unremarkable. Histological examination of the pancreatic cyst shows a rim of foamy cells of unusual type not clearly identifiable as being of pancreatic origin (Fig. 26). Electron microscopy shows that the tumour cells are of the endocrine

## Case 6. Tumour of Stomach

Histology shows a spindle cell tumour (Fig. 28). Electron microscopy shows the focal presence of typical features of smooth muscle differentiation, including myofilaments, patchy cell surface densities, and associated basal lamina (Fig. 29). Despite the variation from cell to cell, the combination of typical features is sufficient to allow confirmation of the diagnosis of leiomyosarcoma.

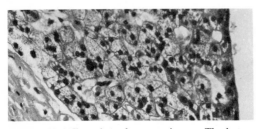

Fig. 26. H & E section of pancreatic cyst. The lumen is on the right and the connective tissue capsule is seen towards the left. The epithelial lining is composed of foam cells with relatively small nuclei.

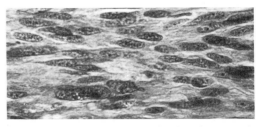

Fig. 28. Case 6. H & E preparation from large gastric tumour. A fairly monotonous spindle cell pattern is evident.

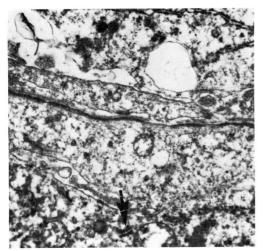

Fig. 29. Case 6. Elements of four cells are seen in this electron micrograph. Cytoplasmic filaments are not identified here, but an adhesion specialisation (arrow) is seen, together with patchy basal lamina and, in the case of one cell, extensive surface densities.

## Case 7. Tumour of Stomach

Histology shows a clear cell pattern (Fig. 30), alternating with ill-defined areas of more spindle cell appearance. Electron microscopy shows typical myofilaments in significant numbers, associated with surface densities and patchy basal lamina (Fig. 31). Micropinocytotic vesicles and focal cellular adhesions are also present. The misleading clear cell appearance of the histology, when

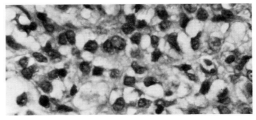

Fig. 30. Case 7. H & E section of polypoid gastric tumour. This area shows an essentially clear cell pattern.

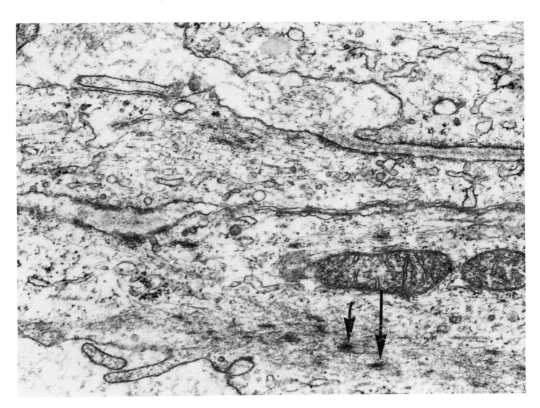

Fig. 31. Case 7. This micrograph demonstrates conspicuous myofilaments with associated fusiform densities (arrows). Cell surface densities and patchy basal lamina are also evident.

associated with these features of smooth muscle differentiation, lead to a confident diagnosis of epithelioid leiomyoma.

## Case 8. Tumour of Small Intestine

Light microscopy shows a poorly differentiated carcinoma (Fig. 32). The appearances are not typical of an intestinal tumour. Electron microscopy shows the typical features of a poorly differentiated squamous cell carcinoma, including

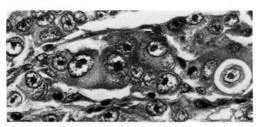

Fig. 32. Case 8. Section, stained H & E, from small intestinal tumour. The appearances are of carcinoma with no specific differentiation.

abundant tonofilaments and large well developed desmosomes (Fig. 33). The diagnosis of secondary squamous cell carcinoma was confirmed at autopsy, which revealed a primary in the lung.

## Case 9. Tumour of Small Intestine

The tumour presented as a segmental thickening of the ileum. Histology shows an unusual malignant infiltrate consisting of plump eosinophilic cells merging deeply with more elongated forms (Fig. 34). The differential diagnosis included plasma cell tumour and muscle tumour. Electron microscopy shows the presence of internally structured inclusions within cisternae of the endoplasmic reticulum (Fig. 35), inconsistent with muscle differentiation. The appearances strongly suggest a plasma cell tumour of an unusual type, with pronounced intracisternal accumulation of secretion product. The nuclear morphology and other features are consistent with this diagnosis.

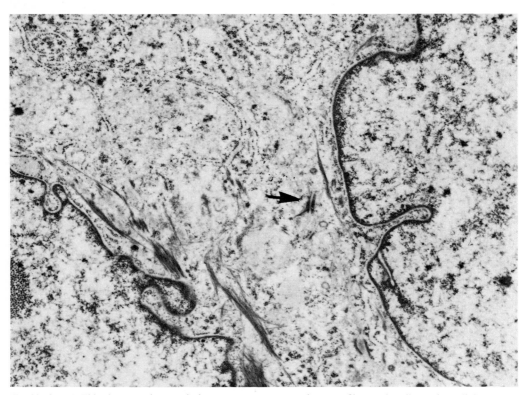

Fig. 33. Case 8. This electron micrograph shows numerous paranuclear tonofilament bundles and a well developed desmosome (arrow).

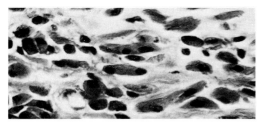

Fig. 34. Case 9. H & E section of small intestinal tumour. Darkly staining elongated cells are admixed with plump cells with plasmacytoid features (Case by courtesy of Dr. G. Slavin, Northwick Park Hospital).

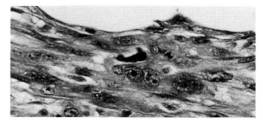

Fig. 36. Case 10. This H & E section shows a malignant spindle cell tumour infiltrating omental fat (top).

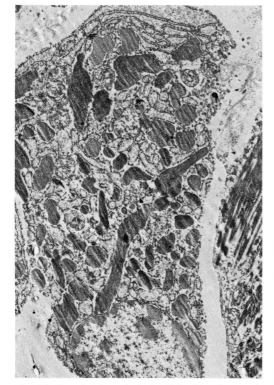

Fig. 35. Case 9. The principal cell in this micrograph is characterised by abundant cisternae of granular endoplasmic reticulum, many of which are filled by internally structured inclusions. The open cisternae at the top of the picture and the nuclear morphology (bottom) are characteristic of a plasma cell.

### Case 10. Tumour of Omentum

Widespread abdominal tumour, but no clear primary site. Histology shows a malignant spindle cell tumour, diagnosed as leiomyosarcoma (Fig. 36). Electron microscopy shows a wide range of ultrastructural specialisation, but with only scanty

evidence suggestive of smooth muscle. Fibroblast-like cells and cells containing lipid droplets are prominent (Fig. 37). In cases such as these, electron microscopy casts some doubt on an otherwise acceptable histological diagnosis, but fails to provide a definitive answer. It seems to us wiser to accept that this case remains unresolved rather than to apply an arbitrary identity

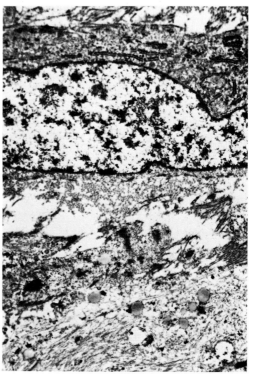

Fig. 37. Case 10. The cell at the top of this electron micrograph shows a basically, fibroblastic pattern of differentiation with, in addition, occasional cell surface densities. In the cell at the bottom, some filaments are seen together with several lipid droplets.

simply on the basis of histology. Detailed ultra-structural analysis (19) of groups of cases like these may eventually lead to a more satisfactory classification than our present understanding permits.

It would be misleading to suggest that cases such as these are numerous, but similar problems of diagnosis must be familiar to any pathologist. While routine prospective study of all gastrointestinal tumours would involve an unacceptably low level of worthwhile results, the judicious use of formalin-fixed tissue and exceptionally of reprocessed tissue from paraffin blocks, provides useful information in many cases which present unresolved problems following conventional histopathological examination.

## ACKNOWLEDGEMENTS

The authors are grateful for the technical assistance of Mr. J. D. Anderson and Mrs. C. Watt and the typing skills of Marion Thomson. They also wish to acknowledge the provision of SEM facilities by the Departments of Ophthalmology and Veterinary Anatomy, Glasgow University and the Department of Metallurgy, University of Strathclyde.

## REFERENCES

1. Abraham, J. L. *Monogr. Pathol.* 1978, *19*, 96–137
2. Almeida, J. D. *New Engl. J. Med.* 1975, *292*, 1403–1405
3. Anderson, J. H. & Withers, R. H. *Scanning Electron Microscopy* 1973, *3*, 566–572
4. Buss, H. & Hollweg, H. G. *Scanning Electron Microscopy 1980/III.* 139–153. SEM. Inc., AMF O'Hare (Chicago), Illinois
5. Carr, K. E., Joffe, S. N., Toner, P. G. & Watt, C. *Scand. J. Gastroenterol.* 1979,*14*, 78–82
6. Carr, K. E., Hamlet, R., Nias, A. H. W. & Watt, C. *Brit. J. Radiol.* 1979, *52*, 485–493
7. Carr, K. E., Hamlet, R., Nias, A. H. W. & Watt C. *J. Microsc.* 1981. In press.
8. Carr, K. E., McLay, A. L. C., Toner, P. G., Chung, P. & Wong, A. *Scanning Electron Microscopy 1980/III.* 121–138. SEM. Inc., AMF O'Hare (Chicago), Illinois
9. Carr, K. E. & Toner, P. G. *Virchows Archs. Abt. B. Zellpathol.* 1972, *11*, 201–210
10. Carr, K. E., Wong, A., Young, D. G., Toner, P. G. & Watt, C. *Scot. Med. J.* 1981. 26, 103–114
11. Carter, H. W. *Scanning Electron Microscopy 1980/III.* 115–120. SEM. Inc., AMF O'Hare (Chicago) Illinois
12. Dobbins, W. O. pp. 253–339 in Trump B. F. and Jones, R. T. (Eds.), *Diagnostic Electron Microscopy Vol. I.* Wiley, New York, 1978
13. Egawa, J. & Ishioka, K. *Acta Radiol. Oncol. Radiol. Phys. Biol.* 1978, *17*, 414–422
14. Ferguson, A., Carr, K. E., McDonald, T. & Watt, C. *Digestion.* 1978, *18*, 56–63
15. Friberg, L. G. *Effects of Irradiation on the Small Intestine of the Rat.* 1980, Thesis, Lund University
16. Hamlet, R., Carr, K. E., Toner, P. G. & Nias, A. H. W. *Brit. J. Radiol.* 1976, *49*, 624–629
17. Johannessen, J. V. *Electron Microscopy in Human Medicine.* Vols. 1–12. McGraw Hill Inc., New York. 1979
18. McLay, A. L. C. & Toner, P. G. pp. 241–261 in Anthony, P. P. and MacSween, R. N. M. (Eds.), *Recent Advances in Histopathology*, Vol. *11*, Churchill-Livingstone, London, 1981
19. McLay, A. L. C. & Toner, P. G. *Investigative and Cell Pathology*, 1981. In press
20. Marsh, M. N., Brown, A. C. & Swift, J. A. pp. 26–45 in Booth, C. C. and Dowling, R. H. (Eds.), *Coeliac Disease.* Churchill-Livingstone, London. 1970
21. Nabeyama, A. & Leblond, C. P. *Am. J. Anat.* 1974, *140*, 147–166
22. Owen, R. L. *Gastroenterology*, 1977, *72*, 440–451
23. Schreiber, D. S., Trier, J. S. & Blacklow, N. R. *Gastroenterology*, 1977, *73*, 174–183
24. Toner, P. G. & Carr, K. E. pp. 203–272 in Hodges, G. M. and Hallowes, R. C. (Eds.), *Biomedical Research Applications of Scanning Electron Microscopy.* Vol. I. Academic Press, London, 1979
25. Toner, P. G. & Carr, K. E. pp. 1–24, in Sircus, W. and Smith, A. N. (Eds.), *Scientific foundations of Gastroenterology.* William Heinemann Medical Books Ltd. London, 1980
26. Toner, P. G., Carr, K. E. & Al. Yassin, T. M. pp. 85–207, in Johannessen (Ed.), *Electron Microscopy in Human Medicine.* Vol. 7. Digestive System. McGraw-Hill. New York, 1980
27. Trump, B. F. & Jones, R. T. *Diagnostic Electron Microscopy.* Vols. 1–3, Wiley, New York, 1978

# Nesidiodysplasia and Nesidioblastosis of Infancy

## Ultrastructural and Immunohistochemical Analysis of Islet Cell Alterations With and Without Associated Hyperinsulinaemic Hypoglycaemia

V. E. GOULD, V. A. MEMOLI, L. E. DARDI & N. S. GOULD

Rush Medical College, Rush-Presbyterian-St. Lukes Medical Center and
Michael Reese Medical Center, Chicago, Illinois, USA

The pancreata of hyperinsulinaemic, hypoglycaemic infants, having the anatomic anomalies characterised as 'nesidioblastosis', were compared with age matched control infants by light microscopy, and electron microscopy. While the hyperinsulinaemic infants showed an apparent increase in total endocrine volume compared with control infants, the light microscopic alterations of topographic maldistribution of endocrine cells, irregularly defined islets and intermingling of endocrine with exocrine elements were common to both hypoglycaemic and control groups. In at least one control case, the total endocrine cell volume was comparable to that seen in hypoglycaemic infants and was not associated with endocrine dysfunction. The ratios of insulin: somatostatin: glucagon cells in hypoglycaemic infants were similar to those of control infants. The results of both immunohistochemistry and electron microscopy gave strong indications of endocrine cells containing more than one immunoreactive peptide and heterogenous granule populations respectively. Ultrastructurally, 'composite' cells with features of both exocrine and endocrine differentiation were found with some frequency in two hypoglycaemic infants.

These findings are discussed in the light of current notions of gastroentero-pancreatic endocrine system development. We conclude that 'nesidioblastosis' as currently defined is not the anatomic substratum of infantile hyperinsulaemic hypoglycaemia. We propose the term 'nesidiodysplasia' to encompass the apparently increased and possibly maldistributed and/or malregulated endocrine cells associated with the clinical manifestations of hyperinsulinaemic hypoglycaemia. The precise relationship between the presumed anatomic abnormalities and abnormal insulin secretion remains to be clarified by further investigations.

*V. E. Gould, M.D., Rush Medical College, Rush-Presbyterian-St. Lukes Medical Center, Chicago, Illinois 60612, USA*

As originally defined by Laidlaw, *nesidioblastosis* referred to . . . 'a diffuse and disseminated proliferation of islet cells as a possible cause of hypoglycaemia' (1). Time and increasing usage have broadened that definition which currently comprises features such as islet cell hypertrophy and hyperplasia and giant islets (2, 3). Moreover, nesidioblastosis may also encompass the more restricted designation *beta cell nesidioblastosis* which, in turn has been defined as . . . 'many additional beta cells scattered either singly or in small packets of 2–6 cells . . . separate from the islets and most often seen about the walls of small ducts or in the glandular acini proper' (4, 5, 6).

It was also suggested that the aforementioned single or small clusters were comprised exclusively of beta cells which, lacking contiguity with other pancreatic endocrine cells, were thus liberated from the normal paracrine regulatory mechanisms with resulting mal(hyper)function (7, 8, 9). The designation of '*multifocal ductoinsular proliferation*' was coined by Heitz et al. to describe what they viewed as an unarrested development of the endocrine pancreas progressing beyond the neonatal and early infancy stages (10). Nesidioblastosis, in their estimation, would comprise a spectrum of alterations ranging from the aforementioned multifocal ductoinsular proliferation to focal adenomatosis to adenomas; the common denominator of those changes was thought to be a notable increase in total pancreatic endocrine cell mass though the ratios of beta cells *vis a vis* the other pancreatic endocrine cells were close to normal (10). These investigators suggested that the increased beta cell mass might be the anatomic basis of infantile hyperinsulinaemic hypoglycaemia (10).

In a recent and thorough investigation Jaffe et al. (11) studied the pancreatic morphology of a group of hyperinsulinaemic hypoglycaemic infants by immunohistochemistry and compared it with that of age-matched controls. Their findings in the hypoglycaemic infants indicated two distinct types of alteration: 1) adenomatosis as defined by a rather massive proliferation of endocrine cells comprising at times over 40% of a given area and either displacing or irregularly encompassing exocrine parenchymal elements, and 2) topographic maldistribution of endocrine cells, irregularly defined islets, intermingling of endocrine with exocrine elements, both ductal and acinar, and islet cell hypertrophy. The latter group of changes was designated as 'endocrine cell dysplasia' (11). However, their quantitive analyses indicated that the mean total endocrine area of age-matched controls was not markedly different from that of infants with clinically overt endocrine syndrome (11). Moreover, 'nesidioblastosis' as often defined, was found to be present in the controls and could therefore not be considered to be the anatomic substratum of infantile hyperinsulinaemic hypoglycaemia (11).

During the last few years we have had the opportunity to study the pancreatic morphology in surgical specimens of several cases of infantile hyperinsulinaemic hypoglycaemia with a combination of electron microscopy and immunohistochemical techniques. All our cases with clinically apparent endocrine syndromes displayed the 'diffuse' type of islet cell 'proliferation'. This report descibes our findings and attempts to compare them with our observations in a group of age-matched controls.

We were able to obtain fresh surgical specimens, from the hypoglycaemic infants and autopsy material, from non-hypoglycaemic controls, which were fixed in routine histological fixatives (formalin and Bouin's fluid) and processed for conventional histology (haematoxylin and eosin stain) and immunocytochemistry (indirect peroxidase-anti-peroxidase) (12). The distributions of insulin, glucagon, pancreatic polypeptide (PP), somatostatin, gastrin and VIP were investigated using specific antisera to the peptides.

Using a slightly modified version of Nakane's technique (13, 14, 15), it was possible to localise simultaneously two separate antigens in the same tissue section. 4-chloro-1-naphthol and 3:3-diaminobenzidene were used as chromogens for the first and second immunostains, respectively.

As well as carrying out these light microscopical investigations the ultrastructural appearance of the cells was examined. Material was fixed in 2% s-collidine buffered glutaraldehyde, post-fixed in 1% osmium tetroxide, dehydrated in graded ethanols and embedded in Epon. One μm thick sections were stained with toluidine blue for orientation purposes. Thin sections were cut with diamond knives on an automatic LKB ultramicrotome, mounted upon Formvar-and carbon coated grids and stained with uranyl acetate and lead hydroxide. A minimum of 3 blocks per case were thin sectioned and 60 to 75 photographs taken. Original magnifications ranged from 1,300 to 12,000; from these, photographic enlargements were prepared when required.

Examination of conventional H & E stained slides of pancreas from hypoglycaemic infants revealed no striking abnormalities in the size, number or distribution of islets. In one case the number of islets did not appear to be increased, but their contour was irregular. No adenomas were recognised. Close scrutiny of the sections disclosed variably abundant pale staining cells arranged either singly or in very small groups outside the well-defined islets. Those pale staining cells were irregularly admixed with acinar cells and/or in paraductal locations. The prominence of these findings varied considerably from case to case as well as in different areas of the same case. Notable differences in the distribution of the endocrine cells in different zones of the pancreas were not detected.

Study of comparable H & E sections of the normal controls revealed architectural and cellular features that were similar to those observed in hypoglycaemic infants. Although the number of endocrine cells appeared greater in hypoglycaemic infants, one of the controls displayed what appeared to be a remarkably large total endocrine cell mass.

A rather diffuse distribution of insulin immunoreactive cells was observed in the hypoglycaemic infants (Fig. 1). When within islets, insulin cells were arranged in the pattern seen in adult human islets, i.e. preferentially in the centre. With the exception of one case our sampling did not show notable abnormalities in the size or contour of the islets, nor was their relative location within the lobules noticeably altered.

Numerous, small clusters of insulin cells were scattered throughout the exocrine pancreas and they often appeared in close proximity to small, intralobular and interlobular ducts (Fig. 2). A good proportion of the aforementioned clusters, however, did not consist exclusively of insulin-containing cells. In sections stained for insulin and somatostatin, cells positive for the latter hormone were readily found (Fig. 3). Solitary insulin-containing cells were found, with variable frequency, in periacinar and intracinar locations.

Somatostatin immunoreactive cells were scattered throughout the pancreas in a pattern of distribution similar to that of insulin cells. The relative number of extrainsular somatostatin cells was striking and appeared to be second only to that of the insulin cells. Glucagon-containing cells

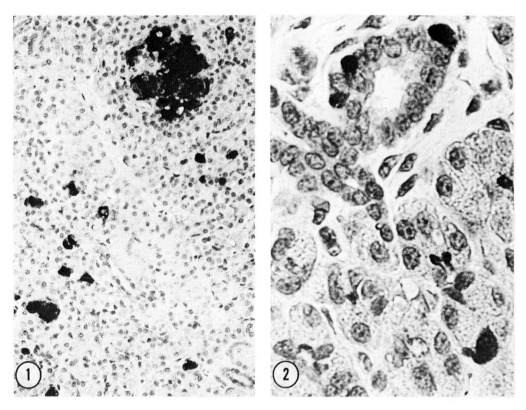

Fig. 1. Hypoglycaemic infant. Immunoperoxidase technique for insulin. Note islet in upper right corner as well as scattered small groups of cells and apparently isolated cells, positive for insulin.    ×135

Fig. 2. Hypoglycaemic infant. Immunoperoxidase technique for insulin. Note immunoreactive cells in interlobular duct and interspersed amidst exocrine parenchyma.    ×575

were observed predominantly within islets where they displayed a propensity for a peripheral position, although 'mantle' islets were not readily found. Human pancreatic polypeptide (HPP) cells were distinctly less abundant than the afore-mentioned; these were located both within and without well defined islets.

It should be noted that the immunohistochemical methods employed did not allow for the dis-

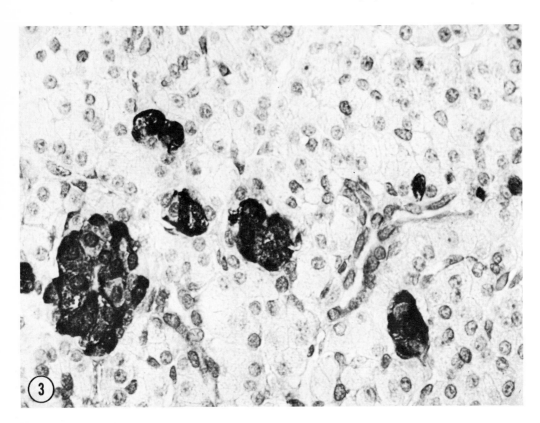

Fig. 3. Hypoglycaemic infant. Combined immunoperoxidase technique for insulin (dark) and somatostatin (light). Note intimate association between both cell types. Also, a number of cells appear 'positive' for both immunostains.  ×450

mentioned. When located outside the islets, they were characteristically found singly and often in association with rather large interlobular ducts (Fig. 4). Vasoactive intestinal polypeptide cells were approximately as frequent as HPP cells but less so than insulin, somatostatin and glucagon cells. VIP cells were most often found singly within islets; however, occasional VIP cells were also found amidst acini and in periductal positions. Nerves within and outside the pancreas were focally positive for VIP. In only one of these hypoglycaemic infants, a few scattered gastrin immunoreactive cells were noted; these were

tribution of 'composite' cells that might contain more than one immunoreactive peptide. Therefore, in assessing selective numbers of endocrine cells in serial sections immunostained for different hormones, the same cell may have been considered more than once. In addition, in double stained sections (insulin, glucagon, insulin and somatostatin) the interrelationships between these cells were, at times, difficult to assess, and the strong suggestion of double immunoreactivity in single cells was evident, as indicated in different contexts by other authors.

In control infants, the basic observations made at the immunohistochemical level pertinent to the distribution and apparent arrangements of endocrine cells were essentially similar to those made in infants with hypoglycaemia. Though the total obviously 'organised islets' and focused predominantly on the endocrine cells located in relation to ducts and acinar tissue. Although extralobular ducts were not abundant in our samples, a number was present and some of those displayed out-

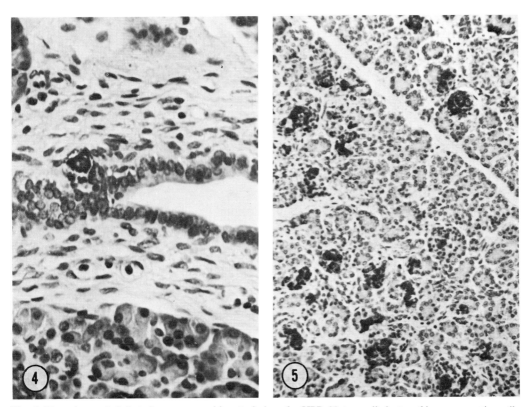

Fig. 4. Hypoglycaemic infant. Immunoperoxidase technique for HPP. Note small cluster of immunoreactive cells closely associated with rather large interlobular duct. ×210

Fig. 5. Control (non-hypoglycaemic) infant. Immunoperoxidase technique for insulin. Notice abundant and widely scattered immunoreactive cells; no islet is seen in this field. ×135

endocrine cell mass was distinctly higher in the hypoglycaemic infants, one of the controls had a similarly high total endocrine mass (Fig. 5). Relative number of somatostatin cells appeared to be slightly lower than in the hypoglycaemic infants. None of the control pancreata displayed gastrin-positive cells.

In hypoglycaemic infants, endocrine cells were readily identified under the electron microscope in literally every low power field. However, we concentrated our observations away from the

pouchings consisting of irregular admixtures of ductal, sustentacular, centroacinar, acinar and endocrine cells.

Within acini, endocrine cells were readily recognisable. They were found predominantly in a basal position applied upon the well defined basal lamina (Fig. 6). Also endocrine cells and cytoplasmic processes of endocrine cells were seen interspersed among exocrine cells closer to, but not in direct contact with, the acinar lumen (Fig. 7). The most frequently observed endocrine

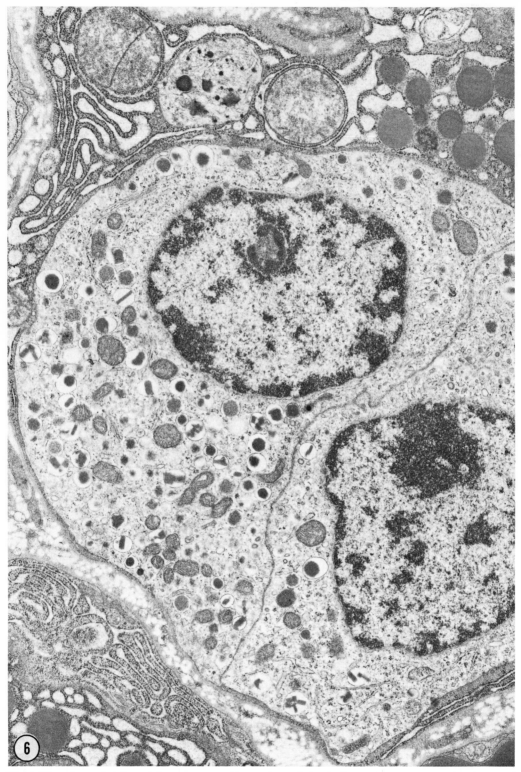

Fig. 6. Hypoglycaemic infant. Acinar structure with exocrine cell clearly discernable in the upper portion of the field. Endocrine cells are conspicious and heterogeneity of their granule populations is evident.   ×17,900

cells displayed typical beta cell characteristics, as indicated by the crystalline cores of their granules. The second most frequently noted cell had granules with very dense and often slightly eccentric cores, whose semilunar halos were either pale or minimally granular (Fig. 8).

differentiation towards the luminal pole while their endocrine features (granules) were distinctly orientated towards the basal or vascular pole (Fig. 11).

In control infant pancreata, endocrine cells were also frequently found admixed with exocrine

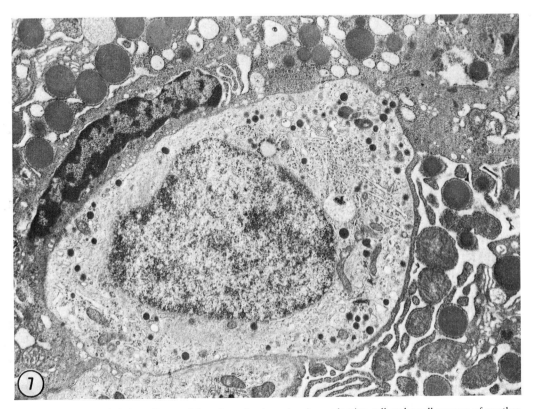

Fig. 7. Hypoglycaemic infant. Tangential section of acinus showing endocrine cell and small process of another endocrine cell almost totally surrounded by exocrine elements.   ×12,650

The most striking ultrastructural finding in two hypoglycaemic infants was the presence of cells displaying a combination of features which included: 1) cells containing granules of both uniformly dense and crystalline cores, and 2) cells with a combination of prominent, parallel arrays of rough endoplasmic reticulum and zymogen granules on the one hand and distinct endocrine features on the other as indicated by the presence of one and occasionally two types of endocrine granules (Figs. 9, 10). These 'composite' cells displayed a distinct polarisation of the exocrine

ductal and acinar structures (Fig. 12). The most frequently noted endocrine cell outside islets was again of the beta type. Composite exocrine and endocrine cells were not identified. However, cells with very heterogenous granule populations were not uncommon.

We can, therefore, summarise our observations made during the study as follows:

1) If nesidioblastosis is defined morphologically as the presence of more or less abundant endocrine cells irregularly admixed with exocrine parenchymal elements, in addition to those endo-

crine cells arranged in true islets, then one may state that nesidioblastosis may be readily found in neonates and young infants with or without an associated clinically apparent endocrine syndrome.

strong suggestion that numerous cells contained more than one immunoreactive peptide.

4) In two hypoglycaemic infants, electron microscopy revealed rather frequent composite or 'intermediate' cells displaying features of

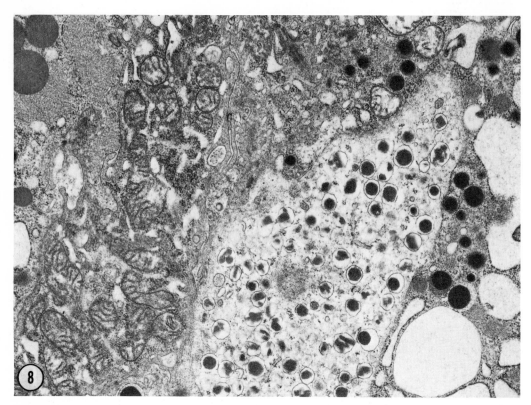

Fig. 8. Hypoglycaemic infant. Acinar structure with portion of exocrine cell discernable in upper left corner. Segments of two endocrine cells are present. Notice B-type cell with pale matrix and granules with crystalline profiles and A-type cell with larger granules, eccentric cores and semilunar halos.   ×20,500

2) The total endocrine cell mass was greater in infants with hypoglycaemia than in the non-hypoglycaemic controls. However, one control case had a total endocrine cell mass comparable with that of any of the hypoglycaemic babies.

3) The most frequently found endocrine cells were of the beta type; however, they were not often found isolated or in 'pure' beta clusters but rather in association with at least one somatostatin and/or glucagon cell. The ratios among endocrine cells remained strikingly similar. Yet, the interpretation of these findings is complicated by methodologic limitations, in particular by the

exocrine and endocrine differentiation and also endocrine cells with variable granule populations.

A critical overview of the literature seems to indicate that the term, and the concept of, nesidioblastosis, including its more recent variants is generally taken to imply a pathologic condition. Moreover, some observers have felt that nesidioblastosis or its variants may indeed account for the syndrome of persistent hyperinsulinaemic hypoglycaemia in infants (4, 5, 6, 7, 10). The pathogenesis of the hyperinsulinaemia was ascribed either to an increase in beta cell mass

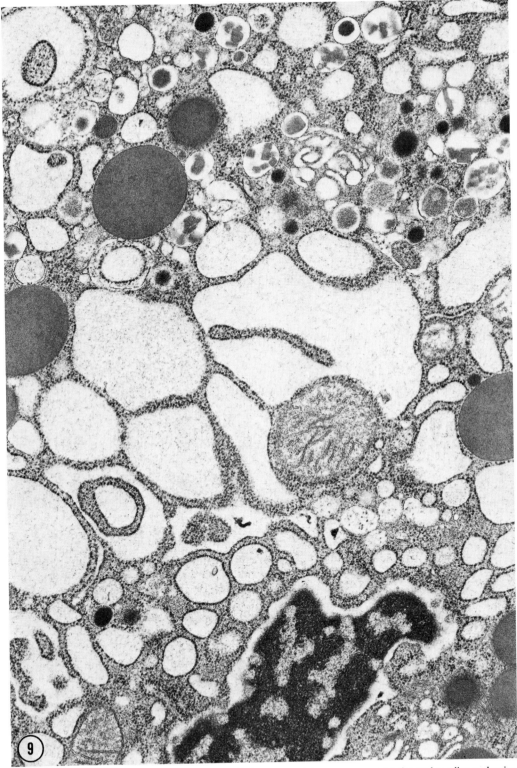

Fig. 9. Hypoglycaemic infant. 'Composite' cell with large conspicious zymogen granules and smaller endocrine granules, some of which display crystalline profiles.   ×29,800

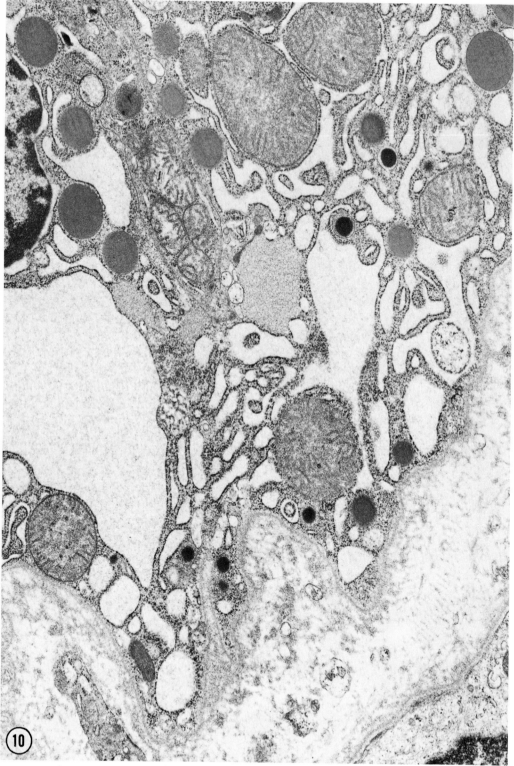

Fig. 10. Hypoglycaemic infant. 'Composite' cell with larger zymogen granules concentrating towards the luminal pole (upper portion of field); smaller, endocrine granules tend to concentrate towards basal pole of cell. ×25,700

(4, 5, 6, 7, 10) or to a relative decrease in soma-tostatin cells (16, 17, 18). However, Jaffe et al. have recently noted that some of the morphologic features included in the definition of nesidioblas-tosis may also be found in non-hypoglycaemic

In addition to the apparent increase in total pancreatic endocrine cell mass, other features included in the definitions of nesidioblastosis have been a) dispersion of endocrine cells amidst exocrine ducts and acini, and, b) small clusters

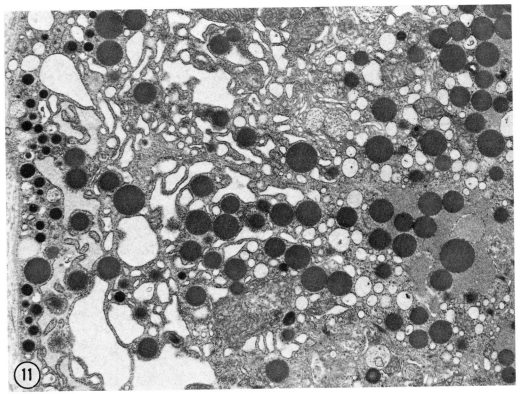

Fig. 11. Hypoglycaemic infant. 'composite' cell; at relatively low magnification. The orientation of the endocrine granules towards the basal pole of the cell is evident.   ×12,100

infants (11). Our findings seem to represent a variation of the aforementioned. We noted that hypoglycaemic infants did have a greater total endocrine pancreatic cell mass than most of the controls. However, that increase was either not as conspicuous as often reported, or, alterna-tively, the 'normal' total mass of pancreatic endocrine cells found in our non-hypoglycaemic controls appeared considerably higher than gen-erally assumed. Moreover, one of our non-hypog-lycaemic controls had a total pancreatic endocrine cell mass comparable to that found in several hypoglycaemic infants.

consisting exclusively or predominantly of beta cells. However, with regard to these features, again we feel that they cannot be viewed as unmistakably pathological for they may be readily found to a greater or lesser extent in a broad spectrum of controls that did not exhibit any apparent endocrine disturbance.

Those apparent discrepancies are not easily explicable. Several speculative notions may be advanced. One may suggest that our current immunohistochemical methods and/or the bat-teries of available antibodies applied to these studies do not reflect faithfully the complexities

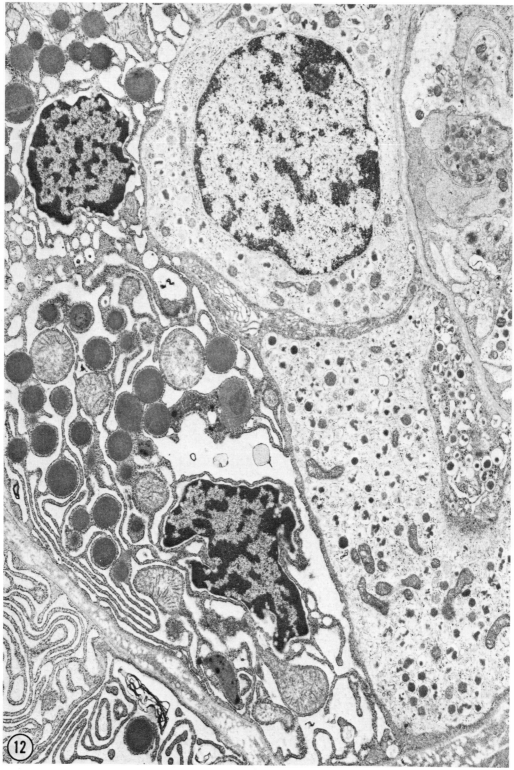

Fig. 12. Control (non-hypoglycaemic) infant. Note acinar structure with obvious exocrine cells intimately admixed with endocrine elements.   ×13,800

of the endocrine cell populations present in the pancreata of hypoglycaemic babies. It would seem that, in addition to the peptide hormones generally accepted as the 'normal' complement for the human pancreatic islet, i.e. insulin, glucagon, somatostatin and HPP, other related materials may also be demonstrated immunohistochemically such as VIP, gastrin and met-enkephalin. We remain uncertain as to the possible significance of these observations. The presence of immunoreactive gastrin is particularly puzzling since it was found in only two hypoglycaemic infants; moreover, the known heterogeneity of gastrin further complicates this matter. Although we have not confirmed the decrease of somatostatin cells in relation to insulin cells suggested as a possible factor in the pathogenesis of hyperinsulinism (16, 18, 19), we cannot, however, exclude the existence of subtle and incompletely understood abnormalities in insular cell secretion and paracrine regulation as possible mechanisms operative in hypoglycaemic infants (20, 21, 22).

Another factor that may help explain the lack of a notable difference between the endocrine pancreas of hypoglycaemic infants and those of our age-matched controls may be attributed to the very nature of the controls used. We have excluded from the control group, infants with endocrine or metabolic disturbances and those with conditions, or born to a mother with conditions, known to be associated with islet cell anomalies. The only possible exception is that of control case 2 considered to have been a 'near miss SIDS' (Sudden Infant Death Syndrome). The insular cell mass in this infant was rather low and therefore, we did not confirm the possible relationship between nesidioblastosis and SIDS (23). Yet, we must consider that the pancreata used as controls did not derive from healthy infants, and, therefore, a variety of poorly understood factors may have influenced the status of their pancreatic endocrine tissue without it being reflected in a clinical hormonal syndrome.

Considerations on the developmental anatomy of the endocrine panceas may shed some light as to the significance of nesidioblastosis; and, thus, as has recently been suggested, the question may be posed as to which cell is truly a nesidioblast

(11). The traditionally held embryological notion has been that the endocrine pancreas arises from exocrine ducts which in turn derive from the primitive gut, an endodermal organ. As the APUD cell system concept was being developed and a possible unifying hypothesis as to its derivation was considered, it was suggested that the pancreatic endocrine cells might be neural crest migrants to the intestine (24). However, several re-evaluations have concluded that the endocrine pancreatic cells though displaying APUD characteristics and members of the dispersed neuroendocrine system are most likely endodermal derivatives, and that they develop in close relationship with the exocrine components of that viscus (17, 25). In some invertebrates, insulin cells are in fact found in the mucosa of the alimentary canal where they co-exist with zymogen (exocrine pancreas) secreting cells (26). In rather primitive vertebrates such as lampreys and hagfish, insulin and somatostatin cells are present in the alimentary canal mucosa only in their larval forms, whereas in the adult forms, they migrate into closely apposed 'islets', though even in adult hagfish some insulin and somatostatin cells are present in the bile duct mucosa. However, in adult forms of both species, zymogen cells remain as part of the alimentary canal proper, and therefore, it has been stated that the endocrine pancreas develops as a separate organ from the gastrointestinal mucosa even before its exocrine counterpart (26). The finding in the pancreas of hypoglycaemic infants of composite or acinar-endocrine cells in various combinations made both by us and previous investigators (4, 11) would suggest the possible existence of a dynamic process whereby acinar or ductal cells may, under the influence of unknown stimuli, become endocrine. Moreover, it seems possible that the said process may be operative well beyond the neonatal period, and, the fact that some infants with hyperinsulinaemic hypoglycaemia remain persistently so even after total excision of the pancreas, suggests the possibility that endocrine cells in other locations (?GI mucosa) may alter their secretory pattern and 'turn' to the production of insulin. The 'instability' of endocrine cells in the pancreas throughout life, and the relatively high number of somatostatin cells in infants have been recently discussed (27).

We conclude that *nesidioblastosis*, as currently defined, is not the anatomic substratum of infantile hyperinsulinaemic hypoglycaemia; and, furthermore, that *nesidioblastosis*, as a constellation of morphologic features, may be either associated with a variety of non-endocrine disease processes or may even be part of the 'normal' spectrum of pancreatic development during the neonatal, and early infancy periods. Since no evident relationship seems to exist between nesidioblastosis and hyperinsulinaemia of infancy, the inadequacy of the term to encompass the functional component alluded to becomes apparent. Therefore, we propose the application of the term *nesidiodysplasia* which would include the apparently increased and possibly maldistributed and/or malregulated endocrine and composite cells associated with a clinically demonstrable malfunction (hyperinsulinaemic hypoglycaemia in these cases) although the precise relationship between the two elements of the definition remain to be clarified by future investigations.

## ACKNOWLEDGEMENTS

We gratefully acknowledge the assistance of Drs. D. Baldwin, Jr., R. Chance, J. Lechago and L. Levitsky for their invaluable cooperation and/or for the supply of materials. Special thanks are due to Ms. M. Baerwaldt, Miss T. A. Saucedo and Mrs. S. Velasco for technical and secretarial assistance.

This investigation was partly supported by the Otho S. A Sprague Memorial Fund.

## REFERENCES

1. Laidlaw, G. F. *Am. J. Pathol.* 1937, *14*, 125–139
2. Kloeppel, G., Altenaehr, E., Reichel, W., Willig, R. & Freytag, G. *Diabetologia* 1974, *10*, 245–252
3. Misugi, K., Misugi, N., Sotos, J. & Smith, B. *Arch. Pathol.* 1970, *89*, 208–220
4. Becker, K., Wendel, U., Pryzyrembel, H., Tsotsalas, M., Muentefering, H. & Bremer, H. J. *Eur. J. Ped.* 1978, *127*, 75–89
5. Grampa, G., Gargantini, L., Grigolato, P. G. & Chiumello, G. *Am. J. Dis. Child* 1974, *128*, 226–231
6. Yakovak, W. C., Baker, L., Hummeler, K. *J. Ped.* 1971, *79*, 226–231
7. Hirsch, H. J., Loo, S., Evans, N., Crigler, J. F., Filler, R. M. & Gabbay K. H. *New Engl. Med.* 1977, *296*, 1323–1326
8. Raptis, S., Escobar-Jimenez, F., Rosenthal, J., Ditschuneit, H. H. & Pfeiffer, E. J. *Clin. Endocrinol. Metab.* 1977, *44*, 1088–1093
9. Taniguchi, H., Utsumi, M., Hasegawa, M., Kobayashi, T., Watanabe, Y., Makimura, H., Sakoda, M. & Baba, S. *Diabetes* 1977, *26*, 700–702
10. Heitz, P. U., Kloeppel, G., Haecki, W. H., Polak, J. M. & Pearse, A. G. E. *Diabetes* 1977, *26*, 632–642
11. Jaffe, R., Hashida, Y. & Yunis, E. J. *Lab. Invest.* 1980, *42*, 356–365
12. Sternberger, L. A. *Immunochemistry*, Prentice-Hall, Englewood Cliffs, New Jersey, 1974
13. Nakane, P. K. *J. Histochem. Cytochem.* 1968, *16*, 557–560
14. Nakane, P. K. & Kawaoi, A. *J. Histochem. Cytochem.* 1974, *22*, 1084–1091
15. Nakane, P. K., *Methods in Enzymology* 1975, *37*, 133–134
16. Bishop, A. E., Polak, J. M., Garin-Chesa, P., Timson, C. M., Bryant, M. G. & Bloom, SR. *Diabetes* 1981, *30*, 122–126
17. Pictet, R. L., Rall, L. B., Phelps, P. & Rutter, W. J. *Science* 1976, *191*, 191–192
18. Soevik, O., Vidnes, J. & Faulkner, S. *Acta Pathol. Microbiol. Scand.*, (A) 1975, *83*, 155–156
19. Kloeppel, G., Altenaehr, E. & Henke, B. *Virchows Arch. (Path. Anat.)*, 1975, *366*, 223–226
20. Lawrence, T. S., Beers, W. H., & Gilula, N. B. *Nature* 1978, *272*, 501–506
21. Meda, P., Halban, P., Perrelt, A., Renold, A. E. & Orci, L. *Science* 1980, *209*, 1026–1028
22. Unger, R. H., Dobbs, R. E. & Orci, L. *Ann. Rev. Physiol.* 1978, *40*, 307–343
23. Polak, J. M., Aynsley-Green, A., Bloom, S. R. & Wigglesworth, J. S. *Scand. J. Gastroenterol.* 1978, *13*, (Suppl, 149) 143 (Abst.)
24. Pearse, A. G. E. & Polak, J. M. *Gut* 1971, *12*, 783–788
25. Le Douarin, N. M. in *Gut Hormones*, Ed. Bloom, S. R. Churchill Livingston, Edinburgh, 1978, 49–56
26. Falkmer, S., Oestberg, Y. & Van Noorden, S. in *Gut Hormones*, ed. Bloom, S. R., Churchill Livingston, Edinburgh, 1978, 57–63
27. Orci, L., Stefan, Y., Malaisse-Lagae, F. & Perrelet, A. *Lancet*, 1979, *1*, 615–616

# ADDENDUM

# Nesidiodysplasia and Nesidioblastosis of Infancy
## *An Addendum*

V. E. GOULD, V. A. MEMOLI, L. E. DARDI & N. S. GOULD

Department of Pathology, Rush Medical College
& Rush-Presbyterian-St. Luke's Medical Center, Chicago, IL 60612, USA

*Addendum* March 1982

Further studies carried out since the original text was prepared as well as review of other investigations suggest the need for the reiteration, restructuring and possible amplification of some of the views and concepts therein expressed.

We have studied the pancreata of two additional infants aged 4 and seven months with hyperinsulinaemic hypoglycaemia. The methodology was identical to the one used in the early text and the results obtained were basically comparable. Again, when pancreata of age matched controls were studied, small clusters of endocrine cells were identified intimately intermingled with exocrine pancreas components; these controls did not have hyperinsulinaemic hypoglycaemia. One of the controls had a total endocrine cell mass which was clearly lower than that of the hypoglycaemic infants but that was not the case with the remaining control. These observations suggest again that while a massive increase in total endocrine cell mass may indeed be related to the hyperinsulinaemic hypoglycaemia, a 'moderate increase' in endocrine cells and their dissemination and diffuse admixture with exocrine ducts and acini—i.e. nesidioblastosis—should not necessarily be viewed as the anatomic substratum of hyperinsulinaemic hypoglycaemia and might indeed reflect physiologic phenomena. A similar view to the effect that 'some degree of nesidioblastosis is thus physiologic in infants' has also been recently expressed by Barrett Damhs et al. (1). Accordingly, the proposed term *nesidiodysplasia* would more accurately reflect those non-neoplastic structural and functional anomalies of the pancreas whenever manifested by an endocrine syndrome.

We have extended our studies to encompass adult pancreata. In several pancreata obtained at autopsy from cases without primary or secondary pancreatic diseases and with no clinical evidence of endocrine abnormalities, immunohistochemical studies showed the focal presence of small groups of endocrine cells intermingled with acinar elements as well as endocrine cells budding of ducts of various sizes. Similar—and apparently more frequent—findings were made when studying surgical specimens showing chronic pancreatitis in the vicinity of pancreatic or ampullar carcinomas. These observations would indicate that the adult pancreas is also capable of forming abundant insular cells from exocrine ducts and acini, and that this capability may be expressed in relation to a spectrum of unknown stimuli including physiologic ones. It is noteworthy that similar morphologic observations were made over half a century ago (2).

With regard to the composite exocrine-endocrine cells described in two of our hyperinsulinaemic hypoglycaemic infants, we might add that we have again observed them by electron microscopy in a few pancreata of infants and adults. They were particularly conspicuous in a case of pancreatic carcinoma thus suggesting that multidirectional differentiation may not be an uncommon phenomenon in epithelial neoplasms (3). Some of those intermediate or 'amphicrine' cells are remarkably similar to those described and schematically drawn by Feyrter in 1938 (4).

## REFERENCES

1. Barrett Damhs B, Landing BJ, Blaskovics M, Roe, TF. Hum Pathol 1980, 11, 641–649
2. Otani S. Am J Pathol 1927, 3, 123–134
3. Gould VE, Memoli VA, Dardi LE. J Submicrosc Cytol 1981, 13, 97–115
4. Feyrter F. Ueber diffuse endokrine epitheliale Organe. Johann Ambrosius Barth (Verlag), Leipzig, 1938, 53–57

# H$_2$ Receptor Antagonists: Ultrastructure of Canine Parietal Cells after Long Term Treatment with Ranitidine

G. AINGE & D. POYNTER
Pathology Division, Glaxo Group Research, Ware, Herts, UK

The ultrastructure of the parietal cell was studied in dogs given massive doses of a new H$_2$ blocker, ranitidine, for up to one year. No toxic changes were detected. The pharmacological activity of the drug was reflected in the structure of the parietal cell where inhibition led to stimulated cells remaining in the resting state. Such cells quickly regained secretory activity once inhibition ceased.

Key-words: dogs; electron microscopy; H$_2$ receptor antagonists; hydrochloric acid; parietal cell; ranitidine; stomach

D. Poynter Ph.D., F.R.C.Path., Pathology Division, Glaxo Group Research Ware, Herts, UK

Ranitidine is a potent new selective H$_2$ receptor antagonist discovered in the laboratories of Glaxo Group Research. It inhibits histamine-induced gastric acid secretion (2) and also secretion induced by 2 deoxy-D-glucose and food in dogs (4). Following the first demonstration in man of its effect on gastric acid secretion by Woodings, Dixon, Harrison, Carey and Richards (19) many workers have attested to its efficacy and found that it is a powerful therapeutic agent for the treatment of peptic ulceration in man (11).

$$(CH_3)_2NCH_2 \quad O \quad CH_2SCH_2CH_2NHCNHCH_3$$
$$\overset{\|}{CHNO_2}$$

Ranitidine

Before any new medicine is made available it is necessary to minimise any potential risk and part of this exercise involves a deliberate attempt to assess the toxic nature of the compound. During the course of our studies we have treated dogs with ranitidine for long periods of time at very high doses. These animals were subjected to a range of clinical, biochemical and haematological examinations and eventually a complete post mortem was carried out on each one, followed by the histopathological examination of 35 representative tissues.

In our studies on ranitidine special attention was given to the stomach and in particular to the parietal cell since it is the eventual target cell. Thus it is necessary to show that potent and prolonged H$_2$ blockade will not induce any significant pathological changes in these cells.

Although we are not aware of any reports on parietal cell ultrastructure after long term treatment with ranitidine there are many published accounts of its normal ultrastructure throughout the secretory cycle (1, 5, 7, 10, 15, 16).

When parietal cells are resting they show a large number of cytoplasmic tubulovesicles and a small canalicular surface area. When stimulated to secrete acid, the number of tubulovesicles is reduced and the canalicular surface area is increased. It is generally accepted that the parietal cell proceeds through three distinct stages during its secretory cycle (6, 9). These stages are shown in Fig. 1.

In the normal stomach it might be expected that parietal cells are present in all three stages of the cycle. Clearly, however, physiological influences affect the degree to which any stage predominates in the gastric gland and some parietal cells show transitional stages.

In order to study the normal sequence of par-

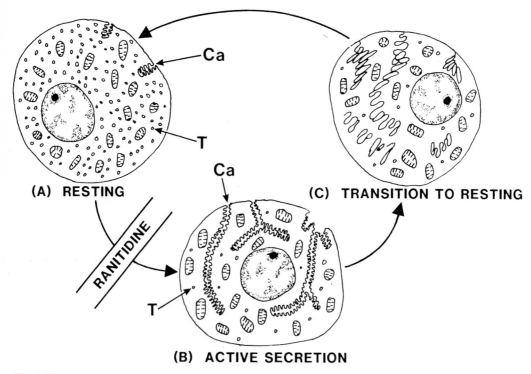

**(A) RESTING**

**Ca**

**RANITIDINE**

**T**

**Ca**

**(B) ACTIVE SECRETION**

**(C) TRANSITION TO RESTING**

Fig. 1. The secretory cycle of the parietal cell.
(A) The resting parietal cell is characterised by numerous cytoplasmic tubulovesicles (T) and a few secretory canaliculi (Ca) with microvilli. During active secretion (B) the tubulovesicles (T) are depleted at the expense of a great increase in the size of the secretory canaliculi (Ca). After acid secretion has ceased (C) the canaliculi collapse, lose their microvilli and are thought to reform the numerous tubulovesicles of the resting cell.

ietal cell ultrastructure we studied dogs with both full and empty stomachs. Having established the normal sequence we studied dogs both under the influence of the inhibiting effect of ranitidine and after inhibition had ceased.

Since particular attention was being given to the parietal cell it was thought necessary to define and, as far as possible quantify certain criteria which might conceivably indicate ranitidine-induced effects. Thus we decided to assess the secretory apparatus, to examine the extent of apoptosis, to examine and count the numbers of lysosomes and multivesicular bodies and to assess the structure and number of mitochondria.

## MATERIALS AND METHODS

### Preparation of specimens

Forty-nine dogs were studied and the details

of their treatment are given in Table I. Dogs received oral daily doses of ranitidine of 25mg, 100mg or 225mg/kg over 1 month, 6 months or 1 year. The dose level of those dogs receiving 225mg/kg/day for 1 year was raised to 450mg/kg/day for the last 5 weeks of treatment. For each period of treatment additional dogs were dosed with a placebo to serve as controls. In all, 31 dogs received ranitidine and 18 received a placebo. At sacrifice a small piece of stomach corpus mucosa from the greater curvature was removed from each animal and fixed in phosphate-buffered 2% glutaraldehyde. The remainder of the stomach was fixed in 10% buffered formaldehyde.

Most dogs received their last dose of ranitidine 18–24 hours before sacrifice. However, some dogs received their last dose of ranitidine 4 hours before sacrifice and in the case of those animals

Table I. Structure of parietal cell secretory apparatus in dogs after placebo or ranitidine treatment

**Placebo-treated dogs**

| Stomach condition | Number of dogs | Structure of canaliculi | Extent of canalicular membrane | Number of tubulovesicles |
|---|---|---|---|---|
| Empty | 5 | closed | + | +++ |
| | 1 | slightly patent | + | +++ |
| | 1 | slightly patent | ++ | +++ |
| | 1 | patent | ++ | +++ |
| | 1 | patent dilated | ++ | +++ |
| | | closed | +++ | + |
| Full | 2 | closed | +++ | + |
| | 1 | collapsed | +++ | + |
| | 1 | collapsed | +++ | 0 |
| | 1 | collapsed or closed | +++ | ++ |
| | 1 | closed or slightly patent | ++ | ++ |
| | 1 | closed or collapsed | ++ | +++ |

**Ranitidine-treated dogs**

| Stomach condition | Dose and duration of ranitidine treatment | Time (before sacrifice) of last dose | Number of dogs | Structure of canaliculi | Extent of canalicular membrane | Number of tubulovesicles |
|---|---|---|---|---|---|---|
| Empty | 100 mg/kg/day 1 month | 18–24 hrs | 2 | closed | + | +++ |
| | 25 mg/kg/day 6 months | 18–24 hrs | 6 | closed | + | +++ |
| | 100 mg/kg/day 6 months | 18–24 hrs | 3 | slightly patent | + | +++ |
| | | | 1 | patent | ++ | +++ |
| | | | 1 | patent | ++ | ++ |
| | | | 1 | closed | + | +++ |
| | 25 mg/kg/day 1 year | 24 hrs | 2 | slightly patent | + | +++ |
| | | 4 hrs | 1 | closed | + | +++ |
| | | | 1 | patent | + | +++ |
| | 225–450 mg/kg/day 1 year | 5–8 days | 2 | slightly patent | + | +++ |
| | | | 1 | slightly patent | ++ | +++ |
| Full | 100 mg/kg/day 1 month | 18–24 hrs | 1 | closed or collapsed | +++ | + |
| | | | 1 | collapsed | +++ | + |
| | 25 mg/kg/day 1 year | 24 hrs | 2 | collapsed | +++ | + |
| | | 4 hrs | 1 | patent | ++ | +++ |
| | | | 1 | closed or patent | + | + |
| | 225–450 mg/kg/day 1 year | 5–8 days | 2 | closed or collapsed / collapsed | +++ / +++ | ++ / ++ |
| | | | 1 | collapsed | +++ | + |
| | | | 1 | closed or collapsed | +++ | ++ |

treated for 1 year at 225–450mg/kg/day, a period of 5–8 days elapsed between the last dose and sacrifice. This treatment enabled animals to be studied both during $H_2$ receptor blockade and after the inhibition had ceased.

The dogs were either starved overnight before sacrifice or after an overnight fast they were allowed access to their normal daily quantity of food one hour before sacrifice. This enabled specimens of corpus mucosa to be obtained from animals with either an empty or a full stomach.

From formaldehyde-fixed stomach, haematoxylin and eosin stained sections were prepared from corpus and antral regions and examined by light microscopy.

All glutaraldehyde-fixed specimens were post-fixed in phosphate-buffered 1% osmium tetroxide, processed, and embedded in Spurr's resin. From each specimen, sections approximately 50 nm thick were cut from the middle area of the gastric glands. Each section had a surface area of approximately 0.5 mm × 0.5 mm. After staining with uranyl acetate and lead citrate, all parietal cells in the sections were examined with an AEI 801 electron microscope. All studies were made on coded specimens by one electron microscopist.

### Study of Secretory Apparatus

Subjective assessments of the extent of canalicular membranes and number of tubulovesicles were made by scoring on a scale from 1 to 3. The appearance of the canalicular membranes was also recorded.

### Study of Apoptosis (single cell shrinkage necrosis)

Ten randomly chosen parietal cells from specimens of dogs treated for 1 year were photographed and electron micrographs were prepared at a magnification of × 8000. Using these electron micrographs the number of parietal cells exhibiting apoptosis was counted. Such cells were almost invariably adjacent to cells of normal appearance. A typical example is shown in Fig. 2.

### Study of Lysosomes and Multivesicular Bodies

Using electron micrographs (× 8000 magnification) of the 10 randomly chosen parietal cells, (from dogs treated for 1 year) the number of lysosomes and multivesicular bodies present in cells was counted.

### Study of Mitochondria

A subjective assessment of the structure of mitochondria was made. In addition a stereological analysis of mitochondria was made on specimens from dogs treated for 1 year. The first ten parietal cells encountered in the sections which showed nuclei and did not exhibit features of apoptosis were photographed. Photomicrographs were prepared of these cells at a standard magnification of × 6250. Using a lattice with intersections spaced at a distance of 1 cm, a count was made of intersections covering mitochondria and also of intersections covering the complete cell, according to the methods of Weibel (18). Volume density (Vv) of mitochondria was calculated from the formula:

$$Vv = \frac{Pi}{PT}$$

Where Pi = number of intersections covering mitochondria, PT = total intersections covering the cell.

The error inherent in the method was calculated after repeating the counts on 30 randomly chosen photomicrographs from the study.

## RESULTS

### Light Microscopy

No changes were seen in the corpus and antral regions of stomach attributable to ranitidine treatment.

### Secretory apparatus

The ultrastructural appearance of the secretory apparatus of parietal cells is given in Table I. No differences in the secretory apparatus attributable to duration of placebo treatment, or to time of last dose of placebo were noted. The results for placebo-treated dogs are therefore presented in Table I without regard to these variables.

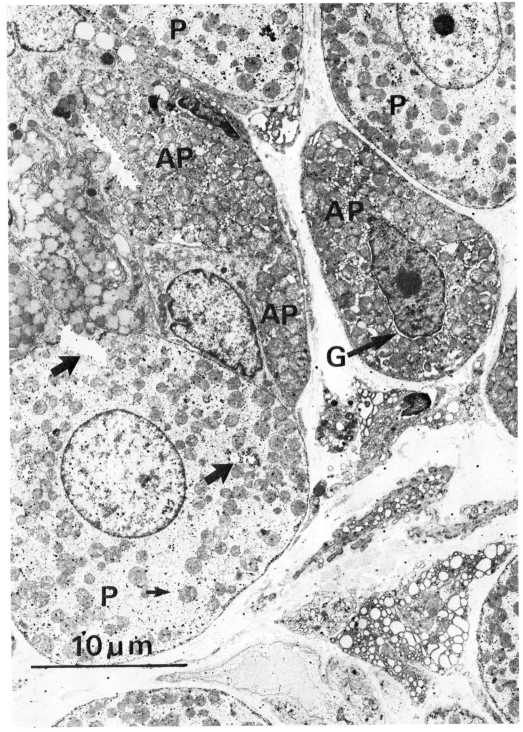

Fig. 2. Parietal cells from empty stomach placebo-treated dog. Several normal parietal cells (P) are adjacent to three cells exhibiting apoptosis (AP). Normal parietal cells are characterised by small canaliculi (➤) and numerous tubulovesicles (→). Parietal cells showing apoptosis are characterised by enlarged mitochondria and increased electron density of cytoplasmic membranes. A gap is seen between the nucleus and cytoplasm of apoptotic cells (G).

(a) empty stomach, small closed canaliculi and numerous tubulovesicles.

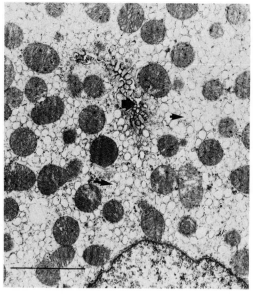

(b) empty stomach, small patent canaliculi and numerous tubulovesicles.

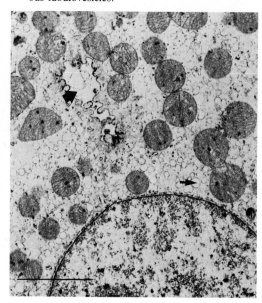

(c) full stomach, large closed canaliculi and a few tubulovesicles.

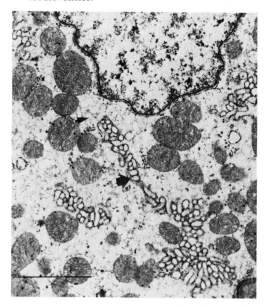

(d) full stomach, collapsed canaliculi.

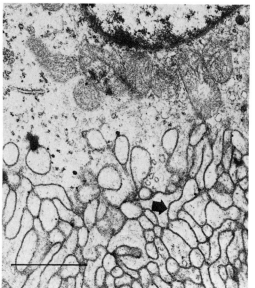

Fig. 3. Parietal cells from placebo treated dogs. Canaliculi (➤,), tubulovesicles (→). Bar represents 5 μ.

## Placebo-treated dogs with empty stomachs

Placebo-treated dogs with empty stomachs showed parietal cells with closed canaliculi or canaliculi exhibiting varying degrees of patency (Figs. 3a and b). Microvilli lined the canalicular membranes and were most abundant in closed canaliculi whilst in patent canaliculi they were generally fewer in number and were shorter in length. Most commonly the canaliculi in these control dogs were small, closed and few in number (Fig. 3a). Tubulovesicles were almost invariably abundant in the cytoplasm.

## Placebo-treated dogs with full stomachs

In placebo-treated dogs with full stomachs the extent of the canalicular membrane was greatly increased (Figs. 3c and d).

Individual canaliculi appeared much larger than in dogs with empty stomachs and were almost invariably closed with abundant microvilli or appeared tightly closed with no distinct microvilli (described as collapsed in Table 1). Figs. 3c and d show typical results. In Fig. 3c the canaliculi are tightly closed with interdigitating microvilli. In Fig. 3d the canaliculi are again tightly closed but no microvilli are present. This latter appearance probably results from the collapse of canaliculi so that plasma membranes of the canaliculi lie adjacent to each other and occlude the lumen. In Fig. 3d each apparent canalicular membrane is in reality composed of two closely apposed plasma membranes.

Only in one dog were slightly patent canaliculi seen. In these full stomach dogs generally few tubulovesicles were seen and in the case of one dog none were observed.

There was, therefore, a clear trend towards a small canalicular membrane and abundant tubulovesicles in empty stomach placebo-treated dogs and a trend towards large canalicular membrane and few tubulovesicles in full stomach dogs. However, the results were not absolute in this respect and one empty stomach dog was seen with parietal cells showing a large canalicular area and few tubulovesicles. In addition one of the full stomach dogs showed abundant tubulovesicles.

## Ranitidine-treated dogs with empty stomachs

In the empty stomach dogs treated with ranitidine the appearance of parietal cell canaliculi and tubulovesicles was similar to placebo-treated empty stomach dogs irrespective of the time of the last dose of ranitidine (Figs. 4a and b). The characteristic small canaliculi lined with microvilli were observed and the cytoplasm contained abundant tubulovesicles.

## Ranitidine-treated dogs with full stomachs

In all full stomach ranitidine-treated dogs receiving their last dose 18 hours or more before sacrifice extensive canalicular membranes were seen in parietal cells. The canaliculi were either closed with abundant microvilli (Fig. 4c) or closed with no microvilli (collapsed). There were few tubulovesicles in the cytoplasm of such cells. The appearance of the cells was therefore similar to that seen in placebo-treated full stomach dogs.

Only in the two dogs with full stomachs which received their last dose of ranitidine four hours before sacrifice was any effect of ranitidine on parietal cell ultrastructure seen. These cells were characterised by a small amount of canalicular membrane, individual canaliculi being small, few in number and either closed (Fig. 4d) or patent. In the parietal cells of one of these dogs abundant tubulovesicles were seen whereas in cells from the other dog few tubulovesicles were observed.

*Apoptosis*

The light microscopy examination of the stomachs revealed no increase in apoptosis. The results of the electron microscopical examination of cells for apoptosis are given in Table II.

A varying number of parietal cells from the dogs showed apoptosis. Sometimes none were seen in sections from a particular dog. On other occasions all 10 cells photographed showed apoptosis as a condensation of electron-dense chromatin in the nucleus particularly adjacent to the nuclear membrane. At the same time a distinct gap was present between the nuclear membrane and the surrounding cytoplasm (Fig. 2). Increased electron density of cytoplasmic components and enlarged mitochondria were often noted in such cells.

(a) 18–24 hrs after last dose, empty stomach, small closed canaliculi and numerous tubulovesicles.

(b) 4 hrs after last dose, empty stomach, small patent canaliculi and numerous tubulovesicles.

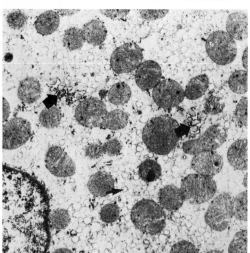
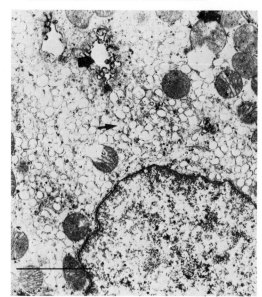

(c) 18–24 hrs after last dose, full stomach, large closed canaliculi and numerous tubulovesicles.

(d) 4 hrs after last dose, full stomach, small closed canaliculi and numerous tubulovesicles.

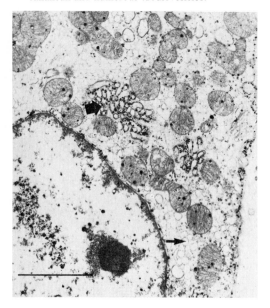
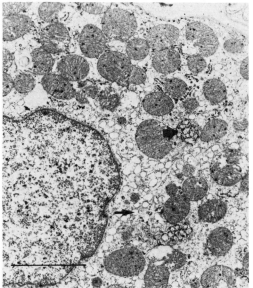

Fig. 4. Parietal cells from ranitidine treated dogs. Canaliculi (➤), tubulovesicles (→). Bar represents 5 μ.

Table II. Results of examination of parietal cells for apoptosis and presence of multivesicular bodies and lysosomes

| Treatment | No. of dogs examined (10 cells from each dog) | No. of cells showing apoptosis | | No. of multivesicular bodies in ten cell sections | | No. of lysosomes in ten cell sections | |
|---|---|---|---|---|---|---|---|
| | | Median | Range | Median | Range | Median | Range |
| Placebo for 1 year | 8 | 1.5 | 0–8 | 13.5 | 3–34 | 40 | 13–52 |
| 25 mg/kg/day for 1 year | 8 | 1 | 0–6 | 9.5 | 6–26 | 33 | 10–46 |
| 225 mg/kg/day for 1 year | 7 | 3 | 1–10 | 10 | 5–29 | 37 | 14–60 |

The number of cells exhibiting apoptosis in the stomach specimens was not related to the treatment of the animals and no statistical analysis was considered necessary.

*Lysosomes and multivesicular bodies*

The results of the examination of cells for presence of lysosomes and multivesicular bodies are given in Table II.

The number of lysosomal structures present in cell sections varied between 0 and 13 and the number of multivesicular bodies/cell section varied between 0 and 7. There is no evidence that the numbers of lysosomes and multivesicular bodies were related to treatment and therefore no statistical analysis was performed.

*Mitochondria*

The subjective assessment of the structure of mitochondria revealed no alterations which were related to ranitidine treatment. The results of the stereological analysis of mitochondrial volume density are given in Table II. Since the volume densities were normally distributed the data was analysed using analysis of variance. Neither of the two ranitidine-treated groups showed significant ($P<0.05$) differences in mitochondrial volume density when compared to the control animals (Dunnett's test). When the data were analysed separately for empty and full stomach, again no significant differences were revealed. Furthermore the time of last dosing did not significantly affect the mitochondrial volume density.

DISCUSSION

It is clear that ranitidine has no adverse effect on dog parietal cell structure even after doses as high as 225–450mg/kg/day for as long as one year.

When dogs which had been treated for one year at 25 mg/kg/day were dosed 3 hours before a meal and killed one hour after it the only changes attributable to ranitidine were that the parietal cell, instead of showing secretory changes appeared like a resting cell even when being stimulated by a full stomach. Work carried out on these and other dogs by Daly and Carey (3)

Table III. Mean volume density of mitochondria (% of cell volume) in 10 parietal cells after ranitidine treatment of dogs for 1 year

| Stomach condition | Control | | 25 mg/kg Ranitidine | | 225 mg/kg Ranitidine | | Error standard deviation* |
|---|---|---|---|---|---|---|---|
| | Dog No. | Volume density | Dog No. | Volume density | Dog No. | Volume density | |
| Empty Stomach | 231 | 28.8 | 239 | 33.7 | 256 | 29.8 | |
| | 232 | 33.6 | 240 | 36.7 | 259 | 29.2 | |
| | 235 | 32.9 | 243 | 37.1 | 260 | 26.7 | |
| | 236 | 36.3 | 244 | 34.1 | | | |
| Mean | | 32.9 | | 35.4 | | 28.5 | 2.3 |
| Full Stomach | 233 | 39.3 | 241 | 28.6 | 257 | 33.7 | |
| | 234 | 35.2 | 242 | 33.4 | 258 | 32.4 | |
| | 237 | 31.2 | 245 | 30.4 | 261 | 30.9 | |
| | 238 | 28.8 | 246 | 36.9 | 262 | 38.5 | |
| Mean | | 33.6 | | 32.3 | | 33.9 | 3.9 |
| Overall Mean | | 33.3 | | 33.9 | | 31.6 | |

* The error standard deviation is the variation between dogs which cannot be attributed to treatment or stomach condition. It includes a component due to variation in counting (calculated from repeat counts on 30 photomicrographs) as well as a component due to differences among animals.

showed that after 48 weeks dosing at 25mg/kg/day at least 90% inhibition of acid secretion was achieved 4 hours after the last dose. The resting parietal cells observed therefore reflect the pharmacological inhibition brought about by $H_2$ receptor blockade in these animals. Ranitidine then blocks the parietal cell in such a way that it cannot change from the resting stage to the active secreting stage (Fig. 1). After treatment for one year the parietal cell can still be inhibited but 24 hours after a last dose, in response to food the cell shows an ultrastructure characteristic of active acid secretion. (Figure 4c).

Placebo-treated dogs with empty stomachs show considerable variations in the ultrastructure of their parietal cells. Canaliculi may be closed or show varying degrees of patency. Nevertheless, the parietal cell secretory apparatus in empty stomach dogs shows a trend towards a small canalicular membrane area and a large number of cytoplasmic tubulovesicles.

In full stomach placebo-treated dogs variation again is seen. However, a clear trend is apparent

in the secretory apparatus; cells most commonly have a large canalicular surface area and few tubulovesicles.

These findings for empty and full stomach dogs are similar to those of other workers' (1, 5, 6, 7, 9, 10, 15, 16) on resting cells and cells stimulated to secrete acid by various agents. The variability in parietal cell ultrastructure was elegantly demonstrated by Zalewsky and Moody (21). In a critical stereological study of dog parietal cells they showed that 5.7% of cells from resting gastric mucosa appeared in the secretory phase and 13.6% of cells retained their resting configuration after stimulation by histamine.

A common finding in our full stomach dogs was the presence of extensive canalicular membrane devoid of microvilli which appeared to be composed of canaliculi which had collapsed. Such membranes were seen in 4 out of the 8 placebo-treated dogs with full stomachs and in 8 out of the 10 ranitidine-treated dogs with full stomachs. Previous workers (6, 9) have shown that such membranes are characteristic of cells returning from active secretion to the resting phase (Fig. 1c).

Stables and Daly (17) using continuous intra-gastric titration presented data on acid secretion of our beagle dogs after a test meal. Acid secretion reached a maximum 30 minutes after ingestion of the test meal and remained elevated for one hour after that. Our finding of collapsed canaliculi in many dogs one hour after ingestion of a meal suggests that parietal cells only secrete acid for a limited period and then return to the resting stage. If this is the case then other parietal cells would need to take over the role of secretion to maintain the maximum acid output measured by Stables and Daly (17).

Using another $H_2$ receptor antagonist, cimetidine, Pillay, Somers, Booyens, Moshal and Bryer (14) studied two patients referred for upper gastrointestinal endoscopy. They noted a dramatic appearance of autophagic vacuoles in parietal cells after one hour of treatment (14) although this was reduced in extent after one year (13). However Zalewsky and Moody (21) in their careful study of dogs saw no such effect of cimetidine one hour after an infusion of the antagonist. Furthermore, Nielsen, Madsen and Christiansen (12) in a recent study of eleven duodenal ulcer patients saw no such changes after 8 weeks of cimetidine treatment although the therapy did appear to reduce the canalicular surface density of parietal cells.

In view of the variability of parietal cell ultrastructure it is possible that Pillay et al (13, 14.) were studying cells unrepresentative of the population of parietal cells. Variation may be more marked and include distinctly abnormal cells in patients referred for endoscopy.

Studies on the action of UK-9040 a gastric secretory inhibitor based on a modification of the $H_1$ blocker triprolidine were published in 1977 by Hamer, Price and Baron (8). They examined, by electron microscopy, gastric biopsies from treated dogs before and after stimulation and found that 70% of the parietal cells remained in the resting stage.

The scheme of events in apoptosis was well described by Wyllie (20). The frequency of apoptosis must be such as to balance the rate of cell production. So, should ranitidine produce an increase in individual cell necrosis or lead to a population of secretory cells whose life cycle is prolonged then this would be reflected in the incidence of apoptosis seen. In the former case there is no doubt that such changes may be detected by light microscopy. Some years ago we discovered in our pharmacological laboratories a compound which led to a considerable decrease in gastric acid secretion. The treatment of dogs with this compound at a level of 30 mg/kg/day for 4 weeks produced a definite increase in apoptosis. It was obvious in histological sections. No such changes were seen with ranitidine.

The studies described here have shown that the long term treatment of dogs with very high doses of ranitidine has not induced pathological changes in the parietal cell. The inhibition of secretion is reflected in parietal cells predominantly having the appearance of cells in the resting condition. Once inhibition has ceased the cells are again capable of a secretory response.

## ACKNOWLEDGEMENTS

We would like to thank Mr J Blacker for technical assistance and Mrs. D Newton and Miss G Leccacorvi for secretarial assistance.

## REFERENCES

1. Adkins, R. B., Ende, N. & Gobbel, W. G. *Surgery* 1967, *62*, 1059–1069
2. Bradshaw, J., Brittain, R. T., Clitherow, J. W., Daly, M. J., Jack, D., Price, B. J & Stables, R. *Br. J. Pharmac.* 1979, *66*, 464
3. Daly, M. J. & Carey, P. Personal communication
4. Daly, M. J., Humphray, J. M. & Stables, R. *Gut* 1979, *20*, A914
5. Forte, T. M., Machen, T. E. & Forte, J. G. *Gastroenterology*, 1975, *69*, 1208–1222
6. Forte, T. M., Machen, T. E. & Forte, J. G. *Gastroenterology* 1977, *73*, 941–955
7. Frexinos, J., Carballido, M., Louis, A & Ribet, A. *Dig. Diseases*, 1971, *16*, 1065–1074
8. Hamer, D. B., Price, A. B. & Baron, J. H. *Gut* 1977, *18*, 91–98
9. Helander, H. F. & Hirschowitz, B. I. *Gastroenterology* 1972, *63*, 951–961
10. Helander, H. F. & Hirschowitz, B. I. *Gastroenterology* 1974, *67*, 447–452
11. Misiewicz, J. J. & Sewing, K. F. *Scand. J. Gastroenterol. Suppl.* 1981, in press

12. Nielsen, H. O., Madsen, P. E. R. & Christiansen, L. A. *Scand. J. Gastroenterol.* 1980, *15*, 793–797

13. Pillay, C. V., Moshal, M. G. & Booyens, J. *S. Afr. med. J.* 1979, *55*, 992–993

14. Pillay, C. V., Somers, S., Booyens, J., Moshal, M. G. & Bryer, J. V. *S. Afr. med. J.* 1977, *51*, 915–919

15. Rosa, F. *Gastroenterology* 1963, *45*, 354–363

16. Sedar, A. W. & Friedman, M. H. F. *J. biophys. biochem. Cytol.* 1961, *11*, 349–363

17. Stables, R. & Daly, M. J. *Agents and Actions* 1980, *10*, 191–192

18. Weibel, E. R. *Stereological Methods Vol. 1* Academic Press. London and New York 1979.

19. Woodings, E. P., Dixon, G. T., Harrison, C., Carey, P. & Richards, D. A. *Gut* 1980, *21*, 187–191

20. Wyllie, A. H. *J. clin. Path.* 1974, *27*, Suppl. 7. 35–42

21. Zalewsky, C. A. & Moody, F. G. *Gastroenterology* 1977, *73*, 66–74

# Long Term Effects of H$_2$-Receptor Antagonists (Cimetidine and Ranitidine) on the Human Gastric and Duodenal Mucosa

A. RIBET, D. BALAS, M. J. BASTIE, F. SENEGAS-BALAS,
J. ESCOURROU, G. BOMMELAER & L. PRADAYROL
Inserm U 151, C.H.U. Rangueil, 31054 Toulouse Cedex, France;
Service de Gastro-Enterologie—C.H.U. Rangueil 31054 Toulouse Cedex, France;
Service d'Histologie—C.H.U. Limoges, 87032 Limoges Cedex, France

Cytological effects of two H$_2$-receptor antagonists on the gastric and duodenal mucosa were studied during therapy of active duodenal ulcer (D.U.) in man. After endoscopic diagnosis (day 0), subjects were treated with cimetidine or ranitidine and re-examined on day 30. Only subjects with healed D.U. on day 30 were retained in this study. Gastric, pyloric and duodenal endoscopic biopsies were taken and treated for further morphometrical analysis both by light and electron microscopy. The use of the immunoperoxidase technique allowed evaluation of G and D cell populations. Kinetic parameters in proliferative zones were measured after *in vitro* incubation of biopsies with $^3$H-thymidine.

No differences could be seen between the two H$_2$-receptor antagonists. Increase of tubulovesicles and decrease of canaliculi in parietal cells are closely related to the inhibitory effect of these drugs on acid secretion. However secretory capacities of parietal cells are preserved since the whole membrane (tubulovesicle + canaliculi surface) remained constant. The collapsed aspect of the tubulovesicles on day 30 and the presence of connections between the tubulovesicle membrane, with both vesicle and canaliculi membrane, could support the theory of osmotic membrane expansion during parietal cell acid secretion.

H$_2$-receptor antagonists have been shown to be trophic in duodenal mucosa: both villi and microvilli area are increased. Confirming these findings, the proliferative compartment in the intestinal crypts was shown to be enlarged. No variation of G cell number could be seen in the antral mucosa; clear intracytoplasmic granules were increased in D.U. on day 0 but were not further modified on day 30. Somatostatin cells in the antral mucosa were increased after H$_2$-receptor antagonists. Antral labelling index decreased. These last findings associated with the lack of G cell variations, suggest the presence of a possible paracrine modulation in the gastric and duodenal mucosa.

*Key-words:* Duodenal mucosa; H$_2$ receptor antagonist; human, gastric mucosa; pyloric mucosa; time factor

*A. Ribet, Groupe de Recherche de Biologie et Pathologie Digestive, Inserm U 151, CHU Rangueil, 31054 Toulouse Cedex, France*

Histamine H$_2$-receptor antagonists are potent inhibitors of gastric acid secretion. Related to the reduction in acid secretion, (or by another unknown mechanism) oral cimetidine improved the success rate of duodenal ulcer (D.U.) healing. However, parietal cell sensitivity is increased in patients with D.U. (35, 54, 60) and no change in secretory parameters has been reported after cessation of cimetidine treatment (1, 2, 7, 8, 66, 67). On the other hand, cimetidine produced in the dog a complete inhibition of histamine stimulated acid secretion and a complete restoration of the resting ultrastructural state of parietal cells (74) but H$_2$-receptor antagonists induced hypertrophy of parietal cells (72) in rats after sustained administration.

A new $H_2$-receptor antagonist, ranitidine, was more potent than cimetidine in reducing gastric acid secretion (10, 21). Ranitidine does not contain the imidazole nucleus of histamine which was thought to be essential since it was also present in the $H_2$-receptor antagonists metiamide and cimetidine.

In this study the preliminary results obtained in an on-going study undertaken to provide more information about long term D.U. therapy in man with $H_2$-receptor antagonists are presented.

As far as the cytological approach is concerned, four areas of inquiry are worthy of investigation:

—Is the secretory sensitivity of parietal cells in D.U. maintained after therapy which may explain relapses?

—Do $H_2$-receptor antagonists mainly act on parietal cells?

—Are there cytological differences seen between the effects of ranitidine and cimetidine?

—Are cytological variations in parietal cells related to secretory inhibition.

Cytological differences between healed and unhealed patients as well as the effect of more prolonged therapy will be investigated and reported elsewhere.

## MATERIAL AND METHODS
### SUBJECTS

Patients with proven endoscopic duodenal ulcer (D.U.) were studied after giving informed consent. Endoscopy had been performed to allow biopsies to be obtained prior to the beginning of treatment (day 0: DO). Then, all patients were randomized into 2 treatment protocols with $H_2$-receptor antagonists. They received either cimetidine (1 g daily) or ranitidine (150 mg twice daily).

A second endoscopic examination was performed one month after treatment (day 30: D 30). Only patients with healed D.U. proven by endoscopic examination were retained in this experiment (1 female, 9 males of ages ranging from 42 to 67 years, mean age: $50 y \pm 9$; cimetidine : n = 5, ranitidine : n = 5).

In all patients, endoscopies were performed after 12 hours of fasting and after administration of diazepam (5–10 mg).

## HISTOLOGICAL TECHNIQUES

Biopsies were obtained on D0 and D30 with a modified endoscope (GIF 1T) in which a special canal allowed us to obtain large biopsies (6 mm × 4 mm). Biopsies were carefully taken in the same biopsy sites for each subject: 6 duodenal fragments, 20 cm below the papilla, in the area of the ligament of Treitz, 6 fragments from the lesser curvature in the antral part of the stomach near the pylorus, 6 gastric fragments from the greater curvature of the body of the stomach mid-way between the gastro-oesophageal junction and incisura. Histologically, the biopsies included the mucosa through to the level of the muscularis mucosae.

For each time and at each biopsy site, 3 samples were taken for light microscopy and 3 samples were taken for electron microscopy. For light microscopy, biopsies were immediately orientated in cold saline (4°C) under a stereoscopic microscope on small watch glasses filled with dental wax and flattened with fine needles so that the connective face was applied to the wax surface. Then the fragments were fixed in Baker's formalin (12 hours). The time lapse between endoscopy and histological fixation never exceeded 5 to 10 minutes. Biopsies were then quickly dehydrated in graded alcohols (4°C) after removal from the watch glasses and embedded in paraffin. Antral and gastric samples were cut at right angle to the mucosal surface. Duodenal fragments were orientated under a Jung horizontal sliding microtome so that the section plane was always perpendicular to the mucosal surface. Sections were cut at different angles ($-22.5° - 0 - +22.5°$) to minimise the variational factors brought about by aleatory angles of incidence (Fig. 1). Histological sections were generally stained using Mallory's technique or Haemalum-eosin safranin.

For ultrastructural studies, biopsies were fixed for 2 hours in cold glutaraldehyde (2% in Sörensen buffer, pH 7.4, adjusted to 420 milliosmoles

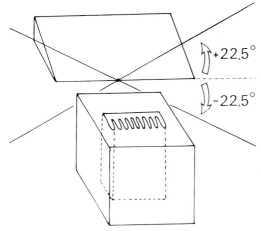

+22.5°

−22.5°

Fig. 1. Duodenal sections were perpendicular to the muscularis mucosae but the 3 sectioning planes were parallel to villi axis.

with sucrose), orientated under a stereoscopic microscope and post-fixed for 1 hour in 2% osmium tetroxide in the same buffer. After dehydration, biopsies were embedded in a mixture of Epon-Araldite. Thin sections were stained with uranyl acetate and lead citrate and examined with an Hitachi H 300 electron microscope.

The morphological findings were further defined by quantitative measurements. All morphological studies were carried out using a double blind method with 2 experimenters.

1) *Gastric mucosa*

*Light microscopy.* The number of parietal cells or chief cells/optical field and the parietal cell/chief cell ratio was calculated. All measurements were performed using a calibrated occular grid lined up to the muscularis mucosa.

*Electron microscopy.* For each subject and in each case, 30 micrographs from the 3 biopsies were used (final magnification: × 10,000, no adjacent slices). In parietal cells, different compartments were measured by Loud method (49, 50): the whole cytoplasmic surface, the surface occupied by tubulovesicles and the surface occupied by the microvilli of the intracellular canaliculi. Microvilli and tubulovesicle surfaces were related to cytoplasmic surface and the two

parameters were expressed as a percent of total relative surface. The microvillus/tubulovesicle ratio was also calculated. Only parietal cells, where both the nucleus and the apex zone were visible, were taken into account.

2) *Antral mucosa*

*Light microscopy.* The number of gastrin and somatostatin cells were evaluated per microscopic field (× 500) in the lower part of the glandular area using an indirect immunoperoxidase technique (3).

The first antiserum was either rabbit antiserum to synthetic gastrin I and II, no. 420051, Calbiochem, San Diego, California, diluted 1 : 30 or rabbit antiserum to pure synthetic somatostatin 28 prepared by L. Pradayrol, and diluted 1 : 100. Somatostatin 28 was synthetized by Dr Wunsch (Munich) (73). The second layer antiserum was peroxidase labelled sheep Fab antirabbit Ig; no. 75111, Institut Pasteur, diluted 1 : 50.

The following controls were used:

—anti-somatostatin-28 serum with added excess synthetic somatostatin-28 followed by peroxidase labelled antiserum;

—anti-somatostatin-28 serum with added excess somatostatin 14 Serono followed by peroxidase labelled antiserum;

—anti-somatostatin-28 serum with added excess pentagastrin;

—peroxidase labelled sheep anti-rabbit (see results).

For each biopsy, G and D cells were counted with a calibrated ocular grid along 10 slices. 5 to 10 counts were made per section. Results were expressed in number of G or D cells/$10^{-2}$ mm².

*Electron microscopy.* The total number of granules in G cells was evaluated, as well as the proportions of dark and clear granules. For each biopsy, 10 to 15 electron micrographs (× 3,000 to 10,000) displaying at least the basal part, the nucleus and the apical cytoplasm of G cells were used. The results were expressed in granules/$10^{-3}$ mm² of cytoplasmic area.

3) *Duodenal mucosa*

*Light microscopy.* Several morphometrical parameters were investigated:

—the number of goblet cells visualized after P.A.S. technique (12 sections/subject, magnification ×100),

—the number of Paneth cells in the bottom of each intestinal crypt (counted for 50 glands sliced along the axis of the glandular lumen, magnification: × 500).

—the increasing rate of villous area (GRv). Since the evaluation of the villous area by a morphometric analysis derived from well-known methods (such as Fisher and Pearson (24)) could not be performed on small biopsies (longitudinal or transverse orientation unknown), this ratio (GRv = P/p) was obtained from the internal perimeter of intestine (P) over the external perimeter (p). For each biopsy, the GRv corresponded to the mean value of the angles previously defined.

—villus height and the number of microvilli were also evaluated.

*Electron microscopy.* The microvillous area of the intestinal brush border was measured at a constant height in the middle part of the intestinal villi (20 micrographs/subject, final magnification: × 25,000). Three parameters were measured: the mean diameter (D), the mean height of each microvillus (h), the mean number of microvilli (N) related to the apex linear unit (l) on columnar cells. Variation in microvillous area was calculated using the formula:

$$GRmv = \frac{\pi DhN^2}{l^2}$$

where the semi-spherical shape at the top of microvilli was neglected.

## KINETIC PARAMETERS

In a parallel test, on 2 volunteers, endoscopic biopsies were taken before and after 3 days of treatment with cimetidine (1 g/day) in the same gastric, pyloric and duodenal zones as previously described. Biopsies were immediately incubated in a shaking water bath at 37°C in 5 ml of Eagle basal medium containing 20 µCi per ml of $^3H$ thymidine (specific activity: 22–26 Ci per mmole). After incubation for 30 minutes, biopsies were washed in unlabelled medium for 30 minutes,

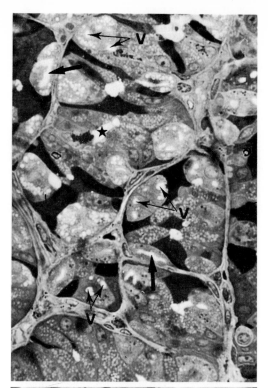

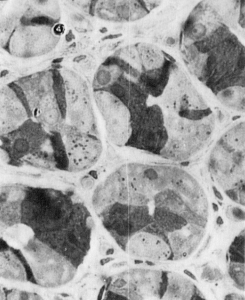

Fig. 2. Morphological aspects of oxyntic glands observed on semi-thin sections. Before treatment with cimetidine (2a) small vacuoles filled the cytoplasm of the parietal cells (V). Clear intracytoplasmic spaces (arrows), correspond to intracytoplasmic canaliculi. Gland lumens, were largely open and connected with cellular canaliculi (*).

After treatment (2b), all these features had disappeared (× 400).

fixed in cold formalin (12 hours) embedded in paraffin and serially sectioned at 4μ. The slides were coated with liquid photographic emulsion (Ilford $L_4$), exposed for 2 weeks, developed and stained with haemalum and periodic acid Schiff method. Labelling index was measured in the specific proliferative zones (300 glands/subject, on 10–20 non-adjacent slices).

Statistical analysis was performed using student 't' test. All data are expressed as mean ± S.E.M.

## RESULTS

*Gastric mucosa.* With both $H_2$-receptor antagonists, neither morphological variations of the surface epithelium, nor modifications of the lamina propria were observed in gastric mucosa.

Only oxyntic glands seemed to be affected. In light microscopy, features of stimulation were surprisingly noted in parietal cells (Fig. 2). Clear clefts or crescents were located in supra-nuclear spaces and could be considered, without doubt, as opened intracytoplasmic canaliculi. Confirming this observation, wide-open canaliculi were seen to be in direct communication with the gland lumen. Other parietal cells exhibited clear microvacuolisations, probably corresponding to swollen mitochondria or lysosomal vacuoles. On the other hand, dilated parietal cells with pyknotic or dilated nuclei were occasionally observed.

All these features, observed on day 0, had completely disappeared on day 30. Most of the parietal cells were then in the resting state and no signs of degenerative processes could be seen.

In conventional light microscope slides and on semi-thin sections, the oxyntic glands did vary in size. The parietal cell/chief cell ratio was not significantly affected nor was the number of parietal cells or chief cells (Table I). Apparent oxyntic gland hypertrophy in duodenal ulcer before treatment is therefore due to the few enlarged degenerative cells and to a slight increase in diameter of some parietal cells in which the intracellular canaliculi are opened.

Confirming the morphometrical analysis in light microscopy, electron microscopy showed the mean cytoplasmic surface of parietal cells between D0 and D30 was unchanged when free parts of canaliculi (deprived of microvilli) were excluded from the area estimation. This surface can be considered as a extra-cellular space. Morphometrical measurement of canaliculi microvillus area and tubulovesicle area showed significant differences between D0 and D30 (Fig. 3). Tubulovesicles were significantly increased on day 30. Reciprocally the microvilli were significantly decreased on D30. Calculation of the microvilli/tubulovesicle ratio verified the significant variation in these two distinct membrane compartments (Fig. 4). However the whole membrane pool involved in the secretory processes of parietal cells—in other words, the sum of microvilli + tubulovesicular surface—did not vary significantly between D0 and D30 (Fig. 4).

For each subject, when individual cell variations were taken into account, important differences were noted between D0 and D30 (Fig. 5). On D0, large discrepancies in the

Table I. Evaluation of the number of parietal cells and chief cells. The ratio between parietal cells and chief cells was also calculated. No significant variations of these parameters could be observed (NS) before (D0) and after treatment (D30).

| Number/optical field | Cimetidine | | Ranitidine | |
|---|---|---|---|---|
| | D0 | D30 | D0 | D30 |
| Parietal cells | 160 ± 7.12 | 161.4 ± 31.2 NS | 166.7 ± 9.58 | 176.5 ± 16.56 NS |
| Chief cells | 257 ± 13 | 197.2 ± 38.9 NS | 227.5 ± 21.46 | 216.5 ± 17.92 NS |
| Parietal cells/Chief cells | 0.631 ± 0.04 | 0.709 ± 0.04 NS | 0.762 ± 0.023 | 0.813 ± 0.015 NS |

microvillus/tubulovesicle ratio were observed on both sides of the mean value. On D30, not only was the mean value lowered but cell variations were also reduced so that nearly all cells were in a resting state.

In addition to the variations seen with the microvilli and canaliculi, degenerative changes in the mitochondria, swelling of the matrix and rarefaction of the mitochondrial cristae, could be seen on D0 in some parietal cells. In other parietal

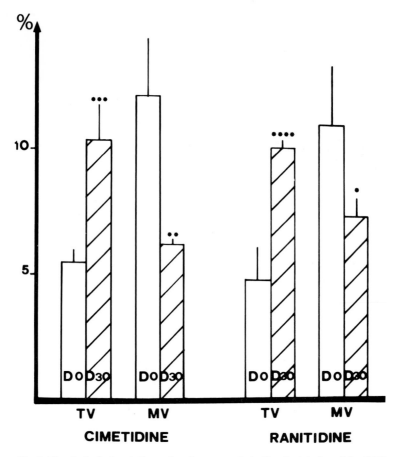

Fig. 3. Morphological variations of surfaces occupied either by tubulovesicles (TV) or microvilli (MV) from the intracellular canaliculi in parietal cells are presented before (D0) and after treatment (D30) with cimetidine and ranitidine
  * significant difference between D0 and D30: $P \leqslant 0.05$
  ** significant difference between D0 and D30: $P \leqslant 0.02$
  *** significant difference between D0 and D30: $P \leqslant 0.01$
  **** significant difference between D0 and D30: $P \leqslant 0.001$

Single micrographs therefore cannot provide a valuable representation of all the morphological variations observed. This was particularly true on day 0. However Figs. 6–8 showed some cytological changes before and after the receptor antagonist treatments.

cells, dilated clear vacuoles filled the latero basal cytoplasm (Fig. 7a). Some of the vacuoles may correspond to lysosomal structures and multivesicular bodies but others seemed to be related to the tubulovesicle compartment (Fig. 7a). Although not accurately counted, secondary

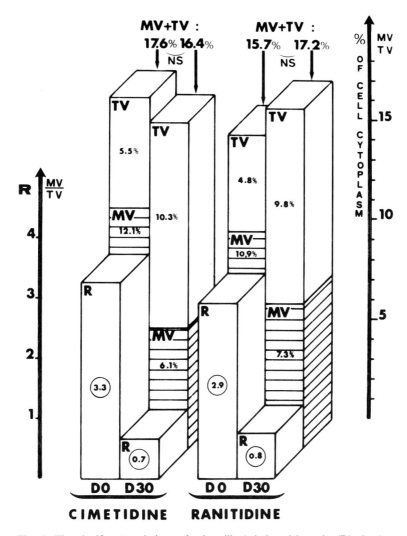

Fig. 4. The significant variations of microvillus/tubulovesicle ratio (R) clearly demonstrated the inhibitory effect of H₂-receptor antagonists on the secretory processes of parietal cells. But the sum:microvilli + tubulovesicle surfaces (TV + MV) did not vary; thus the whole membrane pool involved in the secretory mechanism, was not modified by the two H₂-receptor antagonists tested.

autolysosomes and residual bodies seemed more numerous before treatment (Fig. 6a). Some parietal cells exhibited entire degeneration of the cytoplasmic membranes except for the mitochondria which were still preserved (Fig. 7b). A more interesting cytological observation was the morphological aspect of tubulovesicles on D30 (Fig. 8). They were mostly collapsed with a closely associated limiting membrane, forming concave

pentalaminar structures. A clear hyaloplasmic zone, without any visible content, was located in the concave part of the tubulovesicle. In some cases, marginal parts of tubulovesicles seemed to be undergoing fusion in a very narrow zone. On a few micrographs, features suggesting a connection between tubulovesicles and the limiting membrane of canaliculi could be observed.

    On the other hand, no variations were observed

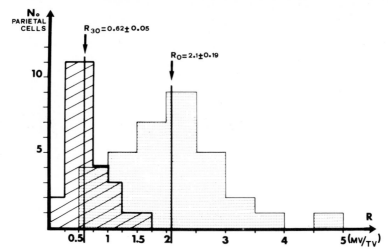

Fig. 5. This figure, illustrates the discrepancies observed between parietal cells for one patient before and after treatment with cimetidine.

in chief cells which did not seem to be affected by treatment with $H_2$ receptor antagonists.

No significant differences were observed between the two $H_2$ receptor antagonists used in this experiment for all the gastric parameters tested.

*Antral mucosa*

No topographic variations were observed at light and electron microscopy.

No significant variation of G cell number was observed using the immuno-peroxidase technique at light microscopy (Table II).

Evaluation of the different granule populations at the electron microscopical level did not reveal any significant variations between D0 and D30. However G cells were mostly filled with clear and intermediate granules (Fig. 9), and the dark granules seemed to us to be fewer in comparison to healthy subjects.

When antiserum raised against synthetic somatostatin-28 was applied in different dilutions (1:30 to 1:200) to sections of antral and duodenal mucosa, incubation time was set at 1 hour at room temperature, staining intensity started to decrease at a higher dilution than 1:100 and completely disappeared at 1:200. Treatment of anti-

Table II. G cells in the antral mucosa: evaluation of different parameters. The cell number/glandular surface and granule population in the cytoplasm were evaluated before (D0) and after treatment (D30) with ranitidine and cimetidine (NS: not significant).

| G Cells | Cimetidine | | Ranitidine | |
|---|---|---|---|---|
| | D0 | D30 | D0 | D30 |
| G-cells number $10^{-2}$ mm$^2$ | 33.3 ± 5.1 | 37.1 ± 7.3 NS | 30.1 ± 8.2 | 34.7 ± 6.3 NS |
| Overall granules $10^{-6}$ mm$^2$ | 9.2 ± 2.7 | 7.1 ± 1.42 NS | 8.9 ± 0.7 | 7.9 ± 1.4 NS |
| Dark granules $10^{-6}$ mm$^2$ | 0.8 ± 0.3 | 0.9 ± 0.6 NS | 1.1 ± 0.5 | 0.6 ± 0.2 NS |
| Clear granules $10^{-6}$ mm$^2$ | 4.8 ± 3.2 | 2.36 ± 0.7 NS | 3 ± 0.4 | 3.1 ± 0.7 NS |

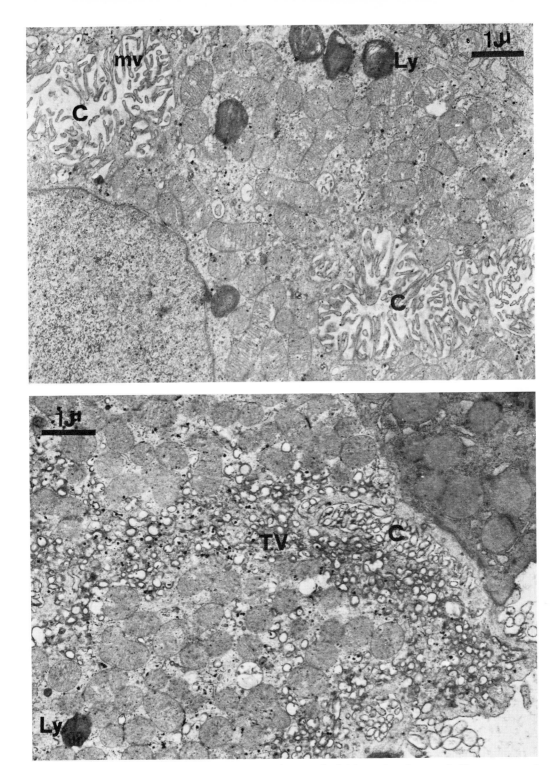

Fig. 6. Before treatment (6a) with the receptor antagonists, canaliculi (c) were largely opened with numerous and extended microvilli.

Intracytoplasmic tubulovesicles were scarce. Lysosomes (Ly) and dense bodies were frequently observed.

After treatment (6b) tubulovesicles (TV) increased and canaliculi decreased.

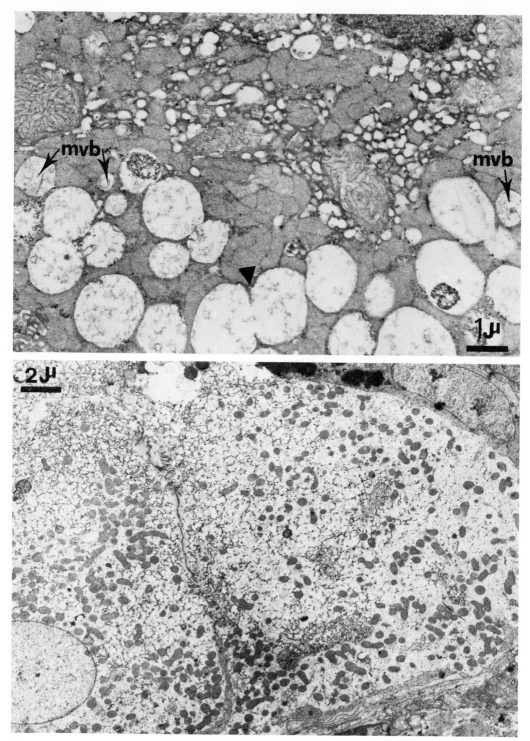

Fig. 7. 7a: Before treatment the intracytoplasmic vacuolisation previously observed at light microscopy (Fig. 2) was also seen at electron microscopy. Some vacuoles could correspond to multivesicular bodies (mvb) but other vacuoles could be dilated tubulovesicles (sometimes interconnected ▲).

7b: Before treatment and particularly in the middle zone of oxyntic glands parietal cells wholly degenerated, could be observed. Only mitochondria could be identified.

serum with synthetic somatostatin-28 (73) or synthetic somatostatin 14 (Serono) abolished all staining. Pentagastrin added to the antiserum had no effect on staining. Although antigen inactivation seemed more potent with somatostatin-28 (73) than with somatostatin-14 on molar basis, the antiserum should be considered as specific against somatostatin-14 and -28 rather than specific against somatostatin-28 alone (i.e. only directed against the sequence 1–14 of somatostatin-28).

The somatostatin antiserum visualised typical endocrine cells in the pyloric glands located preferentially in the middle and basal part of the glands (Fig. 10). These cells occasionally showed connections with the gland lumen. More frequently they were close to the basal lamina with lateral processes parallel to the basal lamina. When the semi-thin/thin section technique was performed, immunostained cells were identified as the D type with round and large (300–330 nm) basal granules, filled with fine and relatively osmophilic particles (Fig. 10b).

Morphometrical analysis, in evaluating somatostatin cell number in antral mucosa showed a significant increase of D cells on D30 after treatment with both $H_2$-receptor antagonists tested (Fig. 11). The somatostatin cell increase was observed in all subjects and seemed more significant after ranitidine. Differences between ranitidine and cimetidine might be attributed to the lesser number of D cells in the ranitidine group. However the differences between ranitidine and cimetidine groups on D0 were not significant (and did not seem to be related to clinical history). In the distal duodenum mucosa, the low number of D cells did not permit quantification.

*Duodenal mucosa*

At the light microscopical level, intestinal villi seemed enlarged and had acquired a more accentuated duodenal aspect with finger-like feature and numerous lateral epithelial foldings. Morphometrical analysis confirmed this (Fig. 12a). The growth ratio of villous perimeter (GRv) was significantly increased with both cimetidine and ranitidine (Fig. 12a). The increase of villous area

was dependent on a significant increase of villus height (cimetidine: $+38.5\%$, $P \leqslant 0.01$, ranitidine: $+22\%$, $P \leqslant 0.05$) without appreciable change in the number of villi.

The number of goblet cells per gland and the number of goblet cells per unit of villus perimeter did not vary significantly. On the other hand the number of Paneth cells, in the bottom of each intestinal crypt, was increased significantly after cimetidine (Table III).

Table III. Paneth cell number in the bottom of each intestinal crypt. (NS: not significant)

| Paneth cells/ glands | Cimetidine | Ranitidine |
|---|---|---|
| D0 | $2.97 \pm 0.40$ | $3.08 \pm 0.56$ |
| D30 | $4.60 \pm 0.10$ | $3.56 \pm 0.56$ |
| | $+55\%\ p < 0.01$ | $+16\%$ NS |

At the electron microscopical level, microvillous area (GRmv) was significantly increased (Fig. 12b). Both the microvillus number (cimetidine: $+22\%$, $P \leqslant 0.01$, ranitidine: $+18\%$, $P \leqslant 0.05$) and the microvillus height (cimetidine: $+33\%$, $P \leqslant 0.02$, ranitidine: $+24\%$, $P \leqslant 0.05$) were significantly increased with a slight decrease of microvillus diameter (Fig. 13). No other cytological variations was observed and electron microscopic observation of the Paneth cells did not give any further information about the hypertrophy or hyperplasia of this cell type.

*Kinetic parameters*

Good preservation of cell structures was obtained using Eagle medium.

Oxyntic mucosa unfortunately was not available for autoradiographic study. Labelling index could only be measured in pyloric and intestinal glands. Counts were performed in the central part of each biopsy to avoid the well known marginal effect, which suggests an increase in cell proliferation. The autoradiographic background was insignificant.

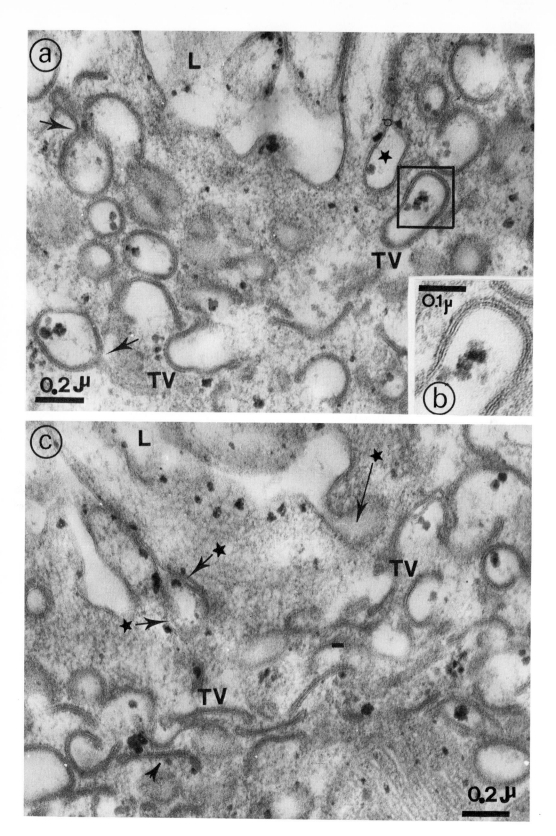

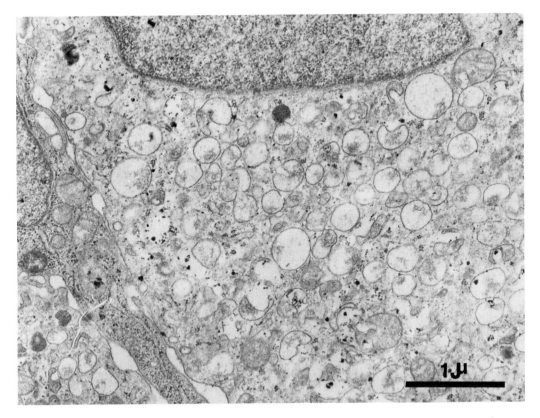

Fig. 9. Ultrastructural aspect of G cell on D 30 for one subject receiving ranitidine. Clear secretory granules were still predominant in number.

Labelling index was significantly decreased on D3 in the pyloric mucosa while it was significantly increased in the duodenal mucosa (Fig. 14).

Moreover, since fine particle emulsion (Ilford L4) was used, silver granules were distinguishable in light microscopy. In the pyloric mucosa, the number of silver granules covering the nuclei were distinctly reduced on day 3 which might be related to a slowing down of S phase in proliferative cells.

## DISCUSSION

This experimental study in man was undertaken in order to provide more information about the cytological effects of H$_2$-receptor antagonists.

Indeed, it seemed important to define relations between the inhibition of acid secretion and the hypothesis of membrane flow during the secretory processes.      According      to      this      hypothesis

---

Fig. 8. These 3 micrographs represent high magnification of tubulovesicles in parietal cells 30 days after H$_2$-receptor antagonist treatment. On Fig. 8a and 8c, near the lumen (L) of intracytoplasmic canaliculi, numerous tubulovesicles (TV) are collapsed and their limiting membrane are closely applied. Clear zones of hyaloplasm are located in the concave part of the collapsed vesicles.

Fig. 8b is an enlargement of surrounded part on 8a: direct contact of the limiting membranes creates multilaminar features with virtual tubulovesicle lumen.

In located zones (➤) tubulovesicles seem to be interconnected (Fig. 8a). Both in Fig. 8a and 8c, infoldings (★) of canalicular membrane could be interpreted as tubulovesicles opened into the lumen and at various degrees of expansion.

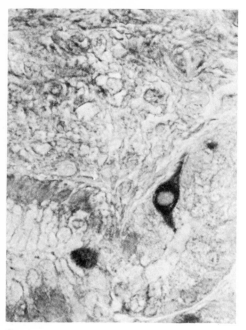

a

(29, 36, 37), the tubulo-vesicular system increases the secretory surface of the canaliculi by eversion or fusion of the tubulovesicles with the plasma membrane. Numerous investigations argue in favour of such a hypothesis. Good correlations between tubulovesicle/canaliculus equilibrium and the variation of gastric potential differences or gastric secretion (4, 32, 33, 38, 68) have been seen. Direct observations of isolated gastric glands using aminopyrine and acridine orange, point to the conclusion that the site of acid secretion is indeed the membrane of parietal cell canaliculi (6–10). However cytological variations during secretory processes may be osmotically induced and do not imply membrane fusions but simply the expansion of collapsed tubulo-vesicles already branched out with the canalicular system (6). This last hypothesis seems attractive since no complex membrane translocations should be involved either during the first step of stimulation

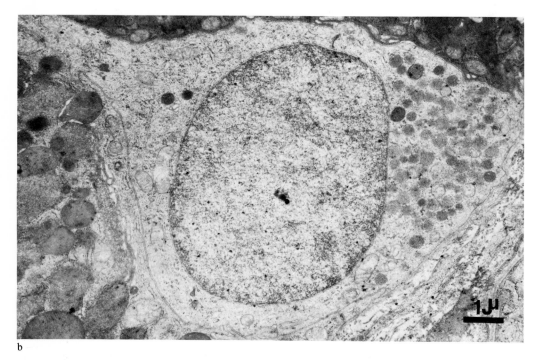

b

Fig. 10. 10a: Endocrine cells were labelled with antiserum to somatostatin-28. Two cytoplasmic processes could be seen: one process reached the gland lumen, another expansion was directed towards the basal lamina (× 400)
    10b: endocrine cell observed on day 30 after raniditine. Numerous slightly osmiophilic and large granules (330 nm) suggest this is a D cell.

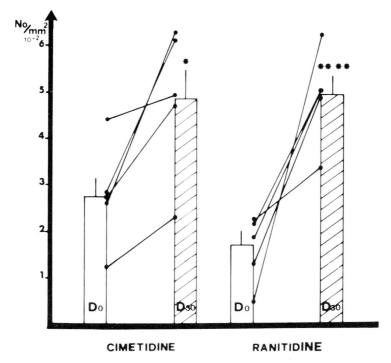

Fig. 11. The variation in number of somatostatin cells is visualized on histograms. Individual variations are also presented (points and lines) for each subject.
  * significant difference between D0 and D30 P ≤ 0.05
*** significant difference between D0 and D30 P ≤ 0.001

or during the reconstitution of the tubulovesicular compartment concommitant to the fall in acid secretion as previously suggested (62).

Thus H₂-receptor antagonists, eliciting potent inhibition of acid secretion, could represent a valuable method of observing membrane movement in parietal cells. Moreover other cytological effects should be investigated to explain the positive action of H₂-receptor antagonists in peptic ulcer therapy since these drugs have been suspected of posessing cytoprotective effects (9).

The main results presented in this paper can be briefly summarized in 5 points.

1) No important difference between the two H₂-receptor antagonists were detected.

2) After treatment with H₂-receptor antagonists, tubulovesicle number is increased in parietal cells while microvilli of the intracellular canaliculi are decreased, giving a striking decrease in the microvillus/tubulovesicle ratio.

3) Absence of variation in the G cells but an increase in the number of D cells.

4) Increase of microvillous and villous area in the duodenum.

5) The labelling index was increased in duodenal mucosa and decreased in antral mucosa.

All these points will be discussed separately.

Ranitidine has been shown to be more potent than cimetidine in reducing gastric acid secretion (10, 17, 21, 42, 43, 58, 64, 65). In addition ranitidine is chemically different from other H₂-receptor antagonists (cimetidine; metiamide) since ranitidine does not contain the imidazole nucleus of histamine. Cytological analysis did not permit us to observe differences between the two antagonists. Thus all other results will be discussed without discrimination between ranitidine and cimetidine.

Variation of tubulovesicles and microvilli in parietal cells can be directly related to the inhi-

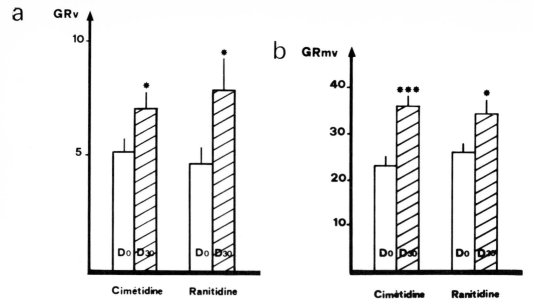

Fig. 12. Quantitative evaluation of the absorptive area in the distal duodenum. On Figure 12a are represented variations of the growth ratio of villus perimeter (GRV).

On Figure 12b are represented variations of the growth ratio of micro villous area (GR mv)

* significative differences between D0 and D30 $P \leqslant 0.05$

*** significant difference between D0 and D30 $P \leqslant 0.01$

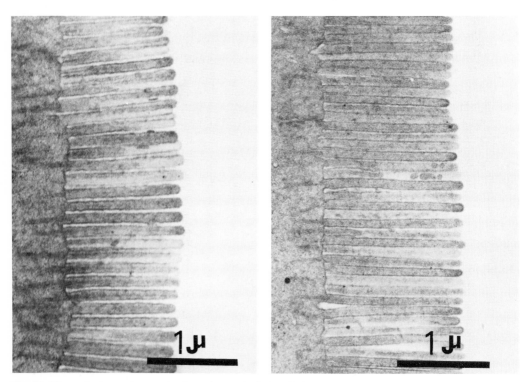

Fig. 13. These electron micrographs show the cytological variations of duodenal brush border microvilli in the middle zone of intestinal villi.

In comparison to D0 (Fig. 13a) the number of microvilli is increased on day 30 (Fig. 13b). Microvillus height is also increased and the diameter is slightly decreased after cimetidine treatment.

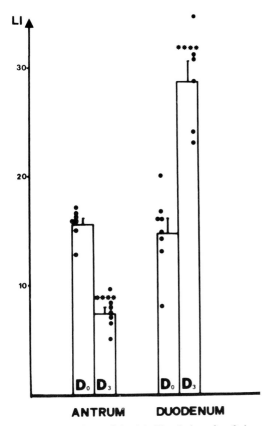

**ANTRUM    DUODENUM**

Fig. 14. Variations of the labelling index after 3 days treatment with cimetidine. Compared to day 0 (before treatment), labelling index on day 3 is significantly decreased in the antral mucosa and significantly increased in the duodenum.

Since only 2 subjects could be taken in this experiment, mean values of the labelling index obtained for each biopsy (black points on the histograms) were pooled and used for statistical analysis.

**** significant differences between D0 and D30 $P \leqslant 0,001$

bition of gastric secretion (28, 29, 32, 33, 36, 37, 62). However, more striking are the discrepancies observed on D0 in parietal cells from D.U. subjects. Since all patients were in a fasting condition, most cells should have been in a resting state (and variations between D0 and D30 could be expected to be small) as has previously been observed in healthy subjects (29). It is now obvious that a great number of parietal cells were in stimulated condition on D0, but increased parietal cell sensitivity in patients with

active D.U. has been previously reported (35, 54, 60). It is also possible that endoscopic examination stimulates parietal cells in D.U. Nevertheless, the efficiency of the H₂-receptor antagonists is demonstrated by D30 since all the parietal cells were in a basal condition (Fig. 4) with microvillus/tubulovesicle ratio always less than unity thus showing that the tubulovesicles had become the predominant compartment. On the other hand, if H₂-receptor antagonists can maintain parietal cells in a resting condition, secretory potency may be preserved as the total membranes involved in parietal cell secretion (Fig. 4) are not significantly modified. This observation agrees with the findings of other authors (7, 8, 34, 66) who reported the absence of any change in pentagastrin stimulated acid secretion after cessation of cimetidine treatment and the maintenance of parietal cell mass sensitivity after cimetidine induced healing of D.U. (1, 2).

If increased sensitivity of oxyntic mucosa represents one invoked factor in the physiopathology of duodenal ulcer, the absence of important modification of parietal cells on D30 could explain possible relapses of ulceration after cessation of H₂-receptor antagonist treatment.

Numerous tubulovesicles were collapsed after cimetidine treatment. The clear zone located against the concave part of tubulovesicles was devoid of visible structures. This zone does not correspond to an extracellular space, connected with the glandular lumen, since this zone is in direct continuity with other part of the cell hyaloplasm (Fig. 8). Such features could be explained as an osmotic phenomenon either during fixation and histological processing or before histological treatment. Since the modifications of tubulovesicles are predominantly observed after H₂ receptor antagonists, the latter hypothesis seems more satisfying. Perhaps H₂-receptor antagonists facilitate the formation of collapsed vesicles.

In some cases, tubulovesicles are inter-connected (Fig. 8). Continuity between the virtual spaces limited by vesicle membrane is therefore possible. Moreover tubulovesicles connections with the membrane of parietal cell canaliculi are also visible with various degrees of expansion of the tubulovesicular content (Fig. 8).

Though these findings require investigation, they may be related to the hypothesis of an osmotic mechanism (6–19) where collapsed tubules having few contacts with the canalicular membrane could expand directly, thus forming canaliculi without necessitating membrane cycling or multiple fusions as has been previously postulated (28, 29, 32, 33, 36, 37, 62).

Confirming previous findings (48), the G-cell number in the antral mucosa did not vary significantly. It is now thought however, that biopsy specimens cannot provide a good estimation of the G cell mass (41) even if biopsies are taken from the same zone.

A true antral gastrin cell hyperplasia in D.U. (56) is probably an uncommon syndrome, and the increased serum gastrin level in duodenal ulcer can be explained by the higher functional activity of G cells both on D0 and D30. The number of dark granules is decreased and empty or pale granules are predominant (Fig. 9). This result is concordant with previous observations (16). Thus the low density of secretory granules could be related to the secretory phase of the G-cell cycle (5, 15, 27) and could confirm the higher activity of G cells in D.U. On the other hand G-cell granule population is unchanged after treatment with $H_2$-receptor antagonists. This result, already observed (52), cannot be related to the increased level of post prandial gastrinaemia found by different authors (11, 13, 23, 25, 26, 31, 47, 59, 63, 67, 71).

For D cells like the G cells, validity of the counts on biopsy specimens should be re-assessed, however only small changes were observed in the D cell count between the different subjects, between different zones in the same biopsy and between non-adjacent sections.

Somatostatin cells were significantly increased in the antral mucosa after $H_2$-receptor antagonists. Different hypotheses, needing further investigations, can be suggested 1) direct action of $H_2$-receptor antagonists on somatostatin cells, or (more probably) indirect action. 2) The lack of $H^+$ feed back-inhibition after treatment with cimetidine or ranitidine might induce more significantly increased gastrin levels than those observed (11, 13, 23, 25, 26, 31, 47, 59, 63, 67,

71). In our own experiments (not shown), after a defined test meal, the difference of gastrin level increase is not significant between D0 and D30. Topographic distribution and different aspects of D type cells (12, 58) have suggested possible paracrine effects of somatostatin in locally controlling G-cell secretory processes (20, 44, 45). Hyperplasia and hypertrophy of D cells could then represent an adaptative mechanism, one which has not been studied and which merits subsequent investigations both in healthy and DU subjects. However, because of the variability of D-cell populations and the small number of subjects in this study, further work will be required to reach a firm conclusion.

$H_2$-receptor antagonist treatment was shown to increase both villous area and microvillous area in the distal duodenal segment (Fig. 12). Such a trophic effect, not observed in the proximal duodenum after 1 years treatment (53, 55), was unexpected but could surely facilitate duodenal ulcer healing. Several mechanisms can be invoked to explain these findings. Pain relief, better nutritional conditions, stress decrease during treatment could be general factors. Since $H_2$-receptor antagonists are potent inhibitors of acid secretion, a decrease of brush border desorption or a decrease of cell desquamation may also be involved although the labelling index increased in the duodenal crypt (Fig. 15). Thus increased cell proliferation is probably the more relevant factor. Causes of this phenomenon are not clear. Perhaps the increase of post prandial gastrin levels after $H_2$-receptor antagonists could represent a more potent iterative stimulus which enhances cell proliferation as mediated by positive action of gastrin on DNA and RNA synthesis (14, 18, 22, 30, 39, 40, 51, 70).

In the distal duodenum where D cells are few, the trophic action of gastrin could be predominant and could increase cell proliferation. Conversely in the antral mucosa, the trophic effect of gastrin could be modulated by the significant increase of D cell number. In this zone, inhibitory action of somatostatin would be predominant. Indeed this last regulatory peptide would represent the antral chalone (69, 46).

Therefore $H_2$-receptor antagonists seem to act

as trophic factors in the distal part of the duo-denum, but in order to be certain that this effect is really important in D.U. healing it will be necessary to observe kinetic parameters in the elective zone of D.U., i.e. the first duodenum (Indeed D cells are more numerous in the first duodenum and the trophic effect could be inhibited in this zone).

In conclusion, good correlation was obtained between cytological variations in parietal cells and the inhibition of acid secretion during duo-denal ulcer therapy with H₂-receptor antagonists in man. A positive action of H₂ receptor antag-onists on duodenal mucosa was also observed. The possible paracrine influence of somatostatin in the antral mucosa and tubulovesicle expansions were also suggested but need further investigation.

Cytological investigations may bring new infor-mation either during prolonged therapy with H₂-receptor antagonists or following cessation of treatment. Moreover H₂-receptor antagonist therapy could represent a suitable tool for observ-ing cytological events occurring during the secre-tory process in parietal cells.

## REFERENCES

1. Aadland, E. and Berstad, A. *Scand. J. Gastroent.* 1978, *13*, 193–197
2. Aadland, E. and Berstad, A. *Scand. J. Gastroent.* 1979, *14*, 111–114
3. Avrameas, S. and Therny, C. K. T. *Immunochem-istry* 1971, *8*, 1175–1179
4. Baldi, F., Salera, M., Ferrarini, F., Millazzo, G., Miglioli, M. & Barbara, L. *Scand. J. Gastroenterol.* 1980, *15*, 171–176
5. Bastie, M. J., Balas, D., Sénégas-Balas, F., Ber-trand, C., Pradayrol, L., Frexinos, J. & Ribet, A. *Scand. J. Gastroent.* 1979, *14*, 35–48
6. Berglindh, T., Dibona, D. R., Ito, S. and Sachs, G. *Am. J. Physiol.* 1980, *238*, G165–G176
7. Binder, H. J., Cocco, A., Crossley, R. J., Finkel-stein, W., Font, R., Friedman, G., Groarke, J., Hughes, W., Johnson, A. F., McGuigan, J. E., Summers, R., Vlahcevic, R., Wilson, E. C. & Win-ship, D. H. *Gastroenterology,* 1978, *74*, Suppl., 380–388
8. Bodemar, G. and Walan, A. *Lancet* 1978, *1*, 403–407
9. Bommelaer, G. and Guth, P. H. *Gastroenterology,* 1979, *77*, 303–308
10. Bradshaw, J., Brittain, R. T., Clitherow, J. W.,

11. Daly, M. J., Jack, D., Price, B. J. & Stables, R. *Brit. J. Pharmac.* 1979, *66*, (3), 464 p.
11. Brodgen, R. N., Heel, R. C., Speight, T. M. & Avery, G. S. *Drugs* 1978, *15*, 93–131
12. Buchan, A. M. J. & Polak, J. M. *Invest. Cell Pathol* 1980, *3*, 51–71
13. Buchanan, K. D., Spencer, J., Ardill, J. & Ken-nedy, T. L. *Gut* 1978, *19*, A–437
14. Casteleyn, P. P., Dubrasquet, M. & Willems, G. *Digestive Diseases* 1977, *22*, 798–804
15. Creutzfeldt, W., Track, N. S., Creutzfeldt, C & Arnold, R. pp. 197–211, in Thompson J. C. (eds.), *Gastrointestinal Hormones*, University of Texas Press: Austin, 1975b
16. Creutzfeldt, W., Arnold, R., Creutzfeldt, C. & Track, N. S. *Gut* 1976, *17*, 745–754
17. Daly, M. J., Humphray, J. M., & Stables, R. *Gut,* 1979, *20*, (10), A 914
18. Dembinski, A. B. and Johnson, L. R. *Endocrinol-ogy* 1979, *105*, 769–773
19. Dibona, D. R., Ito, S., Berglindh, T. & Sachs, G. *Proc. Natl. Acad. Sci. U.S.A.* 1979, Physiological Sciences, *12*, 6689–6693
20. Dockray G. J. & Gregory, R. A. *Proc. R. Soc. Lond. Biol* 1980, *210*, (1178), 151–164
21. Domschke, W., Lux, G. & Domschke, S. *Gastro-enterology* 1980, *79*, (6), 1267–71
22. Enoch, M. R. & Johnson L. R. *Am. J. Physiol.* 1977, *232*, E 223–E228
23. Feldman, M., and Richardson C. T. *Adv. Intern. Med.* 1978, *23*, 1–24
24. Fisher, R. B. and Parson, D. S. *J. Anat.* 1950, *84*, 272–282
25. Forrest, J. A. H., Fettes, M. R., Lidgard, G. P., McLoughlin, G. P. & Heading, R. C. *Gut.* 1978, *19*, A440–441
26. Forrest, J. A. H., Fettes, M. R., McLoughlin, G. P. & Heading, R. C. *Gut* 1979, *20*, 404–407
27. Forssman, W. G. & Orci, L. *Z Zellforsch.* 1969, *101*, 419–432
28. Forte, T. M., Machen, T. E. & Forte, J. G. *Gas-troenterology* 1977, *73*, 941–955
29. Frexinos, J., Carballido, M., Louis, A. & Ribet, A. *Biol et Gastro-Enterol.* 1971, *1*, 57–70
30. Hansen, O. H., Pedersen, T., Larsen, J. K. & Rehfeld, J. F. *Gut,* 1976, *17*, 536–541
31. Hansky, J., Stern, A. I., Korman, M. G. and Waugh, J. *Dig. Dis. Sci.* 1979, *24*, 468–470
32. Helander, H. F. & Hirschowitz, B. I. *Gastroenter-ology* 1972, *63*, 951–961
33. Helander, H. F., *Gastroenterology* 1976, *71*, 1010–1018
34. Hetzel, D. H., Hansky, J., Shearman, D. J. C., Korman, M. G., Hecker, R., Taggart, G. J., Jack-son, R. & Gabb, B. W. *Gastroenterology* 1978, *74* Suppl, 389–392
35. Isenberg, J. I., Grossman, M. I., Maxwell, V. & Walsch, J. H. *J. Clin. Invest.* 1975, *55*, 330–337
36. Ito, S. and Schofield, G. C. *J. Cell Biol.* 1974, *63*, 364–382
37. Ito, S. pp. 705–741 in Code, C. F., Heidel, W. (eds.), *Handbook of Physiology, Alimentary canal II.* American Physiological Society Washington, 1967

38. Ivey, K. J., Tarnawski, A., Sherman, D., Krause, W. J., Ackman, K., Burks, M. & Hewett, J. *Gut* 1980, *21*, 3–8
39. Johnson, L. R. *Gastroenterology* 1977, *72*, 788–792
40. Johnson, L. R., *World J. Surg.* 1979, *31*, 477–486
41. Keuppens, F., Willems, G., De Graef, J. & Woussen-Colle, M. C. *Ann. Surg.* 1980, *19*, (3), 276–281
42. Konturek, S. J., Obtulowicz, W., Kwiecie, N. N., Sito, E., Oleksy, J. and Miszozuk-Jamska, B. *Dig. Dis. Sci.* 1980, *25*, 737–743
43. Konturek, S. J., Obtulowicz, W., Kwiecien, N., Sito, E., Mikos, E. & Oleksy, J. *Gut* 1980, *21* (3), 181–186
44. Larsson, L. I., Goltermann, N., De Magistris, Rehfeld, J. F. & Schwartz, T. W. *Sciences* 1979, *205*, 1393–1395
45. Larsson, L. I. *Invest. Cell Pathol.* 1980, *3*, 73–85
46. Lehy, T., Gres, L. & Bonfils, S., *Digestion* 1979, *19*, (2), 99–109
47. Logan, R. F. A, Forrest, J. A., McLoughlin, G. P., Lidgard, G. & Heading, R. C. *Digestion* 1978, *18*, 220–226
48. Lombardo, L. pp. 113–120 in P. E. Luchelli (ed.), *Proceedings of cimetidine Symposium*, 1978
49. Loud, A. V. *J. Cell Biol.* 1962, *15*, 481–487
50. Loud, A. V., Barany, W. C. and Pack, B. A. *Lab Invest.* 1963, *14*, 258–270
51. Majumbar, A. P. and Goltermann, N. *Digestion* 1979, *19*, 144–147
52. Mortensen, N. J. M. *Annals, of the Royal College of surgeons of England* 1980, *62*, 462–469
53. Moshal, M. G., Spitaels, J. M. & Bhoola, R. S. *Afr. Med. J.* 1977, *52*, 760–763
54. Petersen, H. and Myren, J. *Scand. J. Gastroent.* 1975, *10*, 705–714
55. Pillay, C. V., Moshal, M. G., Bryer, J. V. and Boogens, J., *S. Afr. Med. J.* 1977, *52*, 1082–1085
56. Polak, J. M., Stagg, B. and Pearse, A. G. E. *Gut* 1972, *13*, 501–512
57. Polak, J. M. and Bloom, S. R., pp. 15–30, in Rehfeld, J. H. (ed.), *Gastrin and the Vagus*, Academic Press, 1979
58. Peden, N. R., Saunders, J. H. B. & Wormsley, K. G. *Lancet*, 1979, *1*, 690–692
59. Richardson, C. T. *Gastroenterology* 1978, *74*, 366–370
60. Roland, M. *Scand. J. Gastroent.* 1975, *10*, 603–608
61. Sachs, G., Rabon, E., Chang, H. H., Schackmann, R., Sarau, H. M. & Saccomani, G. pp. 347–360 in Bonfils, S., Fromageot, P. & Rosselin, G., (eds.), in *Hormonal Receptors in Digestive Tract Physiology*, Elsevier, New York, 1977
62. Schofield, G. C., Ito, S., & Bolender, R. P. *J. Anat.* 1979, *128*, 669–692
63. Sewing, K. F., Hagie, L., Ippoliti, A. F., Isenberg, J. I., Samloff, I. H. & Sturdevant, R. A. *Gastroenterology* 1978, *74*, 376–379
64. Sewing, K. F., Billian, A. & Malchow, H. *Gut* 1980, *21*, 750–752
65. Simon, B., Dammann, H. G., Müller, P. & Kather, H. *Dtsch Med Wochenschr* 1980, *105*, 1753–1755
66. Spence, R. W., Celestin, L. R., McCornick, D. A., Owens, C. J. & Olivier, J. M. pp. 116–136 in Creutzfeldt, W. (ed.). *Cimetidine. Proceedings of an International Symposium on Histamine $H_2$ Receptor Antagonist. Excerpta Medica*, Amsterdam, 1978
67. Spence, R. W., Celestin, L. R., McCornick, D. A. & Owens, C. I. pp. 153–169 in Wastell, C. & Lance, P. (ed.). *Cimetidine: the Westminster Hospital Symposium*. Churchill Livingstone, Edinburgh, New-York, 1978.
68. Tarnawsky, A., Ivey, K. J., Krause, W. J., Sherman, D., Burks, M. and Hewett, J. *Lab. Invest.* 1980, *42*, 420–426
69. Thomas, W. E. G. *Medical Hypotheses* 1980, *6*, 919–927
70. Tomkins, G. M. & Gelehrter, T. D. pp. 1–20 in Litwack, G. (ed.), *Biochemical actions of hormones*, vol II, New York Press, 1972
71. Wilcox, L. L., *Clin. Res.* 1977, *25*, 320 A
72. Witzel, L., Halter, F., Olah, A. J. & Häcki, W. H. *Gastroenterology* 1977, *73*, 797–803
73. Wünsch, E., Moroder, L. Gemeiner, M., Jaeger, E., Ribet, A., Pradayrol, L. & Vaysse, N., *Z. Naturforsch,* 1980, *35b*, 911–919
74. Zalewsky, C. A. & Moody, F. G. *Gastroenterology* 1977, *73*, 66–74

Autonomic Nerves of the Gut

# Development of the Intrinsic Innervation of the Gut

P. COCHARD & N. M. LE DOUARIN

Institut d'Embryologie du CNRS et du Collège de France, 49 bis, Avenue de la Belle-Gabrielle, 94130 Nogent-sur-Marne, France

The quail-chick chimera system has been used to study the ontogeny of the enteric nervous system. By the isotopic and isochronic grafting of fragments of the neural primordium between quail and chick embryos, the pattern of migration of the precursor cells of the enteric ganglia could be determined. The intrinsic innervation of the gut was shown to arise from precise levels of the neural axis, while other axial levels of the neural crest gave rise to sympathetic chains and the adrenal medulla. The normal appearance and subsequent development of cholinergic and peptidergic traits in enteric ganglioblasts were studied using biochemical and histochemical methods. The initial expression of these phenotypic characters was detected early in development and followed a rostro-caudal pattern along the gut. The mechanisms governing the chemical differentiation of enteric neurons were investigated through various experimental procedures. Changing the pattern of crest cells migration in the embryo demonstrated that the fate of the precursor cells of the autonomic nervous system is not irreversibly determined in the crest. For example, cholinergic enteric neurons can develop from any given level of the neural crest. The decisive role of environmental factors arising from non-neuronal tissues on neurotransmitter phenotypic expression in autonomic ganglioblasts was evidenced by in vivo culture experiments on the chick chorioallantoic membrane. Extraintestinal migration of neural crest cells and the presence of central preganglionic fibres are not required for the differentiation of enteric ganglia. The gut mesenchyme, by itself, constitutes an appropriate environment for the development of cholinergic characters in crest cells. Factors regulating expression of the adrenergic phenotype in neural crest cells were also studied. Dorsal mesodermal structures are not the only substrates in which adrenergic differentiation can occur. However, the role of the notochord in eliciting the expression of this phenotype appears essential. The existence in the mammalian gut of a population of cells that transiently express a variety of adrenergic characters suggests that initial appearance and persistence of this phenotype are regulated by different factors.

*P. Cochard, Institut d'embryologie du CNRS et du Collège de France, 49 bis Avenue de la Belle-Gabrielle, 94130 Nogent-sur-Marne, France*

## INTRODUCTION

The development of the enteric nervous system and of the sympathetic innervation of the gut depends entirely on a transitory embryonic structure, the neural crest. The neural crest arises from the lateral ridges of the neural plate and after an extensive migration in the developing embryo, neural crest cells differentiate into a variety of cell types. Among the neural crest derived structures are bones, cartilages and dermis in the face, endocrine and paraendocrine elements, all the pigment cells of the body except those of the retina and practically all the cells of the peripheral nervous system, including neurons and supportive cells of the autonomic nervous system (see reviews by Hörstadius, 37; Weston, 85 and Le Douarin, 53–55).

Considerable effort has been focused in recent years to elucidate the mechanisms which underly the transformation of undifferentiated and apparently identical neural crest cells into the various cell types constituting the autonomic nervous system.

As for other parts of the autonomic nervous system, the formation of the intrinsic innervation of the gut raises several problems concerning the migratory behavior and differentiation capabilities of presumptive enteric neurons as well as the regulation of neurotransmitter phenotypic expression in enteric neuroblasts. In our laboratory a series of researches have been devoted to the ontogeny of enteric innervation. They were based on the use of a stable cell marking technique (50–52) and have led to significant advances in our knowledge. The embryological origin and the migration pathways of enteric neuron precursors have been determined; the degree of commitment of neural crest cells prior to their migration and the role of the environment in the acquisition of a specific neuronal phenotype have been examined in a series of experiments involving in vivo and in vitro transplantations of neural crest cells and neural crest derivatives.

In addition, the biochemical and structural modifications taking place along the course of the development of enteric nerve cells have been studied through the use of appropriate biochemical and cytochemical markers.

## A. *The origin of enteric ganglioblasts*

Although enteric ganglia have long been recognised to derive from the neural crest, the precise level of origin along the neural axis of their precursor cells and the migration pathways they follow have been a controversial matter. Some authors considered the vagal level of the neural primordium to be the only source of enteric ganglia (87–90) while others attributed a role in their constitution to the trunk neural anlage as well (1, 2, 5–8, 45, 80, 81–83).

As a prerequisite to the analysis we undertook of the mechanisms controlling autonomic nerve cell differentiation it was necessary to reinvestigate the question of their origin in normal development by using the quail-chick chimera system (58, 59).

The principle of this technique is based on differences in nuclear structures in the quail and chick species. Whereas in chick cell nuclei heterochromatin is distributed in several chromocentres, in the quail in contrast, it is highly condensed in a large mass associated with the nucleolus. Chimeric bird embryos can be constructed in ova by grafting neural primordia of quails into chicks or vice versa; identification of the grafted cells within host tissues is then possible at the light microscope level after DNA staining by the Feulgen-Rossenbeck technique (Fig. 1), and also at the electron microscope level whatever the duration of the chimeric association (50–52).

Isotopic and isochronic grafts of small fragments (corresponding to a length of four to six somites) of quail neural primordium into chick embryos were systematically performed along the whole length of the neural axis. The developmental stages of host and donor embryos were always identical and varied according to the level elected for the operation to ensure that neural crest cells had not started migrating at the time of the intervention. Thereafter, grafted crest cells were observed on serial sections of the digestive tract. A correspondence was established between the level of the graft and the definitive localisation of ganglion cells. Since these operations do not significantly disturb the course of development, the results give a reliable picture of normal ontogenetic processes. This allowed us to establish a fate map of the enteric ganglia and other autonomic structures on the neural crest (Fig. 2).

The intrinsic innervation of the gut was shown to arise from two different levels of the neural axis. The main contribution to enteric ganglia comes from the vagal region of the neural primordium, specifically corresponding to the level of somites 1 to 7. The neural crest from this region gives rise to all ganglion cells of both myenteric and submucous plexuses in the preumbilical gut, and to most of them in the post-umbilical intestine. The latter also receives a contribution, although somewhat discrete, from the lumbosacral level of the neural primordium, located posterior to the level of the 28th somite. This part of the neural axis is also the main source of the cells which constitute the nerve of Remak (59, 76).

Thus it appears that the cervical and dorsal parts of the neural primordium, located between somites 7 to 28, do not provide the developing gut with ganglionic cells. In fact, it was observed that neural crest cell migration in the trunk region

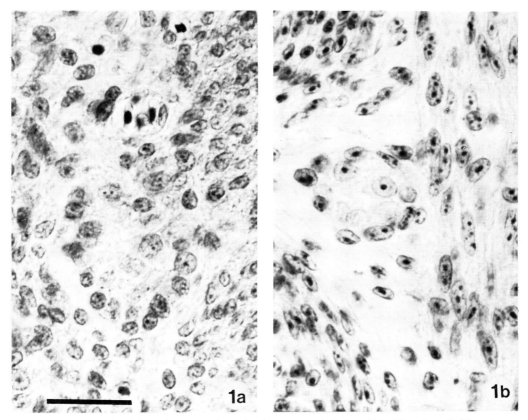

Fig. 1. Enteric ganglia of the submucous plexus in the rectum of 13-day chick (a) and quail (b) embryos. Feulgen-Rossenbeck's staining shows one or two large clumps of nucleolar heterochromatin in quail nuclei, while in the chick the chromatin is evenly distributed in the nucleoplasm with small dispersed chromocenters. Bar represents 20 μm.

was strictly confined to the doral mesenchymal region derived from the somites and intermediate cell mass. Except for the Schwann cells that followed the nerve bundles to the periphery, neural crest derivative distribution was restricted to the sensory and sympathetic chain ganglia, the aortic and adrenal plexuses and the adrenomedullary cords. No cells were ever found in the mesonephros or the gonads, but of more importance is the fact that they did not penetrate the dorsal mesentery.

At the vagal level of the neural primordium, neural crest cells migrate massively in a ventral direction, into the mesodermal wall of the foregut. The duration of crest cell emigration from the neural primordium was investigated by performing isotopic and isochronic grafts at progressively older stages. The migration of crest

cells from the vagal level starts around the 9–10 somite stage and is most active before the 13-somite stage. However crest cells still leave this region of the neural primordium until the 14–16 somite stage. Thereafter, they undergo a long cranio-caudal migration in the splanchnopleural wall of the gut down to the rectum. During the migration process, neural crest cells appear dispersed within the loose mesenchymal tissue. A precise timing of the migration was established. At stage 17 of Hamburger and Hamilton (32), i.e. at $2\frac{1}{2}$ days of incubation, vagal neural crest cells are dispersed within the mesenchyme of the fore-gut. One day later, at stage 20, they have reached the level of the hepatopancreatic ducts. At about 5 days of incubation the front of the migration is observed at the level of the umbilicus. The colorectum is not fully colonised before 8

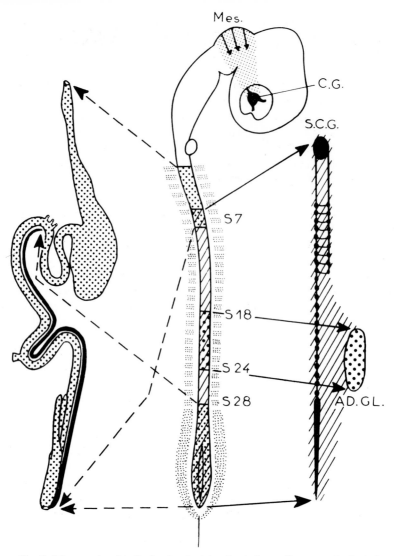

Fig. 2. Diagram showing the levels of origin of enteric ganglia, sympathetic chains and plexuses and ciliary ganglion on the neural crest. The vagal level of the neural crest (from somites 1–7) provides all the enteric ganglia of the preumbilical gut and contributes to the innervation of the post-umbilical gut. The lumbosacral level of the neural crest gives rise to the ganglion of Remak and some ganglion cells of the postumbilical gut. The ciliary ganglion arises from the mesencephalic crest. The sympathetic chain and plexuses are derived from the entire length of the neural crest posterior to the 5th somite, and the adrenomedullary cells originate from the level of somites 18–24. ADLG, adrenal gland; SCG, superior cervical ganglion; S, somite; RG, ganglion of Remak; CG, ciliary ganglion; Mes, mesencephalic crest.

days. Our results are in agreement with the observations of Allan and Newgreen (4) who followed the progression of enteric precursor cells by transplanting defined portions of the gut of chick embryos on the chorio-allantoic membrane (CAM) and by looking subsequently for the presence of nerve cells in the explants.

Migration of neural crest cells from the lumbosacral region to the postumbilical intestine has been observed in the two kinds of grafts, i.e. quail neural primordium into chick embryo and vice versa. The presumptive neuroblasts of the lumbosacral region do not invade the gut wall before 7–8 days of incubation (59).

As mentioned above, the main parasympathetic structure arising from the lumbosacral crest is the ganglion of Remak. The ontogeny of this ganglion found only in birds, has been the subject of a detailed study by Teillet (76). The primordium of the ganglion of Remak was selectively labelled by means of a graft of quail neural primordium at the lumbosacral level of a chick embryo, (76). Subsequently, the complex consisting of colorectum plus mesorectum containing the labelled primordium of the Remak ganglion was taken from the chimeric host at 5 days of incubation and grafted onto the CAM of a chick host for 10 days. Passage of ganglioblasts from the ganglion of Remak to the gut was observed, indicating that at least part of the lumbosacral ganglionic supply to the hind gut intramural innervation migrated through the ganglion of Remak, in which crest cells stop for a while before undertaking the last part of their ventral progression.

B. *Ontogenetic appearance of neurotransmitters and neurohumoral factors in the enteric nervous system*

From observations in recent years, based on pharmacological, histochemical, biochemical and immunohistochemical grounds, the diversity of neuronal cell types in the enteric nervous system has been well documented (see 10, 25, 27 and this supplement). In particular, an increasing number of neurotransmitter candidates have been identified in the gut plexuses. Apart from classical neurotransmitters such as acetylcholine (ACh) (18) and noradrenaline (NA) (65), putative transmitter substances include 5-hydroxytryptamine (28, 29, 86), adenosine-5'-triphosphate (9) and a number of neuropeptides: substance P, somatostatin, vasoactive intestinal polypeptide (VIP), enkephalin, gastrin-cholecystokinin and their tetrapeptide, neurotensin and bombesin (see 25, 35 for references).

Although relatively few studies have been so far devoted to the development of neurotrans-

mitters in enteric plexuses, it has been shown that the various substances that have been identified appear according to a sequential pattern.

In chick and quail embryos, the appearance and development of cholinergic traits have been followed in the intestine, using biochemical and histochemical techniques (73). The marker enzymes of cholinergic neurons, choline acetyltransferase (CAT) and acetylcholinesterase (AChE) are detectable soon after the appearance of enteric ganglioblasts in a given region of the gut, i.e. at 6 and 7 days of incubation in the chick duodenum and hind-gut, respectively, thus recapitulating the antero-posterior migration of enteric neuron precursor cells within the gut. CAT specific activity increases rapidly thereafter and reaches a maximum at 14 days in the duodenum and 19 days in the colorectum. Similar observations have been made in the quail. Thus it seems that cholinergic traits appear early and develop very rapidly in intramural ganglia.

On the other hand, the uptake of $^3$H-5-hydroxytryptamine, used to detect the presence of enteric serotonergic neurons, cannot be demonstrated in the chick duodenum before day 8–9 of incubation (20). Thus the ontogeny of cholinergic neurons precedes that of serotonergic nerve cells. The extrinsic adrenergic innervation of the gut is evidenced, either chemically (44) or through the transmitter uptake mechanism specific of adrenergic axons (20) from day 12. A similar ontogenetic sequence of neurotransmitters has been reported in the gut of mammalian embryos (30, 70).

The developmental patterns of peptide-containing nerves have been studied in embryonic mammalian (11, 33, 48, 49, 62) and avian guts (23, 56, 75).

It must be pointed out that experimental conditions for such studies vary greatly among workers. Thus the definition of a specific time of appearance of a given peptide in nerve cells also relies upon the sensitivity inherent to each technique. Nevertheless, it seems that the expression of peptidergic traits in enteric neurons occurs much later than that of the cholinergic metabolism (48, 75).

In chick and quail embryos, VIP and substance

P immunoreactivities appear sequentially along a cranio-caudal gradient from day 9 in the quail and day 10 in the chick. Substance P and VIP immunoreactive fibers are first visible in the fore gut and at 12 days extent over the whole length of the gut. VIP immunoreactive cell bodies are first observed in the oesophagus at day 9 in the quail embryo and day 10 in the chick embryo. The first substance P-containing nerve cell bodies are detected in 13-day-old quail and 14-day-old chick embryo (23).

To determine the origin of peptide-containing nerves, fragments of various parts of the digestive tract were transplanted on the CAM soon after the completion of neural crest cell migration (23). In agreement with the results of in vitro culture experiments of the embryonic mammalian gut (24, 38, 72), peptidergic neurons and nerve fibres developed in these conditions, indicating their intrinsic origin.

An interesting observation in these experiments is that a greater number of VIP- and substance P-immunoreactive neurons appeared in grafted guts as compared to control guts of the same age, suggesting that the potentiality to produce peptides is more widespread among enteric neurons than it seems to be in normal conditions. Similar observations have been reported in the cultured mouse embryonic gut (72).

The lack of central innervation for enteric ganglia in grafted guts might be responsible for the accumulation of peptides in cell bodies and nerve fibres.

Regardless of the mechanisms involved, the important number of peptide-containing neurons reinforces the idea that cholinergic and peptidergic functions may coexist in certain neurons, as it has been demonstrated for other peripheral and central nerve cells (see 36).

## C. Determination of transmitter function in developing neuroblasts

The variety of physiologically and morphologically distinct neural crest derivatives raises several questions about the mechanisms which control determination and differentiation of neural crest cells.

One aspect of this problem concerns the heterogeneity of the neural crest with respect to its fate as cholinergic parasympathetic and enteric neurons on the one hand and adrenergic sympathetic and paraganglionic cells on the other hand. Crest cells at each level of the neural axis could already be determined to a specific neurotransmitter metabolism before migration. Another alternative would be that they are pluripotent when they leave the neural primordium. In this case, the environment in which they become localised would orientate their differentiation to a specific cell type. The problem of the commitment and of the developmental capabilities of crest cells has been investigated through various experimental procedures.

1. *Multipotentiality of the autonomic precursor population along the neural axis.* In the first series of experiments, neural primordia were transplanted heterotopically between quail and chick embryos. Neural crest cells of the adrenomedullary region, grafted at the vagal level, were able to colonise the gut (which they never do in normal development) and gave rise to functional cholinergic enteric ganglia. In the same way, presumptive enteric ganglioblasts from the vagal region of the neural primordium, when transplanted into the adrenomedullary area populated the adrenal gland and differentiated into adrenomedullary cells (57, 60).

An interesting observation was made in this last series of experiments. Some quail cells from the grafted vagal neural rudiment participated in the formation of enteric ganglia in the ileum and large intestine of the chick host. Since orthotopic grafting experiments showed that crest cells in the adrenomedullary region never normally penetrate the dorsal mesentery, a special migration pathway followed by these hind-brain crest cells cannot be invoked to explain this result. A possible alternative resides in the fact that at the cephalic level, the crest cell population is much more numerous than in the trunk. Therefore, after having filled all the available sites of arrest during their ventral migration in the dorsal mesenchyme, crest cells, subsequently, migrate further and colonise the gut. However at the present stage of our investigations no satisfactory answer can be given to this question.

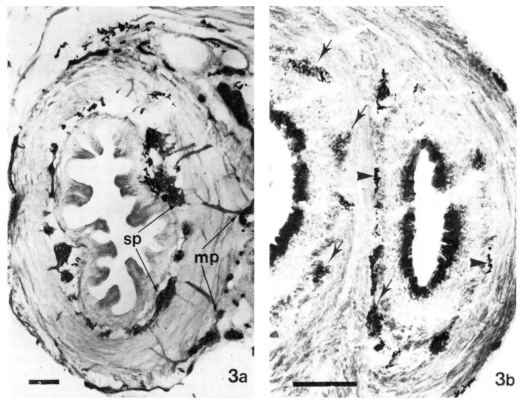

Fig. 3. Association of the quail vagal (a) and trunk (b) neural crest with the aneural colorectum of a chick (see Fig. 4). Culture of the explants for 8 days on the CAM of a chick: (a) well organised submucous (SP) and myenteric (MP) plexuses showing a strong AChE activity developed in the gut. (b) intense ChE reaction is evident in the cytoplasm of enteric ganglion cells (arrows). Note also the presence of pigment cells at the level of the nerve plexuses (arrow heads) Bars represent 100 μm.

Nevertheless, as far as crest cell colonisation of the adrenal gland and of the gut are concerned, the experiments reported above demonstrate that preferential pathways characterise the adreno-medullary as well as the vagal level of the neural axis, leading the cells to differentiate into adreno-medullary cells and enteric ganglia respectively. Consequently, the phenotypic expression of crest cells appears to be regulated by the environment they encounter after leaving the neural primordium. Moreover, the capacity to produce enteric ganglia, adrenergic neurons and paraganglionic cells is not confined to the areas from which they originate during the normal process of embryogenesis, but appears to be a property of all regions of the neural primordium tested so far.

2. *Influence of tissue environment on the chemical differentiation of autonomic neurons.* The non-commitment of autonomic precursor cells to their metabolic option (cholinergic or adrenergic) being demonstrated, we have concentrated on the analysis of the epigenetic influences that regulate transmitter choice after the onset of crest cell migration.

At first, we asked the question as to whether the environmental differentiating signals act on neural crest cells during their migration or when they are settled in their definitive location. In particular, it was of interest to know whether significant changes occurred in enteric neuron precursor cells during the extraintestinal phase of their migration or when they were settled in the gut itself. Experimental conditions were devised to suppress the phase of migration and to see what kind of transmitter the neuron would synthesise in this case.

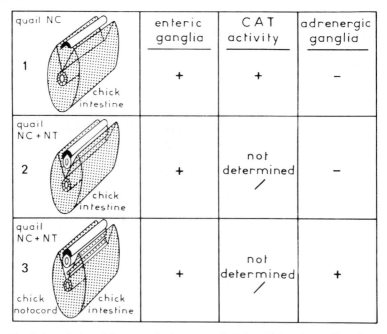

| quail NC<br>chick intestine | enteric<br>ganglia | CAT<br>activity | adrenergic<br>ganglia |
|---|---|---|---|
| **1** | + | + | − |
| quail<br>NC + NT<br>chick intestine<br>**2** | + | not<br>determined<br>/ | − |
| quail<br>NC + NT<br>chick notocord   chick intestine<br>**3** | + | not<br>determined<br>/ | + |

Fig. 4. Association of the aneural colorectum of a 5-day chick embryo with various dorsal trunk structures of 2-day embryos. (1) chick intestine plus quail neural crest (NC); (2) chick intestine plus quail neural crest and neural tube (NT); (3) chick intestine plus quail neural crest, neural tube, and chick notochord. Cholinergic ganglia develop in all cases. Adrenergic ganglia differentiate only in explants containing the notochord.

As described above, crest cells reach the hind gut at 7–8 days of incubation only. Thus the colorectum remains totally devoid of intrinsic innervation if it is removed from the embryo before this stage and subsequently cultured on the CAM (73). In different series of experiments, the aneural colorectum was associated with the neural primordium, i.e. neural tube plus neural crest, or with the neural crest alone, from vagal and trunk levels. The associated tissues were grafted for 7 to 15 days on the CAM. In all instances, we were able to show that enteric ganglia, exhibiting intense AChE activity, developed apparently normally, forming well organised myenteric and submucous plexuses (Fig. 3). In addition, when the crest alone was placed in the association, significant levels of CAT were measured in the explants (Fig. 4), irrespective of the level of the neural axis from which it was taken (73). In contrast, catecholamine (CA)-containing cells were never detected in the associations (73, 77). Furthermore, it was recently demon-strated by a physiological assay that the colorectum grown in similar conditions with the vagal neural anlage showed non-adrenergic, non-cholinergic inhibitory nervous activity, in addition to the expected cholinergic excitatory responses (64).

These results indicate that the initial phase of migration that the neural crest cells undergo to reach the gut has no significant influence in their orientation toward cholinergic metabolism. Moreover, the initial expression of the cholinergic phenotype seems independent of any influence of central nerve fibres since in the total absence of the spinal cord rudiment the autonomic neuronal precursors differentiate into neurons exhibiting significant levels of CAT and AChE activity. More likely is the alternative explanation that the environment of the gut itself is solely responsible for their cholinergic differentiation. On the other hand the gut mesenchyme is unable to provide appropriate conditions for the expression of the adrenergic phenotype.

The influence of tissue environment on adrenergic cell differentiation was analysed by several authors, again with the aim of determining if specific cues are received by sympathetic neuron precursor cells during their migration or in their sites of arrest.

Precursors of adrenergic cells migrate ventrally from the neural primordium, in close vicinity to the neural tube, notochord and somitic mesenchyme. In the chick embryo, CA are not detectable before and during this dorso-ventral migration but appear at 3.5 days of incubation in sympathoblasts after they have aggregated to form the primary sympathetic chains (3, 15, 19, 69). Similarly, using specific antisera directed against enzymes responsible for the biosynthesis of CA, it was shown in the rat embryo that noradrenergic characters were undetectable in the neural crest or in migrating crest cells. Tyrosine hydroxylase (TOH), dopamine-$\beta$-hydroxylase (DBH) and CA first appeared simultaneously at 11.5 days of gestation, soon after the aggregation of neuroblasts into the primitive sympathetic anlage (13, 14, 71, 78).

In experiments involving culture of trunk neural crest in association with various tissues on the CAM, Cohen (15) concluded that the future site of sympathoblast aggregation was not primordial in eliciting catecholaminergic cell differentiation. Thus crest cells expressed the adrenergic phenotype in response to environmental signals encountered during migration. In addition, he also showed that the somitic mesenchyme was essential in this process, cardiac or limb bud mesenchymes being unable to promote the appearance of CA-containing cells.

The importance of dorsal trunk structures, namely ventral neural tube, notochord and somites, in the expression of adrenergic traits was further examined by Norr (66) in in vitro organ cultures. Cellular contacts between somitic mesenchyme and neural crest were found to be necessary for the development of catecholaminergic cells. However, the somitic mesenchyme acquired its inductive capacity only after being previously conditioned by the neural tube and the notochord.

These results, and the fact that sympathoblasts develop in close vicinity of the notochord, prompted us to see whether this structure could, by itself, promote adrenergic cell differentiation (77). The aneural colorectum, taken from a chick embryo at 5 days of incubation, well before its colonisation by neural crest cells, was associated with the quail neural primordium from vagal or trunk levels and cultured on the CAM for 2 to 10 days.

As in experiments reported above (Figs. 3 and 4) crest cells migrated into the gut and constituted well developed myenteric and submucous plexuses, but never expressed the adrenergic phenotype. In some cases, however, CA-containing cells were found at some distance of the gut wall, along blood vessels of the CAM, but appeared in significant numbers only several days after the beginning of the graft.

In contrast, association of the notochord in the explant resulted in the appearance of groups of catecholaminergic cells along the developing circular muscle layer of the gut (Figs. 4 and 5). These cells were already present after 2 to 3 days of grafting (Fig. 6) and could still be evidenced 10 days after the beginning of the graft. We observed that there was a direct relationship between the occurrence of CA-containing cells in close vicinity of the gut wall and the amount of notochordal material included in the graft. In initial experiments a single fragment of notochord was grafted. Adrenergic cells developed along the gut wall in about 25% of the grafts (77). Additional experiments showed that the association of several fragments of notochord, or of a longer piece of this structure, increased the number of positive cases up to 80% (Cochard, Teillet and Le Douarin, unpublished results).

These findings do not confirm the exclusive ability of somitic and intermediate cell mass derived mesenchymes to induce adrenergic cell differentiation, as previously suggested (15, 66) since this process can occur in the splanchnopleural mesenchyme of the gut and in the CAM. On the other hand, the fundamental role of the notochord is demonstrated by its ability to promote the appearance of the adrenergic phenotype in an ectopic environment such as the gut mesenchyme where it is not normally expressed.

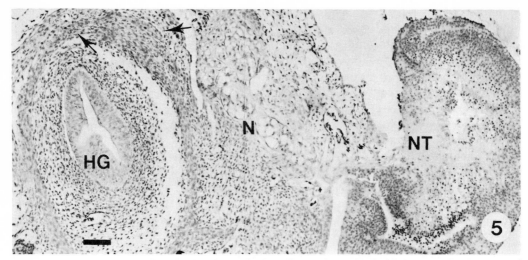

Fig. 5. Association of the quail cervicodorsal neural primordium and notochord with the aneural colorectum of a chick. Culture of the explant for 3 days on the chick CAM. The notochord (N) is found between the hind-gut rudiment (HG) and the neural tube (NT). Neural crest cells, having presumably migrated past the notochord, develop into enteric ganglia (arrows). Bar represents 100 μm.

In support of the preceding findings an interesting observation was made in the gut of mammalian embryos. As described above, CA and their synthesizing enzymes first appeared in cells of the primitive sympathetic anlage of the rat embryo at 11.5 days of gestation. In addition, immunoreactive cells for TOH and DBH (which also contained CA) were detected at this stage in the gut mesenchyme. However the adrenergic phenotype was only transiently expressed in these cells since they were not detected after the 14th gestational day (13, 14, 78, 79). To further characterise these cells and to study their fate, transmitter uptake experiments were performed (41). Those transitory adrenergic cells exhibited a high affinity uptake process specific for NA. Moreover, a population of cells with a similar transmitter uptake system was demonstrated in the gut at later stages, up to 17.5 days of gestation, suggesting that the disappearance of the catecholaminergic cells was not due simply to their death, but, more likely, that they lost some of their adrenergic traits, i.e. the capacity to synthesise CA, although keeping for several days the ability to take up NA.

Transient adrenergic cells with a similar developmental time course have also been found in the gut of the mouse embryo but we were unable to detect such cells in the avian gut (Cochard and Le Douarin, unpublished observations).

The time of appearance, morphology and location of these cells strongly suggest their neural crest origin. Their resemblance to sympathoblasts is further accentuated by the fact that they respond to nerve growth factor (43) and glucocorticoids (40) by expressing their CA synthetic activity at a higher level and for longer periods of time. It is thus possible that they express transiently the adrenergic phenotype as a result of interactions with the somite-notochord-neural tube complex that they meet during their dorso-ventral migration. However CA metabolism cannot be maintained in cells which home to the gut possibly because of the lack of the appropriate stimulation.

In any case, these observations indicate that the initial expression and the further maintenance of the adrenergic phenotype are regulated by different factors.

CONCLUSIONS

The experimental data reported in this article show that the intrinsic innervation of the gut arises

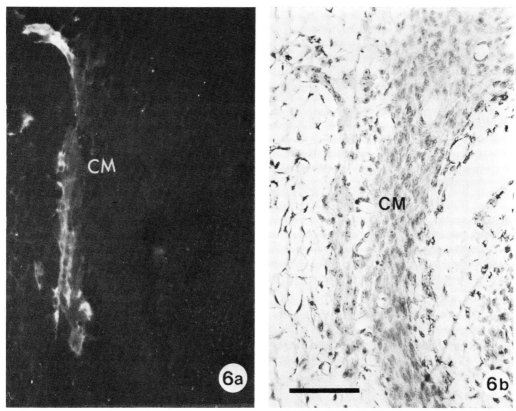

Fig. 6. Same experiment as in Fig. 5(a) already 3 days after the beginning of the graft groups of CA-containing cells, evidenced by the formaldehyde-induced-fluorescence technique, are found along the circular muscle layer of the gut (CM) at the level of the myenteric plexus (b) the same section, stained by Feulgen-Rossenbeck's technique, shows that adrenergic cells are of quail origin. Bar represents 50 μm.

from well defined areas of the neural crest. However, considerable homogeneity actually exists in the differentiating potentialities of the crest cell population and, in fact, the myenteric and submucous plexuses can be formed by cells of the cephalic or truncal level of the crest just as well as by their normal vagal precursors. Specific migration pathways lead the neural crest cells into the gut and other parts of the body and the sites of arrest for the precursors of the autonomic nervous system, for instance in the gut or in the adrenal medulla, are recognised equally well by crest cells arising from any region of the neural axis.

The in vivo experiments have shown that the microenvironment that neural crest cells meet during or at the end of their migration is of critical importance in influencing their ultimate phenotype. Moreover, such experiments have provided significant indications concerning the nature of the tissues or organs responsible for the regulation of the chemical differentiation of autonomic neurons.

The gut mesenchyme is, by itself, an appropriate environment for the differentiation of cholinergic neurons. As stated earlier in this review, enteric neuroblasts express cholinergic properties soon after they stop migrating. An early cholinergic mechanism has also been demonstrated in other parasympathetic ganglia (12, 47, 61) as well as in sympathetic (17, 34, 39, 68) and sensory ganglia (42, 63) and appears to be a general characteristic of differentiating neuroblasts (22). In fact, recent evidence in our laboratory indicates the presence of cholinergic traits at even earlier stages, in the neural crest itself. We have been able to show that mesencephalic crest cells in the process of migration convert $^3$H-choline to $^3$H-acetylcholine and that this transformation is due to CAT (74). Moreover, trunk crest cells that have migrated within the somitic environment also express cholinergic properties (21). Finally recent observations indicate the presence of AChE in crest cells from all axial levels, before and during their migration (Cochard, Coltey, Massoulié and Le Douarin, unpublished results). It is not known whether all or only some of the crest cells are concerned by the cholinergic metabolism. Nevertheless, assuming that an early cholinergic system exists in presumptive autonomic neurons, the influence of the environment on the cholinergic differentiation could not be considered any more as an inductive process. Cholinergic neurons would rather result from the stabilisation and increase of already acquired properties, via factors released by the environment (see the review by Patterson, 67).

As far as the adrenergic differentiation is concerned, it seems now clear that the expression of this phenotype depends upon a stimulus produced by trunk axial tissues, the notochord and neural tube being of decisive importance in the initiation of this process.

The ultimate isolation and characterisation of the factors involved in the regulation of neurotransmitter phenotypic expression can only be achieved by an in vitro approach.

Manipulation of the fluid environment in which dissociated neurons from the newborn rat superior cervical ganglion are growing has been shown to influence the choice of transmitter they synthesise. These elegant experiments (reviewed by Patterson, 67) have revealed the existence of a soluble factor, mediating the conversion of an adrenergic to a cholinergic phenotype. Its purification and biochemical characterisation are currently in progress (84). Moreover, during the switch in transmitter metabolism in culture, neurons with both adrenergic and cholinergic functions have been identified in single-cell cultures (26, 46).

The morphological and biochemical differentiation of neural crest cells grown in various culture conditions are currently studied in our laboratory. Neural crest cells cultured in the virtual absence of cells from other embryonic structures achieve a certain degree of biochemical differentiation characterised by the synthesis of ACh and CA, thus confirming the bipotentiality of the crest cell population along the neural axis (21, 91). The amount of neurotransmitter synthesised can be increased by co-culturing crest cells with a variety of embryonic tissues. In this respect, it is interesting to note that hind-gut mesenchyme is the only tissue able to stimulate ACh synthesis in mesencephalic crest cells in the presence of fetal calf serum, while somitic mesenchyme is the most effective stimulator of adrenergic differentiation in truncal crest cultures. The composition of the culture medium is also of importance in regulating the ratio of ACh to CA production in a given culture: horse serum was found to stimulate ACh synthesis, while foetal calf serum preferentially enhanced CA production. These studies, together with those of other workers (16, 31; see also the review by Le Douarin, 55) also confirm that the chemical differentiation of the autonomic neuroblasts is highly dependent upon the environment in which they grow and strongly suggests that direct intercellular contact with non-neural tissues might not be essential for regulating neurotransmitter synthesis.

## ACKNOWLEDGEMENTS

This work was supported by the CNRS, DGRST and by NIH research grant RO1 DEO 4257 03 CBY.

## REFERENCES

 1. Abel W. Proc R Soc Edinb 1909, 30, 327–347
 2. Abel W. J Anat Physiol, Paris 1912, 47, 35–72
 3. Allan IJ, Newgreen DF. Am J Anat 1977, 149, 413–421
 4. Allan IJ, Newgreen DF. Am J Anat 1980, 157, 137–154
 5. Andrew A. J Anat 1964, 98, 421–428
 6. Andrew A. J Anat 1969, 105, 89–101
 7. Andrew A. J Anat 1970, 107, 327–336
 8. Andrew A. J Anat 1971, 108, 169–184
 9. Burnstock G. Pharmac Rev 1972, 24, 509–581
10. Burnstock G. pp 406–414 in Burnstock G, Gershon MD, Hökfelt T, Iversen LL, Kosterlitz HW, Szur-

szewski JH (eds). Neurosciences Research Program Bulletin, vol 17, Non-adrenergic, noncholinergic autonomic neurotransmission mechanisms. Cambridge, The MIT Press 1979

11. Chayvialle SA, Myata M, Rayford PI, Thompson JC. Gastroenterology 1980, 79, 837–843
12. Chiappinelli V, Giacobini E, Pilar G, Uchimura H. J. Physiol 1976, 257, 749–766
13. Cochard P, Goldstein M, Black IB. Proc Natl Acad Sci USA 1978, 75, 2986–2990
14. Cochard P, Goldstein M, Black IB. Develop Biol 1979, 71, 100–114
15. Cohen AM. J Exp Zool 1972, 179, 167–182
16. Cohen AM. Proc Nat Acad Sci USA 1977, 74, 2899–2903
17. Coughlin MD, Dibner MD, Boyer DM, Black IB. Develop Biol 1978, 66, 513–528
18. Dale HH. J Mt Sinai Hosp 1937, 4, 401–415
19. Enemar A, Falck B, Hakanson R. Develop Biol 1965, 11, 268–283
20. Epstein ML, Sherman D, Gershon MD. Develop Biol 1980, 77, 22–40
21. Fauquet M, Smith J, Ziller C, Le Douarin NM. J Neurosci 1981, 1, 478–491
22. Filogamo G, Marchisio PC. Neurosci Res 1971, 4, 29–64
23. Fontaine-Perus J, Chanconie M, Polak JM, Le Douarin NM. Histochemistry 1981, 71, 313–323
24. Franco R, Costa M, Furness JB. Naunyn Schmiedebergs Arch Pharmacol 1979, 307, 57–63
25. Furness JB, Costa M. Neurosci 1980, 5, 1–20
26. Furshpan EJ, MacLeish PR, O'Lague PH, Potter DD. Proc Natl Acad Sci 1976, 73, 4225–4229
27. Gershon MD. Ann Rev Neurosci 1981, 4, 227–272
28. Gershon MD, Dreyfus CF. pp 197–206 in Brooks FP, Evers PW. (eds). Nerves and the Gut. CB Slack and NJ Thorofare 1977
29. Gershon MD, Dreyfus VM, Pickel VM, Joh TH, Reis DJ. Proc. Natl Acad Sci US 1977, 74, 3086–3089
30. Gershon MD, Thompson EB. J Physiol (London) 1973, 234, 257–278
31. Greenberg JH, Schrier BK. Develop Biol 1977, 61, 86–93
32. Hamburger V, Hamilton HL. J Morphol 1951, 88, 49–92
33. Helmstaedter V, Taugner CM, Feurle GA, Forssman WG. Histochemistry 1977, 53, 35–41
34. Hill CE, Hendry IA. Neurosci 1977, 2, 741–750
35. Hökfelt T, Johansson O, Ljungdahl A, Lundberg JM, Schultzberg M. Nature 1980a, 284, 515–521
36. Hökfelt T, Lundberg JM, Schultzberg M, Johansson O, Ljungdagk A, Rehfeld J. pp 1–24 in Costa E, Trabucchi M (eds). Neural peptide and neuronal communication, Adv Biochem Psychopharmacol 22, Raven Press, NY 1980b
37. Hörstadius S. Oxford University Press, London and New York 1950
38. Jessen KR, Van Noorden D, Bloom SR, Burnstock G. Nature 1980, 283, 391–393
39. Johnson M, Ross D, Meyers M, Rees R, Bunge R, Wakshöll E, Burton H. Nature 1976, 308–310
40. Jonakait GM, Bohn MC, Black IB. Science 1980, 210, 551–553
41. Jonakait GM, Wolf J, Cochard P, Goldstein M, Black IB. Proc Natl Acad Sci USA 1979, 76, 4683–4686
41. Karczmar AG, Nishi S, Minota S, Kindel G. Gen Pharmacol 1980, 11, 127–134
43. Kessler JA, Cochard P, Black IB. Nature 1979, 280, 141–142
44. Konaka S, Ohashi H, Okada T, Takewaki T. Brit J Pharmacol 65, 257–260
45. Kuntz A. The autonomic nervous system. London, Baillière, Tindall and Cox, pp 117–134
46. Landis SC. Proc Natl Acad Sci 1976, 73, 4220–4224
47. Landmesser L, Pilar G. Fiedn Proc 1978, 37, 2016–2022
48. Larsson LI. Histochemistry 1977, 54, 173–176
49. Larsson LI, Fahrenkrug J, Schaffalitzky de Muckadell OB, Sundler F, Hakanson R, Rehfeld JF. Proc Nat Acad Sci USA 1976, 73, 3197–3200
50. Le Douarin N. Bull Biol Fr Belg 1969, 103, 435–452
51. Le Douarin N. Ann Embryol Morph 1971, 4, 125–135
52. Le Douarin N. Develop Biol 1973, 30, 217–222
53. Le Douarin N. Med Biol 1974, 52, 281–319
54. Le Douarin N. Current Topics in Developmental Biology 1980, 16, 31–85
55. Le Douarin NM. 1982, Cambridge University Press, in press
56. Le Douarin NM, Fontaine-Pérus J. pp 107–118 in Bloom SR, Polak JM (eds). Gut Hormones, 2nd edition, Churchill Livingstone 1981
57. Le Douarin NM, Renaud D, Teillet MA, Le Douarin GH. Proc Natl Acad Sci USA 1975, 72, 728–732
58. Le Douarin N, Teillet MA. C.R. Acad Sci 1971, 273, 1411–1414
59. Le Douarin N, Teillet MA. J Embryol exp Morph 1973, 30, 31–48
60. Le Douarin N, Teillet MA. Develop Biol 1974, 41, 162–184
61. Le Douarin NM, Teillet MA, Ziller C, Smith J. Proc Natl Acad Sci USA 1978, 75, 2030–2034
62. Lehy T, Gres L, Ferreira de Castro E. Cell Tissue Res 1979, 198, 325–333
63. Marchisio PC, Consolo S. J Neurochem 1968, 15, 759–764
64. Newgreen DF, Jahnke I, Allan IJ, Lewis Gibbins I. Cell Tissue Res 1980, 208, 1–19
65. Norberg KA. Int J Neuropharmacol 1964, 3, 379–382
66. Norr SC. Develop Biol 1973, 34, 16–38
67. Patterson PH. Ann Rev Neurosci 1978, 1, 1–17
68. Ross D, Johnson M, Bunge R. Nature 1977, 267, 536–539
69. Rothman TP, Gershon MD, Holtzer H. Dev Biol 1978, 65, 322–341
70. Rothman TP, Ross LL, Gershon MD. Brain Res 1976, 115, 437–456
71. Rothman TP, Specht LA, Gershon MD, Joh TH, Teitelman G, Pickel VM, Reis DJ. Proc Natl Acad Sci USA 1980, 77, 6221–6225
72. Schultzberg M, Dreyfus C, Gershon MD, Hökfelt T, Elde RP, Nilsson G, Said S, Goldstein M. Brain Res 1978, 155, 239–248

73. Smith J, Cochard P, Le Douarin NM. Cell Diff 1977, 6, 199–216
74. Smith J, Fauquet M, Le Douarin NM. Nature 1979, 282, 853–855
75. Sundler F, Alumets J, Fahrenkrug J, Hakanson R, Schaffalitzky de Muckadell OB. Cell Tissue Res 1979, 196, 193–201
76. Teillet MA. Wilhelm Roux's Arch 1978, 184, 251–268
77. Teillet MA, Cochard P, Le Douarin NM. Zoon 1978, 6, 115–122
78. Teitelman G, Baker H, Joh TH, Reis DJ. Proc Natl Acad Sci USA 1979, 76, 509–513
79. Teitelman G, Joh T, Reis DJ. Brain Res 1978, 158, 229–234
80. Uchida S. Acta Sch med Undiv Kioto 1927, 10, 63–136
81. Van Campenhout E. C.R. Ass Anat Amsterdam, XXVe réunion 1930, pp 74–78
82. Van Campenhout E. Arch Biol Paris 1931, 42, 479–507
83. Van Campenhout E. Phys Zool 1932, 5, 333–353
84. Weber MJ. J Biol Chem 1981, 256, 3447–3453
85. Weston JA pp 41–114, in Abercrombie M, Brachet J, King T. (eds). Advances in Morphogenesis, Academic Press, New York 1970
86. Wood JD, Mayer CJ. J Neurophysiol 1979, 42, 582–593
87. Yntema CL, Hammond WS. J Exp Zool 1945, 100, 237–263
88. Yntema CL, Hammond WS. Biol Rev Cambridge Phil Soc 1947, 22, 344–359
89. Yntema CL, Hammond WS. J Comp Neurol 1954, 101, 515–541
90. Yntema CL, Hammond WS. J exp Zool 1955, 129, 375–414
91. Ziller C, Smith J, Fauquet M, Le Douarin NM. Prog Brain Res 1979, 51, 59–74

# On the Ultrastructure of the Enteric Nerve Ganglia*

G. GABELLA
Dept of Anatomy, University College London,
Gower Street, London, England

This brief article reviews some aspects of the ultrastructure of the enteric ganglia which have been brought to light by electron microscopy. The ganglion neurons are surrounded by a vast neuropil in which axons, dendrites and glial cells with their processes are tightly packed together. Blood vessels and connective tissue do not penetrate into the ganglia but lie outside them. The exclusion of connective tissue from the ganglia takes place during embryonic development and is complete soon after birth. By ultrastructural criteria it has proven difficult to classify neuronal cell types, in spite of the differences in their functional specializations and their projections. The glial cells are rich in gliofilaments and have processes which are firmly anchored to the surface of the ganglion. Glial cells outnumber ganglion neurons and probably confer structural stability to the ganglia and at the same time allow substantial changes in the shape of the ganglia and in the arrangements of its elements to occur when the adjacent muscle layers contract. Numerous specialized contacts are found between vesicle-containing nerve endings and glial cell bodies or glial processes. The question of how freely substances diffuse inside a ganglion, along the narrow spaces between processes and cell bodies, remains to be answered. Since parts of the surface of many neurons are directly covered by the basal lamina of the ganglion and by connective tissue, certain substances of the interstitial space may have direct access to the nerve cells. Investigations on the intraganglionic nerve endings have provided several classifications of axonal types, mainly based on the appearance of their vesicles. However, these classifications are tentative and are in many respects still uncertain. The great majority of endings originate from intrinsic neurons and synaptic specializations are commonly encountered.

G. Gabella, Dept of Anatomy, University College London, Gower Street, London, England

When the structure of the intestinal innervation began to be studied by electron microscopy, it came as no surprise that it was extremely varied and complex. All the morphological studies during nearly a century had clearly pointed to this conclusion, and there has never been any doubt that the nervous system of the gut is special in many respects and lies in a class quite different to the nerves of other viscera and blood vessels. Nerves are abundantly distributed through the whole wall of the gastro-intestinal tract, but the brain of the system are the nerve ganglia of the submucosal and the myenteric plexus, situated in the submucosa and within the muscle coat.

The ganglia of the myenteric plexus are connected by nerve strands and form a mesh which extends without interruptions from the oesophagus to the terminal part of the large intestine. The plexus has a characteristic pattern in each portion of the gastrointestinal tract, but in the transition zones (e.g. between oesophagus and stomach, or stomach and duodenum, or ileum and caecum, or duodenum and bile duct) it extends without discontinuity from one segment to the other. The ganglia are not always well individualized. Where they are large and numerous (e.g. in the guinea-pig proximal colon) they merge with each other forming a sort of fenestrated neuronal sheet; conversely, ganglia can be scattered along nerve strands which run circumferentially, parallel to the circular musculature (e.g. in the rat ileum). Single neurons can be found in the strands of the plexus. The plexus is

* A more detailed survey of the topics covered in this article can be found in a review paper by the same author in Physiology of the Gastrointestinal Tract, edited by L. R. Johnson, 1981, pp 197–241, Raven Press, New York.

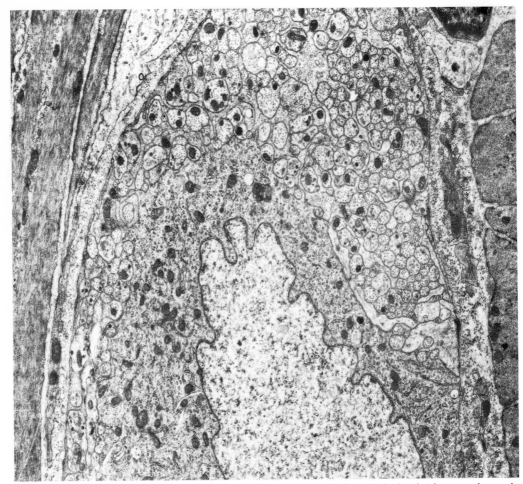

Fig. 1. Electron micrograph of the myenteric plexus of a guinea-pig. To the right is the circular musculature, in transverse section, to the left the longitudinal musculature, in longitudinal section. The ganglion displays a nerve cell with a crenated nucleus. In an area the cell membrane reaches the surface of the ganglion and is directly apposed to the basal lamina (bottom right). The neuron is surrounded by a neuropil with numerous neurites and glial processes. Around the ganglion are collagen fibrils and processes of interstitial cells. Magnification: 10,700 ×.

confined to the space between circular and longitudinal muscle layers, where presumably certain mechanical conditions prevail. It makes its appearance as a plexus during the embryonic life at the outer surface of the circular layer before a longitudinal muscle differentiates; the latter develops at a later stage and covers the outer surface of the plexus and the circular muscle.

Viewed in the electron microscope, the ganglia of the myenteric plexus display a compact structure with tightly packed cells and cell processes (Fig. 1). The ganglia are well separated from the muscle cells, and connective tissue, capillaries, fibroblasts, interstitial cells and other cell types lie outside them (Figs. 1, 2). There are rare exceptions to this arrangement in larger animal species, such as cat, man and sheep, where some of the largest ganglia may contain minute septa of connective tissue cutting across the ganglia. In the guinea-pig myenteric plexus the exclusion of the connective tissue from the plexus takes place gradually during development. In late embryonic stages "islands" of collagen fibrils are still found inside some ganglia, and they disappear only after

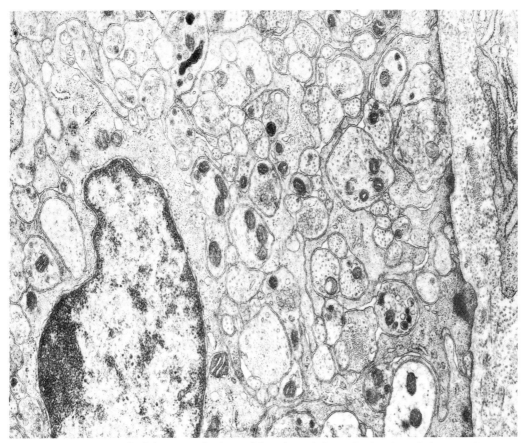

Fig. 2. Electron micrograph of the myenteric plexus of the guinea-pig ileum. Section through the neuropil. A glial cell (rich in gliofilaments and with a nucleus of characteristic appearance) and several neural and glial processes are visible. Collagen and a basal lamina invest the ganglion. At the surface of the ganglion there are vesicle-containing nerve endings and glial processes. The latter display conspicuous electron dense material which is penetrated by gliofilaments. Magnification: 19,500 ×.

birth. In embryonic ganglia there are numerous direct appositions of muscle cells and elements of the ganglia. These appositions disappear too, while the amount of connective tissue surrounding the ganglia increases, but occasionally muscle cells directly abutting on the ganglion surface can still be found in adult animals.

The two major cell types within the ganglia are ganglion neurons and glial cells. Their morphology is distinctive and characteristic in light micrographs (Fig. 3) and in low-power electron micrographs (Figs. 1, 2). The shape of the cell, the size and texture of the nucleus, the electron density of the cytoplasm allow an immediate distinction of the two cell types. (The occurrence of other cell types, such as interstitial cells and possibly microglial cells within the ganglia is very rare and will not be discussed here.) The ratio of glial cells to neurons is particularly high in the myenteric plexus of the guinea-pig ileum; in the ganglia alone the glial cells are twice as numerous as ganglion neurons, and many more glial cells are found in the connecting strands. Glial cells appear relatively less numerous in the submucosal ganglia of the same region, and in the plexuses of other regions of the gut of the guinea-pig and other species, but they always outnumber nerve cells.

Because of their position between the muscle layers, the ganglia of the myenteric plexus are greatly affected by the mechanical activity in the

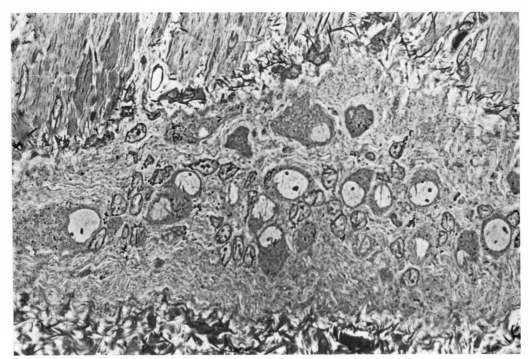

Fig. 3. Ganglion of the myenteric plexus of the rabbit caecum. Plastic section stained with thionine. The ganglion neurons are recognized by their dark cytoplasm and their large, vacuolar nucleus. The glial cells show only the nucleus, which is small and dark, and they outnumber the ganglion neurons. Collagen fibres and interstitial cells are interposed between the muscle layer and the ganglion. Magnification: 620 ×.

muscle, and this is clearly shown in their appearance. There are other intramural ganglia in the body, e.g. in the trigone of the bladder, in the atrial myocardium, in the musculature of the tongue, but these ganglia are well encapsulated and not so closely associated with the adjacent musculature and, therefore, less directly influenced by its contractile activity. To some extent this is also true of the submucosal ganglia, whereas the myenteric ganglia reflect in their changeable shape the degree of contraction in the surrounding muscle layers. In the fully distended intestine (e.g. in a segment of the distal colon around a fecal pellet) the ganglia are spread out and can measure only about 15 μm in thickness (Fig. 4); the neurons are flattened and arranged in a thin cell monolayer. Conversely, in the maximally contracted intestine (e.g. in a segment of the distal colon between two fecal pellets) the ganglia become 2–3 times thicker, their width is reduced and the neurons lie side by side and tend to form

a palisade (Fig. 4). It is not known whether this "message" of the myenteric ganglia produced by the contraction of the adjacent muscles does affect the neuronal activity, but the occurrence of this phenomenon should be kept in mind when considering the inputs to the ganglia.

The perikarya of some neurons are smooth-surfaced, but the majority of them are distinctly irregular in shape with deep invaginations and many cell processes. The myenteric ganglion neurons are plentiful: about 7,200 in every $cm^2$ of the ileum, and twice as many or more in the large intestine (15). By comparison with the guinea-pig, the neurons are more densely packed in smaller animal species (e.g. the mouse) and less densely packed in larger animal species (e.g. sheep and man), although the total number of neurons is somewhat related to the total volume of the intestinal musculature (10). This vast neuronal population is heterogeneous in all respects. Even a crude parameter such as the cell size varies

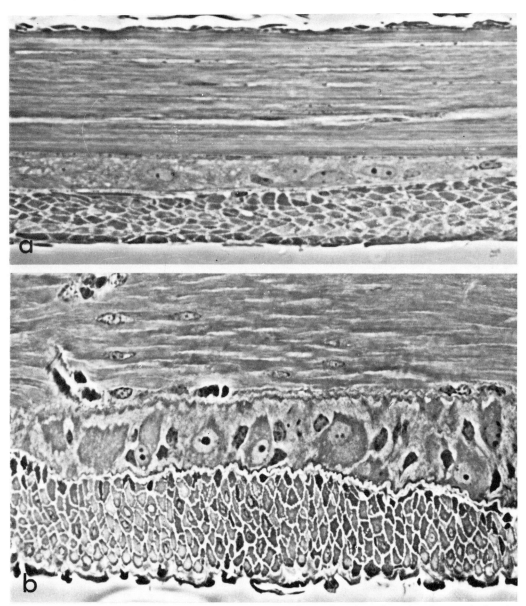

Fig. 4. Transverse sections through adjacent portions of the distal colon of a guinea-pig, photographed at the same magnification. *a.* a distended segment containing a fecal pellet; *b.* a contracted segment from a region between two fecal pellets. Note the difference in appearance of the muscle layers in the two conditions. When the muscle is fully contracted the shape of the ganglia and the arrangement of the neurons is markedly changed. Magnification: 620 ×.

over a wide range: in the myenteric plexus of the rat the areas of the nerve cell profiles span more than one order of magnitude. Increasingly, smaller neurons are more abundant in the small intestine, while a wider range of sizes and more

numerous large neurons are found in the stomach and distal colon, and the largest neurons are characteristic of the caecum (10).

The question of neuronal cell types in the enteric plexuses is obviously one of paramount

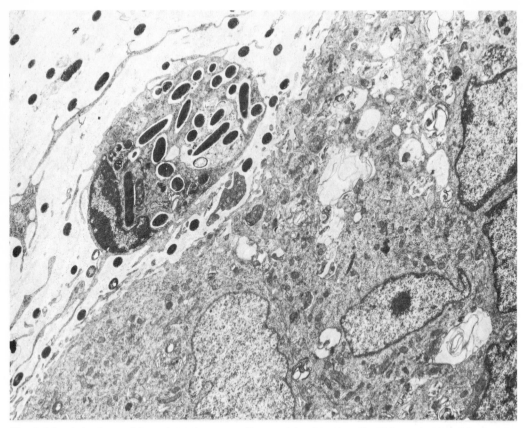

Fig. 5. Myenteric plexus of the guinea-pig caecum. From a strip of taenia coli which was incubated in vitro for 48 hr and was invaded by bacteria. Bacteria heavily infiltrated the muscle and the spaces around the ganglia. In the micrograph bacteria are visible in the top right corner, around the myenteric ganglion and inside a macrophage. In these experimental conditions, however, bacteria did not penetrate into the ganglia in spite of a certain disruption of the ganglionic fine structure related to the long incubation time. Magnification: 6,600 ×.

importance. Morphological classifications of the enteric neurons have been put forward ever since the end of the last century. In more recent times observations on the variability of the neuronal morphology and tentative classifications have been produced by several electron microscopists (3, 8, 9, 20, 21, 23). In spite of these efforts the question of neuronal cell types and their morphological correlates remains open. We are probably still lacking the proper descriptive bases on which a classification of neuronal types can be built. There are, of course, other forms of classification of the enteric neurons based on electrical properties and chemical composition. The recent developments of immunofluorescence studies on serotonine-containing neurons and

peptide-containing neurons are reported in other papers in this issue (see Bishop et al.; Furness et al.; Gershon et al.). They provide the most successful attempt, so far, at sorting out subpopulations of neurons and unravelling their projections. The electrophysiological studies have recognized two types of neurons: type 1 or S-neurons and type 2 or AH-neurons (characterized by a long-lasting hyperpolarization) (22). However, it has been shown that the two types cannot be clearly distinguished morphologically from one another, at least on the basis of size and shape of the soma and type of processes as identified after intracellular injection of a fluorescent dye (14). These studies are also interesting in that they allow to follow the axonal projections of

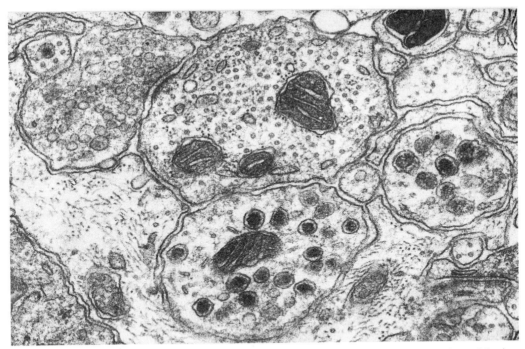

Fig. 6. Myenteric plexus of the proximal colon of a guinea-pig. A nerve ending with small agranular vesicles (top left) synapses on a dendrite; in the latter, mitochondria, microtubules, neurofilaments and endoplasmic reticulum are visible. Endings containing mainly large granular vesicles are also present. Magnification: 57,000 ×.

individual neurons, and have shown for example that there are at least twice as many aborally-directed processes as orally-directed ones (14). More refined data on the axonal projections of populations of neurons, as defined by the presence of a certain peptide, have been obtained by immunohistochemistry on stretch preparations of the guinea-pig ileum (4, 5, 6).

One remarkable feature of the ganglion neurons is that large areas of the surface of the perikaryon and of large dendrites are not covered by a glial sheath but lie directly beneath the basal lamina and the connective tissue surrounding the ganglion (Fig. 1). This arrangement is unique to the intramural ganglia (especially the myenteric plexus), since in other autonomic ganglia the perikarya are fully sheathed by satellite cells (in sympathetic ganglia only small areas of certain dendrites, where they contain clusters of vesicles, are directly exposed to the basal lamina and the connective tissue). Where the neuronal membrane of the myenteric neurons is lined externally by a basal lamina, it is associated with only a minute felt of intracellular microfilaments. On the contrary, the glial processes that reach the ganglion surface and abut on the basal lamina display conspicuous incrustations of electron-dense material which are anchored to the cytoplasmic surface of the cell membrane and receive insertion of large bundles of gliofilaments (11) (Fig. 7). The gliofilaments are a prominent component of the enteric glial cells (Fig. 2). These intermediate filaments are immunologically identical (17) to the gliofilaments found in astrocytes of the central nervous system (2). It has been suggested that the enteric glial cells, on account of their shapes and their richness in gliofilaments, may be important in conferring structural stability to the ganglia and at the same time allowing structural re-arrangement of the ganglia in the course of the muscular contraction (11).

The ganglia are made of nerve cells and of a complex neuropil, a term which includes all the neuronal processes and the glial cells with their

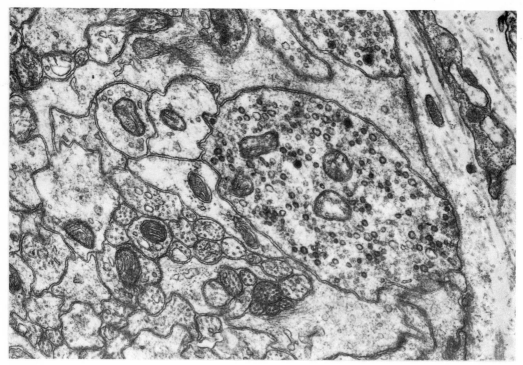

Fig. 7. Myenteric plexus of the guinea-pig caecum. From a strip of taenia coli incubated in vitro in the presence of 6-hydroxy-dopamine. A large nerve ending, partly exposed at the surface of the ganglion, contains numerous synaptic vesicles; most of these have either an electron dense granule or a membrane of enhanced electron density. The appearance of these vesicles is related to the uptake of the "false transmitter" and the ending is therefore interpreted as adrenergic. The nerve ending partly visible at the top shows no granularity and probably contains a different transmitter than the adrenergic ending. Magnification: 31,000 ×.

processes. All these structures are tightly packed together so that only a very narrow intercellular space is left, not unlike what is found in the central nervous system (Figs. 1, 2). For both tissues, however, the exact amount of the intercellular space present in vivo is still uncertain (for a discussion of the possibility that the spaces between cell processes in the central nervous system are much larger than usually thought, see ref. 7). How accessible are the small intercellular spaces of the myenteric ganglia to substances in the extracellular space around the ganglia? They *are* accessible, as can be shown in pharmacological experiments and by the use of extracellular space tracers. However, how easily nutrients and drugs penetrate into the ganglia and diffuse through the narrow spaces of the neuropil remains to be established. It is also not clear which substances gain direct access into the neuronal cell bodies

through the areas of the membrane exposed at the ganglion surface, and which go first through the glial cells. It seems likely that the very texture of the ganglia provides some limitation to the free diffusion of substances through the ganglia. Moreover, when bacteria invade the tissues of a long-term organ bath experiment (e.g. a taenia coli incubated in vitro for 48 hr), the bacteria infiltrate the muscle, are engulfed by muscle cells and phagocytes, and appear very numerous around the ganglia of the myenteric plexus, but are not found inside the ganglia themselves (Fig. 5). Gershon and Bursztajn (12) have recently put forward the interesting idea of a barrier between the blood and the myenteric plexus preventing leakage of tracers from the vasculature and into the plexus. However, the structural bases of this possible entity are not yet very clear. In other experimental conditions tracers penetrate into

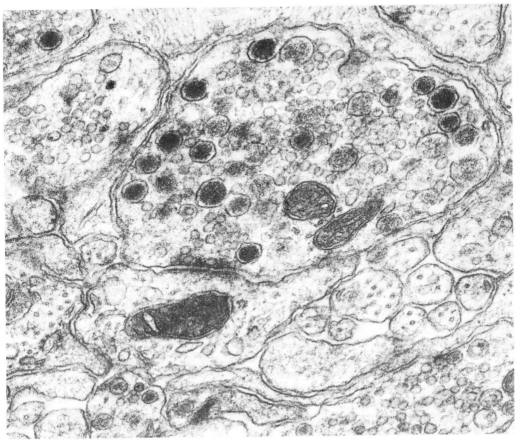

Fig. 8. Myenteric plexus of the proximal colon of the guinea-pig. A small dendrite receives a synapse from a nerve ending. The latter contains mitochondria, small clear vesicles and several large granular vesicles which vary markedly in size and electron density. Magnification: 57,000 ×.

and diffuse through the myenteric ganglia (16). Intramuscular capillaries are usually not fenestrated but in freeze-fracture preparations tight junctions in their endothelial cells are absent or poorly developed (at least in the guinea-pig ileum).

One of the most pressing questions facing the electron microscopists working on the enteric ganglia is that of recognizing and classifying the nerve endings of the neuropil. Since pharmacological studies indicate the occurrence of a variety of neurotransmitters in the enteric ganglia, the question of the morphological correlates of different types of nerve is one of considerable importance. When a classification of nerve endings as seen in the electron microscope is put foward it is assumed that there is a finite number of types of ending, that they are morphologically identifiable, and that they serve different functional roles. It is also generally assumed, although not specifically stated, that the neuronal circuit of the enteric plexuses are constructed according to a totally non-random plan. These assumptions are easily acceptable, although to what extent each of them is correct has not yet been established. In any part of a ganglion vesicle-containing axons are extremely numerous. The great majority of them, irrespective of the type of vesicle contained, are varicosities or ovoid expansion along the length of thin axons. It is likely that the terminal portions of most if not all the axons are beaded in shape and contain a very large number of "endings". The intervaricose segments of an axon can measure as little as 0.1 μm in diameter, and are mainly occupied by micro-tubules. All the nerve endings except a very small percentage of them are intrinsic in origin, i.e. they are axons issued by intramural neurons and are not altered after the extrinsic nerve supply to the gut is severed.

Some nerve endings, but not all, form synaptic junctions on the perikarya or on dendrites or on spines. Clear reciprocal synapses and axo-axonic synapses have not been identified; the occurrence of the axo-axonic synapses, however, cannot be ruled out, since in these ganglia the distinction between axons and dendrites is sometimes dubious and the post-synaptic process cannot always be identified with certainty. Moreover, axons are usually packed into bundles which are surrounded but not penetrated by glial cell pro-cesses, so that they lie close to each other; occa-sionally, nerve endings of different morphology are directly apposed to each other and, although synaptic specializations cannot be seen, the pos-sibility exists of a reciprocal influence. There is no evidence of the presence of electrical synapses, and gap junctions are not found between neuronal elements; some glial cells, however, display a few, small gap junctions. A large number of nerve endings are in contact with a glial cell or a glial process, and some of these endings show clus-tering of vesicles and localized thickening of the cell membrane. These structures cannot be described as synapses, but they represent special-ized axo-glial contacts, the significance of which is at present obscure (10).

The morphology of the nerve endings, in par-ticular their vesicle content, varies so widely that classifications have been and still are extremely difficult and uncertain and should be regarded at best as tentative. From three to eight or more types of endings have been identified by different investigators (1, 3, 8, 9, 21, 23) and still these classifications were not meant to be exhaustive. The morphological variety is slightly smaller if only the endings which form a clear synaptic junction are taken into account. However, those varicosities which lack synaptic specializations may be equally important in the traffic of impulses within the ganglia. Some synaptic endings contain almost exclusively small agranular vesicles, and

they are regarded as cholinergic (Fig. 6). These endings are likely to contain mainly acetylcholine, as their principal neurotransmitter, on the grounds of their structural similarity to cholinergic nerve endings at the motor endplates and in the sphincter pupillae and of the vast amounts of acetylcholine known to be stored and released by the myenteric plexus. These endings, however, are not numerous and cannot account for all the cholinergic endings one expects to find in a gan-glion. Many of the endings containing, beside a majority of small granular vesicles, a substantial number of large granular vesicles are probably also cholinergic. Whether these large granular vesicles contain substances, e.g. neural peptides, which are also released with acetylcholine is an interesting possibility which remains to be proven.

Endings with small granular vesicles are iden-tified as adrenergic on the basis of their structural similarity to adrenergic endings in other organs. They are numerous in the wall of the intestine; the granularity of their vesicles is enhanced by the use of an adrenergic "false transmitter" (Fig. 7); and they are all of extrinsic origin as they disappear after extrinsic denervation of the gut. In the myenteric ganglia the identification of adre-nergic endings by electron microscopy is compli-cated by the presence of other endings which are intrinsic and not adrenergic and have a mor-phology rather similar to adrenergic endings (13, 18). Studies on the sites of uptake of exogen-ous tritiated noradrenaline (10), on permanga-nate fixed tissues (19) and on the uptake of an adrenergic "false transmitter" (13, 18) suggest that the adrenergic endings of the myenteric plexus are mainly located near the surface of the ganglia.

Nerve endings in which large granular vesicles predominate are numerous in the myenteric plexus, especially in the large intestine. Various types of large granular vesicles can be distin-guished morphologically and some endings seem to contain a fairly uniform population of large granular vesicles. On this basis several types of endings have been described (3). Other endings contain a collection of large granular vesicles, heterogeneous in size and electron density, and their appearance is so characterstic that they probably constitute a neuronal cell type (9). All the nerve endings rich in large granular vesicles which form synaptic contacts contain in the immediately pre-synaptic area only small agranular vesicles (9) (Fig. 8).

In conclusion, the question of the morphological classification of nerve endings within the enteric plexuses remains considerably uncertain. Some types of nerve endings have been identified, others will soon be, particularly as immunochemical techniques are now successfully used at ultrastructural level (see Bishop et al., this issue). However, a somewhat skeptical attitude as regards the possibility of finding in the electron microscope the morphological correlates of the functionally different neuronal types and of the different nerve endings, it is not unreasonable. There are several other aspects of the ganglion structure (e.g. location of synapses, extent and pattern of dendritic arborization, origin of axons, distribution of varicosities, neuro-glial relations) which are also relevant to understanding its function and deserve further investigation.

## REFERENCES

1. Baumgarten HG, Holstein AF, Owman, CH. Z. Zellforsch 1970, 106, 376–397
2. Bignami A, Eng LF, Dahl D, Uyeda CT. Brain Res 1972, 43, 429–435
3. Cook RD, Burnstock G. J. Neurocytol 1976, 5, 171–194
4. Costa, M, Furness JB, Buffa R, Said SI. Neuroscience 1980, 5, 587–596
5. Costa M, Furness JB, Llewllyn-Smith IJ, Cuello AC. Neuroscience 1981, 6, 411–424
6. Costa M, Furness JB, Llewellyn-Smith IJ, Davies B, Oliver, J. Neuroscience 1980, 5, 841–852
7. Cragg B. Tissue & Cell 1980, 12 63–72
8. Fehér E, Vajda J. Acta morphol Acad Sci Hung 1972, 20, 13–25
9. Gabella G. J. Anat 1972, 111, 69–97
10. Gabella G. Int Rev Cytol 1979, 59, 129–193
11. Gabella G. Neuroscience 1981, 6, 425–436
12. Gershon MD, Bursztajn S. J. comp Neurol 1978, 180, 467–487
13. Gordon-Weeks PR. Neuroscience 1981, 6, 1793–1811
14. Hodgkiss HP, Lees GM. In: Gastrointestinal Motility (ed by J Christensen) 1980, 111–117, New York, Raven Press
15. Irwin DA. Am J Anat 1931, 49, 141–166
16. Jacobs JM. J Neurocytol 1977, 6, 607–618
17. Jessen KR, Mirsky R. Nature 1980, 286, 736–737
18. Llewellyn-Smith IJ, Wilson AJ, Furness JB, Costa M, Rush RA. J Neurocytol 1981, 10, 331–352
19. Manber L, Gershon, MD. Am J Physiol 1979, 236, E738–E745
20. Richardson KC. Am J Anat 1958, 103, 99–136
21. Taxi J. Ann Sci Nat Zool 1965, 7, 413–674
22. Wood JD. In: Physiology of the Gastrointestinal Tract (ed by LR Johnson) 1981, 1.37, New York, Raven Press
23. Yamamoto M. Arch histol jap 1977, 40, 171–201

# Serotonergic Neurotransmission in the Gut

M. D. GERSHON
Dept. of Anatomy and Cell Biology, Columbia University College of Physicians and Surgeons, 630 West 168th Street, New York, New York 10032, USA

Serotonin (5-hydroxytryptamine; 5-HT) was first suggested to be a neurotransmitter in the enteric nervous system (ENS) by Gershon, Drakontides, and Ross in 1965 (38); however, it has not been until recently that 5-HT has finally satisfied all of the criteria necessary for proof of its transmitter role. 5-HT has now been shown by biochemical, histochemical, and immunocytochemical techniques to be present in enteric neurons. The amine has also been demonstrated to be released from stimulated enteric neurons by a $Ca^{+2}$-dependent mechanism. The enteric neurons that contain 5-HT synthesize the amine from the dietary amino acid L-tryptophan. A specific, high-affinity uptake mechanism for 5-HT is another feature of enteric serotonergic neurons and probably serves as an inactivating mechanism for the amine. Physiologically, evidence derived by Wood and Mayer (103) from studies with intracellular microelectrodes indicates that 5-HT mimics the action of the transmitter responsible for eliciting slow epsps in one of the types of enteric neuron (the AH cell). In addition, Julé has determined that enteric serotonergic neurons are involved in the descending suppression of vagal excitation of the gut that accompanies peristalsis (67). Since the neurons that contain 5-HT survive for extended periods of time in organotypic tissue culture, it is clear that they are intrinsic to the gut itself. It may now be assumed, therefore, that there are enteric serotonergic neurons. Questions now arise as to their role in gastrointestinal function and the cellular biology of this neuronal class.

*M. D. Gershon, M.D., Dept of Anatomy and Cell Biology, Columbia University College of Physicians and Surgeons, 630 West 168th Street, New York, New York 10032, USA*

Although the enteric nervous system (ENS) is more accessible to the probes of researchers than is the central nervous system (CNS), less is known about the intrinsic neurons of the gut and their interconnection than about the brain. This paradox has resulted, in part, from the vastly greater amount of research that has been done on the CNS than on the ENS. In fact, the paucity of research on the ENS has led one writer, reviewing the subject of its pharmacology, to call the ENS, "the forgotten nervous system" (77). Another factor, however, was the view of the ENS that prevailed until recently, that it is simply a collection of parasympathetic relay ganglia that are interposed in the vagal and sacral nervous pathways to the smooth muscle of the bowel (72). This view not only was stultifying as far as research was concerned, it led investigators to denigrate the independence of the ENS from central control and the sophisticated neurally mediated behaviors of the gut that are dependent on the ENS (34, 40). This, in turn, directed attention away from the fact that there are many interneurons in the ENS and many different types of neuron (26, 34, 40). It is now apparent that the ENS is a large and complex nervous system (26), that it is capable of autonomous patterns of activity, and that it contains at least ten different kinds of neuron, many if not all of which are also present in the CNS (26, 34, 40).

## Transmitter identification in the ENS

The current climate of awareness of the diversity of enteric neuronal phenotypic expression has greatly diminished the reluctance of investigators to accept a variety of putative enteric neurotransmitters. In 1965, however, when a neurotransmitter action for serotonin (5-hydroxytryptamine; 5-HT) was first proposed (38), the climate was different. At that time, acetylcholine (ACh) and norepinephrine (NE) were both known to be enteric neurotransmitters and it was not apparent why the gut needed more. Since 1965, the evidence in favor of 5-HT as an enteric neurotransmitter has increased and 5-HT has now satisfied all of the criteria necessary for transmitter identification (34, 40). This evidence for 5-HT was not easy to amass; many observations provoked controversy and some remain controversial today. Certainly, if it has become easier to accept that there are serotonergic neurons in the ENS, the question raised in 1965 about why these neurons are needed has still not been answered.

In identifying a neurotransmitter it is generally agreed that five points must be satisfied (61). (i) The proposed substance should be present in the neurons in question. Generally, the neurotransmitter is synthesized in those neurons; however, there is no reason why a neuron could not use a substance as a transmitter that it takes up. For example, the sympathetic nerves of the pineal gland contain 5-HT as well as norepinephrine (NE) (33). They synthesize NE but their 5-HT store is apparently the result of uptake of 5-HT released in high concentration by pinealocytes. Conceivably, such indirect loading of neurons could provide them with a store of a compound that might, if released by nerve stimulation, evolve a neurotransmitter function. (ii) The suspected transmitter should be released by nerve stimulation, probably by a $Ca^{+2}$-dependent mechanism (73). (iii) The putative neurotransmitter should mimic in all respects the action of the naturally released substance. (iv) An effective means of inactivating the proposed transmitter should be demonstrated. Enzymatic breakdown, a re-uptake mechanism into the presynaptic nerve, and an uptake by the postsynaptic cell or by surrounding glia are examples of processes that might serve to augment diffusion as a means of reducing the concentration of the transmitter in the synaptic cleft. (v) Finally, parallel pharmacological antagonism should be demonstrated for the action of the putative transmitter and nerve stimulation.

*Enteric neurons contain 5-HT*

Historically, the most difficult of these points to satisfy for 5-HT was the first, to prove that enteric neurons actually contain the amine. As is also true of enteric neuropeptides, 5-HT is a constituent of mucosal enteroendocrine cells (enterochromaffin, or EC cells) as well as of the ENS (23, 81). The mucosal concentration of 5-HT is much greater than the concentration of 5-HT in the deeper layers of the bowel that contain the cells of the ENS (24, 48, 50, 68). As a consequence, it was possible for some investigators either to ignore the extramucosal 5-HT, or to assume that it was somehow derived from material released from the EC cells of the mucsoa (68). The ENS, moreover, cannot be dissected free of other tissues for biochemical analysis. It is therefore necessary to use a histochemical approach to demonstrate 5-HT within enteric neurons. This, however, is difficult to do because 5-HT is much harder to locate by standard procedures for formaldehyde- or glyoxylic acid-induced histofluorescence than are catecholamines. Consequently, unless pharmacological means are used to eliminate the histofluorescence of NE and to increase the 5-HT concentration in the ENS, and extreme reaction conditions are also employed (19, 28, 81), the histofluorescence of 5-HT cannot be visualized in situ in enteric neurons (3, 4, 13, 21). Although many central serotonergic neurons and their processes require procedures similar to those used for the gut before they too become histochemically demonstrable (1, 2), the difficulty encountered with histofluorescence led many investigators to remain skeptical of 5-HT as an enteric neuronal constituent (13). In fact, the possibility was raised that enteric neurons might contain some indolic compound other than 5-HT (13).

The problems with histofluorescence have now been overcome. When the gut is grown in organotypic tissue culture, even for several weeks, intrinsic neurons survive (19, 20) while, for the most part, EC cells do not. Mucosa-free preparations can also be grown. The histofluorescence of 5-HT can readily be demonstrated in cultured enteric neurons even without recourse to pharmacological amplification of stored 5-HT (19). Their survival in culture indicates that the neurons of the ENS that contain 5-HT are intrinsic to the gut itself. More recently, 5-HT has been demonstrated in neurons and processes of the myenteric plexus by immunocytochemical techniques (H. Steinbusch, reported at the International Meeting, "Le Neurone Serotoninergique", Marseilles, France, 1980; M. Costa and J. Furness,

reported at the Tenth Annual Meeting of the Society for Neuroscience, Cincinnati, Ohio, November, 1980). Immunoreactive 5-HT (Fig. 1) first appears in myenteric neurons during prenatal life (T. P. Rothman and M. D. Gershon, personal observations). It can therefore now be concluded that neurons of the myenteric plexus contain 5-HT. Costa and Furness estimate that these neurons comprise less than 5% of the total neuronal population (personal communication).

It seems likely that the 5-HT present in enteric neurons is synthesized there. Enteric neurons have been found immunocytochemically to contain material that cross reacts with an antibody to tryptophan hydroxylase (the rate limiting enzyme in 5-HT's biosynthesis) purified from raphe nuclei (39). Moreover, both mucosa-free preparations of guinea pig longitudinal muscle with adherent myenteric plexus and cultures containing myenteric neurons but not EC cells synthesize $^3$H-5-HT from its radioactive precursor, $^3$H-L-tryptophan (19). In fact, the myenteric plexus actually manifests a saturable, high-affinity uptake mechanism for L-tryptophan (19, 35, 63). This uptake is a temperature-sensitive, $Na^+$-dependent, energy-requiring process. Uptake of L-tryptophan is competitively inhibited by other neutral amino acids (affinities: tryptophan > phenylalanine > isoleucine > leucine), but not by acidic or basic amino acids (35). A subset of perikarya and neurites of the myenteric plexus has been shown by dry-mount radioautography to be responsible for the uptake of $^3$H-L-tryptophan (Fig. 2) (35). Labeling of these structures persists, even when protein synthesis is inhibited by cycloheximide (0.1 mM). It remains to be demonstrated whether the enteric neurons specialized to take up L-tryptophan are the same ones that synthesize and store 5-HT.

Myenteric neurons not only take up L-tryptophan, convert it to 5-HT and contain 5-HT, they also appear to produce a specific protein that adapts them for 5-HT storage. Enteric neurons resemble central serotonergic neurons in that they both contain a specific serotonin-binding protein (SBP) (65, 91, 92, 93, 94). This protein from brain, gut and also thyroid (where 5-HT is stored in the neural-crest-derived parafollicular cells)

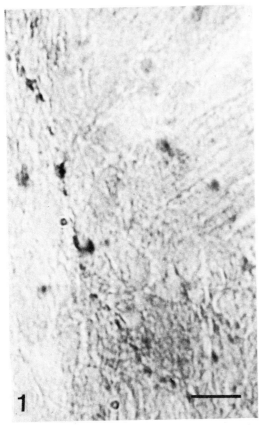

Fig. 1. A single varicose serotonergic axon traverses the field of this 10 μm cryostat section of fetal mouse intestine (gestational day 17). The tissue was treated with antiserum to 5-HT prepared by Dr. H. Steinbusch. Immunoreactivity was demonstrated using peroxidase-antiperoxidase. No immunoreactivity was seen when sections were treated with primary antiserum that had been absorbed with 5-HT. The immunoreactive fiber is within the myenteric plexus. The marker = 10 μm.

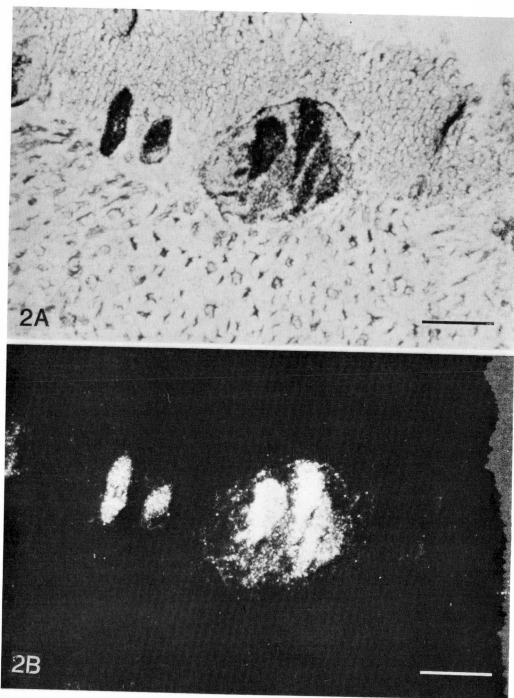

Fig. 2. A dry mount radioautograph of guinea pig myenteric plexus labeled by ³H-L-tryptophan. Dissected longitudinal muscle and adherent myenteric plexus were incubated in vitro for 30 minutes with ³H-L-tryptophan (50 μM) and cycloheximide (100 μM). Tissue was frozen at −155°C, dried and embedded in epoxy resin. One-μm sections were cut and subjected to radioautography. ³H-L-tryptophan has labeled some myenteric neurons and neuritic processes. The markers = 25 μm. A. Brightfield microscopy. B. Indirect (vertical) dark-field microscopy.

has similar properties (5, 91). The neuronal SBP differs from other proteins that bind 5-HT that can be isolated from non-neural cells, such as mast cells, platelets, or EC cells. In the brain, SBP appears to be a component of the synaptic vesicles of serotonergic neurons and is transported proximo-distally in axons by fast axonal transport (90). In the gut, SBP is present in the dissected innervated myenteric plexus, develops during ontogeny at about the same time as other phenotypic markers of serotonergic neurons (65, 83), and is released from the gut by electrical stimulation in a $Ca^{+2}$-dependent manner (64). The cytosol-marker protein, lactic acid dehydrogenase, is not similarly released; therefore it seems probable that enteric SBP is released by exocytosis. This release, in turn, implies that SBP is stored in vesicles. The role of SBP may be to reduce the osmotic pressure within the synaptic vesicles of serotonergic neurons by binding 5-HT. The dissociation constants of the 5-HT-SBP complex of about $10^{-10}$ M and $10^{-7}$ M under intracellular conditions indicate that, until the protein is saturated with 5-HT, little free amine would exist in a small storage vesicle in equilibrium with SBP (48). On the other hand, $Na^+$ and $Ca^{+2}$ markedly inhibit the binding of 5-HT by SBP. At the time of exocytosis, therefore, release of free 5-HT would be accomplished because the 5-HT-SBP complex would be exposed to extracellular $Na^+$ and $Ca^{+2}$ and would dissociate. The extracellular free 5-HT might then diffuse to its receptors or be subject to axonal re-uptake and possible recycling.

*5-HT is released from stimulated enteric neurons*

A number of early experiments provided evidence that stimulation of enteric nerves would lead to release of 5-HT. For example, Paton and Vane in 1953 (80) and Bülbring and Gershon in 1967 (9) reported that vagal or electrical stimulation released 5-HT from isolated guinea pig or mouse stomachs. Paton and Vane, noted that the stomach contracted when the vagus nerves were stimulated and thus they speculated that the 5-HT release they measured might have resulted from mechanical stimulation of the mucosa. Pres-

sure is an excellent releaser of mucosal 5-HT (8). Bülbring and Gershon (9), however, tried to eliminate mechanical effects by stimulating the vagus nerves in the pressure of atropine to prevent gastric contraction. They also attempted to avoid mucosal release of 5-HT by asphyxiating the mucosa prior to stimulation. They detected a release of 5-HT from the stomach by electrical stimulation despite these precautions; this release, moreover, was blocked by tetrodotoxin. Still, the released 5-HT was detected by bioassay and its $Ca^{+2}$-dependence was not evaluated. These results, therefore, are only as reliable as the 5-HT receptors of the bioassay preparation. They detect a substance that acts in the assay as does 5-HT. Other investigators have also reported from time to time the release of a substance from enteric nerves that acts on various intestinal preparations like 5-HT (15, 25, 86). Always worrisome in these experiments, even if one believes that the various assays are responding specifically to 5-HT, is the possibility that enteric nerves release 5-HT they have picked up secondarily, perhaps as a result of experimental manipulation, from the mucosa. This problem might be especially severe in experiments such as those of Bülbring and Gershon (9), where the mucosa was asphyxiated. 5-HT released during that process might have been taken up by nerves that later released the amine when they were stimulated.

The problems of identifying the source of released amine does not apply if enteric nerves are preloaded with $^3$H-5-HT before they are stimulated (64, 88). Enteric nerves of the myenteric and submucosal plexuses take up $^3$H-5-HT (37, 42, 81) and can be selectively labeled (see below). Thus, preparations can be stimulated in which all $^3$H-5-HT is present in neurons or their processes (64). These preparations release $^3$H-5-HT when stimulated electrically (64, 88); this release is inhibited by tetrodotoxin, high $Mg^{+2}$- or $Ca^{+2}$-free solutions (64). As noted earlier, the release of $^3$H-5-HT is accompanied by the release of SBP (64). Enteric nerves, therefore, can release 5-HT and they do so, probably by exocytosis, in a manner that is consistent with 5-HT's being a neurotransmitter. $^3$H-5-HT, however, is an exogenous substance. The specificity of measurements of [3]H-5-HT release, consequently, is that of the uptake mechanism. If [3]H-5-HT is taken up only by serotonergic neural elements and if, after uptake, [3]H-5-HT mixes with endogenous 5-HT stores, then assay of [3]H-5-HT release is a good, relatively simple procedure to use to study the regulation of the 5-HT release mechanism. Obviously, however, for purposes of transmitter identification, release of endogenous 5-HT from stimulated enteric nerves must be shown.

In the course of experiments with [3]H-5-HT, a barrier to the transmural passage of the radioactive amine from mucosa to serosa was found (49, 50). In these experiments segments of the guinea pig small intestine were everted, or turned inside out, and perfused in vitro through their newly created serosal lumen. When [3]H-5-HT was added to the mucosal surface, little radioactivity reached the serosal perfusate. Radioautographic examination of the perfused gut showed labeling of mucosal enteroendocrine cells but no labeling of neuronal structures. On the other hand, if [3]H-5-HT was added to the fluid perfusing the serosal lumen, radioautographic labeling was found in both myenteric and submucosal plexuses but little or no labeling of enteroendocrine cells occurred (49, 50, 64). 5-HT, therefore, apparently cannot pass readily from mucosa to serosa. The radioautographic data indicate that the transmural barrier to [3]H-5-HT must lie either within the mucosa or between the mucosa and submucosa. The existence of this barrier is probably necessary to protect the neurons of the ENS from the high concentrations of mucosal 5-HT that would probably bathe them in its absence. EC cells seem constantly to release 5-HT (96). 5-HT is highly active on enteric neurons (7, 8, 9, 10, 14, 29, 59, 62, 103) and, whatever the physiological role of 5-HT may turn out to be, it is doubtful that the ENS could function normally if constantly exposed to a medium containing a high concentration of 5-HT. In fact, 5-HT has different actions on the peristaltic reflex depending on which surface of the gut the amine is applied to (8, 10). Mucosal application stimulates the reflex by activating intrinsic enteric afferent nerve fibers, while the serosal application of 5-HT blocks peristalsis through its disruptive action on the myenteric plexus.

The barrier to the transmural passage of 5-HT makes it possible to measure the release of endogenous 5-HT from the ENS (49, 50). The perfused, everted preparations of small intestine are convenient to use for this purpose. 5-HT released from the serosal surface cannot, because of the 5-HT barrier, be of mucosal origin. Electrical stimulation releases endogenous 5-HT from the serosal surface of the gut and this release is abolished in the absence of $Ca^{+2}$ (49, 50). More 5-HT is released by electrical stimulation than metabolites of the amine. As is true of other transmitters, newly taken up 5-HT is preferentially released by nerve stimulation. The release of 5-HT also appears to be modulated by sympathetic nerves in the bowel and by NE (36). Since a pronounced increase in the rate of release of 5-HT from the serosal surface of the rabbit small intestine has been found to accompany peristaltic activity, it seems likely that 5-HT neurons are involved in peristalsis (56).

### 5-HT mimics actions of enteric nerves

It has been known for some time from pharmacological experiments that 5-HT activates enteric ganglia (7, 9, 14, 29, 32). Application of 5-HT stimulates cholinergic neurons, releasing ACh (98) that in turn causes the contraction of the longitudinal (32) and circular layers of smooth muscle (14, 57). Intrinsic inhibitory neurons are also stimulated by 5-HT (9, 14, 17, 25, 32). These pharmacological observations, however, do not constitute mimicry of the effects of nerve stimulation, although they are consistent with the idea that the intrinsic enteric serotonin-containing neurons are interneurons. Electrophysiological studies, however, have confirmed that 5-HT does activate enteric neurons (15, 16, 86). More recently, 5-HT has been demonstrated to precisely mimic the action on a subset of enteric neurons of transmitter released by stimulating an interganglionic connective containing fibers leading to the ganglion being recorded from (102, 103). The cells of this subset are known as type 2 or AH neurons (58, 75) (Fig. 3). Action potentials in this cell type are characterized by

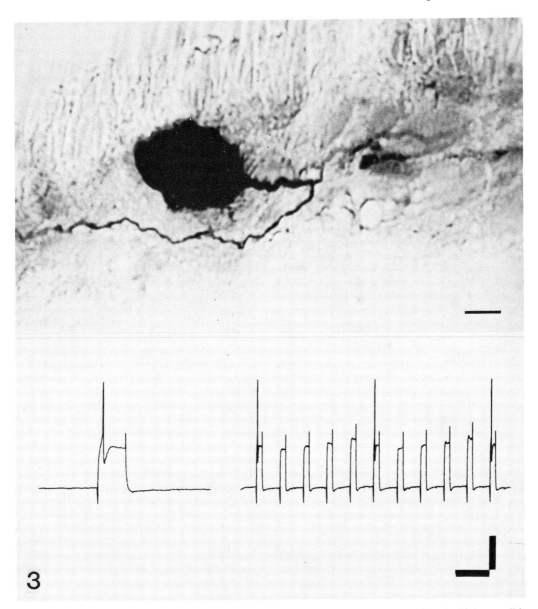

**3**

Fig. 3. A. An AH cell in the guinea pig myenteric plexus that has been intracellularly injected with horseradish peroxidase. The cell has a rounded perikaryon and a single process, probably its axon, that bifurcates. Other, non-injected ganglion cells are barely visible in this thin plastic section. The marker = 10 μm. B. Intracellular depolarizing current injection provokes a single spike (left). Subsequent injections of constant current pulses (right) reveal that a decreased membrane resistance follows the spike for a prolonged period of time. Until the cell recovers, it is refractory and subsequent injections of constant current pulses do not elicit spikes. The decreased membrane resistance is due to a $Ca^{+2}$-activated increase in $K^+$ conductance that is also responsible for the cell's after-hyperpolarization (54). Calibration = 20 mv; left—400 msec; right—2 sec.

a prolonged after-hyperpolarization of the AH, that renders the neuron relatively inexcitable. It is likely that the rising phase of the spike in AH cells is associated with the movement of $Ca^{+2}$ into the cells (60, 76, 78). This inward movement of $Ca^{+2}$ has been postulated to activate a $K^+$ conductance that is responsible for the after-hyperpolarization (54). Stimulation of an interganglionic fiber tract evokes a slow epsp in AH cells that is associated with an increased membrane resistance and abolition of the after-hyperpolarization (102, 103). These actions of the slow epsp increase the probability that AH cells will fire action potentials repetitively. The iontophoretic application of 5-HT to AH cells that manifest the slow epsp precisely mimics the naturally evoked potential (55, 103). Membrane conductance changes are the same and, in addition, both the effects of the iontophoretic application of 5-HT and the neurally evoked slow epsp are antagonized by 5-HT desensitization or by the addition of methysergide. Other substances, such as substance P, also have actions on AH cells that resemble those of 5-HT (69, 70); however, unlike the slow epsp, the action of substance P is not antagonized by methysergide or 5-HT desensitization (53), nor is the slow epsp abolished in preparations desensitized to substance P (J. Wood, reported at the Tenth Annual Meeting of the Society for Neuroscience, Cincinnati, November 1980). Although a peptidase, chymotrypsin, does antagonize the slow epsp (74), that agent's pharmacology is unknown. Only 5-HT, therefore, mimics all actions of the naturally released transmitter and shows a parallel sensitivity to pharmacological antagonists. It is possible, since different investigators elicit slow epsp's in AH cells by stimulating in somewhat different ways (North and co-workers stimulate the surface of a ganglion while Wood and collaborators stimulate an interganglionic connective), that one type of stimulation activates serotonergic fibers preferentially, while another mainly stimulates substance P-ergic axons. If so, then conceivably both 5-HT and substance P may mediate a slow epsp in AH neurons.

While 5-HT thus mimics the effects of nerve stimulation on a cellular level, little is known about what the function of enteric serotonergic neurons might be. The release of 5-HT from the serosal surface of the rabbit intestine during peristalsis (56) suggests that serotonergic neurons increase their activity at this time and thus participate in the peristaltic reflex. Reports in the literature indicate that partial depletion of 5-HT in animals receiving the tryptophan hydroxylase inhibitor, parachlorophenylanine (PCPA), interferes with gastrointestinal motility (6, 85, 100, 101). PCPA treatment also makes the gut supersensitive to 5-HT (89), an effect that might be expected from a drug that chronically depletes an enteric neurotransmitter (89). Probably the best-documented function linked to enteric serotonergic neurons is the neural inhibition of vagally evoked excitatory junction potentials that accompanies the descending inhibitory phase of the peristaltic reflex in the colon (67). This blockade, elicited by increasing intraluminal pressure, can be suppressed by depleting 5-HT with PCPA. This action of PCPA appears to be specific and due to its inhibition of tryptophan hydroxylase, because its blockade of junction potential suppression can be overcome by injection of additional L-tryptophan, and reproduced by inhibiting the conversion of 5-hydroxytryptophan to 5-HT. The suppression of vagally evoked excitatory junction potentials during descending peristaltic relaxation is, moreover, potentiated and prolonged in duration by inhibition of the 5-HT re-uptake mechanism. The descending phase of the peristaltic reflex, therefore, involves a neural inhibition of potentially competing cholinergic excitation of the bowel, as well as the activation of intrinsic neurons that relax the intestinal smooth muscle (11, 12, 67). 5-HT seems to be one of the neurotransmitters of the interneurons of the myenteric plexus that are involved in at least the excitatory-suppressive component of the reflex.

*Inactivation of 5-HT: the re-uptake process*

The observation that inhibition of 5-HT uptake potentiates its neurotransmitter action (67) suggests that 5-HT re-uptake into enteric neurites is the mechanism for inactivation of the amine. Enteric neurites do take up 5-HT and they become radioautographically labeled by ³H-5-hydroxytryptophan (38, 43, 44) or by ³H-5-HT (81). The uptake of ³H-5-HT by enteric neurites is a saturable, temperature-dependent process, with a $K_m$ of about 0.7 μM (37). Metabolic energy is required for 5-HT uptake and the uptake is also inhibited by ouabain (37). Ionic requirements of the 5-HT uptake mechanism are relatively precise; the uptake is $Na^+$-dependent (37) and is inhibited as a logarithmic function of the $K^+$ concentration (42). Uptake of ³H-5-HT is also depressed when the ambient $Ca^{+2}$ concentration is low (0 mM) or high (12 mM). Affinity of indolic compounds for the 5-HT uptake site is much reduced in compounds that have no alkyl amino

side chain, in which the amino group is methylated, or that have no 5-hydroxyl group on the indolic ring (42). Compounds such as 6-hydroxytryptamine (6-HT) or 5,6- and 5,7-dihydroxytryptamine (5,6-DHT; 5,7-DHT) competitively inhibit the uptake of ³H-5-HT and are transported into neurites by the 5-HT uptake mechanism (42, 46).

The formaldehyde-fluorophore of 6-HT has a higher fluorescent yield than that of 5-HT (66). 6-HT, therefore is useful for demonstrating enteric serotonergic neurities by histofluorescence (91). 5,7-DHT is a neurotoxin that causes lesions to form in enteric serotonergic neurites (46). At short times after administration of 5,7-

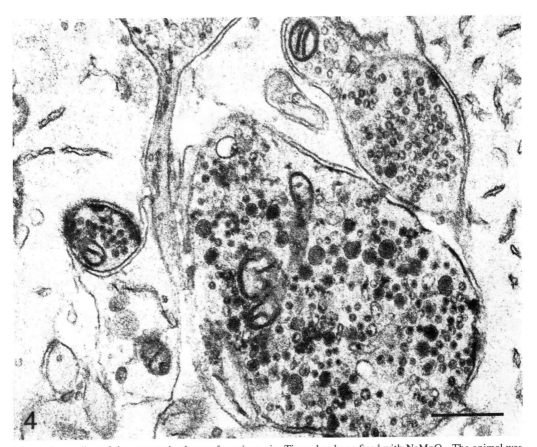

Fig. 4. A ganglion of the myenteric plexus of a guinea pig. Tissue has been fixed with $NaMnO_4$. The animal was injected with 5,7-DHT following pretreatment with desmethylimipramine and methysergide. Tissue was fixed 2 hours after administration of 5,7-DHT. The neurotoxin has loaded terminals that are distinguished by large and small synaptic vesicles filled with electron-dense material. Electron-dense material also coats the cytoplasmic face of the presynaptic plasma membrane of the 5,7-DHT-loaded varicosities. The marker = 0.5 μm.

DHT ultrastructural examination of aldehyde/ OsO$_4$-fixed myenteric plexus reveals, within affected varicosities, membrane delimited regions, characterized by extremely electron-dense cytoplasm and aggregates of recognizable synaptic vesicles. After several hours varicosities that have taken up 5,7-DHT degenerate and are phagocytized by surrounding glial cells. In order to use 5,7-DHT as a specific neurotoxin for enteric serotonergic varicosities it is necessary to pretreat animals with desmethylimipramine to prevent uptake of 5,7-DHT by noradrenergic axons, and with methysergide to protect animals from the 5-HT-mimetic actions of 5,7-DHT. When tissue that has been fixed with NaMnO$_4$ or KMnO$_4$

instead of aldehyde/OsO$_4$ is looked at by electron microscopy, then the 5,7-DHT that has entered serotonergic varicosities is visible (45) (Fig. 4). Dense material fills synaptic vesicles and appears on the cytoplasmic face of presynaptic membranes. The loaded terminals contain a mixture of small vesicles (mean diameter 58.5 ± 0.06 nm) and large vesicles (mean diameter = 116.7 ± 2.7 nm), both of which contain electron opaque cores. The small vesicles of 5,7-DHT-loaded terminals are larger than the small granular vesicles of noradrenergic axons (also identifiable in permanganate-fixed material) and the 5,7-DHT-loaded varicosities contain many more large synaptic vesicles than do noradrenergic varicosities

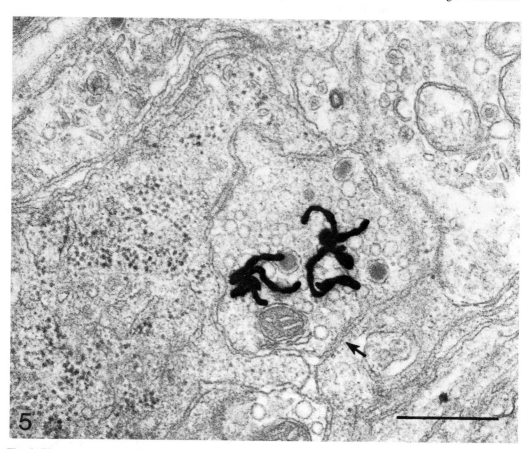

Fig. 5. Electron microscopic radioautographic localization of $^3$H-5-HT. Tissue has been subjected to aldehyde/ OsO$_4$ fixation. A labeled varicosity in the myenteric plexus of a mouse contains small lucent and large dense-cored vesicles and forms a synaptic membrane specialization (arrow). The labeled synapse is axosomatic. The animal had been subjected to chemical sympathectomy with 6-hydroxydopamine 1 day prior to intraperitoneal injection of $^3$H-5-HT. No axons label if similarly treated animals are injected with $^3$H-NE. Labeled varicosities, therefore, are serotonergic. The marker = 0.5 μm.

(105 vesicles per mm$^2$ vs. 6 vesicles per mm$^2$). As a consequence, the myenteric plexus from animals treated appropriately with 5,7-DHT and fixed with NaMnO$_4$ before degeneration begins (1–2 hours after administering the neurotoxin) is doubly labeled for electron microscopy. Serotonergic (loaded) and noradrenergic terminals can both be recognized and each can be distinguished from the other. Varicosities that load with 5,7-DHT persist after chemical sympathectomy with 6-hydroxydopamine while varicosities of the type recognized as noradrenergic disappear.

Terminals identified as serotonergic in the myenteric plexus from animals treated with 5,7-DHT and fixed with NaMnO$_4$ have an appearance that is similar to terminals identified in aldehyde/OsO$_4$-fixed material as serotonergic by electron microscopic radioautography with $^3$H-5-HT (Fig. 5). In both cases the labeled varicosities contain a similar mixture of large and small synaptic vesicles; however, in the absence of 5,7-DHT, or permanganate, the small vesicles have electron-lucent cores. Both techniques,

5,7-DHT/NaMnO$_4$ and $^3$H-5-HT/radioautography, reveal a population of serotonergic axon terminals that preferentially contacts cell bodies and proximal dendrites of the postsynaptic neurons. Both radioautography and treatment with 5,7-DHT permit at least some serotonergic perikarya (Fig. 6) to be identified as well as axons. Although initial radioautographic studies did not reveal labeling of cell bodies by $^3$H-5-HT, longer exposures to $^3$H-5-HT, more extensive examination of the myenteric plexus, and the extension of the radioautographic technique to electron microscopy have permitted labeled cell bodies to be identified (Fig. 7). After 5,7-DHT administration and permanganate fixation, affected cells can be distinguished by amorphous deposits of electron-dense material in their cytoplasm, damage to intracellular membranes, and the presence of dense-cored vesicles.

The question arises in dealing with a neurotransmitter re-uptake mechanism as to how specific the process is. This question assumes particular importance in interpreting studies that use

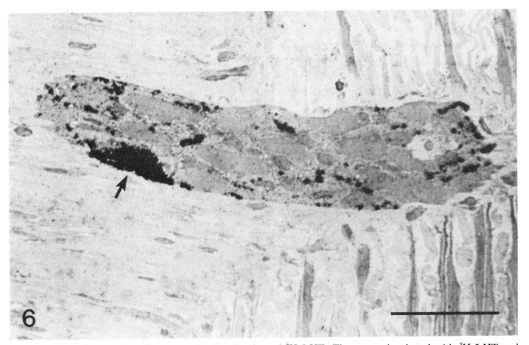

Fig. 6. Light microscopic radioautographic localization of $^3$H-5-HT. Tissue was incubated with $^3$H-5-HT and desmethylimipramine. A ganglion of the guinea pig's myenteric plexus is shown. It contains one labeled neuronal perikaryon on the edge of the plexus (arrow) and many labeled neurites. The marker = 50 µm.

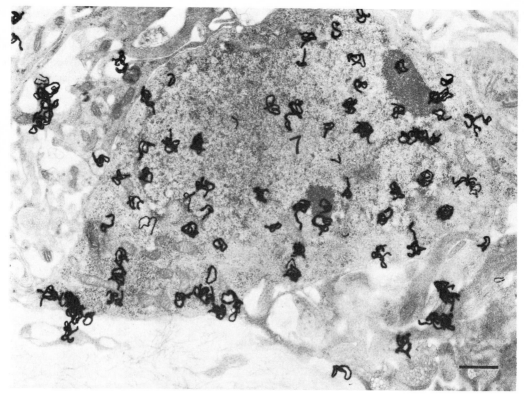

Fig. 7. Electron microscopic radioautographic localization of $^3$H-5-HT. A ganglion cell is labeled in the myenteric plexus of a guinea pig. The dissected longitudinal muscle and myenteric plexus were incubated as described for Fig. 6. In vitro incubation has caused separation of processes in the neuropill of the myenteric plexus; however, cellular preservation remains good. The labeled neuron shows nuclear labeling. The marker = 1.0 μm.

uptake as a phenotypic or anatomical marker for a given type of neuron. Specifically, it is important to know if $^3$H-5-HT, 5,7-DHT or 6-HT are taken up exclusively by serotonergic neural elements in the ENS or whether other types of enteric axon also become labeled by these substances. Noradrenergic axons are the enteric neurites to worry about in this regard because they are known to be capable of taking up exogenous amines including 5-HT (18, 95); however, the affinity of noradrenergic axons for 5-HT is very low in comparison to their affinity for NE (95). The nonspecific noradrenergic uptake of $^3$H-5-HT can easily be prevented, therefore, by incubating tissues in the presence of an excess of unlabeled NE (10 to 100 times the concentration of 5-HT). NE does not compete with 5-HT for uptake by enteric serotonergic neurites and does not decrease uptake

of $^3$H-5-HT (37, 83). Noradrenergic neurites are clearly not responsible for the bulk of the uptake of $^3$H-5-HT by the ENS. Chemical sympathectomy does not reduce the uptake of $^3$H-5-HT (37, 42) and, during ontogeny, the enteric uptake of $^3$H-5-HT precedes that of $^3$H-NE by a wide margin in both rabbits (83) and guinea pigs (47, 51). The uptake of 5-HT, moreover, is not lost when the gut is grown for up to 3 weeks in organotypic tissue culture (20). On the other hand, the entirely extrinsic noradrenergic neurites degenerate in these cultures, so that the cultures contain no immunocytochemically demonstrable dopamine beta hydroxylase (87) and fail to take up $^3$H-NE (20). The 5-HT uptake mechanism also persists in gut that has been extrinsically denervated (27). It can be concluded, therefore, that the neurons responsible for $^3$H-5-HT uptake are neither sympathetic nor noradrenergic. The gut contains no other non-serotonergic neurons known to be able to take up $^3$H-5-HT, 6-HT, or 5,7-DHT.

The pharmacological sensitivity of the enteric 5-HT uptake process is similar to that of the CNS (42). Desmethylimipramine is a fine inhibitor of NE uptake but has little action against 5-HT. Chlorimipramine is a better enteric 5-HT uptake inhibitor but also releases the amine (41). The most selective inhibitor of the uptake of 5-HT by the ENS, and one that does not also release 5-HT, is fluoxetine (41).

Enteric serotonergic neurons, recognized by histofluorescence or radioautography with $^3$H-5-HT, appear to be present in all vertebrates (4, 52, 99). The neurons are probably also found in cephalochordates (84) although not in echinoderms or tunicates (52). Serotonergic neurons have also been detected in the human bowel (82). Interestingly, unlike noradrenergic and cholinergic neurites, the processes of enteric serotonergic neurons fail to grow into the aganglionic segments of bowel of patients with congenital megacolon. Instead, serotonergic neurites in ganglia above these regions sprout and form neuromas at the superior boundary of the aganglionic zone. Recently, evidence has been accumulating that indicates that peripheral serotonergic neurons may be located at other sites, besides the ENS. Examples of such additional locations include the superior cervical ganglion (97), the pancreas (71, 79), and the nodose ganglion (30).

*Conclusions*

Until recently a great deal of the work on enteric serotonergic neurons was done to test the hypothesis that these neurons exist. It seems reasonable to conclude at this time that there are intrinsic serotonergic neurons in the ENS and that they are one of an expanding list of known enteric interneurons. 5-HT, for example, releases other enteric neurotransmitters such as ACh (98) and vasoactive intestinal polypeptide (VIP) (22). Much more needs to be learned about the cellular biology of enteric serotonergic neurons and the ways in which these neurons are similar to or different from their counterparts in the CNS. A more complete answer to the question of what enteric serotonergic neurons do is also necessary. This latter need is not likely to be fully satisfied until better antagonists of the neural actions of 5-HT in the ENS become available. In the gut there are both neural and muscular receptors for 5-HT and these receptors differ from one another (12, 13, 14, 17). Methysergide is a good antagonist of 5-HT's action on muscle, but some neural effects of 5-HT persist even in its presence (17). Phenylbiguanide first mimics and then blocks the action of 5-HT on myenteric neurons of mice but not guinea pigs (14, 17). It seems likely that multiple 5-HT receptors may be found on myenteric neurons, as has proved to be the case for neurons in molluscan ganglia (31). Future research will probably help to better define the enteric neuronal 5-HT receptor(s) (28). The past has thus been interesting and has served to introduce 5-HT as one of the enteric cast of characters. The future promises to be exciting because the stage is now set and the action can unfold.

## ACKNOWLEDGEMENT

Supported by NIH grant NS-12969.

## REFERENCES

1. Aghajanian GK, Asher IM. Science 1971, 172, 1159–1161
2. Aghajanian GK, Kuhar MJ, Roth RH. Brain Res 1973, 54, 85–101
3. Ahlman H, Enerback L. Cell Tissue Res 1974, 153, 419–434
4. Baumgarten HG, Björklund A, Lachenmayer L, Nobin A, Rosengren E. Z Zellforsch 1973, 141, 33–54
5. Bernd P, Nunez EA, Gershon MD, Tamir H. pp 123–132 in MacIntyre I, Szelke M (eds). Molecular Endocrinology. Elsevier/North Holland, Amsterdam, New York, Oxford 1979
6. Breisch ST, Zemlan FP, Hoebel, BG. Science 1976, 192, 382–385
7. Brownlee G, Johnson ES. Br J Pharmacol 1963, 21, 306–322
8. Bülbring E, Crema A. J Physiol (London) 1959, 146, 18–28
9. Bülbring E, Gershon MD. J Physiol (London) 1967, 192, 823–846
10. Bülbring E, Lin RCY. J Physiol (London) 1958, 140, 381–407

11. Burnstock G. pp 406–414 in Burnstock G, Gershon MD, Hökfelt T, Iversen LL, Kosterlitz HW, Szurszewski JH (eds). Neurosciences Research Program Bulletin, Vol 17, Non-adrenergic, Non-cholinergic Autonomic Neurotransmission Mechanisms. MIT Press, Cambridge 1979

12. Costa M, Furness JB. Naunyn-Schmiedeberg's Arch Pharmacol 1976, 294, 47–60

13. Costa M, Furness JB. Biochem Pharmacol 1979, 28, 565–571

14. Costa M, Furness JB. Br J Pharmacol 1979, 65, 237–248

15. Dingledine R, Goldstein A. J Pharmacol Exp Ther 1976, 196, 97–106

16. Dingledine R, Goldstein A, Kendig J. Life Sci 1974, 14, 2299–2309

17. Drakontides AB, Gershon MD. Br J Pharmacol 1968, 33, 480–492

18. Drakontides AB, Gershon MD. Br J Pharmacol 1972, 45, 417–434

19. Dreyfus CF, Bornstein MB, Gershon MD. Brain Res 1977, 128, 125–139

20. Dreyfus CF, Sherman D, Gershon MD. Brain Res 1977, 128, 109–123

21. Dubois A, Jacobowitz DM. Cell Tissue Res 1974, 150, 493–496

22. Eklund S, Fahrenkrug J, Jodal M, Lundgren O, Schaffalitzky de Muckadell OB, Sjöqvist A. J Physiol 1980, 302, 549–557

23. Erspamer V. pp 132–181 in Erspamer V (ed). Handbook of Experimental Pharmacology, Vol 19. 5-Hydroxytryptamine and Related Indolealkylamines. Springer-Verlag, New York 1966

24. Feldberg W, Toh CC. J Physiol (London) 1953, 119, 352–362

25. Furness JB, Costa M. Phil Trans Roy Soc Series B 1973, 265, 123–133

26. Furness JB, Costa M. Neuroscience 1980, 5, 1–20

27. Furness JB, Costa M, Howe RC. pp 367–372 in Eränkö O, Soinila S, Paivarinta H (eds). Histochemistry and Cell Biology of Autonomic Neurons, SIF Cells and Paraneurons. Raven Press, New York 1980

28. Fuxe K, Jonsson G. Histochem 1967, 11, 161–166

29. Gaddum JH, Picarelli ZP. Br J Pharmacol 1957, 12, 323–328

30. Gaudin-Chazal G, Segu L, Seyfreitz N, Puizillou JJ. Neuroscience 1981, 6, 1127–1138

31. Gerschenfeld HM, Paupardin-Tritsch D. J Physiol (London) 1974, 243, 427–456

32. Gershon MD. Br J Pharmacol 1967, 29, 259–279

33. Gershon MD. pp 573–623 in Brookhart JM, Mountcastle VB, Kandel ER, Geiger SR (eds). Handbook of Physiology. Section 1. The Nervous System. Vol 1. Cellular Biology of Neurons. Am Physiol Soc, Bethesda, Maryland 1977

34. Gershon MD. Ann Rev Neurosci 1981, 4, 227–272

35. Gershon MD. Proc Eighth Int Cong Pharmacol, Tokyo, July 1981, p 397

36. Gershon MD. pp 285–298 in Grossman MI, Brazier MAB, Lechago J (eds). Cellular Basis of Chemical Messnegers in the Digestive System. Academic Press, New York 1981

37. Gershon MD, Altman RF. J Pharmacol Exp Ther 1971, 179, 29–41

38. Gershon MD, Drakontides AB, Ross LL. Science 1965, 149, 197–199

39. Gershon MD, Dreyfus CF, Pickel VM, Joh TH, Reis DJ. Proc Natl Acad Sci, USA 1977, 74, 3086–3089

40. Gershon MD, Erde SM. Gastroenterology 1981, 80, 1571–1594

41. Gershon MD, Jonakait GM. Br J Pharmacol 1979, 66, 7–9

42. Gershon MD, Robinson RG, Ross LL. J Pharmacol Exp Ther 1976, 198, 548–561

43. Gershon MD, Ross LL. J Physiol (London) 1966, 186, 451–476

44. Gershon MD, Ross LL. J Physiol (London) 1966, 186, 477–492

45. Gershon MD, Sherman D. Anat Rec 1981, 199, 92A–93A

46. Gershon MD, Sherman D, Dreyfus CF. J Comp Neurol 1980, 190, 581–596

47. Gershon MD, Sherman D, Gintzler AR. J Neurocytol 1981, 10, 271–296

48. Gershon MD, Tamir H. pp 37–50 in Haber B, Gabay S, Issidorides M, Alivisatos S. (ed). Serotonin. Plenum Publishing Co, New York 1981

49. Gershon MD, Tamir H. pp 285–298 in Grossman MI, Brazier MAB, Lechago J (eds). Cellular Basis of Chemical Messengers in the Digestive System. Academic Press, New York 1981

40. Gershon MD, Tamir H. Neuroscience 1981, in press

51. Gintzler AR, Rothman TP, Gershon MD. Brain Res 1980, 189, 31–48

52. Goodrich JT, Bernd P, Sherman DL, Gershon MD. J Comp Neurol 1980, 190, 15–28

53. Grafe P, Mayer CJ, Wood JD. Nature (London) 1979, 279, 720–721

54. Grafe P, Mayer CJ, Wood JD. J Physiol (London) 1980, 305, 235–248

55. Grafe P, Wood JD, Mayer CJ. Brain Res 1979, 163, 349–352

56. Gwee MCE, Yeoh TS. J Physiol (London) 1968, 194, 817–825

57. Harry J. Br J Pharmacol Chemother 1963, 20, 399–417

58. Hirst GDS, Holman ME, Spence I. J Physiol (London) 1974, 236, 303–326

59. Hirst GDS, Silinsky EM. J Physiol (London) 1975, 251, 817–832

60. Hirst GDS, Spence I. Nature (London) 1973, 243, 54–56

61. Iversen LL. p 406 in Burnstock G, Gershon MD, Hökfelt T, Iversen LL, Kosterlitz HW, Szurszewski JH (eds). Neurosciences Research Program Bulletin, Vol 17. Non-adrenergic, Non-cholinergic Autonomic Neurotransmission Mechanisms. MIT Press, Cambridge 1979

62. Johnson SM, Katayama Y, North RA. J Physiol (London) 1980, 304, 459–479

63. Jonakait GM, Gintzler AR, Gershon MD. J Neurochem 1979, 32, 1387–1400

64. Jonakait GM, Tamir H, Ginzler AR, Gershon MD. Brain Res 1979, 174, 55–69

65. Jonakait GM, Tamir H, Rapport MM, Gershon MD. J Neurochem 1977, 28, 277–284
66. Jonsson G, Fuxe K, Hamberger B, Hökfelt T. Brain Res 1969, 13, 190–195
67. Julé Y. J Physiol (London) 1980, 159, 361–368
68. Juorio AV, Gabella G. J Neurochem 1974, 221, 851–858
69. Katayama Y, North RA. Nature (London) 1978, 274, 387–388
70. Katayama Y, North RA, Williams JT. Proc R Soc Lond Ser B 1979, 206, 191–208
71. Koevary SB, McEvoy RC, Azmitia EC. Am J Anat 1980, 159, 361–368
72. Kuntz A. The Autonomic Nervous System (4th ed) Lea & Febiger, Philadelphia 1953
73. Llinas RR, Steinberg IZ. pp 565–574 in Llinas RR, Heuser JE (eds). Neuroscience Research Program Bulletin, Vol 15, Depolarization-Release Coupling Systems in Neurons. MIT Press, Cambridge, 1977
74. Morita K, North RA, Katayama Y. Nature (London) 1980, 287, 151–152
75. Nishi S, North RA. J Physiol (London) 1973, 231, 471–491
76. North RA. Br J Pharmacol 1973, 49, 709–711
77. North RA. Trends in Pharmacol Sci 1980, 1, 434–442
78. North RA, Nishi S. pp 303–307 in Bülbring E, Shuba MF (eds). Physiology of Smooth Muscle. Raven Press, New York 1976
79. Nunez EA, Gershon P, Gershon MD. Am J Anat 1980, 159, 347–360
80. Paton WDM, Vane JR. J Physiol (London) 1963, 165, 10–46
81. Robinson R, Gershon MD. J Pharmacol Exp Ther 1971, 178, 311–324
82. Rogawski MA, Goodrich JT, Gershon MD, Touloukian RJ. J Pediat Surg 1978, 13, 608–615
83. Rothman TP, Ross LL. Gershon MD. Brain Res 1976, 115, 437–456
84. Salimova N. Dokl Acad Sci USSR 1978, 242, 939–941
85. Saller CF, Stricker EM. J Pharm Pharmacol 1978, 30, 646–647
86. Sato T, Takayanagi I, Takagi K. Jap J Pharmacol 1974, 24, 447–451
87. Schultzberg M, Hökfelt T, Nilsson O, Terenius L, Rehfeld JF, Brown M, Elde R, Goldstein M, Said S. Neuroscience 1980, 5, 689–744
88. Schulz R, Cartwright C. J Pharmacol Exp Ther 1974, 190, 420–430
89. Schulz R, Cartrwight C. Fed Proc 1974, 33, 502a
90. Tamir H, Gershon MD. Neurochem 1979, 33, 35–44
91. Tamir H, Gershon MD. J Physiol (Paris) 1981, 77, in press
92. Tamir H, Huang IL. Life Sci 1974, 14, 83–93
93. Tamir H, Klein A, Rapport MM. J. Neurochem 1976, 26, 871–878
94. Tamir H, Kuhar MJ. Brain Res 1975, 83, 164–172
95. Thoa HB, Eccleston D, Axelrod J. J Pharmacol Exp Ther 1969, 169, 69–73
96. Toh CC. J Physiol (London) 1954, 126, 248–254
97. Verhofstad AAJ, Steinbusch HWM, Penke B, Varga J, Joosten HWJ. Brain Res 1981, 212, 39–49
98. Vizi VA, Vizi ES. J Neural Transmission 1978, 42, 127–138
99. Watson AHD. Cell Tissue Res 1979, 197, 155–164
100. Weber LJ. Biochem Pharmacol 1970, 19, 2169–2172
101. Welch AS, Welch BL. Biochem Pharmacol 1968, 17, 699–708
102. Wood JD, Mayer CJ. J Neurophysiol 1979, 42, 569–581
103. Wood JD, Mayer CJ. J Neurophysiol 1979, 42, 582–593

# Peptidergic Nerves

A. E. BISHOP, G-L. FERRI, L. PROBERT, S. R. BLOOM* & J. M. POLAK
Histochemistry Unit, Dept. of Histochemistry and Dept. of Medicine*
Hammersmith Hospital, London W12 0HS, UK

In recent years the autonomic nervous system has been shown to consist of nerves containing a number of different neurotransmitter substances; a system far more complex than was originally thought. It has been demonstrated that a large part of the autonomic nervous system contains peptides, and that, in the gut, these nerves form a major complex that infiltrates the entire length and breadth of the tract.

The detailed study of this peptidergic system has been facilitated by the development of specialised immunocytochemical methods, which have yielded information on the distribution and morphology of the various types of nerve. Thus, the distribution of these nerves can often be seen to parallel what is known about the actions of individual peptides.

The majority of peptidergic nerves are intrinsic to the gut, forming, with the other intrinsic nerves, what appears to be a largely autonomous unit. This enteric system can be visualised as a "minibrain", under the general influence of the central nervous system but able to function, to a certain extent, by itself. The consequences of a breakdown in the normal functioning of this system can be seen in a number of gut diseases.

*J. M. Polak, Histochemistry Unit, Dept of Histopathology, Hammersmith Hospital, London W12 0HS, UK*

Although the autonomic nervous system was classically considered to be bipartite, the first suggestion of the existence of non-cholinergic, non-adrenergic autonomic nerves came as long ago as Langley's era, in 1898 (47), when he found that stimulation of the vagus nerve causes gastric relaxation. At the time it was thought by certain workers that there may be some sympathetic fibres in the vagus. However, it was soon suspected that this was not the case when the pattern of response was found to differ from that obtained after adrenergic nerve stimulation. Later, when blockers of adrenergic transmission became available it was possible to show that the effect is not due to adrenergic nerves (28).

The finding, in 1963 (11), of inhibitory junction potentials in the musculature of the guinea pig gut led Burnstock to postulate the existence of non-adrenergic inhibitory autonomic nerves. He later put foward his theory that purine nucleotides act as neurotransmitters in this type of nerve (12). The first suggestion, based on morphological evi-

dence, of the existence of gut peptidergic nerves emerged in 1970 when Baumgarten described autonomic fibres with an ultrastructural profile which did not appear to correspond to that of either cholinergic or adrenergic nerves (1). These fibres contained large, electron dense vesicles, which differed from the agranular vesicles found in cholinergic nerves and the small, electron dense granules in adrenergic fibres. These "new" nerves were called p (for peptidergic)-type, because of the similarity they bore to the peptidergic nerves of the hypothalamic-hypophyseal system. The insight Baumgarten had in recognising the peptidergic characteristics of these nerves was made apparent in 1975 when substance P was localised, by two independent groups (6, 62), to autonomic fibres in mammalian gut.

Since then, detailed morphological and physiological analysis of gut peptidergic nerves has been carried out and still continues. Presented below is an account of the current status of knowledge of the peptidergic nervous system of the gut.

## TECHNOLOGY

Immunocytochemistry, at the light and electron microscopical levels, has provided the major means for the study of the morphology and distribution of the peptidergic nervous system. Since its first application in 1955 (16), immunocytochemistry has evolved into an accurate investigative procedure, providing invaluable information. Over the years, many advances have been made, mainly due to modifications of the basic techniques of Coons, Leduc, Connolly (16) and Sternberger (76) as well as the production of specific antisera appropriate for immunocytochemistry and the development of new fixation procedures (81). Immunocytochemistry, however, can not be used in isolation. Parallel quantitative data, obtained by radioimmunoassay of tissue extracts, as well as chemical analysis of the peptides under study, must be carried out to validate fully all immunocytochemical findings. In addition, conventional histological and ultrastructural examination of all tissues is of prime importance.

There are two areas in immunocytochemistry which have presented particular difficulties. One concerns the specificity of the antisera and the other the fixation and preparation of tissue.

### Antisera

The problem of immunostaining of unrelated antigens has largely been countered by the use of standard controls (76) and will, hopefully, be erased completely when monoclonal antibodies become generally available. The production by each lymphocyte of a single antibody has been made use of by hybridising lymphocytes with myeloma cells in order to obtain an indefinite supply of antibodies of a single clone (54). This work is at an early stage but obviously has enormous potential value in many fields.

In addition to producing single antibody populations, careful consideration is needed of the structure of the antigen recognised by the antibody. A single antibody species will probably recognise a sequence of six or seven amino acids at most, and therefore cannot be considered specific for an entire peptide molecule of twenty amino acids or more. In order to obtain an immunostain which is as specific as is currently possible to achieve, antibodies must be used which have been raised against various defined portions of the peptide molecule.

There are two main reasons why the use of a range of region-specific antisera is so important. Firstly, several peptides have regions of their molecular structure which are similar to those of otherwise distinctly different peptides. Secondly, it has long been known that a peptide can exist in more than one molecular form. A good example of this is CCK which occurs in the gut in at least two forms (17). One form, CCK 34 (amino acids) is found in cells in the mucosal epithelium. The octapeptide at the carboxyl terminal of this molecule (CCK-8) can also be found in cells but it is this form which predominates in autonomic nerve fibres of the gut (17). Obviously, antibodies directed against the mid-portion of the molecule or the amide terminal will not detect neuronal CCK-8.

Some of the disagreement concerning whether or not a certain peptide occurs in the gut autonomic innervation has centered on the fact that it can be detected, by the same anitserum, in one species but not in another. Clearly, this may also reflect differences in molecular forms. This may be the case with somatostatin, which has been found in gut nerves in mammals other than man (34). As somatostatin has a cyclic form, it appears that the mid-portion of the molecule reacts with the antibodies as the two ends are "hidden". If the molecular forms found for example in guinea pig and rat gut differ in the mid-portion from that present in human gut then this would explain why human somatostatin-containing nerves have yet to be described.

### Tissue preparation

Different centres have developed their own fixation procedures for tissues undergoing immunocytochemistry. However, a major advance has been the use of cross-linking, bifunctional reagents, which preserve the full antigenicity of the peptide molecules without altering the general morphology of the tissue (63). P-benzoquinone has been found to be particularly suitable for

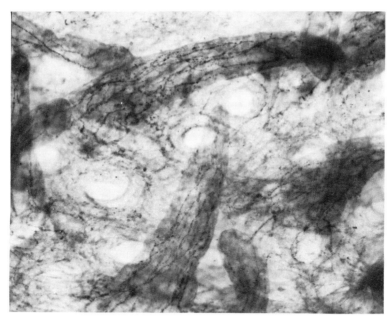

Fig. 1. Separated lamina propria from human ileum. Substance P immunoreactive nerve fibres can be seen around the base and along the length of the villi (×163).

fixation of tissue in which peptidergic nerves are to be immunostained (3). Tissue is fixed by immersion in a solution of p-benzoquinone and cryostat sections are then cut and immunostained.

Separated layers of the gut wall can also been immunostained and, in animals, this method has been used successfully in combination with experimental surgical procedures to obtain information on the projections of peptidergic fibres (27). Recently, a technique for the layer separation of the human gut was achieved, providing whole mount preparations for immunostaining (26). This technique has the particular advantage of enabling examination of the three dimensional arrangement of the peptidergic neural network and will provide an important investigative tool in human gut pathology. Using this method it is possible to demonstrate that, for example, in the lamina propria of human gut, different substance P fibres run in a plane at right angles to the villi, encircle the base of the villi and project up into each villus (Fig. 1).

*Gut neuropeptides*

It is not and may never be, possible to produce a complete list of peptides which occur in the gut autonomic innervation. Not only is the list continually being added to but there appears to be a level of disagreement amongst researchers as to whether all peptides reported to be in nerves actually occur in this location. Table I shows those peptides which are generally considered, at the moment, to be present in the autonomic innervation of the gut of mammals, and others for which this localisation has yet to be fully established.

The research into the chemical characteristics of these peptides is far too extensive to be fully reported here. Table II, therefore, provides a summary.

Table I. Gut neuropeptides (reference).

Vasoactive intestinal polypeptide (VIP) (70)
Substance P (75)
Enkephalin (45)
Bombesin (51)
Somatostatin (7)
Neurotensin (30)
Thyrotrophin releasing hormone (TRH) (20)
Cholecystokinin octapeptide (CCK-8) (18)
Motilin (40)

Table II. Chemical Characteristics.

| Peptide | Molecular variant | No. of amino acids | Molecular weight | Sequence similarities |
|---|---|---|---|---|
| Bombesin | Amphibian | 14 | 1620 | Substance P |
| | Porcine | 27 | 2806 | Ranatensin |
| | Chicken | 27 | 2841 | Litorin |
| CCK-8 | Octa- | 8 | 1143 | Gastrin/CCK family |
| Enkephalin | Leu$^5$ | 5 | 574 | |
| | Met$^5$ | 5 | 556 | Endorphin |
| Motilin | Porcine | 22 | 2700 | 2 forms in gut and plasma |
| Neurotensin | Human | 13 | 1673 | Xenopsin |
| Substance P | Bovine | 11 | 1348 | Physalaemin |
| | | | | Eledoisin |
| TRH | Ovine | 3 | 362 | Not known |
| VIP | Porcine | 28 | 3326 | Secretin |
| | | | | Glucagon |
| | | | | PHI |

*Actions*

These peptides all have numerous actions. For the sake of brevity the reader is referred, in Table I, to articles on each individual peptide.

*Motility.* Many of the peptides are involved, either directly or indirectly, in the control of gut motility. VIP nerves are thought to form the main non-adrenergic, inhibitory neural circuit (27). Certainly, VIP has an inhibitory effect and has been shown to relax isolated muscle strips in organ baths (14). The enkephalins also reduce gut motility. They appear to slow the transit rate by inhibiting the release of acetylcholine (82) and by reducing the firing of neurons in the myenteric plexus (59). Conversely, substance P (37) and CCK (80) stimulate muscle activity. It is not yet clear whether or not the effect of substance P is direct as although it does have some effect on muscle cells (83), it also modulates cholinergic and adrenergic transmission (30). CCK causes contraction of guinea pig ileum in what is thought to be an indirect manner involving cholinergic nerves (80).

There have been several reports of the effects of TRH (thyrotropin-releasing hormone) on the gut but fewer reporting its neuronal localisation. In man, for example, TRH inhibits gastric motility induced either by distention or hypoglycaemia (19). The mainly inhibitory effects of TRH in man are not seen in rat or dog (56), where the peptide causes contraction of smooth muscle.

Several other peptides have actions on gut motility but are not widely accepted as being neurotransmitters. For example, somatostatin inhibits many gut functions including motility (7) but it has not been shown, in many mammalian species, whether this effect is mediated by peptide of cellular or neuronal origin. The motor simulatory effects of motilin are well described (39) but there are few, isolated reports of its occurrence in nervous tissues (57). Most, if not all, of the peptide is probably produced by mucosal cells. Intravenous administration of neurotensin causes inhibition of peristaltic waves in human small intestine (68) but as it has only, so far, been found in very few nerves in the rat (73), it is likely that the endogenous neurotensin having this effect is also produced mainly by endocrine cells, which are present in large numbers in the ileum. However, although neurotensin has not been found in nerves in the guinea pig, it causes contraction of the ileum in this species and the effect is blocked by tetrodotoxin (29), indicating that perhaps the complete distribution of neurotensin containing nerves has yet to be revealed.

Blood flow in the gut is likely to be controlled to a significant extent by peptidergic nerves. Both of the neuropeptides found in the largest concentrations in the gut, VIP and substance P, have the same effect on the circulatory system and cause vasodilation (70, 75). VIP has been cited as being the neurotransmitter in the reflex hyperaemia of the gut which follows mechanical or chemical stimulation (21). It is released during such stimulation (25, 42) and administration of VIP causes an increase in blood flow matching that which occurs after mechanical or chemical stimulation (22). Recently, it was postulated that the release of VIP during this induced vasodilation is mediated by serotonin (5-HT) produced by enterochromaffin cells (21). The effect of serotonin on VIP nerves may be paracrine but the possibility that the nerves may be in direct contact with the cells has been previously suggested (66).

*Secretion.* (a) Endocrine. Few neuropeptides have been reported as acting on the endocrine cells of the gut. Bombesin and somatostatin, however, modulate the release of a number of gastrointestinal hormones (50, 7). Bombesin is known as the universal releaser because of the variety and extent of its stimulatory actions, whilst conversely, somatostatin is known as the universal inhibitor. Thus, they have an entirely antagonistic relationship; bombesin stimulates the release of hormones and somatostatin inhibits it. So far, bombesin has been shown to cause the release of gastrin, motilin, neurotensin, CCK and enteroglucagon from the gut, as well as pancreatic polypeptide and insulin from the pancreas. Somatostatin, on the other hand; inhibits the release of these peptides. Bombesin and somatostatin may present an example of a delicately balanced "pull-push" system controlling not only hormone release by the gut but also exocrine secretion (65).

(b) Exocrine secretion. The release of gastric acid is stimulated and inhibited by bombesin (50) and somatostatin (7), respectively. It remains to be seen into how many other systems this antagonistic relationship extends.

One of the most powerful stimulators of exocrine secretion, from the gut, pancreas or salivary gland, is VIP (70). The potency of its actions in the gut is clearly seen in the Verner-Morrison (VIPoma) syndrome, characterised by water diarrhoea, where VIP is produced by a tumour and released to give high levels of the peptide in the circulation (8). Removal of the tumour restores normal concentrations of circulating VIP and the diarrhoea ceases. Administration of VIP to experimental animals in similar quantities as those which occur in the syndrome reproduce the classical features of watery diarrhoea and hypokalaemia (55). Subsequent infusion studies in man have shown that VIP does cause active secretion of both water and electrolytes from the bowel, possibly by activating adenylate cyclase, leading to an increase of c-AMP concentrations (45).

*Trophism.* It has been known for some time that the autonomic innervation is involved in the trophic maintenance of the gut. Neural stimulation increases mitotic activity (78) whilst denervation slows cell turnover (46).

The trophic effect of peptidergic nerves specifically has yet to be demonstrated. There is some evidence that certain neuropeptides act on cell turnover in the gut. For example, bombesin may have a direct or indirect effect on the gut. Its activity as a trophic agent has been shown in both the exocrine and endocrine pancreas, where it causes hyperplasia (50). It may have similar effects on the gut. In addition, the capacity of bombesin to simulate release of other peptides may give it an indirect effect, for example by releasing enteroglucagon, which is widely considered to be a major factor in the regulation of intestinal mucosal growth (6). In a similar way, somatostatin may inhibit release of enteroglucagon and, thus, have an anti-trophic effect. It has also been reported to decrease cell proliferation in the rat gut (49).

*Sensory system*

Very little is known about the sensory innervation of the gut. However, additional information has become available with the finding that substance P may be a sensory neurotransmitter (61). The discovery of substance P in neurons of spinal ganglia (35) was an early indication that it may have such a function. Substance P is now known to be present in primary sensory afferents and evidence is accumulating to show that it is involved in peripheral nociception (64).

Capsaicin, the active ingredient of red pepper, has proved to be extremely useful in the investigation of the role of substance P as a neurotransmitter. This chemical releases substance P from sensory terminals and, so, depletion of the peptide after capsaicin application provides a simple marker for substance P-containing sensory fibres (75).

In the gut, it has been reported that capsaicin does not alter the substance P content, which suggests that there are no substance P containing sensory fibres (36). However, these findings remain unconfirmed. It may be that sensory fibres containing the peptide form only a small part of the total population of substance P nerves in the gut. If this is so, then it may not be easy to recognise a relatively small depletion of peptide content. A recent report, shows that there are a number of substance P-containing sensory fibres around blood vessels in the gut. These are capsaicin-sensitive and have previously been shown to have an extrinsic origin (reported at "Brain-Gut Axis" Symposium. Florence 1981, by Dr. J. B. Furness).

## ORIGIN OF PEPTIDERGIC FIBRES

### (a) Extrinsic

The extrinsic autonomic nervous supply to the gut arises from the vagus nerve and sacral spinal outflow and from prevertebral sympathetic ganglia. Several peptides can be demonstrated in these inputs. Substance P, enkephalin, VIP and somatostatin have all been found in the vagus, where ligation studies show that these are transported towards the periphery (79).

A large proportion of the principal ganglion cells of the inferior and superior mesenteric ganglia and the coeliac ganglion contain somatostatin (32). Also sensory fibres containing substance P may project to the gut via sympathetic ganglia (33). Although the exact contribution made to gut peptidergic innervation by these extrinsic fibres has not yet been fully established, the greater part of the peptidergic innervation is known to arise from intrinsic neurons.

### (b) Intrinsic

It has been established by experimentation that in the pig (53), guinea pig (41) and mouse (72) gut, at least, the vast majority of the peptidergic nerves have an intrinsic origin. The peptidergic

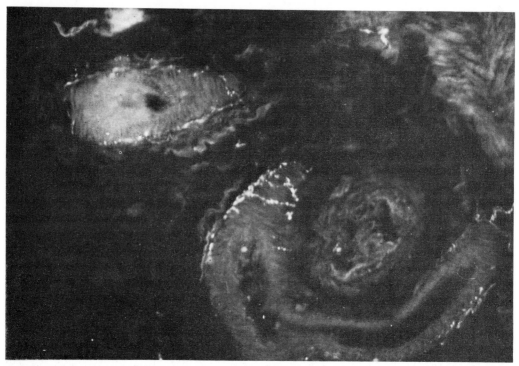

Fig. 2. VIP immunoreactive nerve fibres in association with blood vessels in the sub-mucosa of human ileum (×220).

nerves, with other intrinsic autonomic fibres, appear to form an autonomous unit in the gut, which receives relays from outside but can continue functioning when these influences are disturbed, e.g. gut motility is not significantly altered following extrinsic denervation. It is only when this "minibrain" itself is damaged that the mechanism really ceases to run smoothly. This can be seen clearly in examples of gut disease where peptidergic nerve abnormalities occur (see Pathology).

## DISTRIBUTION

### Light microscopy

Peptidergic nerves are found along the entire length of the gastrointestinal tract and are present in each layer of the gut wall. Localisation of gut peptidergic nerves by immunocytochemistry has revealed a high degree of correlation between the distribution of each type of nerve and what is known about the actions of each peptide. This is well illustrated by the distribution of VIP nerves.

In man, and several other mammalian species, VIP nerves are the most abundant of all peptidergic fibres. In accordance with its three main actions in the gut, i.e. vasodilation, muscle relaxation and stimulation of water and electrolyte secretion, VIP nerves are found around blood vessels and, mostly in the circular muscle coat and mucosa. The close association of VIP nerves with blood vessels can be seen in all areas of the gut. They encircle the muscles surrounding arterial vessels (Fig. 2) and form fine meshworks around capillaries in, for example, the lamina propria.

The stimulation of secretion by VIP may be mediated by direct release from nerve fibres on to cells in the mucosal epithelium. There has been a preliminary report of a direct contact between VIP nerves and epithelial cells (69). In addition, epithelial cells are known to have VIP receptors, which are coupled with adenylate cyclase stimulation (45). Another possible functional relationship which may be mediated by direct contact between VIP nerves and mucosal cells is that

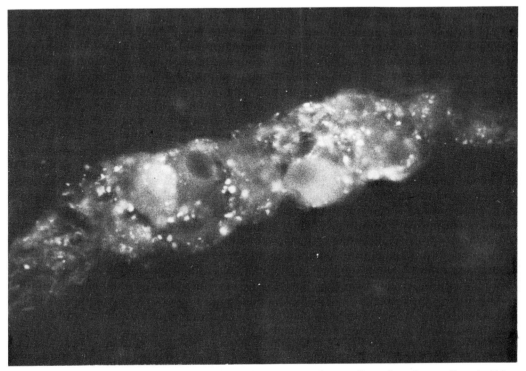

Fig. 3. Sub-mucous plexus in rat colon containing VIP immunoreactive ganglion cells and nerve fibres ($\times 404$).

between VIP and serotonin (21), previously mentioned in the section on Actions.

Ganglion cells containing VIP are found, in most mammals, predominantly in the sub-mucous plexus (40) (Fig. 3). This distribution fits well with the peptide's role as a stimulator of secretion as it was previously known that this plexus supplies the mucosal innervation.

Conversely, most substance P neuronal cell bodies occur in the myenteric plexus (40) and this is the site where the majority of substance P fibres are found (Fig. 4). The high ratio of substance P fibres in the myenteric plexus is in agreement with its postulated role as a transmitter of excitatory interneurons within this plexus rather than the sub-mucous plexus (43). No effects of substance P on the neurons in the sub-mucous plexus have been described. Substance P fibres are also present in larger numbers in the circular muscle coat, where they may act directly to increase contractions. The substance P fibres which are frequently seen around blood vessels may mediate the function of the peptide as a vasodilator (75)

or, as has recently been suggested, they may have a sensory function.

Enkephalin containing fibres, in keeping with the peptide's role as an inhibitor of neuronal activity (59), are found mainly in the myenteric plexus. In man, scattered fibres can also be found in the circular muscle coat (Fig. 5) and muscularis mucosae.

Somatostatin nerves have been described in the gut of the guinea pig and rat (73), where they are found mainly in the two ganglionated plexuses. Sparse fibres can also be seen in the circular muscle. Rodents are the only mammals shown so far to have CCK nerves in the gut (73). Although the rat has more CCK-8 containing nerves than the guinea pig, they are only found in very small numbers in this species. These fibres are present predominantly in the circular muscle coat. Low numbers of neurotensin containing nerves have also been described in the circular muscle and myenteric plexus of the rat gut (73).

By separately culturing neurons from the two ganglionated plexuses of the guinea pig gut, it has

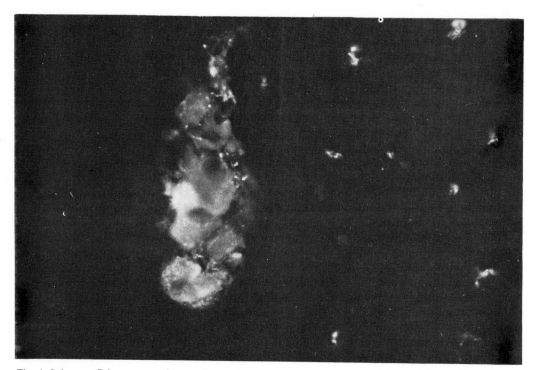

Fig. 4. Substance P immunoreactive ganglion cells in the myenteric plexus of guinea pig colon (×266).

been possible to show that there are peptidergic connections between them (40). Immunostaining of cultures of submucosal ganglion cells revealed only VIP fibres and conversely cultures of the myenteric plexus revealed only substance P containing fibres. Thus the VIP fibres found in the myenteric plexus and the substance P fibres found in the sub-mucous plexus may represent interconnections running across the muscle coat. The possibility of the fibres seen in each plexus originating from an extrinsic source seems unlikely as it has been shown that virtually all the peptidergic innervation of the guinea pig gut is intrinsic.

*Co-existence.* Prior to the discovery of the gut peptidergic nervous system, there was a period of great excitement when reports were made of the co-existence of peptides in the same cell. With the development of more advanced technology and the acquisition of further knowledge, new evidence emerged suggesting that the co-existence is usually between structurally related pepides, e.g. ACTH and endorphin in the pitui-

tary (48), rather than completely different peptides. It has been reported, however, that dissimilar substances such as peptides and amines co-exist in cells of certain species (31).

As yet, there has been only one report of two peptides occurring in the same peripheral autonomic nerve. These peptides were somatostatin and cholecystokinin/gastrin (73). Conversely, co-existence of peptides and classical neutrotransmitters has been described a number of times. The first description was that of somatostatin in a proportion of principal adrenergic ganglion cells in the guinea pig (32). Also, in the superior cervical ganglion of the rat, small numbers of ganglion cells were found to contain both noradrenaline and enkephalin (74). More recently, VIP has been shown to be present in nerve fibres in feline exocrine glands which can be demonstrated by the histochemical method for staining acetylcholinesterase and it was suggested from this evidence that VIP and acetylcholine may co-exist in these fibres (52). The significance of the acetylcholinesterase staining has been a matter of dispute for

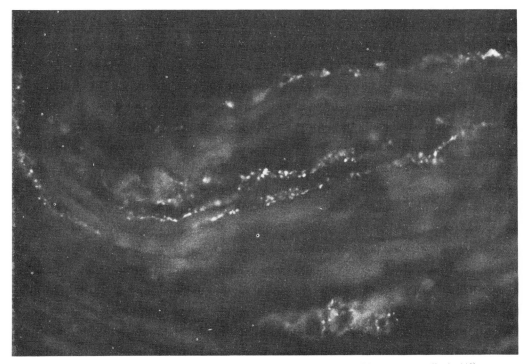

Fig. 5. Few, fine enkephalin immunoreactive nerves in the circular muscle of human appendix (×440).

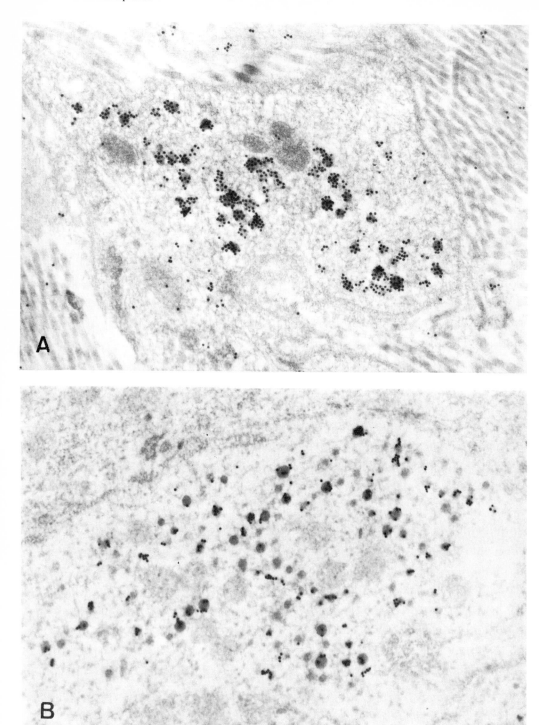

Fig. 6. (A) Secretory granules in a nerve of the guinea pig colon immunostained using the immuno-gold staining method (×45K). (B) Secretory granules in a similar tissue to that in (A), immunostained for VIP using the immuno-gold staining method (×45K).

some time, as many workers feel that the method does not stain cholinergic nerves specifically. Moreover, acetylcholinesterase has been shown to hydrolyse substance P, suggesting that it might also function as a peptidase (13). Support for the light microscopical evidence for co-storage of VIP and acetycholine has been provided by ultrastructural studies where VIP was localised, using the peroxidase-anti-peroxidase method, to fibres which also contained small, agranular vesicles, like those found typically in cholinergic nerves (42). As the authors of this work point out, the concept of the co-existence of these two neurotransmitters and their differential or combined release is certainly an attractive one and might help to explain some observed physiological anomalies (e.g. the two part vasodilatory response in the salivary gland following parasympathetic stimulation).

*Electron microscopy*

Use of the electron microscope provided the first morphological suggestion of the existence of peptidergic nerves in the gut (1). Baumgarten described non-adrenergic, non-cholinergic nerves with large (85–160 nm) electron dense granules, which he called p- (for peptidergic) type. Six years after Baumgarten's report, in 1976, Cook and Burnstock observed that the autonomic nerves of the gut represent a heterogeneous population and they described at least 8 separate ultrastructural profiles (15).

Subsequent electron microscopical studies have reported the occurrence of p-type fibres in a number of systems but it was not until the advent of immunostaining at the electron microscopical level that it became possible to show that peptides are actually present in p-type granules. Using a colloidal gold labelling method, both substance P and VIP have been immunostained in p-type nerve fibres (67). However, analysis of the size of the granules containing the two peptides shows that they, in fact, form a heterogeneous group. This finding, thus, fully supports the observations made by Cook and Burnstock.

Substance P nerves contain round neurosecretory granules of medium electron density which measure 85 nm, on average (Fig. 6a). These gran-

ules have a clear halo between the core and the limiting membrane and correspond to those classified by Cook and Burnstock as type 5b. VIP is found in larger (98 nm) granules (Fig. 6b), in nerves which may be those of type 5c. These fibres also contain small, agranular vesicles intermingled with the VIP granules.

There is, in addition, a number of p-type nerves which are not immunostained by antisera to either substance P or VIP. These main contain other peptides known to occur in nerves of the gut.

## PATHOLOGY

The pathology of gut peptidergic nerves has not been extensively studied in the past. Changes in the concentrations of peptides have been reported in certain isolated diseases, but it has been only recently that the involvement of peptidergic nerves in human gut pathology has received more attention.

Due to its highly integrated organisation, any lesion of the intrinsic nervous system of the gut would be expected to affect the peptidergic innervation. Thus, in congenital aganglionosis, it follows that there should be a depletion of peptidergic nerves. In specimens from children, a reduction in peptidergic innervation has been found, by immunocytochemistry (Fig. 7) and radioimmunoassay, which appears to be in proportion to the length of the aganglionic segment (5). The hyperplasia of cholinergic (9) and adrenergic (2) nerves in this disease is thought to be due to extrinsic fibres which, during development, undergo extensive ramifications as they "search" for intrinsic neuronal cell bodies with which to synapse. The finding of a lack of peptidergic nerves in aganglionic human bowel supports the theory that the majority of peptidergic nerves are instrinsic. Conversely, the minimal contribution made by extrinsic peptidergic fibres is reflected by the absence of a peptidergic nerve hyperplasia, like that seen with cholinergic and adrenergic nerves.

The effect of the loss of peptidergic innervation is made apparent by the clinical features of the disease. The most important feature of congenital aganglionosis is the constriction which forms in

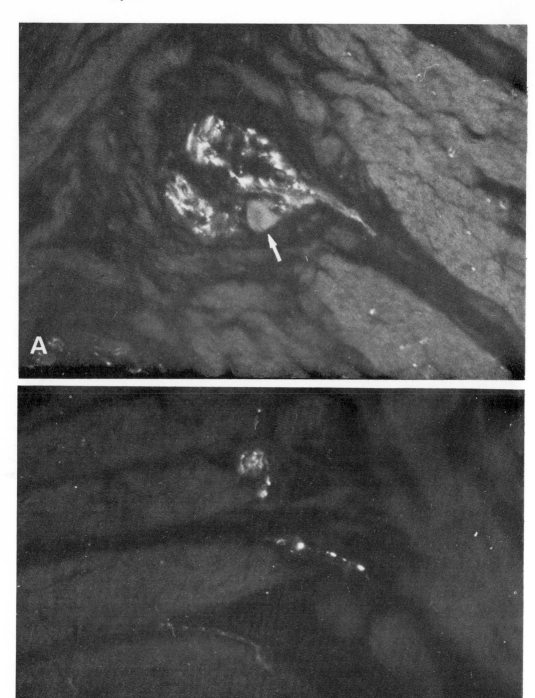

Fig. 7. (A) Substance P immunoreactive nerves and a single immunoreactive ganglion cell (arrow) in the myenteric plexux of normal neonatal human colon (×270). (B) Sparse substance P immunoreactive nerves in a similar region to that in (A) taken from a child with aganglionic bowel (×270).

the aganglionic region of the bowel. As the larger part of the peptidergic innervation probably forms most of the inhibitory nervous supply, its absence may leave the inherent excitation of the circular muscle coat uncontrolled, leading to constriction. The resulting chronic constipation is further promoted by the lack of normal VIP induced secretion from the bowel.

Depletion of peptidergic nerves also occurs when reduction of intrinsic innervation is acquired rather than congenital, as seen in Chagas' disease. This disease is a result of infestation with Trypanosoma cruzi which causes, by an unknown mechanism, degeneration of intramural neurons and the development of megabowel (most commonly megacolon and megaoesophagus). In rec-

tal biopsies from Chagasic patients low levels of peptidergic innervation and peptide content (Fig. 8) were found, whether the biopsies were taken from patients with megaoesophagus or megacolon (51). This indicates the diffuse nature of the gut lesion. Preliminary investigation of resected specimens of large bowel show that there is a varied pattern of peptidergic nerve loss, reflecting the different degrees of neuronal degeneration found along the length of the bowel.

The contribution made by the peptidergic abnormalities to the development of the gastrointestinal malfunction observed in Chagas' disease may well be similar to that in Hirschsprung's disease.

In Crohn's disease, a reverse situation appears to occur. There is a striking increase in VIP nerves in the gut wall and the total content of VIP in surgical specimens is increased by more than 100% (Fig. 9) in comparison not only with normal bowel but also samples from ulcerative colitis

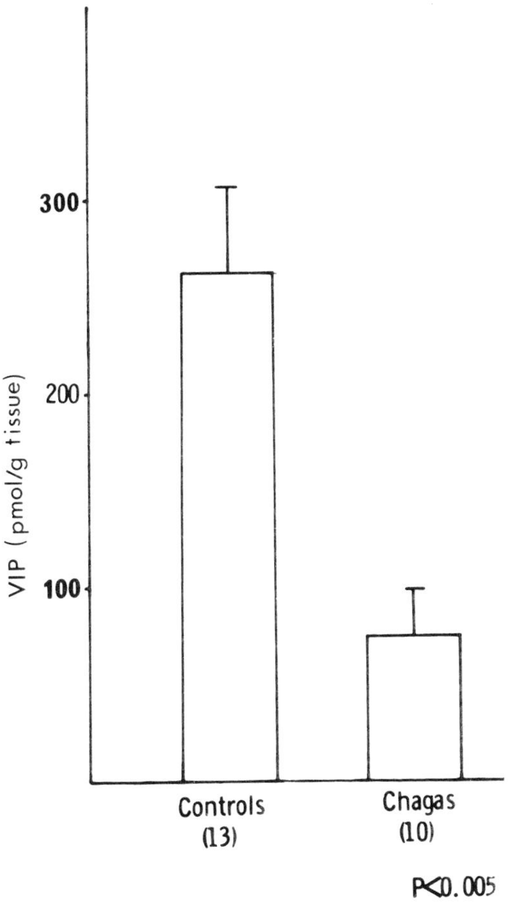

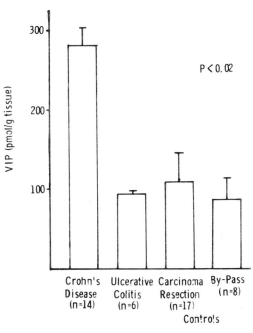

Fig. 8. Concentrations of VIP, as measured by radioimmunoassay of tissue extracts, in rectal biopsies from normal controls and patients with Chagas' disease.

Fig. 9. Concentrations of VIP, as measured by radioimmunoassay of tissue extracts, in surgical specimens from patients with Crohn's disease, ulcerative colitis. These are compared with normal bowel from patients undergoing resection for carcinoma or by-pass for obestity.

patients (4). If these nerves were fully functional and releasing their peptide content to the mucosal epithelium, watery diarrhoea would be expected to develop. However, despite a consistent VIP nerve hyperplasia in this disease, severe diarrhoea is not a typical clinical feature. The possibility of a non-functional VIP nerve hyperplasia is supported by the appearance of individual fibres. They are enlarged, thickened and distorted, perhaps as a result of some form of damage.

As the abnormalities of VIP innervation and bowel content were found only in Crohn's disease and not in the other major inflammatory bowel condition, ulcerative colitis, this difference may form the basis of a useful diagnostic tool. This possibility was investigated by examination of a series of endoscopic rectal biopsies from patients with Crohn's disease affecting or not involving the rectum, ulcerative colitis, active or quiescent, and normal controls (60). The characteristic hyperplasia of morphologically abnormal VIP nerves was found only in tissue from patients with Crohn's disease. Some less marked increased were observed in cases of ulcerative colitis with very severe inflammatory changes which reached the submucosal layer but the fibres were normal in appearance. These methods may therefore have applications in the differential diagnosis of inflammatory bowel diseases.

## FUTURE

Research into gut peptidergic innervation is expanding at a phenomenal rate, with new developments being made in a number of different areas. Below are two areas of major interest which hold promise for the future.

### New peptides

In the past few years alone at least four previously unrecognised regulatory peptides with a possible neuronal localisation have been discovered. In the Karolinska Institute, Sweden, a method of C-terminal amide fragmentation has revealed the existence of two important peptides (77). One is PHI, *p*eptide of intestinal origin with *h*istidine at the N-terminal end and *i*soleucine at the C-terminal amide end. This peptide has cer-

tain features in common with peptides of the secretin-glucagon family (which includes VIP). Like VIP, PHI increase C-AMP activity, relaxes smooth muscle and has also been shown to bind the VIP receptors on cells. The other recently discovered peptide is PYY (tyrosine at both the N- and C-terminal ends) which has some characteristics in common with neurotensin and pancreatic polypeptide.

Two "new" regulatory peptides have also been found by Erspamer and co-workers in Italy. These are called dermorphin (10) and sauvagine (23). Dermorphin has opiate effects which are far more potent than those exhibited by any previously investigated mammalian endorphin, whilst sauvagine causes vasodilation and the release of ACTH.

As these peptides have yet to be localised in mammalian gut, it remains to be seen if any or all of them will be found in the autonomic nerves. Undoubtedly there will be still more newly discovered peptides to be localised in the not too distant future.

### "Brain specific" proteins

An area of research which is already yielding useful information is the localisation in the gut of proteins which were originally thought to be specific to the brain. An example is neuron specific enolase which is found not only in all autonomic nerves but also in endocrine cells (24). The localisation of this enzyme therefore provides a unique means for the simulateneous demonstration of the nervous and endocrine systems of the gut (Fig. 10). Other proteins appear to be specific markers for glial cells, e.g. S-100 (38). Thus, there are currently available markers of neuronal and glial components which can be used in several ways in the study of the enteric nervous system, particularly as some of these proteins are enzymes in the glycolytic pathway and may also be markers of functional activity.

An obvious application for these markers is in pathology. Immunostaining of neuron specific enolase, for instance, gives an immediate assessment of the overall state of the nervous and endocrine systems, the individual components can then be "dissected out" by subsequent histochem-

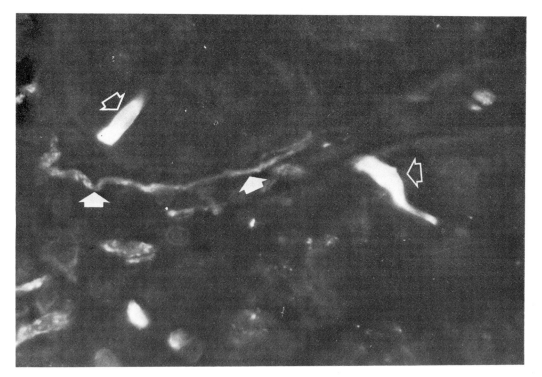

Fig. 10. NSE immunoreactive endocrine cells (open arrows) and nerve fibres (closed arrows) in human colonic mucosa (×313).

ical and immunocytochemical stains. Specific areas where such an approach will prove useful include the diseases which were mentioned in the section of pathology.

## CONCLUSIONS

The autonomic nervous system can no longer be considered bipartite in nature. It is now established that there is at least one further division and a wealth of evidence indicates that peptides are neurotransmitters in the majority of these non-adrenergic, non-cholinergic nerves.

The highly integrated network of peptidergic nerves forms a major component of the enteric nervous system. This component has a predominately intrinsic origin and seems to be largely autonomous. It is when damage occurs to the intrinsic system itself that malfunction occurs, as can be seen in a number of diseases.

The exponentially growing amount of information available on the peptidergic nerves of the gut has yet to be fully assimilated to produce a clear understanding of not only the functions of these nerves but also the complex relationships which exist between the various components of the enteric nervous system. However, if the current rate of expansion continues, it should not be long before the physiology and pathophysiology of the gut ceases to be so enigmatic.

## ACKNOWLEDGEMENTS

This work was supported by funds from the Medical Research Council (UK) and Janssen Pharmaceuticals.

G-LF is a research fellow from the Department of Medicine, University of Bologna, Italy, receiving financial support from the British Council.

LP is the holder of an MRC studentship.

REFERENCES

1. Baumgarten HG, Holstein AF, Owman CH. Z Zellforsch 1970, 106, 376–397
2. Bennett A, Garrett JR, Howard ER, Brit Med J 1968, 1 487–489
3. Bishop AE, Polak JM, Bloom SR, Pearse AGE. J Endocrinol 1978, 77, 25–26
4. Bishop AE, Polak JM, Bryant MG, Bloom SR, Hamilton, S. Gastroenterol 1980, 79, 853–860
5. Bishop AE, Polak JM, Lake BD, Bryant MG, Bloom SR. Histopath (in press) 1981
6. Bloom SR. Gut 1972, 13, 520–523
7. Bloom SR. Gastroenterology 1978, 75, 145–147
8. Bloom SR, Polak JM, Pearse AGE. Lancet 1973, ii, 14
9. Bodian M, Carter CO, Ward BCK. Lancet 1951, i, 302–309
10. Broccardo M, Erspamer V, Falconieri Erspamer G, Improta G, Linari G, Melchiorri P, Montecucchi PC. Br J Pharmacol 1981, 73, 625–631
11. Burnstock G, Campbell G, Bennett M, Holman ME. Nature (London) 1963, 200, 581–582
12. Burnstock G, Campbell G, Satchell DG, Smythe A. Brit J Pharmacol 1970, 40, 668–688
13. Chubb IW, Hodgson AJ, White GH. Neurosci 1980, 5, 2065–2075
14. Cocks T, Burnstock G. Euro J Pharmacol 1979, 54, 251–259
15. Cook RD, Burnstock GJ. J. Neurocytol 1976, 5, 171–194
16. Coons AH, Leduc EH, Connolly JM. J Exp Med 1955, 102, 49–60
17. Dockray GJ. pp 43–48 in Bloom SR, Polak JM (eds), Gut Hormones. 2nd ed Churchill Livingstone, Edinburgh 1981
18. Dockray GJ. pp 228–239 in Bloom SR, Polak JM (eds), Gut Hormones 2nd ed. Churchill Livingstone, Edinburgh 1981
19. Dolva LO, Stadaas J. Scand J Gastroenterol 1979, 14, 419–423
20. Dolva LO, Stadaas J, Hanssen KF. pp 445–448 in Bloom SR, Polak JM (eds), Gut Hormones, 2nd ed. Churchill Livingstone, Edinburgh 1981
21. Eklund Q, Fahrenkrug J, Jodal M, Lundgren O, Schaffalitzky de Muckadell OB, Sjoquist A. J Physiol (Lond) 1980, 302, 549–557
22. Eklund S, Jodal M, Lundgren O, Sjoqvist A. Acta Physiol Scand 1979, 105, 461–468
23. Erspamer V, Falconieri Erspamer G, Improta G, Negri L, De Castiglione R, Naunyn-Schmiedeberg's Arch Pharmacol 1978, 303, 133–138
24. Facer P, Polak JM, Marangos PJ, Pearse AGE. Proc Roy Microscop Soc 1980, 15, 113–114
25. Fahrenkrug J, Haglund U, Jodal M, Lundgren O, Olbe L, Schaffalitzky de Muckadell OB. J Physiol (Lond) 1978, 248, 291–305
26. Ferri GL. Harris A, Probert L, Buchan AMJ, Marangos PJ, Adrian TE, Ghatei MA, Bloom SR, Polak JM. Gut In Press
27. Furness JB, Costa M, Franco R, Llewellyn-Smith IJ. in Costa E, Trabucchi M. (eds), Neural peptides and Neuronal communication. Raven Press, New York 1980

28. Greeff K, Kasperat H, Oswald W. Arch Exp Pathol Pharmakol (Naunyn-Schmiedeberg's) 1962, 243, 528–545
29. Hammer RA, Leeman SE. pp 290–299 in Bloom SR, Polak JM, (eds), Gut Hormones 2nd ed. Churchill Livingstone, Edinburgh 1981
30. Hedqvist P, Von Euler US, pp 89–95 in Von Euler US, Pernow B, (eds). Substance P. Raven Press, New York 1977
31. Heitz Ph, Polak JM, Kasper M, Timson CM, Pearse AGE. Histochem 1977, 50, 319–325
32. Hokfelt T, Elfvin LG, Elde R, Schultzberg M, Goldstein M, Luft R. Proc Natl Acad Sci USA 1977, 74, 3587–3591
33. Hokfelt T, Elfvin LG, Schultzberg M, Goldstein M, Nilsson G. Brain Res 1977, 132, 29–41
34. Hokfelt T, Johansson O, Efendic S, Luft R, Arimura A, Experientia 1975, 31/7, 852–854
35. Hokfelt T, Kellerth JO, Nilsson G, Pernow B. Science 1975, 190, 889–890
36. Holzer P, Gamse R, Lembeck F. Euro J Pharmacol 1980, 61, 303–307
37. Holzer P, Lembeck F. Naunyn-Schmiedeberg's Arch Pharmacol 1978, 307, 257–264
38. Hyden H, McEwen B. PNAS 1966, 55, 354
39. Itoh Z. pp 280–289 in Bloom SR, Polak JM, (eds), Gut Hormones, 2nd ed. Churchill Livingstone, Edinburgh 1981
40. Jessen KR, Polak JM, Van Noorden S, Bloom SR, Burnstock G. Nature 1980, 5745, 391–393
41. Jessen KR, Saffrey MJ, Van Noorden S, Bloom SR, Polak JM, Burnstock G. Neurosci 1980, 5, 1717–1735
42. Johansson O, Lundberg JM. Neurosci 1981, 6, 847–862
43. Katayama Y, North RA. Nature (Lond) 1978, 274, 387–388
44. Konturek SJ. pp 432–440 in Bloom SR, Polak JM, (eds), Gut Hormones 2nd ed. Churchill Livingstone, Edinburgh 1981
45. Laburthe M, Mangeat P, Marchis-Mouren G, Rosselin G. Life Sci 1979, 1931–1938
46. Lachat JJ, Goncalves RP. Cell Tiss Res 1978, 192, 285–297
47. Langley JN. J Physiol (Lond) 1898, 23, 407–414
48. Larsson LI pp 151–157 in Grossman MI, Brazier MAB, Lechago J, (eds), Cellular Basis of Chemical Messengers in the Digestive System. Academic Press, New York 1981
49. Lehy T, Dubrasquet M, Bonfils S. Digestion 1979, 9, 99–109
50. Lezoche E, Basso N, Speranza V. pp 419–424 in Bloom SR, Polak JM, (eds), Gut Hormones 2nd ed. Churchill Livingstone, Edinburgh 1981
51. Long RG, Bishop AE, Barnes AJ, Albuquerque RH, O'Shaughnessy DJ, McGregor GP, Bannister R, Polak JM, Bloom SR. Lancet 1980, i, 559–562
52. Lundberg JM, Hokfelt T, Schultzberg M, Uvnas-Wallensten K, Kohler C, Said SI. Neurosci 1980, 4, 1539–1559
53. Malmfors G, Leander S, Brodin E, Hakanson R, Holmin T, Sundler F. Cell Tiss Res 1981, 214, 225–238

54. Milstein C, Galfre G, Secher DS, Springer T. Cell Biology International Reports 1979, 3, 1–16
55. Modlin IM, Bloom SR, Mitchell SJ. Experientia 1978, 34, 535–536
56. Morley JE, Steinbach JH, Feldman EI, Travis ES. Life Sci 1979 24, 1059–1066
57. Nagai K, Yanaihara C, Shimizu F, Kobayashi S, Fujita T. Reg Peptides 1980, Suppl 1, 578
58. Nilsson G, Larsson LI, Hakanson R, Brodin E, Pernow B, Sundler F. Histochem 1975, 43, 97–99
59. North RA, Williams JT. Nature 1976, 264, 460–461
60. O'Morain C, Bishop AE, Levi AJ, Peters TJ, Bloom SR, Polak JM. Gastroenterol 1981, 80, 1234
61. Otsuka M, Konishi S. pp 207–214 in Von Euler US, Pernow B, (eds), Substance P. Nobel Symposium (vol 37). Raven Press, New York 1977
62. Pearse AGE, Polak JM. Histochem 1975, 41, 373–375
63. Pearse AGE, Polak JM. Histochem J 1975, 7, 179–186
64. Polak JM, Bloom SR. Peptides Suppl (in press) 1981
65. Polak JM, Bloom SR. In press in Fink G Whalley LJ, (eds), "Neuropeptides-basic and clinical aspects". Proceedings of the eleventh Pfizer Symposium. Churchill Livingstone, Edinburgh 1981
66. Polak JM, De Mey J, Bloom SR. In Vanhoutte, E, De Clerck, F, (eds), Proc Workshop "5-hydroxy-tryptamine in peripheral reactions". Raven Press, New York (in press) 1981
67. Probert L, De Mey J, Polak JM. Gut (in press) 1981
68. Rosell S. Proc of the Int Union of Physiol Sciences XXVIII International Congress Budapest 1980, 14, 228
69. Rosselin GE. pp 137–143 in Bloom SR, Polak JM, (eds), Gut Hormones (2nd ed). Churchill Livingstone, Edinburgh 1981
70. Said SI. pp 379–384 in Bloom SR, Polak JM, (eds), Gut Hormones, 2nd ed. Churchill Livingstone, Edinburgh 1981
71. Schaffalitzky de Muckadell OB, Fahrenkrug J, Holst JJ, Lauritsen KB. Scand J Gastroenterol 1977, 12, 739–799
72. Schultzberg M, Dreyfus CF, Gershon MD, Hokfelt T, Elde RP, Nilsson G, Said S, Goldstein M. Brain Res 1978, 155 239–248
73. Schultzberg M, Hokfelt T, Nilsson G, Terenius L, Goldstein M, Said S. Neurosci 1980, 5, 689–744
74. Schultzberg M, Hokfelt T, Terenius L, Elfvin LG, Lundberg JM Brandt J, Elde RP, Goldstein M. Neurosci 1979, 4 249–270
75. Skrabanek P, Powell D. Substance P (vol 2). Churchill Livingstone, Edinburgh 1980
76. Sternberger, LA. Immunocytochemistry (2nd ed). John Wiley & Sons, New York 1979
77. Tatemoto K, Mutt V. Nature 1980, 285, 417–418
78. Tutton PJM. Cell Tiss Kinet 1974, 7, 125–136
79. Uvnas-Wallensten K. In Grossman MI, Brazier MAB, Lechago J, (eds), Cellular Basis of Chemical Messengers in the Digestive System. Academic Press, New York 1981
80. Vizi ES, Bertaccini G, Impicciatore M, Mantovani P, Zseli J, Knoll J. Naunyn-Schmiedeberg's Arch Pharmacol 1974, 285, 233–243
81. Van Noorden S, Polak JM. pp 80–89 in Bloom SR, Polak JM, (eds), Gut Hormones 2nd ed. Churchill Livingstone, Edinburgh 1981
82. Waterfield AA, Smockum RWJ, Hughes J, Kosterlitz HW, Henderson G. Euro J Pharmacol 1977, 43, 107–116
83. Yau WM. Gastroenterol 1978, 74, 228–231

# Detection and Characterisation of Neurotransmitters, Particularly Peptides, in the Gastrointestinal Tract

J. B. FURNESS*, M. COSTA*, R. MURPHY*, A. M. BEARDSLEY*, J. R. OLIVER*,
I. J. LLEWELLYN-SMITH*, R. L. ESKAY†, A. A. SHULKES‡, T. W. MOODY¶ & D. K. MEYER†
* Centre for Neuroscience and Departments of Medicine, Human Morphology and Physiology, Flinders University; † Laboratory of Clinical Science, NIMH, Bethesda; ‡ Department of Surgery, Austin Hospital, Melbourne; ¶ Department of Biochemistry, George Washington University, Washington, DC

There are now about twelve substances, many of them peptides, that are thought to act as neurotransmitters in the enteric nervous system. Most of the studies of peptides have relied on immunochemical methods for their detection. However, difficulties arise in these studies because of the close similarities between peptides. Related peptides can be grouped in several ways according to similarities of origin, function, effects in bioassays and amino acid sequences. Peptides with the same function in different species, and only slight differences in amino acid sequence, have been called isopeptides. Peptide families that have sequences of amino acids in common, but do not necessarily have similar functions are described. In the guinea-pig small intestine, used as a model, the concentrations of fourteen nerve-related peptides and amines are compared. The actual chemical natures of the peptides are discussed. It is concluded that nerves containing authentic leu- and met-enkephelin, somatostatin and substance P are present. VIP in guinea-pig enteric nerves is different from the porcine standard. Peptides similar to authentic CCK8 and amphibian skin bombesin are present. Angiotensin and neurotensin-like peptides shown immunohistochemically are not the authentic peptides. In the longitudinal muscle plus myenteric plexus, most neuropeptide concentrations are in the range of 10–500 pmole/g. The exception is met-enkephalin (1,300 pmole/g). The amine transmitters have considerably higher concentrations, noradrenaline having a concentration of about 3,500 pmole/g and acetylcholine $1-2 \times 10^5$ pmole/g.

*J. B. Furness, Dept. of Human Morphology, Flinders University Medical School, Flinders Medical Centre, Bedford Park, SA 5042, Australia*

For many years only two transmitters were accepted to be present in intestinal nerves: noradrenaline and acetylcholine. However, during the 1960's it was recognised that an inhibitory substance other than noradrenaline was released from certain nerves (4, 13, 14, 60), that excitation of the muscle could be caused by the release of something other than acetylcholine (1, 2) and that 5-hydroxytryptamine could possibly be a gastrointestinal neurotransmitter (11, 42). More recently the number of proposed transmitter substances in the digestive system has grown dramatically, particularly with the discovery of neuropeptides (see 31, 33).

The first substantial indication that peptides might transmit information from enteric nerves came from immunohistochemical studies showing the presence in the nerves of peptides that resembled somatostatin (45), enkephalin (23), substance P (66, 70) and vasoactive intestinal polypeptide (9, 57). Evidence that most of these nerve fibres came from intrinsic nerve cell bodies was soon gathered (e.g. 74, 75).

A general review of the evidence for many of the proposed intestinal transmitters is available (33). The particular cases of ATP (12), 5-HT (41) and VIP (24, 32) have been separately reviewed. In this article some of the general problems of transmitter identification in the enteric nervous system will be dealt with, particular attention being given to the neuropeptides.

*Criteria for transmitter identification*

Lists have often been made of the criteria that are claimed to be required for a substance to be a neurotransmitter. These criteria usually specify that the substance is found in and synthesised by the nerve, that it is released when the nerve is active, that it is removed by enzymatic degradation or uptake into a cell, and that drugs can be found that have parallel actions on transmission and on the action of the compound. These extended lists of criteria have been criticised (33, 68, 79). In fact, if a transmitter is defined as a substance that, when released by activation of a nerve, has an acute effect on an adjacent cell, then the only essential criteria to be met are that it is indeed released and indeed has the appropriate effect. Synthesis, degradation and other criteria merely list properties that are associated with many transmitters but are not necessary requirements for their being transmitters. For example, an amino acid transmitter may be taken up from the interstitial fluid rather than synthesised by the neuron. Likewise, termination of the transmitter's action could be by receptors assuming a refractory state or merely by diffusion from the site of action rather than through enzymatic degradation or uptake mechanisms.

*Problems in the enteric nervous system*

In studies that resulted in the identification of acetylcholine and noradrenaline as peripheral transmitters, it was possible to choose experimental situations in which nerves could be stimulated at a distance from the site of transmitter release and in which a relatively 'pure' response to stimulation could be obtained. Even in the central nervous system, neurons of one or other chemical type are gathered together and may have, to some extent, separate projection pathways. In the intestine, the nerve cell bodies are grouped in small ganglia that are distributed at frequent intervals along its length. However, the different chemical types of neurons are not grouped in the intestine, but each enteric ganglion

represents a collection of many types, as if a random sample were taken from the total population (58). In some cases, the overall proportion of a particular cell type is so low that it is not present in all ganglia. Likewise many types of nerve terminal are present in each ganglion, and with histochemical methods an apparently homogenous supply is often seen, although functional connections made within the ganglia are presumed to be selective. Because of this distributed presence of nerve cell bodies and terminals, and because of the number of different potential transmitters, it is not possible to provide a selective electrical stimulation of a single nerve type. It may be that selective chemical stimuli will eventually be discovered, but none are known at present.

However, even with electrical stimuli that affect many nerve types at once the consequent release of a particular peptide can be measured and it

Table I. Grouping of peptides

| | |
|---|---|
| *Isopeptides* | Peptides with the same biological roles but slight differences in amino acid composition, e.g. isopeptides of vasopressin and of gastrin. |
| *Closely related peptide families* | Peptides with similar sequences of amino acids and with similar effects in bioassays, but with different biological functions and usually with different cells or tissues of origin, e.g. the substance P-related tachykinins and bradykinin-related peptides from different species and classes. |
| *Loosely related peptide families* | Peptides with some sequences of amino acids in common, and hence possible immunological similarity, but with differences in their biological roles and effects in bioassays, e.g. secretin and glucagon. |
| *Co-derived peptides* | Peptides with different sequences and biological activities derived from the same precursor molecule, e.g. the peptide derivatives of pro-opiocortin. |

Table II. Examples of grouping of peptides

*Isopeptides*: e.g. Vasopressins

Arg-Vasopressin (man + most mammals)  Cys-Tyr-Phe-Gln-Asn-Cys-Pro-Arg-Gly-NH$_2$

Lys-Vasopressin (pig)  Cys-Tyr-Phe-Gln-Asn-Cys-Pro-Lys-Gly-NH$_2$

e.g. Gastrins
Gastrin II (man)     Gln-Gly-Pro-Trp-Leu-Glu-Glu-Glu-Glu-Glu-Ala-Tyr(SO$_4$)-Gly-Trp-Met-Asp-Phe-NH$_2$
Gastrin II (pig + dog)   Gln-Gly-Pro-Trp-Met-Glu-Glu-Glu-Glu-Glu-Ala-Tyr(SO$_4$)-Gly-Trp-Met-Asp-Phe-NH$_2$

*Closely related peptide families*: e.g. Tachykinins

| | | |
|---|---|---|
| Substance P | (Mammalian) | Arg-Pro-Lys-Pro-Gln-Gln-Phe-Phe-Gly-Leu-Met-NH$_2$ |
| Physalaemin | (Amphibian) | Pyr-Ala-Asp-Pro-Asn-Lys-Phe-Tyr-Gly-Leu-Met-NH$_2$ |
| Phyllomedusin | (Amphibian) | Pyr-Asn-Pro-Asn-Arg-Phe-Ile-Gly-Leu-Met-NH$_2$ |
| Uperolein | (Amphibian) | Pyr-Pro-Asp-Pro-Asn-Ala-Phe-Tyr-Gly-Leu-Met-NH$_2$ |
| Eledoisin | (Octopus) | Pyr-Pro-Ser-Lys-Asp-Ala-Phe-Ile-Gly-Leu-Met-NH$_2$ |
| Kassinin | (Amphibian) | Asp-Val-Pro-Lys-Ser-Asp-Gln-Phe-Val-Gly-Leu-Met-NH$_2$ |

*Loosely related peptide families*: e.g. Secretin—related peptides

| | | | | |
|---|---|---|---|---|
| Secretin | (27 amino acids) | His-Ser -Asp- | Gly-Thr-Phe-Thr-Ser- | Glu-Leu - - - - |
| Glucagon | (29 amino acids) | His-Ser -Gln- | Gly-Thr-Phe-Thr-Ser- | Asp-Tyr - - - - |
| GIP | (43 amino acids) | Tyr-Ala-Glu- | Gly-Thr-Phe-Ile-Ser- | Asp-Tyr - - - - |
| VIP | (28 amino acids) | His-Ser -Asp- | Ala-Val-Phe-Thr-Asp- | Asn Tyr - - - - |

*Co-derived peptides*: e.g. Derivatives of pro-opiocortin

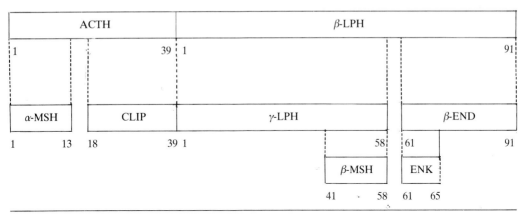

Examples of the four groupings defined in Table I are given. Similarity in amino acid sequences is emphasised by underlining or by enclosing the groups of amino acids. Deviations from common sequences are marked by underlining thus:~. As an example of co-derived peptides, part of the sequence of pro-opiocortin is illustrated. The peptides that are included in this molecule are adrenocorticotropic hormone (ACTH), lipotropins ($\beta$ and $\gamma$-LPH), melanocyte stimulating hormones ($\alpha$ and $\beta$ MSH), $\beta$-endorphin ($\beta$-END), methionine enkephalin (ENK) and corticotropin-like intermediate peptide (CLIP). Note that there are at least 6 known biologically active peptides in pro-opiocortin (ACTH, $\alpha$-MSH, $\beta$-LPH, $\beta$-MSH, $\beta$-END and met-ENK).

can be tested whether the release is dependent on action potential propagation or the presence of ions such as calcium, or if it is modified by drugs.

*Peptide presence, chemical identity and the grouping of related peptides*

The evidence for the presence of peptides in intestinal nerves rests heavily on immunochemical (histochemical and immunoassay) observations. However, by themselves these studies only indicate that the endogenous peptide has a sequence of amino acids that is similar to part of the sequence of the peptide against which the antibody preparation was raised (this problem applies to both monoclonal antibodies and antisera raised in whole animals).

Peptides can be grouped in a number of ways which indicate similarities between them (Tables I and II). These groupings emphasise some of the experimental problems that are encountered in studying neuropeptides. In general, each peptide hormone or peptide neurotransmitter has sequences of amino acids that do not appear to influence its biological activity and a sequence on which the biological activity of the peptide depends. Thus we have two problems 1) the determination of the true chemical nature of the peptide that has been identified immunologically and 2) the identification of the part of the molecule that is responsible for its biological effects.

In considering the identification of peptides as transmitters (or hormones) it is the *biological* activity that is most important. The term *isopeptides* can be introduced to describe peptides that may vary in their amino acid composition by substitution or deletion but which have essentially the same biological roles. Thus lys-vasopressin and arg-vasopressin both perform the biological function of vasopressin and, although it might sometimes be desirable to distinguish between them by species of origin, functionally they are isopeptides. Likewise, the peptides that perform the biological function of gastrin in different mammals, although they vary in their amino acid composition, are isopeptides of gastrin.

Peptides can also be grouped in families that share sequences of amino acids but have different biological roles (Tables I and II). It is possible that members of such families have evolved from common ancestral peptides (20, 77). Some structurally related peptides form what can be called *close families*—not only do they have amino acid sequences in common, but they also have similar effects in biological assay. This is not to say they have similar functions; indeed in most cases they do not. An example of a close peptide family is

the tachykinins (6, Table II). These include substance P, physalaemin and eledoisin which have widely different species and cellular origins but interact with the same receptors in a bioassay. *Loose peptide families* comprise groups of peptides that share sequences of amino acids but do not share (or share only to a small extent) actions on the same sets of receptors either in vivo or in bioassay. Thus peptides can have in common, to greater or lesser extents, biological activities and amino acid groupings.

A further difficulty for the investigator is the existence of several peptides, each with potential biological activity, as part of a larger molecule. The best known example is pro-opiocortin, a molecule that contains ACTH, MSH, endorphin and enkephalin (Table II). A single neuron containing pro-opiocortin can be stained using antisera directed against the different biologically active peptides that are part of pro-opiocortin (10, 40). This gives no indication, however, whether the individual peptides are released as chemical messengers by the neuron.

Thus, the presence of immunoreactivity for a certain peptide in a nerve does not necessarily mean the same peptide is present, nor does it mean that the peptide which is contained in the nerve has a similar biological role or can act on similar receptors to the immunogen. Furthermore, even if the amino acid sequence for the immunogen and the tissue antigen are similar, the tissue antigen sequence may be buried in a larger molecule along with other biologically active peptides.

Finding a neuropeptide by immunochemical methods is only the first step. It is necessary to determine the true amino acid sequence of the peptide, its biological effects and the conditions under which it is released. For most of the peptides in the enteric nervous system we are at the first step or little beyond it.

### Peptides in the guinea-pig small intestine

The small intestine of the guinea-pig has been used as a model to study peptide nerves, and to provide a standard reference point with which to compare other areas and species. Immunohistochemical studies are being used to document the cellular distribution of the different peptides in this area of intestine (15, 16, 37, 52, 75) and the projections of individual peptide and amine neurons are also being determined (17, 18, 30, 34, 36). Intracellular micro-electrode studies have been made of the actions of the peptides in guinea-pig myenteric ganglia (55, 56, 67, 80, 81). There are a number of studies of the effects of peptides on the movements of the guinea-pig small intestine. On the other hand, there are few studies in this or other species of the effects of neural peptides on mucosal transport. Evaluation of the effects of peptides on intestinal blood flow have been confined, for the most part, to cat and dog.

In view of the substantial work on the guinea-pig small intestine, a comparison of apparent peptide and amine concentrations in the different layers has been made (Table III). The concentrations of the two amine transmitters, acetylcholine and noradrenaline, are substantially greater than those of the peptides which, with the exception of met-enkephalin, have concentrations in the longitudinal muscle/myenteric plexus below 500 pmole/g (noradrenaline is >3,000 pmole/g, acetylcholine > 80,000 pmole/g). Dopamine and adrenaline in the intestine appear to be partly in the noradrenergic nerves and partly in an unidentified non-vesicular compartment; neither of these amines is considered likely to be a neurotransmitter in the intestine (33, 47).

In the cases of four of the peptides that have been assayed (met-enkephalin, leu-enkephalin, somatostatin and substance P) it seems likely that the authentic peptide is present. Met-enkephalin and leu-enkephalin extracted from the intestine co-elute with the authentic peptides on Sephadex G15 and on thin layer chromatography using silica gel plates and furthermore the eluted materials have effects in bioassay that are blocked by the opiate receptor antagonist naloxone (48). Extracted somatostatin co-eluted with the authentic peptide in high pressure liquid chromatography using both reverse phase and molecular seive conditions (31). Substance P from the nerves in the guinea-pig intestine acts through the same receptors as authentic substance P (27). It also co-elutes with authentic substance P on reverse

phase high pressure liquid chromatography (authors' unpublished results). All the extracted immunoreactive material elutes with the authentic peptide on Sephadex G15 (46).

The amino acid sequence of vasoactive intestinal polypeptide (VIP) determined for an extract of pig intestine (65) is probably the sequence for enteric neural VIP in that species because the peptide appears to be present in neural rather than endocrine tissue (see discussion in 32). In the guinea-pig intestine the sequence probably differs from that in pig. The major component of immunoreactive VIP in guinea-pig extracts elutes earlier than porcine VIP on CM Sephadex, although it elutes in the same position on Sephadex G50 columns (51). Thus VIP in guinea-pig enteric nerves appears to be of similar molecular weight, but is more acidic than porcine VIP. Antisera that are directed against different parts of porcine VIP indicate the presence of widely different concentrations of VIP in guinea-pig intestine (51, Table III). Guinea-pig VIP is seen very poorly with an antiserum (L25) directed against N-terminal regions of porcine VIP, and is also seen poorly with antiserum 7913 that is sensitive to mid or C-terminal parts of porcine VIP (37). Thus guinea-pig VIP might have a number of differences from porcine VIP. The true concentration of guinea-pig VIP is likely to be at least that determined using antiserum R501, the antiserum that reacts most strongly with guinea-pig VIP.

Bombesin concentrations in guinea-pig intestine are similar when determined with antiserum 1078 (51) and with antiserum BN/TWM used in the present work (for characterisation of BN/TWM see 63). Both antisera were raised against amphibian skin bombesin and recognise amino acid groups of its C-terminal. Separation by chromatography using Sephadex G50 indicates the presence of two forms of bombesin, one similar to the amphibian tetradecapeptide (64% of activity) and a larger form in nerves of guinea-pig small intestine (51). With reverse phase high pressure liquid chromatography, a small form that eluted with synthetic amphibian bombesin was detected (unpublished results of the authors). Both radioimmunoassay and immunohistochem-

Table III. Comparison of apparent concentrations of peptides and amines in guinea-pig small intestine

| Substances | Concentration (pmole/g · wet · wt) | | | | References |
|---|---|---|---|---|---|
| | LM/MP | SM | Mucosa | W.W. | |
| Angiotensin | <0.07 | <0.07 | <0.07 | <0.07 | Present work |
| Bombesin | 32.0 ± 4.1 (6) | 29.6 ± 4.0 (6)† | <1.5 | 6.4 ± 0.5 (9) | Hutchison et al. (51) |
| | 32.6 ± 1.0 (9) | 15.8 ± 0.7 (9) | <0.2 | | Present work |
| CCK-8 | 14.1 ± 2.2 (6) | 10.4 ± 1.2 (6)† | 5.2 ± 1.1 (6) | | Hutchison et al. (51) |
| | 7.3 ± 1.2 (6) | 6.4 ± 0.2 (6) | 2.2 ± 0.4 (6) | 2.4 ± 0.8 (6) | Present work |
| Enkephalin (Met) | 1350 ± 110 (6) | 1040 ± 150 (6) | 100 ± 10 (6) | 820 ± 90 (6) | Present work |
| | 410 ± 50 (4) | | | | Hughes et al. (48) |
| Enkephalin (Leu) | 130 ± 20 (6) | 100 ± 20 (6) | 6.3 ± 0.8 (6) | 38 ± 3 (6) | Present work |
| | 151 ± 16 (4) | | | | Hughes et al. (48) |
| Neurotensin | <0.02 | <0.02 | 8.0 ± 0.6 (4) | 5.0 ± 0.2 (4) | Present work |
| Somatostatin | 172 ± 9 (5) | 239 ± 20 (5) | 132 ± 16 (5) | 160 ± 16 (5) | Furness et al. (38) |
| Substance P | 240 ± 12 (9) | 135 ± 5 (9) | 33 ± 1 (5) | 87 ± 3 (5) | Present work |
| | 369 ± 42 (7) | | 32 ± 5 (6) | 173 ± 14 (10) | Holzer et al. (46) |
| | 356 ± 67 (18) | | | | Franco et al. (28) |
| VIP* R501 | 135 ± 34 (6) | 119 ± 5 (6)† | 83 ± 10 (6) | 104 ± 7 (6) | Hutchison et al. (51) |
| 5603 | 39 ± 5 (6) | 24 ± 2 (6)† | 21 ± 6 (6) | 25 ± 3 (6) | Hutchison et al. (51) |
| L25 | <1 | <1 | <1 | <1 | Hutchison et al. (51) |
| 7913 | 6.2 ± 1.9 (8) | 1.7 ± 0.4 (8) | 3.3 ± 0.9 (8) | | Present work |
| Acetylcholine | 190000 ± 18000 (6) | | | 47000 ± 3400 (6) | Paton & Zar (69) |
| | 81200 ± 12300 (6) | | | | Hutchison et al. (50) |
| Noradrenaline | 3900 ± 400 (10) | 11500 ± 800 (10) | | | Howe et al. (47) |
| | 3100 ± 300 (10) | | | | Juorio & Gabella (53) |
| Dopamine | 340 ± 70 (10) | 560 ± 90 (10) | | | Howe et al. (47) |
| | 390 ± 65 (10) | | | | Juorio & Gabella (53) |
| Adrenaline | 160 ± 20 (10) | 250 ± 25 (10) | | | Howe et al. (47) |
| 5-HT | 460 ± 60 (6) | | $3.6 \times 10^6 \pm 0.4 \times 10^6$ (9)‡ | | Robinson & Gershon (72) |
| | 620 ± 110 (11) | | | | Juorio & Gabella (53) |

The values are given in terms of equivalents. That is, in referring to a peptide concentration, the concentration of peptide-like material is expressed as the amount of authentic peptide which, if present in the tissue, would give equivalent displacement in radioimmunoassay. Values are means ± standard errors of the mean with the number of determinations in brackets. In the cases of the enkephalins, somatostatin, substance P, acetylcholine, noradrenaline, dopamine, adrenaline and 5-HT, the authentic substances are believed to be present. Compounds similar to the standards for bombesin, CCK8 and VIP appear to be present. A neurotensin-like compound is present in the mucosa. Angiotensin-II-like material seen by immunohistochemistry is not recognized as similar to authentic angiotensin-II in RIA.

* The codes refer to different antisera used to determine VIP concentrations.　† The circular muscle was included with the submucosa.　‡ The circular muscle and submucosa were included with the mucosa.

Abbreviations: LM/MP, longitudinal muscle and myenteric plexus combined. This usually includes some strands of circular muscle; SM, submucosa; W.W., whole wall.

ical studies indicate that bombesin-like activity is not contained in mucosal endocrine cells of the guinea-pig small intestine. Neural bombesin from guinea-pig intestine thus seems to be quite similar to the 14 amino acid peptide isolated from amphibian skin. Whether a large form similar to porcine gastric mucosal bombesin (61) is present has yet to be determined.

There have been some differences in the conclusions reached by different investigators who have examined material with gastrin and/or cholecystokinin-like immunoreactivity in the intestine. Gastrin and CCK share the same C-terminal pentapeptide amide, and the differences in interpretation concern whether there is any gastrin (G17) present and whether CCK-like immunoreactive material is primarily the C-terminal octapeptide of CCK (CCK8) or the common C-terminal tetrapeptide (CCK/G4) (see 21, 33, 51 for discussion). Recent RIA determinations of column fractions of extracts from guinea-pig intestine suggest that there is little or no G17 or CCK/G4 in enteric nerves in this species and that the major form is similar in charge and molecular weight to sulphated CCK8 (51). There does not seem to be any significant amount of non-sulphated CCK8. Results reported in the present work (Table III) were obtained using antiserum R5 (3). These values are lower than those obtained by Hutchison et al (1981) with antiserum L48. Both antisera were raised in rabbits against synthetic sulphated CCK8. It is possible that the extraction procedure used in the present studies with R5 (neutral boil followed by acidification with 3% acetic acid) was less effective than for the L48 determinations (neutral boil) (see 51).

Nerves showing histochemical immunoreactivity for neurotensin have been reported in the guinea-pig and rat intestine (75). However, other investigators specifically state that they have been unable to detect reactive nerves in the intestine (43, 78), although they, like others, detected enteric endocrine cells with neurotensin-like activity. In the present work we have used an antiserum (SK NT4) raised in rabbits against authentic neurotensin. No neurotensin was detected in the nerve containing layers of the

intestine, although neurotensin was readily detected in the mucosa (Table III). In our experiments, this means that the concentration in the nerve-containing layers was less than 0.02 pmole/g. The substance which showed histochemical immunoreactivity for neurotensin (75) was therefore probably not authentic neurotensin.

It has been reported that some intestinal nerves show angiotensin-II-like activity immunohistochemically (39). We have confirmed this observation, showing angiotensin-II-like activity in a considerable proportion, about 30%, of neurons in the guinea-pig myenteric plexus. The labelling is not random; it is of a specific set of neurons that send processes only in an oral direction. However, attempts to demonstrate any angiotensin-like activity in extracts of the guinea-pig small intestine have so far failed (Table III). The antiserum used for this assay has been previously characterised (62). It has a threshold for detection of angiotensin-II of less than 10 fmole. With this assay angiotensin-II could be detected in plasma and 90% of angiotensin II added to the intestine before the extraction was recovered and detected by radioimmunoassay. Therefore it seems unlikely that the numerous intestinal neurons containing a substance that cross-reacts with angiotensin-II contain the authentic peptide. Until an assay for the angiotensin-II-like material in enteric nerves is discovered it will not be possible to determine its true nature.

*Release of neuropeptides*

In order to detect release of peptides from enteric nerves, direct measurement of peptide levels in perfusates, superfusates or bathing media can be made. Alternatively, indirect evidence of release can be obtained by examining the pharmacology of transmission from nerves. Some of the peptides are present in both nerves and endocrine cells, hence experiments need to be designed to ensure that the released peptide that is detected originated from nerves. There is some direct and some indirect evidence for the release from enteric nerves, in response to their activation, of enkephalin (49, 71, 76), substance P

(27, 64) and vasoactive intestinal polypeptide (7, 22, 25, 26, 73). These experiments imply that these enteric neuropeptides are released when action potentials invade the terminals and that under admittedly artificial conditions they are released in sufficient quantity to have effects on the gastrointestinal tract.

*Mimicry*

If a substance is released as a neurotransmitter, exogenous application of that substance should mimic the effect of neurotransmission when it is applied to the same field of receptors with the same time course and in the same concentration. Approximating these conditions is not possible in the intestine. The axons of enteric nerves that supply muscle, nerve cells and the epithelium have long varicose sections from which, it is believed, the transmitter is released to interact with a number of effector cells (e.g. 5, 29). There may be differences between the receptors close to the axon varicosities and extra-junctional receptors further away as seems to be the case at other autonomic junctions (e.g. 8, 19, 44). These differences are both in local sensitivity, with junctional receptor areas being more sensitive, and in pharmacology, with drugs that are antagonists at extra-junctional receptors not necessarily antagonising the action of the transmitter at the junctional receptors. In the intestine, there is at present no possibility of mimicking the natural pattern of release of transmitter by applying a compound in an organ bath or by infusing it through the vascular bed. The most that might be expected is that the exogenously applied compound might affect the tissue in the same direction as does the activation of nerves, that is, both should cause secretion or both relaxation and so on. Furthermore, if an antagonist is found for the exogenously applied compound, it would also be expected to antagonise transmission, although not necessarily to the same extent.

Other observations indicate that it is not a simple matter to mimic transmission from peptide-containing nerves with exogenous peptide. First, there are many sites at which an exogenous peptide might act and second, there may be several nerve pathways in which a particular peptide is involved (see 36). Because of these and other complexities, few of the possible roles of the peptide pathways have been explored.

Nevertheless, there are indications that substance P might be a transmitter at neuro-neuronal junctions in the myenteric plexus. At some of these junctions, slow excitatory postsynaptic potentials (slow EPSPs) can be recorded (54, 82). Substance P also causes slow depolarisations (56). Both the slow EPSP and substance P depolarisations are associated with an increase in membrane resistance, and both are reduced in the presence of chymotrypsin, a proteolytic enzyme that degrades substance P (64). Thus substance P mimics the slow excitatory potentials in some myenteric neurons and, because it is known to be present in and released from nerves in the myenteric plexus, it is possible that substance P is an excitatory transmitter in this situation.

VIP has been suggested to be a transmitter released from enteric inhibitory nerves, and in many parts of the gastrointestinal tract it has been shown to cause relaxation (32). The relaxation caused by VIP is generally slower than that caused by stimulation of the enteric inhibitory nerves. However, a more substantial reason to doubt that VIP is the transmitter is that it no longer mimics after certain drug treatments. It has been shown that chymotrypsin substantially reduces the effect of VIP, without altering the response to stimulation of enteric inhibitory nerves and that apamin antagonises transmission from the nerves without affecting the action of VIP (59). Moreover, when receptors for VIP are desensitised by repeated exposure to the peptide, the effectiveness of transmission is not diminished)(83).

CONCLUSIONS

The foregoing discussion indicates that it is not possible to identify the neuropeptides in the intestine from immunochemical criteria alone. However, by using chromatographic separation and immunoassay, in some cases with a variety of antisera, it is possible to conclude that authentic leu- and met-enkephalin, authentic somatostatin and authentic substance P are present in nerves of the guinea-pig intestine. This means that possible functions of nerves containing these peptides may now be deduced from considerations of their distributions and projections and of the effects of the peptides. Further studies of the conditions under which these peptides are released are required.

Guinea-pig VIP appears to have significant structural differences from porcine VIP which has been used as a standard. It is possible that the receptors for VIP in guinea-pig are also slightly different from those in pig. Cholecystokinin-like and bombesin-like peptides in guinea-pig enteric nerves seem to be similar to or identical with CCK8 and amphibian skin bombesin respectively. The angiotensin-like and neurotensin-like material that is revealed by immuno-histochemical means appear to be substantially different from authentic angiotensin II and neurotensin in radioimmunoassay. Until a biochemical assay for these substances is discovered, their isolation, purification and chemical characterisation will not be possible.

## ACKNOWLEDGEMENTS

This work was supported by grants from the National Health and Medical Research Foundation of Australia and from the Utah Foundation. Part of the work was done during the tenure of a Fulbright Fellowship awarded to J. B. Furness. We should like to thank Dr. J. H. Walsh, who provided antibody 7913, and Dr. M. Beinfeld, who provided antibody R5, for their generosity. We are grateful for the able assistance of Venetta Esson, Bob Long and Pat Vilimas. Don Mayor is thanked for his helpful discussion of the manuscript.

## REFERENCES

1. Ambache N, Freeman MA. J Physiol 1968, 199, 705–727
2. Ambache N, Verney J, Zar MA. J Physiol 1970, 207, 761–782
3. Beinfeld MC, Meyer DK, Eskay RL, Jensen RT, Brownstein MJ. Brain Res 1981, 212, 51–57
4. Bennett MR, Burnstock G, Holman ME. J Physiol 1966, 182, 541–558
5. Bennett MR, Rogers DC. J Cell Biol 1967, 33, 573–596
6. Bertaccini G. Pharmacol Rev 1976, 28, 127–177
7. Bloom SR, Edwards AV. J Physiol 1980, 299, 437–452
8. Bolton TB. Proc R Soc B 1976, 194, 99–119
9. Bryant MG, Polak JM, Modlin I, Bloom SR, Albuquerque RH, Pearse AGE. Lancet 1976, 1, 991–993
10. Bugnon C, Bloch B, Lenys D, Fellmann D. Cell Tiss Res 1979, 199, 177–196
11. Bülbring E, Gershon MD. J Physiol 1967, 192, 823–846
12. Burnstock G. pp 3–32 in Baer HP, Drummond GI (eds), Physiological and Regulatory Functions of Adenosine and Adenine Nucleotides, Raven Press, New York 1979
13. Burnstock G, Campbell G, Bennett M, Holman ME. Int J Neuropharmacol 1964, 3, 163–166
14. Burnstock G, Campbell G, Rand MJ. J Physiol 1966, 182, 504–526
15. Costa M, Cuello AC, Furness JB, Franco R. Neuroscience 1980, 5, 323–331
16. Costa M, Furness JB, Buffa R, Said SI. Neuroscience 1980, 5, 587–596
17. Costa M, Furness JB, Llewellyn-Smith IJ, Cuello AC. Neuroscience 1981, 6, 411–424
18. Costa M, Furness JB, Llewellyn-Smith IJ, Davies B, Oliver J. Neuroscience 1980, 5, 841–852
19. Dennis MJ, Harris AJ, Kuffler SW. Proc R Soc B 1971, 177, 509–539
20. Dockray GJ. Ann Rev Physiol 1979, 41, 83–95
21. Dockray GJ, Vaillant C, Hutchison JB. pp 215–230 in Grossman MI, Brazier MAB, Lechago J. (eds.), Cellular Basis of Chemical Messengers in the Digestive System. Academic Press, New York and London 1981
22. Edwards, AV, Bircham PMM, Mitchel SJ, Bloom SR. Experientia 1978, 34, 1186–1187
23. Elde R, Hökfelt T, Johansson O, Terenius L. Neuroscience 1976, 1, 349–351
24. Fahrenkrug J. Digestion 1979, 19, 149–169
25. Fahrenkrug J, Galbo H, Holst JJ, Schaffalitzky de Muckadell, OB. J Physiol 1978, 280, 405–422
26. Fahrenkrug J, Haglund U, Jodal M, Lundgren O, Olbe L, Schaffalitzky de Muckadell OB. J Physiol 1978, 284, 291–305
27. Franco R, Costa M, Furness JB. Naunyn-Schmiedeberg's Arch Pharmacol 1979, 306, 185–201
28. Franco R, Costa M, Furness JB. Naunyn-Schmiedeberg's Arch Pharmacol 1979, 307, 57–63
29. Furness JB, Costa M. Ergebn D Physiol 1974, 69, 1–51
30. Furness JB, Costa M. Neurosci Lett 1979, 15, 199–204
31. Furness JB, Costa M. Neuroscience 1980, 5, 1–20
32. Furness JB, Costa M. pp 391–406 in Advances in Peptide and Hormone Research, vol. 1. Raven Press, New York 1982
33. Furness JB, Costa M. in Bertaccini G (ed.), Handbook of Experimental Pharmacology, Springer, Heidelberg 1982
34. Furness JB, Costa M. Neuroscience 1982, in press
35. Furness, JB, Costa M, Franco R, Llewellyn-Smith IJ. Adv Biochem Psychopharmacol 1980, 22, 601–617

36. Furness JB, Costa M, Llewellyn-Smith IJ. Peptides 1982 (in press)
37. Furness JB, Costa M, Walsh JH. Gastroenterology 1981, 80, 1557–1561
38. Furness JB, Eskay RL, Brownstein MJ, Costa M. Neuropeptides 1980, 1, 97–103
39. Fuxe F, Hökfelt T, Said SI, Mutt V. Neurosci Lett 1977, 5, 241–246
40. Gainer H, Loh YP, Russell JT. Prog Biochem Pharmacol 1980, 16, 60–68
41. Gershon MD. Ann Rev Neurosci 1981, 4, 227–272
42. Gershon MD, Drakontides AB, Ross LL. Science 1965, 149, 197–199
43. Helmstaedter V, Taugner C, Feurle GE, Forssmann WG. Histochemistry 1977, 53, 35–41
44. Hirst GDS, Neild TO. J Physiol 1981, 313, 343–350
45. Hökfelt T, Johansson O, Efendic S, Luft A, Arimura A. Experientia 1975, 31, 852–854
46. Holzer P, Emson PC, Iversen LL, Sharman DF. Neuroscience 1981 (in press)
47. Howe PRC, Provis JC, Furness JB, Costa M, Chalmers JP. Clin Exp Pharm Physiol 1981 (in press)
48. Hughes J, Kosterlitz HW, Smith TW. Br J Pharmacol 1977, 61, 639–647
49. Hughes J, Kosterlitz HW, Sosa P, Br J Pharmacol 1978, 63, 397P
50. Hutchinson M, Kosterlitz HW, Gilbert JC. Eur J Pharmacol 1976, 39, 221–235
51. Hutchison JB, Dimaline R, Dockray GJ. Peptides 1981, 2, 23–30
52. Jessen KR, Saffrey MJ, Van Noorden S, Bloom SR, Polak JM, Burnstock G. Neuroscience 1980, 5, 1717–1735
53. Juorio AV, Gabella G. J Neurochem 1974, 22, 851–858
54. Katayama Y, North RA. Nature 1978, 274, 387–388
55. Katayama Y, North RA. J Physiol 1980, 303, 315–323
56. Katayama Y, North RA, Williams JT. Proc R Soc Lond B 1979, 206, 191–208
57. Larsson LI, Fahrenkrug J, Schaffalitzky de Muckadell O, Sundler F, Håkanson R, Rehfeld JF. Proc Natl Acad Sci USA 1976, 73, 3197–3200
58. Llewellyn-Smith IJ, Furness JB, Wilson AJ, Costa M. pp in Elfvin LG (ed.), Autonomic Ganglia. John Wiley, New York 1982
59. Mackenzie I, Burnstock G. Eur J Pharmacol 1980, 67, 255–264
60. Martinson J. Acta Physiol Scand 1965, 64, 453–462
61. McDonald TJ, Jornvall H, Nilsson G, Vagne M, Ghatei M, Bloom SR, Mutt V. Biochem Biophys Res Comm 1979, 90, 227–233
62. Meyer DK, Eisenreich M, Nutto D. Clinical Science 1979, 57, 401–407
63. Moody TW, Pert CB. Biochem Biophys Res Comm 1979, 90, 7–14
64. Morita K, North RA, Katayama Y. Nature 1980, 287, 151–152
65. Mutt V, Said SI. Eur J Biochem 1974, 42, 581–589
66. Nilsson G, Larsson LI, Håkanson R, Brodin E, Pernow B, Sundler F. Histochemistry 1975, 43, 97–99
67. North RA, Katayama Y, Williams JT. Brain Res 1979, 165, 67–77
68. Orrego F. Neuroscience 1979, 4, 1037–1057
69. Paton WDM, Zar MA. J Physiol 1968, 194, 13–33
70. Pearse AGE, Polak JM. Histochemistry 1975, 41, 373–375
71. Puig MM, Gascon P, Graviso GL, Musacchio, JM. Science 1977, 195, 419–420
72. Robinson RG, Gershon MD. J Pharmacol Exp Ther 1971, 178, 311–324
73. Schaffalitzky de Muckadell OB, Fahrenkrug J, Holst JJ. Gastroenterology 1977, 72, 373–375
74. Schultzberg M, Dreyfus CF, Gershon MD, Hökfelt T, Elde RP, Nilsson G, Said SI, Goldstein M. Brain Res 1978, 155, 239–248
75. Schultzberg M, Hökfelt T, Nilsson G, Terenius L, Rehfeld J, Brown M, Elde R, Goldstein M, Said SI. Neuroscience 1980, 5, 689–744
76. Schulz R, Wüster M, Simantov R, Snyder S, Herz A. Eur J Pharmacol 1977, 41, 437–438
77. Stewart JM, Channabasavaiah K. Federation Proc 1979, 38, 2302–2308
78. Sundler F, Håkanson R, Hammer RA, Alumets A, Carraway R, Leeman S, Zimmerman EA. Cell Tiss Res 1977, 178, 313–321
79. Werman R. Comp Biochem Physiol 1966, 18, 745–766
80. Williams JT, Katayama Y, North RA. Eur J Pharmacol 1979, 59, 181–186
81. Williams JT, North RA. Brain Res 1979, 175, 174–177
82. Wood JD, Mayer CJ. Neurophysiol 1979, 42, 569–581
83. Yahasaki O, Nabata H, Sasaki N, Yanagiya I. Proc Eighth Int Cong Pharmacol 1981, 1, 759

# Innervation of the Muscularis Mucosa in the Canine Stomach and Colon

F. ANGEL, P. F. SCHMALZ, K. G. MORGAN, V. L. W. GO &
J. H. SZURSZEWSKI
Dept of Physiology and Biophysics and Dept of Pharmacology,
Mayo Medical School, Rochester, Minnesota 55905, USA

A preliminary report is presented of studies into the innervation of the canine muscularis mucosa. In vitro experiments have investigated the mechanical response to electrical stimulation and the release of gut peptides known to modulate gastrointestinal function. Exogenous substance P increased tone and amplitude of phasic contractions while neurotensin and vasoactive intestinal polypeptide (VIP) relaxed the muscularis mucosa. Immunoreactive VIP was released into the superfusate during transmural electrical stimulation of the antrum while VIP and substance P were present in superfusate from the colon. The significance of these findings has been discussed briefly.

*J. H. Szurszewski, Ph.D., Dept of Physiology and Biophysics, Mayo Medical School, Rochester, Minnesota 55905, USA*

## INTRODUCTION

The muscularis mucosa is a thin band of smooth muscle located at the base of the gastrointestinal mucosa. Compared to the external smooth muscle layers, it has received very little attention. However, the muscularis mucosa probably has great influence on the absorptive and secretory functions of the mucosa because the mucosa sits on this muscle layer and because fingers of muscularis mucosa project into the pits and villi of the mucosa. Because of its strategic location, contraction and relaxation of the muscularis mucosa will alter the mucosal surfaces exposed to luminal content.

The neural control mechanisms in the muscularis mucosa are virtually unknown. Anatomic (1, 10) and pharmacological (4, 5) data suggest that the muscularis mucosa may receive cholinergic and adrenergic nervous input. However, this is, in part, disputed (2). The use of immunohistochemical, fluorescent antibody techniques indicates that this muscle layer contains a number of peptides: substance P, neurotensin and vasoactive intestinal polypeptide (VIP) (6). We are ignorant of any of the effects these peptides might exert on the smooth muscle of the muscularis mucosa.

During the course of a separate series of studies on the circular muscle of the canine antrum (7, 8), we noticed that removal of the mucosa and submucosa from the circular muscle left the muscularis mucosa virtually intact in the "waste" tissue. One of us (K. G. Morgan) initiated a series of studies which led to our present investigations. This report should be considered only preliminary as much more intensive and quantitative studies will be required before the role of peptides as neurotransmitters or modulators in this muscle is understood.

## METHODS AND RESULTS

Strips of muscularis mucosa from the canine stomach and colon were obtained by dissecting off the external muscle coats and completely removing the mucosa. Strips of muscularis mucosa were "strung-up" in a glass-chambered superfusion apparatus. To record isometric ten-

## PREPARATION   OF   MUSCULARIS   MUCOSA
## OF   CANINE   ANTRUM

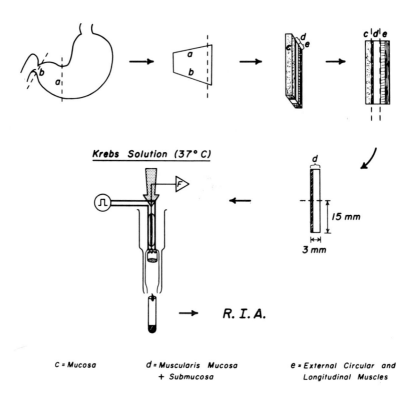

Krebs Solution (37° C)

15 mm

3 mm

R. I. A.

C = Mucosa

d = Muscularis Mucosa
+ Submucosa

e = External Circular and
Longitudinal Muscles

Fig. 1. Schematic representation of method used to obtain strips of muscularis mucosa from the canine stomach. Similar dissection procedures are used to prepare strips of muscularis mucosa from the colon.

sion, one end of the strip was securely anchored to a steel hook; the other end was attached to an isometric force transducer. Intramural nerves were stimulated by two platinum wire electrodes placed parallel to the strip. Modified Krebs solution (8) warmed to 37°C passed continuously over the muscle. The solution was collected in chilled test tubes for radioimmunoassay of several gut peptides known to play a role in modulating gastrointestinal function and known to be present in this muscle layer (6) or adjoining nervous plexuses (Furness, this volume). The experimental set up is illustrated diagrammatically in Fig. 1.

*Muscularis mucosa of canine antrum.* The muscularis mucosa from the antrum exhibited resting tone and spontaneous phasic mechanical activity (Fig. 2). Transmural nerve stimulation induced relaxation and inhibited spontaneous mechanical activity (Fig. 2). This effect was not abolished by atropine ($10^{-6}$ M), phentolamine ($10^{-6}$ M), propranolol ($10^{-6}$ M) (Fig. 3) or methysergide ($10^{-6}$ M), but was abolished by tetrodotoxin ($10^{-6}$ M). These pharmacological experiments suggest that the relaxation induced by electrical stimulation of intramural nerves was not mediated by cholinergic, adrenergic or serotonergic nerves.

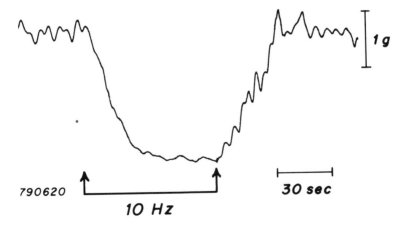

Fig. 2. Effect of transmural electrical nerve stimulation on spontaneous activity of canine gastric muscularis mucosa.

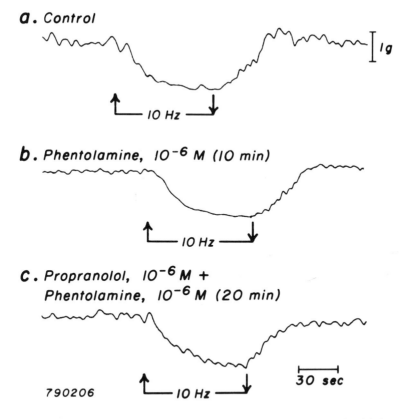

Fig. 3. Response to transmural nerve stimulation in normal Krebs solution (a), in Krebs solution containing phentolamine (b) and in Krebs solution containing phentolamine and propranolol (c). Canine gastric muscularis mucosa.

Of the different peptides studied, only exogenous substance P, neurotensin and vasoactive intestinal polypeptide affected the mechanical activity of the muscle. Substance P increased tone and the amplitude of phasic contractions. Both neurotensin and vasoactive intestinal polypetide relaxed the muscularis mucosa. One of the most interesting observations made was that there was no desensitisation to either peptide even after two hours of stimulation. Of these three peptides, our preliminary results suggest that only immunoreactive VIP was released into the superfusate during transmural electrical nerve stimulation and muscle relaxation. For example, in one experiment, immunoreactive-like VIP increased from <10 to 67 pg/ml during transmural electrical nerve stimulation. All other peptides measured were below the levels of detection. Since exogenous VIP strongly mimicked the response to nerve stimulation and since VIP was elevated in the superfusate during nervous activation, it may be that VIP functions as a neurotransmitter or neuromodulator in the muscularis mucosa.

*Muscularis mucosa of the canine colon.* The muscularis mucosa of the colon exhibited resting tone and spontaneous phasic mechanical activity. Unlike gastric muscularis mucosa, transmural electrical nerve stimulation induced a biphasic response which consisted of a powerful contraction followed by a prolonged relaxation. This biphasic response was abolished by tetrodotoxin ($10^{-6}$ M) but not by either propranolol ($10^{-5}$ M) or phentolamine ($10^{-6}$ M). Atropine ($10^{-6}$ M) and hexamethonium ($10^{-5}$ M) abolished the relaxation only. These results suggest that a much more complex neural wiring is present in colonic muscularis mucosa than in gastric muscularis mucosa. Our preliminary radioimmunological data suggest than only immunoreactive-like VIP and substance P are present in colonic muscularis mucosa. Gastrin-cholecystokinin, bombesin and neurotensin were below the limits of our assays.

Exogenously added substance P and VIP affect mechanical activity. Exogenous substance P induced a strong contraction whereas exogenous VIP induced a relaxation. Furthermore, both immunoreactive VIP and substance P were present in the superfusate during electrical nerve stimulation. In the future, more detailed experiments should indicate if either or both of these peptides function as neurotransmitters or modulators.

## DISCUSSION

The physiology and pharmacology of the smooth muscle of the muscularis mucosa has been virtually neglected. Because of its strategic location below the absorptive and secretory apparatus of the bowel, abnormalities in its behavior may contribute to some bowel diseases. For example, in ulcerative colitis and ileitis, the striking pathological finding is hypertrophy and contraction of the muscularis mucosa (3). This change undoubtedly leads to changes in motility of the muscularis mucosa. Understanding the normal physiological motor pattern of this muscle may be important in understanding its pathophysiological significance in disease states. Also, peptide containing nerves or their postsynaptic receptors in the muscularis mucosa may participate in many gastrointestinal disturbances. For example, peptidergic nerves have been implicated in the pathology of Crohn's disease (9). In this disease, VIP-containing nerves are highly immunoreactive. Our preliminary studies show that the receptor for VIP shows virtually no desensitisation. Consequently high circulating levels of VIP ought to continuously effect the spontaneous mechanical activity of the muscularis mucosa and hence alter normal secretory and absorptive processes. An understanding of the type of peptide receptors and peptidergic nerves present in the muscularis mucosa of the gastrointestinal tract should provide basic information on the significance of peptidergic innervation in diseased states.

## ACKNOWLEDGEMENTS

Supported by HHS Grant AM17238 and the Mayo Foundation.

## REFERENCES

1. Cajal RY. Madrid Consejo Superior de Investigationes Cientificas (Facsimilie reprint of 1911, Paris Edition) 1955, 2, 934–936

2. Gallacher M, Mackenna BR, and McKirdy HC. Br J Pharmacol 1973, 47, 760–764

3. Goulston SJM, and McGovern VJ. Am J Dig Dis 1968, 13, 501–514

4. Kamikawa Y, and Shimo Y. Arch int Pharmacodyn 1979, 238, 220–232

5. King, CE, and Robinson MH. Am J Physiol 1945, 143, 325–335

6. Loren I, Alumets J, Hakansen R and Sundler F. Cell Tissue Research 1979, 200, 179–186

7. Morgan KG, Muir TC and Szurszewski JH. J Physiol (London) 1981, 311, 475–488

8. Morgan KG and Szurszewski JH. J Physiol (London) 1980, 301, 229–242

9. Polak JM, Bishop AE and Bloom SR. Scand J Gastroenterol (Suppl 49) 1978, 13, 144

10. Thorell G. Skand Arch Physiol 1927, 50, 205–282

# Recent Physiological Studies of the Alimentary Autonomic Innervation

A. V. EDWARDS & S. R. BLOOM

The Physiological Laboratory, University of Cambridge, Cambridge CB2 3EG
and the Dept of Medicine, Royal Postgraduate Medical School, Hammersmith Hospital, London W12, UK

The optimum pattern of stimulation of the VIP-ergic fibres in the submaxillary gland of the cat has been investigated by comparing the effects of continuous stimulation at 2 Hz for 10 min with those of stimulation at 20 Hz for 1 sec at 10 sec intervals for the same period. Both the fall in submaxillary vascular resistance (SVR) and release of VIP from the gland are significantly increased when the same total number of impulses is delivered in bursts at the higher frequency. Comparison of submaxillary responses to stimulation in 1 sec bursts, over a wide range of frequencies, has shown that, in atropinised cats, the fall in SVR is linearly related to stimulus frequency over the range 2–60 Hz, and maximal at 80 Hz. In addition, the fall in SVR is linearly related to stimulus frequency over the range 2–60 Hz, and maximal at 80 Hz. In addition, the fall in SVR is linearly related to *log* VIP output from the gland over the whole of the frequency range 2–160 Hz.

Stimulation in 1 sec bursts at 10 sec intervals has also shown that certain non-peptidergic autonomic responses are optimal at much higher stimulus frequencies than has hitherto been supposed on the basis of classical studies employing continuous stimulation. It is concluded that it is no longer justified to assume that autonomic nerve fibres are invariably characterised by low natural discharge frequencies or that they necessarily fire at relatively constant rates. The results obtained using bursts of stimuli also show how differential responses can be obtained in the same tissue simply by varying the stimulus frequency and pattern.

*AV Edwards, The Physiological Laboratory, University of Cambridge, Cambridge CB2 3EG, UK*

Just as the advent of radioimmunological techniques has already revolutionised the study of gastrointestinal endocrinology, so their application to the innervation of the alimentary tract is now leading to a reappraisal of the physiological characteristics of these autonomic nerves. The purpose of this article is to provide a brief review of two aspects of the physiology of the autonomic nerves which supply the alimentary tract and associated glands; namely their release of biologically active peptides, and the optimum pattern of stimulus that can be applied to them.

## PUTATIVE PEPTIDERGIC TRANSMITTERS

### Vasoactive intestinal polypeptide (VIP)

The evidence that peptides are released from autonomic nerve terminals in the alimentary canal, and act as specific transmitters, is most compelling in the case of VIP. The combined results of numerous histochemical studies have shown that VIP is localised to the nerve terminals and that these are distributed widely throughout the gut wall (29, 82, 87). Sundler and his colleagues have shown that the distribution of VIP-ergic neurones is unchanged 1 to 4 months after jejunal autotransplantation in the pig and concluded that the fibres were therefore intrinsic to the gut wall (95) but a small population of VIP-immunoreactive fibres has been identified in the human vagus nerve (91). Nerve fibres exhibiting VIP-immunoreactivity have also been found in the oesophagus (126), gall-bladder (122) pancreas (12, 81, 123) and salivary glands (14, 88, 90, 130).

In each of these tissues VIP is known to exert potent effects, some of which have also been shown to occur in response to stimulation of the autonomic innervation and to be resistant to muscarinic and adrenergic blockade. Thus, in the gastrointestinal tract such non-adrenergic, non-cholinergic responses include gastric relaxation and vasodilatation of the colonic mucosa (48, 49); VIP is a potent gastrointestinal vasodilator agent (74, 110, 125) and also causes gastrointestinal smooth muscle to relax (27, 101). In the oesophagus VIP-ergic nerve fibres may be particularly abundant in the region of the lower oesophageal sphincter (3, 38), which VIP causes to relax (9, 57, 103, 119). VIP also inhibits the normal contractile response of this sphincter to pentagastrin (36, 119). Release of VIP could also explain the inhibitory effect of vagal stimulation on the pyloric sphincter, which occurs when this stimulus is applied during periods of continuous adrenergic stimulation (37). In the gall-bladder VIP has been shown to reduce the tension exerted by the smooth muscle of the wall of the viscus at rest, antagonise its spontaneous contractile activity, inhibit the contractile response to CCK-octapeptide and stimulate the secretion of $Na^+$, and $HCO_3^-$ across the mucosa (73, 99, 109). Secretion of pancreatic juice, with a high $HCO_3^-$ but low enzyme content, in response to preganglionic vagal stimulation, in species such as the pig and horse has long been known to persist after full muscarinic blockade (2, 63, 64). i.v. infusions of VIP produce precisely the same response in cats, pigs and birds (34, 78, 85), and to a lesser extent in dogs (79, 93). The secretory effect of VIP appears to be mediated in the exocrine pancreas by activation of adenylate cyclase (100, 107) as it is in the small intestine (115, 120) in which VIP also produces a watery secretion (45, 80, 94). In species such as the cat and dog, stimulation of the chorda tympani produces an intense vasodilatation in the submaxillary gland (11) which, unlike the secretory response, is resistant to atropine (61) and can be precisely mimicked by VIP (16, 19, 118).

Evidence that VIP is released during stimulation of autonomic nerves was first obtained from investigations of the changes in the concentration of the peptide in portal blood and intestinal lymph in response to stimulation of the peripheral ends of the vagus nerves in anaesthetized animals (13, 17, 22, 23, 40, 48, 49, 50, 112). Under these conditions there is a small rise in the concentration of VIP in the arterial plasma and a larger risk in the portal plasma, whereas stimulation of the peripheral ends of the splanchnic nerves causes a fall in the concentration in both portal and arterial plasma (48). Fahrenkrug, and his colleagues (48) concluded from these results that the VIP-ergic neurones receive a dual innervation with opposing effects. However, VIP is rapidly inactivated in the blood (97), as is evidenced both by the low concentration in which it is normally present in the peripheral plasma and the restricted range within which it varies in response to vagal stimulation at high frequency in both pigs and calves (17, 48). Furthermore, the concentration in the peripheral circulation depends not only on the rate at which the peptide enters the vascular system but also on the rates at which it leaves, and is inactivated within it. At best therefore, changes in the arterial plasma concentration of VIP can only provide a muted and rather reliable index of changes in entry rate. Nor can the entry rate of VIP into the blood be regarded as a reliable guide to the rate at which the peptide is actually released within the tissue of origin, as concomitant vasoconstriction will reduce it and vasodilatation enhance it. The interpretation of changes in the concentration of a peptide in portal blood is further complicated by the absence of any measurements of portal blood flow (48). Yet, even if the flow of venous effluent can be measured and the total outflow of a peptide, such as VIP determined, it may reflect the rate at which that peptide is 'washed out' of the tissue, rather than the rate at which it is released within tissue.

With these considerations in mind, we chose to examine the changes in the concentration of VIP in intestinal lymph, simultaneously with those occurring in arterial plasma in the young calf (17). This decision was taken in the belief that the concentration of VIP in the lymph would provide a more accurate indication, albeit delayed, of the changes in the concentration of the peptide which occur in the extracellular fluid in response to stimulation of the autonomic innervation. The further advantage emerged that VIP is inactivated more slowly in lymph than in plasma and so, by measuring the total dead space and the $\frac{1}{2}$ life of the peptide in the lymph, it was possible to extrapolate back to an estimated mean change in the concentration of the peptide, which must have occurred within the tissue fluid (gastrointestinal ECF). The results of these experiments confirmed the finding that VIP is released within the gastrointestinal tract in response to vagal stimulation (48), but refuted the suggestion that VIP release is inhibited by stimulation of the splanchnic sympathetic innervation because the fall in the concentration of VIP in the arterial plasma during splanchnic nerve stimulation was associated with a pronounced *rise* in the concentration in the intestinal lymph (17, 25). Thus, release of the peptide within the gastrointestinal tract is not inhibited during splanchnic nerve stimulation, but rather the rate at which it is lost into the circulation is reduced, presumably due to vasoconstriction of the splanchnic vascular bed. This conclusion is further supported by the finding that, in the pig, $\alpha$ adrenoceptor blockade, which would abolish the splanchnic vasoconstrictor response to adrenergic stimulation, annuls the usual depression in portal plasma VIP concentration (48).

The finding that release of VIP is not inhibited by adrenergic stimulation is crucial to a proper understanding of the role which VIP probably plays as an autonomic transmitter. The contention that the release of VIP from neural elements within the gastrointestinal tract (or anywhere else) could be enhanced by preganglionic parasympathetic, and inhibited by preganglionic sympathetic stimulation, would be difficult to reconcile with the proposition that VIP is released from a population of postganglionic parasympathetic neurones, and thereby provides an explanation for various of the 'atropine-resistant' responses to parasympathetic stimulation that have been described. That proposition is, however, in complete accord with the conclusion we have drawn, that release of VIP from the gastrointestinal tract is unaffected by stimulation of

the splanchnic nerves, except in so far as the rate at which the peptide passes into the circulation is reduced by adrenergic vasoconstriction (17). These results of experiments in anaesthetized calves have recently been confirmed in conscious calves, in which the peripheral ends of either the splanchnic or vagus nerves have been stimulated below behavioural threshold (18, 20).

In the cat, Fahrenkrug and his colleagues obtained rather stronger evidence that certain non-adrenergic, non-cholinergic gastrointestinal responses were attributable to the release of VIP. Thus, they were able to show that such responses as the increases in intestinal and colonic blood flow, which occur during mechanical stimulation of the intestinal mucosa and electrical stimulation of the pelvic nerves respectively, are accompanied by a significant increase in the concentration of VIP in the venous effluent plasma. The fact that this occurs during vasodilator responses clearly shows that the stimuli are associated with an increase in the total output of VIP from these tissues (48). However, the results of a more recent study suggest that colonic vasodilatation in response to pelvic nerve is due at least in part to the production of some kinin, such as bradykinin, as it is substantially reduced by the administration of Trasylol (54).

More compelling evidence that VIP is released from postganglionic parasympathetic nerve terminals and acts as a transmitter, has been obtained from studies of the responses to stimulation of the chorda tympani in atropinised cats, in which it has been shown to account for the atropine-resistant vasodilatation which occurs in the submaxillary gland (16, 19, 88). This can be summarised as follows:

1) The identification of VIP by immunocytochemical techniques within nerve terminals in the submaxillary gland (14, 88, 90, 91, 127, 130).

2) The peptide is promptly released from the gland in response to stimulation of the parasympathetic innervation, both in the presence and absence of atropine, and release is abruptly curtailed when stimulation is discontinued (Fig. 1a & b). It can be seen from the data illustrated in this Figure that the rise in salivary blood

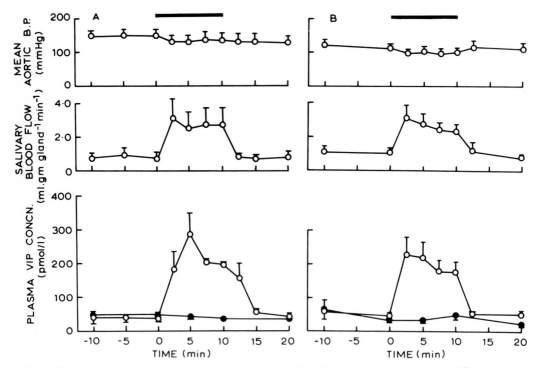

Fig. 1. Changes in mean aortic blood pressure, submaxillary blood flow and submaxillary venous (○) and arterial (●) plasma VIP concentration of anaesthetised cats, in response to stimulation of the chorda tympani at 20 Hz for 10 min (a) in the absence of atropine, n = 4, (b) in the presence of atropine, 1.0 mg/Kg, n = 5. Horizontal bars: duration of stimulus. Vertical bars: S.E. of each mean value. (Bloom & Edwards 1980c, reproduced by kind permission of the Journal of Physiology).

flow must be due to dilatation of blood vessels within the gland as there is no rise in the effective perfusion pressure.

3) Intra-arterial infusions of acetylcholine in doses which, in the absence of atropine, cause pronounced submaxillary vasodilation, have no effect on the release of VIP from the gland (Fig. 2); hence the release of the peptide is not secondary to some muscarinic mechanism.

4) In molar units, VIP is a far more potent vasoactive agent than acetylcholine; comparable vasodilator responses to i.a. VIP at a dose of 6 pmol/min requiring a dose of about 1500 pmol/min acetylcholine (Fig. 2).

5) Intra-arterial infusions of VIP which mimic the rise in the concentration of the peptide in the submaxillary venous effluent plasma during chorda stimulation, also produce an increase

in submaxillary blood flow of the same order of magnitude as that observed during chorda stimulation at the same frequency (Figs. 1 & 2).

6) Unlike the colonic vasodilatation response to pelvic nerve stimulation, which is substantially reduced in the presence of Trasylol (54), the atropine-resistant submaxillary vasodilator response to stimulation of the chorda tympani is unaffected by Trasylol (4, 5). It cannot therefore be attributed to the production of a kinine, such as bradykinin, as has been suggested by Hilton and others (66, 67, 68, 69, 128).

In addition, it has been claimed that the submaxillary vasodilator response to stimulation of the chorda tympani can be blocked in atropinised cats by the administration of antibodies to VIP (88, 89), although apparently this can only be

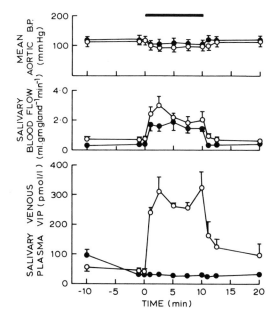

Fig. 2. Changes in mean aortic blood pressure, salivary blood flow and salivary venous plasma VIP concentration of anaesthetized cats in response to intra-carotid infusions of either acetyl choline (●; c1500 pmol/min) or VIP (○; c6 pmol·Kg$^{-1}$ min$^{-1}$; n = 5). Horizontal bar: duration of infusion. Vertical bars: S.E. of each mean value. (Bloom & Edwards, 1980c; reproduced by kind permission of the Journal of Physiology).

achieved during stimulation at a rather low frequency (2 Hz). Even more recently it has been reported that the vasodilator action of VIP on the submaxillary vasculature is blocked by avian pancreatic polypeptide (aPP) (89). If this is so, aPP could prove to be an invaluable tool in the study of the characteristics of this newly discovered transmitter, but the finding has yet to be confirmed and it is not yet known whether aPP blocks actions of VIP elsewhere.

Holst and his co-workers (70) have presented very convincing evidence that release of VIP from postganglionic parasympathetic nerve terminals in the pancreas fully accounts for the atropine-resistant responses to parasympathetic stimulation (51, 52). In these experiments the venous drainage from the head of the pancreas was isolated in anaesthetized pigs, thereby making it possible to quantify changes in the total output of the peptide. After administration of atropine a marked increase in the output of VIP was

associated with the secretion of water and HCO$_3^-$, which occurred in response to vagal stimulation, together with a three-fold rise in pancreatic blood flow. They went on to show that somatostatin caused a parallel suppression of vagally induced release of VIP and the flow of pancreatic juice. As somatostatin had no affect on the exocrine responses of the isolated perfused pig's pancreas to VIP it was concluded that it probably acted by inhibiting the release of VIP from the nerve terminals. Somatostatin has no effect on the release of VIP from nerve terminals in the submaxillary gland of the cat (17), so that such inhibition is not a general characteristic of VIP-ergic nerve terminals. As (51, 52) proposed that both the secretion of water and HCO$_3^-$ by the pancreas, and the vasodilatation that occurs in response to vagal stimulation in atropinised pigs, is attributable to release of VIP, it would have been interesting to know whether somatostatin blocked both or only one of these responses.

The further question whether VIP coexists with other transmitters in the same nerve terminals has also been investigated, particularly in relation to cholinergic nerve terminals using a combination of immunohistochemistry and acetylcholinesterase staining (8, 87, 88, 91). It is reported that 10–15% of the principal ganglion cells in the stellate, L7 and S1 ganglia contain both VIP-like immunoreactivity and intense acetylcholinesterase activity suggesting the presence of VIP in a population of sympathetic cholinergic neurones. In addition, overlapping accumulations of VIP immunoreactivity and acetylcholinesterase staining was observed around a ligation of the sciatic nerve and the patterns of distribution of VIP-immunoreactive and acetylcholinesterase-containing fibres around certain sweat glands and blood-vessels were very similar. Both types of staining disappeared from fibres around sweat glands and skeletal muscle vessels after lumbosacral sympathectomy. VIP-immunoreactivity was also found in other acetylcholinesterase staining neurones in other sympathetic ganglia, and in certain parasympathetic ganglia although it was not a general characteristic of such neurones. Lundberg et al (91) concluded that three different populations of neurone can be distinguished: neurones that are both rich in acetylcholinesterase and also contain a VIP-like peptide, VIP-immunoreactive neurones and neurones rich in acetylcholinesterase but lacking VIP-immunoreactivity. However, as the authors themselves point out, the use of acetylcholinesterase staining in order to identify cholinergic neurones is not totally reliable, as non-cholinergic neurones will respond if incubated for long enough (47, 72). These results can therefore be regarded as suggestive, but not conclusive, evidence that the two transmitters VIP and ACh can coexist in the same nerve terminals.

*Other neuropeptides*

Numerous other neuropeptides have also been identified in nerve fibres in the gastrointestinal tract by immunocytochemical techniques. These include substance P, enkephalin, somatostatin, gastrin/CCK, neurotensin and bombesin (35, 56, 114). As in the case of VIP, substance P-, enkephalin and somatostatin-like immunoreactivity are widely distributed throughout the tract whereas gastrin/CCK- and neurotensin-like immunoreactivity have a more restricted distribution. Neural immunoreactive neurotensin and bombesin has so far been seen only in nerve terminals whereas that to all the other of these peptides has been observed in both the nerve cell bodies and fibres. Schultzberg and her colleagues (114) have mapped out the precise distribution of all these different types of neurone, except those believed to contain bombesin, and also obtained evidence of a somatostatin-like and a gastrin/CCK like peptide in the same neurones. They suggest that this may indicate a common precursor for these two peptides in these particular neurones and observed that each of the substance P-, VIP and enkephalin-like peptides appeared to be present in different populations of nerve cells, which were also distinct from those containing somatostatin and gastrin/CCK-like immunoreactivity. There appears to be a rich distribution of fibres containing bombesin-like immunoreactivity to the gastric mucosa, at least in the rat, with a comparatively sparse supply in the intestinal mucosa of the same species (35). On the other hand, nerve cell bodies in the myen-

teric plexus are provided with an abundant supply of these fibres throughout the gut. Dockray et al. (35) have suggested on the basis of these findings that bombesin-like peptides are neurotransmitters in the gastrointestinal tract, which could play a role in the modulation of mobility and in the release of gastrin. All the available evidence indicates that the gastrointestinal tract contains numerous populations of neurones, each of which contains its own peptide, or mixture of peptides, or even a peptide together with one of the classical autonomic transmitters. Further study of peptidergic mechanisms in the gut therefore seems certain to revolutionise our understanding of the physiology of digestive and absorptive processes in the next few years.

The pancreas also appears to be richly supplied with a peptidergic innervation. In addition to VIP-ergic fibres referred to previously, neurones containing substance P-, enkephalin- and gastrin/CCK-like immunoreactivity have now been described in this organ (81, 105). Interpretation of the precise function of these various fibres is complicated by the fact that each of the peptides in question is known to influence either the endocrine or the exocrine pancreas, or both, in one or more ways (58, 77, 121). Thus, in the case of the islets, substance P stimulates the release of both glucagon and somatostatin (28, 62, 75, 98) and has been found to inhibit and stimulate the release of insulin under different experimental conditions, not only in vivo but also in vitro (28, 62, 75, 92, 98, 111). Studies in various perfused pancreas preparations have shown that VIP is capable of causing release of both glucagon and insulin (62, 85, 113, 124) and strongly potentiates the release of insulin in response to other stimuli, such as glucose and B-adrenergic agonists (1). Various analogues of gastrin/CCK have been shown to release insulin, glucagon, somatostatin & PP (62, 86, 96, 105), the most potent being the terminal tetrapeptide common to both molecules (105). Rehfeld (104) has recently proposed that in the case of CCK, which produces responses from both exocrine and endocrine cells, inappropriate interactions are avoided by the fact that different forms of the molecule are responsible for the different actions and reach the tissue by different routes; actions of CCK on the islets being mediated by CCK4, released from nerve terminals, while those on the acinar cells are mediated by CCK8, which is blood borne.

In the pig, either a small CCK analogue or VIP, or conceivably both, might well turn out to be the transmitter(s) released from some post-ganglionic parasympathetic nerve terminals that supply the islets, as the release of both glucagon and insulin, but not PP, in response to vagal stimulation is now known to be atropine resistant and effectively blocked by hexamethonium (70). In this report those endocrine responses resemble the secretion of water and $HCO_3^-$ from the gland in response to vagal stimulation in the same species (63, 64). In the calf, on the other hand, in which the pancreatic endocrine responses to wide variety of glycaemic stimuli are mediated largely via the parasympathetic innervation (21, 22, 23, 24, 26, 41, 42), the effect of vagal stimulation appears to be completely suppressed by atropine (20). Atropine also completely blocks the release of both insulin and glucagon from the pancreas in response to vagal stimulation in the dog (10, 55, 76, 102) and substantially reduces the rise in plasma insulin concentration which occurs after the administration of exogenous glucose in the baboon (31). The proposition that peptides fulfil the role of a postganglionic transmitter would appear to be insupportable in respect of response to parasympathetic stimulation that are blocked by atropine and responses to sympathetic stimulation that are suppressed by adrenoceptor blockade. Two separate responses which might well prove to be mediated by some peptide or other are the release of pancreatic glucagon in response to stimulation of the splanchnic nerves and stimulation of hepatic glycogenolysis directly via the sympathetic innervation. The former response persists in the presence of phentolamine, propranolol and atropine (15) and the latter is unaffected by dichloroisoproterenol in doses which effectively block the hepatic glycogenolytic response to catecholamines (116). In the case of the liver, it is now known that, whereas catecholamines activate phosphorylase via cyclic AMP, splanchnic nerve stimulation achieves the same result by inhibition of phosphorylase phosphatase

(117). Clearly, if a different intracellular mechanism is activated it is most likely that a different receptor, very possibly responding to a different transmitter, is involved. Further speculation about the precise functions of peptidergic neurones in relation to the endocrine pancreas would appear to be unjustified in our present state of knowledge; the most immediate identifiable need being further information about the extent of species variation.

## OPTIMUM PATTERNS OF ELECTRICAL STIMULATION

Traditionally, autonomic nerves have almost invariably been tested experimentally by means of a continuous stimulus at constant frequency. The results of such experiments have lead to general acceptance of the supposition that maximal autonomic responses occur during stimulation of the efferent nerves at frequencies of up to 20 Hz (65, 108), and results obtained using higher stimulus frequencies have been severely criticised on the grounds that such experiments were unphysiological. However, peptidergic neurones elsewhere, such as those of the tuberoinfundibular system in the basal hypothalamus and those releasing oxytocin in the neurohypophysis, are capable of firing at much higher frequencies (83, 84, 106). In fact the release of physiologically effective amounts of oxytocin appears to be *restricted* to periods when bursts of activity at a high frequency (50–60 Hz) are occurring in neurones of the preoptic and paraventricular nuclei (83, 84). Accordingly, having established that VIP is released from certain post-ganglionic parasympathetic neurones in the submaxillary gland of the cat, where it acts as a transmitter, we have recently undertaken an investigation of the effects of high frequency stimulation in short bursts on submaxillary and various other autonomic responses (4, 39).

*Submaxillary responses to stimulation in bursts*

In these experiments the effects of continuous preganglionic stimulation of the chorda tympani at 2 Hz for 10 min were compared with those of stimulation at 20 Hz for 1 sec at 10 sec intervals for the same period in atropinised cats while Trasylol, which did not itself effect the response, was continually infused intra-arterially at a rate of 500 K.I.U./min in order to minimise inactivation of VIP between the point of release and collection. Both the fall in mean submaxillary vascular resistance (SVR) and the rise in mean VIP output from the gland were significantly increased ($p < 0.1$; $p < 0.2$) when the same total number of impulses were delivered in bursts at the higher frequency (Fig. 3). Both these responses were also consistently increased by stimulating the postganglionic innervation in bursts in the same way in atropinised cats, or by stimulating the preganglionic innervation in bursts in the absence of atropine.

In a further series of experiments the effects of stimulation of the chorda tympani in 1 sec bursts at 10 sec intervals for 2–3 min were investigated over the frequency range 2–160 Hz. The change in mean SVR under these conditions was significantly reduced by the administration of atropine at frequencies between 2 and 20 Hz, but not at higher frequencies. In atropinised cats, the fall in mean SVR was linearly related to stimulus frequency ($r = 0.993$) over the range 2–60 Hz and a maximal response was obtained during stimulation at 80 Hz (Fig. 4). In the same experiments the fall in mean SVR was linearly related to *log* mean VIP output from the gland over the whole of the frequency range 20–160 Hz ($r = 0.998$; Fig. 5). In the absence of atropine, the flow of submaxillary saliva was also found to be linearly related to stimulus frequency between 2 and 40 Hz, when the stimuli were delivered in bursts, and secretion of saliva was maximal at 60 Hz (Fig. 6).

The results of these experiments show that the release of the peptidergic transmitter VIP from peripheral postganglionic parasympathetic neurones is enhanced at high stimulus frequencies, just as the release of various peptides from hypothalamic neurones are. The fact that the change in mean SVR in response to stimulation in bursts was significantly reduced by prior administration of atropine at low stimulus frequencies (2–20 Hz), but not at higher frequencies, shows that physiologically effective amounts of acetylcholine are

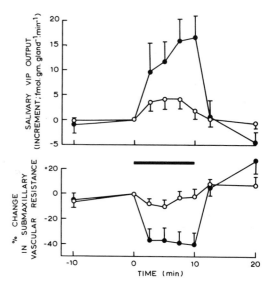

Fig. 3. Comparison of the changes in mean submaxillary vascular resistance (A) and mean submaxillary VIP output (B), in response to preganglionic stimulation of the chorda tympani at either 2 Hz continuously for 10 min (O; n = 7) or at 20 Hz in 1 sec bursts at 10 sec intervals for the same period (●; n = 8). Atropine (0.5 mg/Kg) was given by i.v. injection 10 min prior to stimulation. Horizontal bars: duration of stimulus. Vertical bars: S.E. of each mean value. (Andersson et al. 1981b; reproduced by kind permission of the Journal of Physiology).

released from parasympathetic nerve terminals within the gland at frequencies below those needed to cause effective release of VIP. This conclusion is supported by the earlier observation that the submaxillary vascular response to single stimuli delivered to the chorda tympani is completely blocked by atropine (46) and the finding that, even using continuous stimulation, the vascular response at low frequencies is depressed by atropine whereas that at high frequencies (10–20 Hz) is not (32).

The linearity of the relation between *log* VIP output and the falling mean SVR in atropinised cats, during stimulation of the chorda tympani in bursts (Fig. 5) at frequencies between 20 and 160 Hz is reminiscent of dose/response relations generally over the response range 20–80%. The excellence of the linearity down to an output of less than $5 \, \text{fmol} \cdot \text{gm} \cdot \text{gland}^{-1} \cdot \text{min}^{-1}$ ($r = 0.998$) suggests that the intracarotid infusion of Trasylol effectively prevented significant inactivation of

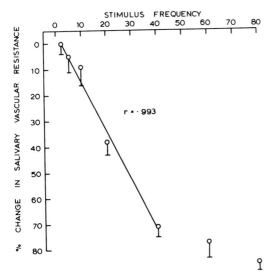

Fig. 4. The relation between mean % change in submaxillary vascular resistance and stimulus frequency in cats treated with atropine (0.5 mg/Kg) in response to preganglionic stimulation of the chorda tympani in 1 sec bursts at 10 sec intervals (n = 6) at each frequency. Vertical bars: S.E. of each mean value. Regression line calculated by method of least squares (r = 0.993). (Andersson et al. 1981b; reproduced by kind permission of the Journal of Physiology).

VIP between the sites of release and collection. It also supports the contention that the vasodilator response is attributable exclusively to release of VIP under these conditions, in which the effect

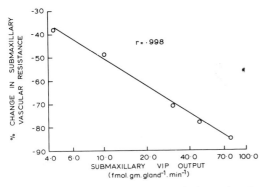

Fig. 5. The relation between mean % change in submaxillary vascular resistance and mean submaxillary VIP output during preganglionic stimulation of the chorda tympani at various frequencies, between 20 and 160 Hz in 1 sec bursts at 10 sec intervals for 2–3 min in atropinsed cats (0.5 mg atropine/Kg). Regression line (r = 0.998) calculated by method of least squares. (Andersson et al. 1981b; reproduced by kind permission of the Journal of Physiology).

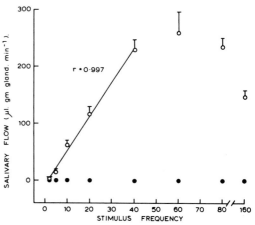

Fig. 6. Comparison of the changes in submaxillary salivary flow, in response to preganglionic stimulation of the chorda tympani, using 1 sec bursts at 10 sec intervals, at various frequencies, in the presence (●) and absence (○) of atropine (0.5 mg/Kg). Regression line calculated by method of least squares (r = 0.997). Vertical bars: S.E. of each mean value where these exceed the size of the symbol. (Andersson et al. 1981b; reproduced by kind permission of the Journal of Physiology).

of acetylcholine had been blocked by atropine and production of bradykinin prevented by administration of Trasylol. Further evidence is provided by the finding that the fall in mean SVR is linearly related to stimulus frequency between 2 and 40 Hz (r = 0.993; Fig. 4), when stimulation is carried out in bursts in atropinised cats. In the absence of atropine the response was found to be non-linear, as one would expect when more than one transmitter contributes to the response and the proportional contribution of each varies with stimulus frequency. Salivary flow, which is known to depend entirely on the release and subsequent muscarinic action of acetylcholine was also linearly related to stimulus frequency over the range 2–40 Hz, when the chorda tympani was stimulated in bursts in the absence of atropine (Fig. 6).

Maximal rates of salivary flow and changes in SVR occur at much lower frequencies during continuous stimulation of the chorda tympani than when 1 sec bursts at 10 sec intervals are employed (see for instance 46 and 131). Furthermore, there is generally a curvilinear relation (approaching a rectangular hyperbola) between the responses of a wide variety of autonomic effectors and the frequency of continuous stimulation of the innervation (30, 108). Stimulation for 1 sec at 10 sec intervals presumably causes the release of substantially less transmitter than would occur if the same frequency were employed continuously; 10% if it happened to be in precise proportion to the total number of impulses delivered in unit time. If the amount of transmitter that the nerve terminals are capable of releasing exceeds the requirements of the effector tissue the receptor sites presumably become saturated during continuous stimulation at frequencies well below those at which the nerve fibres are capable of conducting. Thus, simply by reducing the total amount of transmitter released in unit time, by the device of stimulating intermittently for a comparatively small part of the time available, the effector tissue is enabled to 'follow' the activity of the innervation more faithfully. The response is then seen to be linear over a wide frequency range and peaks at a much higher frequency. The original finding, attributed to Rosenblueth (108) by von Euler (129), that even after cutting a considerable portion of the nerve the maximal response to the effector tissue may be approached provided the frequency of stimulation is increased sufficiently, strongly supports this explanation.

*Responses of other tissues to stimulation in bursts*

The effects of stimulation of the autonomic innervation in bursts have now been investigated in a small number of other tissues. Comparison of the changes in vascular resistance of skeletal muscle in response to stimulation of the sympathetic vasoconstrictor supply in bursts with those to continuous stimulation at the corresponding frequency has revealed no significant difference in response (6). In contrast, Andersson and Järhult (7) have shown that the colonic vascular bed of atropinised cats responds to stimulation of the pelvic nerve in precisely the same way as the submaxillary vascular bed does to stimulation of the chorda tympani. Thus stimulation in bursts at either 20 or 40 Hz for 1 sec at 10 sec intervals produces a substantial increase in the blood flow whereas stimulation at the corresponding continuous frequency (2 or 4 Hz) is totally ineffective (7). These authors have made

the further even more intriguing discovery that another non-cholinergic, non-adrenergic response in the same tissue, contraction of the colonic smooth muscle (53, 71), behaves in the opposite way. Stimulation of the pelvic nerve, in bursts at 10 sec intervals, produces no significant contractile response at any frequency tested over the range 2 to 160 Hz, whereas continuous stimulation at frequencies between 4 and 16 Hz invariably produces a forceful contraction, which is apparently maximal at 8 Hz (7). In this way it is possible to obtain a complete separation between the motor and vascular colonic responses to pelvic nerve stimulation in atropinised cats. This phenomenon has yet to be explained; one obvious possibility is that the two responses depend upon different transmitters and that these are released preferentially at different stimulus frequencies.

Finally, the adrenal medullary response to stimulation of the peripheral end of the splanchnic nerve has been investigated in the calf (39). Calves were employed for these experiments because it is possible to stimulate the splanchnic nerve in unanaesthetised animals of this species, and various anaesthetics have been found to modify this response substantially (43). Calves also have the advantage that the 'adrenal clamp' technique (44) can be employed to quanfity the adrenal medullary output. In these experiments the output of adrenaline was significantly greater in response to stimulation in bursts at frequencies of 40 Hz and below than when the equivalent number of impulses were delivered at a constant rate (p < 0.02). Bursts of stimuli at 70 and at 100 Hz produced a similar output to that obtained in response to continuous stimulation at 7 and 10 Hz, whereas the output in response to bursts at 150 Hz was significantly less than that during continuous stimulation at 15 Hz. The output of noradrenaline was not significantly increased by using bursts of stimuli at any frequency, but was significantly decreased at 70 Hz and above compared with the equivalent constant rate of stimulation. Thus, in this case high frequency activity in bursts in the splanchnic innervation would favour the output of adrenaline from the gland and low frequency tonic activity the output of noradrenaline. The adrenal medulla therefore provides another example of a tissue in which some separation of response can be achieved by this sort of variation in the pattern of autonomic stimulation.

## GENERAL CONSIDERATIONS

The consistent finding that maximal autonomic responses to stimulation at constant rates occur at relatively low frequencies had lead to the widespread belief that a low frequency of discharge is a physiological characteristic of autonomic nerve fibres. This view has been strengthened in the case of the salivary gland by the finding that the highest rates of flow that occur naturally in the conscious animal can be matched by stimulation of the chorda tympani at a constant frequency of 7–8 Hz under anaesthesia (46). However, the choice of a constant as opposed to an intermittent rate of stimulation, which has almost invariably been made in the past, is merely an experimental convenience. We have no way of knowing what the physiological pattern of activity is in the autonomic fibres which supply the salivary gland, but in view of the fact that the afferent stimuli which provoke salivary responses are themselves inconstant, it is difficult to justify the assumption that the activity in these efferent fibres is constant or even approximates to constancy. In order to discover what the physiological pattern of activity is in the chorda tympani, and the rates at which the fibres are capable of discharging naturally, it would be necessary to record the activity of single units, or at most small groups of fibres, in conscious animals in anticipation of, or during, a meal. So far as we are aware no one has overcome the formidable technical difficulties that would be generated by such a protocol. Hagbarth and his colleagues at Uppsala have, however, succeeded in recording from small bundles of sympathetic nerve fibres in the skin of conscious human subjects (33, 59, 60). The results of these extremely elegant studies clearly show that these autonomic nerve fibres discharge naturally in *bursts*, and that the bursts are not synchronous with pulsatile cardiovascular events.

The discovery that certain autonomic nerve terminals contain peptide transmitters in addition to, or possibly instead of, one of the classical transmitters, has stimulated a reassessment of the optimum stimulus pattern for the release of various autonomic transmitters. The results that have so far been obtained show that it is no longer justified to assume that autonomic nerve fibres are always characterised by low natural discharge patterns. They also show that differential responses can be obtained in the same tissue by variation in stimulus frequency. This is due to preferential release of one of two transmitters (VIP) at high frequencies, at least in the submaxillary gland of the cat and probably elsewhere. Unfortunately the capacity to release transmitters, preferentially in this way does not of itself provide any evidence for or against the contention that different transmitters coexist within the same nerve terminal.

## REFERENCES

1. Ahrén B, Lindquist T. Diabetalogia 1981, 20, 1–16
2. Alexander F, Hickson JCD. In Physiology of Digestion and Metabolism in the Ruminant 1970, ed AT Phillipson. Oriel Press, Newcastle upon Tyne
3. Alumets J, Schaffalitzky de Muckadell O, Fahrenkrug J, Sundler F, Håkanson R, Uddman R. Nature 1979, 280, 155–156
4. Andersson P-O, Bloom SR, Edwards AV, Järhult J. J Physiol 1981a 313, 20–21P
5. Andersson P-O, Bloom SR, Edwards AV, Järhult J. J Physiol 1981b (in press)
6. Andersson PO, Järhult J. Personal communication 1981a.
7. Andersson P-O, Järhult J. Acta physiol Scand 1981b (in press)
8. Änggård A, Lundberg JM, Hökfelt T, Nilsson G, Fahrenkrug J, Said S. Acta physiol scand (1979) Suppl 473, 50
9. Beher J, Field S, Marin C. Gastroenterology 1979 77, 1001–1007
10. Bergman RN, Miller RE. Amer J Phys 1973 225, 481–486.
11. Bernard C. Cr hebd Seanc Acad Sci (Paris) 1958, 47, 245–253
12. Bishop AE, Polak JM, Green TC, Bryant MG, Bloom SR. Diabetalogia 1980 18, 73–78
13. Bitar KN, Said SI, Weir GC, Saffouri B, Mahklouf GM. Gastroenterology 1980 79, 1288–1294
14. Bloom SR, Bryant MG, Polak JM, Van Noorden S, Wharton J. J. Physiol 1979 289, 23P
15. Bloom SR, Edwards AV. J Physiol 1978 280, 25–35
16. Bloom SR, Edwards AV. J Physiol 1979 295, 35–36P
17. Bloom SR, Edwards AV. J Physil 1980a, 299, 437–452

18. Bloom SR, Edwards AV. J Physiol (1980b) 308, 39–48
19. Bloom SR, Edwards AV. J Physiol 1980c 300, 41–53
20. Bloom SR, Edwards AV. J Physiol 1981a 315, (in press)
21. Bloom SR, Edwards AV. J Physiol 1981b 314, 37–46
22. Bloom SR, Edwards AV, Hardy RN. J Physiol 1978a 280, 37–53
23. Bloom SR, Edwards AV, Hardy RN. J Physiol 1978b 280, 9–23
24. Bloom SR, Edwards AV, Jarhult J. J Physiol 1980 308, 29–38
25. Bloom SR, Edwards AV, Mitchell SJ. J Physiol 1979 289, 47P
26. Bloom SR, Edwards AV, Vaughan NJA. J Physiol 1974 236, 611–623
27. Bodanszky M, Klausner VS, Said SI. Proc Natl Acad Sci USA 1973 70, 382–384
28. Brown M, Vale W. Endocrinology 1976 98, 819–822
29. Bryant MG, Bloom SR, Polak JM, Albuquerque RH, Modlin F, Pearse AGE. Lancet 1976 1, 991–993
30. Celander O. Acta physiol scand 1954 32, Suppl 116
31. Daniel PM, Henderson JR. Acta endocr (Copenh) 1975 78, 736–745
32. Darke AC, Smaje LH. J Physiol 1972 226, 191–203
33. Delius W, Hagbarth KE, Hongell A, Wallin BG. Acta physiol scand 1972 84, 117–186
34. Dimaline R, Dockray GJ. J Physiol 1979 294, 153–163
35. Dockray GJ, Vaillant C, Walsh JH. Neuroscience 1979 4, 1561–1568
36. Domschke W, Lux G, Domschke S, Strunz U, Bloom SR, Wunsch E. Gastroenterology 1978 75, 9–12
37. Edin R, Ahlman H, Kewenter J. Acta Physiol scand 1979, 107, 169–174
38. Edin R, Lundberg JM, Ahlman H, Dahlström A, Fahrenkrug J, Hökfelt T, Dewenter J. Acta physiol scand 1979 107, 185–187
39. Edwards AV. J Physiol 1981 J Physiol 317, 41–42P
40. Edwards AV, Bircham PMM, Mitchell SJ, Bloom SR. Experientia 1979 34, 1186–1187
41. Edwards AV, Bloom SR. In Gut Hormones 1978, ed SR Bloom, pp 394–405. Edinburgh, Churchill Livingstone
42. Edwards AV, Bloom SR, Järhult J. Front Horm Res 1980 7, 30–40
42. Edwards AV, Furness PN, Helle KB. J. Physiol 1980 308, 15–27
44. Edwards AV, Hardy RN, Malinowska KW. J. Physiol 1974 239, 477–498
45. Eklund S, Jodal M, Lundgren O, Sjöquist A. Acta physiol scand 1979 105, 461–468
46. Emmelin N. In the Handbook of Physiology 1967, Sect 6, Vol II, ed CF Code, pp 595–632. American Physiological Society, Washington DC
47. Eränkö O, Härkönen A. Acta physiol scand 1964 61, 299–300
48. Fahrenkrug J, Haglund U, Jodal M, Lundgren O, Olbe L, Schaffalitzky de Muckadell OB. J Physiol 1978a 284, 291–305
49. Fahrenkrug J, Haglund U, Jodal M, Lundgren O, Olbe L, Schaffalitzky de Muckadell OB. Acta physiol scand 1978b 102, 22A–23A
50. Fahrenkrug J, Galbo H, Holst JJ, Schaffalitzky de Muckadell, OB. J Physiol 1978c 280, 405–422
51. Fahrenkrug J, Schaffalitzky de Muckadell OB, Holst JJ, Lindkaer-Jensen S. Amer J Physiol 1979a 237, E535–E540
52. Fahrenkrug J, Schaffalitzy de Muckadell OB, Holst JJ, Lindkaer-Jensen S. In Gastrins and the Vagus 1979b, ed JF Rehfeld, E Amdrup. Academic Press, London
53. Fasth S, Hultén L, Nordgren S. J Physiol 1980 298, 159–169
54. Fasth S, Hultén L, Nordgren S, Zeitlin IJ. J Physiol 1981 311, 421–429
55. Frohman LA, Ezdinli EZ, Javid R. Diabetes 1967 16, 443–448
56. Furness JB, Costa M. Neuroscience 1980 51, 1–20
57. Goyal RK, Rattan S, Said SI. Nature 1980 288, 378–386
58. Grossman MT. In Endocrinology of the Gut, 1974, ed WY Chey, FP Brooks. Charles B Stack Inc, Thorofare, New Jersey
59. Hagbarth KE, Hallin RG, Hongell A, Torebjörk HE, Wallin BG. Acta Physiol scand 1972 92, 303–317
60. Hallin RG, Torebjörk HE. Acta physiol scand 1974 92, 303–317
61. Heidenhain R. Pflügers Arch 1872 5, 309–318
62. Hermansen K. Endocrinology 1980 107, 256–261
63. Hickson JCD. J Physiol 1970a 206, 275–298
64. Hickson JCD. J Physiol 1970b 206, 299–322
65. Hillarp N-Å. In the Handbook of Physiology, Sect I 1960, ed J Field, HW Magoun, VE Hall. Vol II, pp 999–1006. American Physiological Society, Washington DC
66. Hilton SM. In Polypeptides which affect Smooth Muscles and Blood Vessels, ed M Schachter 1960, pp 258–262. Pergamon Press, London
67. Hilton SM, Lewis GP. J Physiol 1955a 128, 235–248
68. Hilton SM, Lewis GP. J Physiol 1955b 129, 253–271
69. Hilton SM, Lewis GP. J Physiol 1956 134, 471–483
70. Holst JJ, Gronholt R, Schaffalitzky de Muckadell OB, Fahrenkrug J. Acta phys scand 1981 111, 9–14
71. Hultén L. Acta physiol scand 1969 335, 1–116
72. Jacobowitz D, Koelle GB. J pharmac exp Therap 1965 148, 225–237
73. Jansson R, Steen G, Svanvik J. Gastroenterology 1978, 75, 47–50
74. Kachelhoffer J, Eloy MR, Pousse A, Hohmatter D, Grenier, JF. Pflügers Arch 1974 352, 37–46
75. Kaneto A, Kaneko T, Kajinauma H, Kosaka K. Endocrinology 1978 102, 393–401
76. Kaneto A, Miki E, Kosaka K. Endocrinology 1974 95, 1005–1010
77. Konturek SJ. Irish J Med Sci 1978 147, 1–16

78. Konturek SJ, Pucher A, Radecki T. J Physiol 1976 255, 497–509
79. Konturek SJ, Thor P, Dembinski A, Król R. Gastroenterology 1975 68, 1527–1535.
80. Kreys GJ, Barkley RM, Read NW, Fordtran JS. J clin invest 1978 61, 1337–1345
81. Larsson LI. J Histochem Cytochem 1979 27, 1283–1284
82. Larsson L-I, Fahrenkrug J, Schaffalitzky de Muckadell OB, Sundler F, Häkanson R, Rehfeld JF. Proc Natl Acad Sci NY 1976 73, 3197–3200
83. Lincoln DW, Wakerley JB. J Physiol 1972 222, 23–24P
84. Lincoln DW, Wakerley JB. J Physiol 1974 242, 533–554
85. Lindkaer-Jensen S, Fahrenkrug J, Holst JJ, Vagn Nielsen O, Schaffalitzky de Muckadell OB. Amer J Physiol 1978 235, E381–386
86. Lindkaer-Jensen S, Rehfeld J, Holst JJ, Fahrenkrug J, Neilsen OV, Schaffalitzky de Muckadell OB. Amer J Physiol 1980 238, E186–192
87. Lundberg JM Acta physiol scand 1979 Suppl 473, 14
88. Lundberg JM, Änggärd A, Fahrenkrug J, Hökfelt T, Mott V, Proc Natl Acad Sci USA 1980a 77, 1651–1655
89. Lundberg JM, Änggärd A, Hökfelt T, Kimmel J. Acta physiol scand 1980b 110, 199–201
90. Lundberg JM, Hökfelt T, Kewenter J, Petterson G, Ahlman H, Edin R, Dahlstrom A, Nilsson G, Terenius L, Uvnäs-Wallensten K, Said S. Gastroenterology 1979a, 77, 468–471
91. Lundberg JM, Hökfelt T, Schultzberg M, Uvnäs-Wallensten K, Köhler C, Said SI. Neursci 1979b 4, 1539–1559
92. Lundquist T, Sundler F, Ahrén B, Alumets J, Häkanson R. Endocrinology 1979 104, 832–838
93. Mahklouf GM, Said SI, Yan WM. Gastroenterology 1974 66, 737
94. Mailman D. J Physiol 1978 279, 121–132
95. Malmfors G, Häkanson R, Okmian L, Sundler F. J Pediat Surg 1980 15, 53–56
96. Meyer FD, Gyr K, Häcki WH, Beglinger C, Jeker L, Varga L, Kayasseh L, Gillessen D, Stalder GA. Gastroenterology 1981 80, 742–747
97. Modlin IM, Mitchell SJ, Bloom SR. In Gut Hormones 1978, ed SR Bloom, pp 470–474. Churchill Livingstone, London
98. Moltz, JH, Dobbs RE, McCann SM, Fawcett, CP. Endocrinology 1977 101, 196–202
99. Morton IKM, Phillips SJ, Saverymuttu SH, Wood JR. J Physiol 1977 266, 65P.
100. Olinger FJ, Gardner JD. Gastroenterology 1979 77, 704–713
101. Piper PJ, Said SI, Vane JR. Nature 1970 225, 1144–1146
102. Porte D, Girardier L, Seydoux J, Kanazawa Y, Posternak J. J Clin Invest 1973 52, 210–214
103. Rattan S, Said SI, Goyal RK. Proc Soc exp biol Med 1977 155, 40–43
104. Rehfeld J. Amer J Physiol 1981 240, G255–266
105. Rehfeld JF, Larsson L-I, Goltermann NR, Schwartz T, Holst JJ, Jensen SL, Morley JS. Nature 1980 284, 33–38
106. Renaud LP. Brain Res 1976, 105, 59–72
107. Robberecht P, Conlon TP, Gardner JD. J Biol Chem 1976 251, 4635–4639
108. Rosenblueth A. Amer J Physiol 1932 102, 12–38
109. Ryan JP, Ryave J. Amer J Physiol 1978 234, E44–46
110. Said SI, Mutt V. Science 1970 169, 1217–1218
111. Sasaki H. Metabolism 1976 25, 1463–1467
112. Schaffalitzky de Muckadell OB, Fahrenkrug J, Holst JJ. Gastroenterology 1977 72, 373–375
113. Schebalin M, Said SI, Mahklouf GM. Amer J Physiol 1977 232, E197–200
114. Schultzberg M, Hökfelt T, Nilsson G, Torenius L, Rehfeld JF, Brown M, Elde R, Goldstein M, Said S. Neuroscience 1980 5, 689–744
115. Schwartz CJ, Kimberley DV, Sheerin HE, Field M, Said SI. J clin invest 1974 54, 536–544
116. Shimazu T, Amakano A. Biochem biophys Acta 1968 165, 349–356
117. Shimazu T, Amakawa A. Biochem & biophys Acta 1975 835, 242–256
118. Shimazu T, Taira N. Br J Pharmac 1979 65, 683–688
119. Siegel SR, Brown FC, Castell DO, Johnson LF, Said SI. Dig Dis & Sci 1979 24, 345–349
120. Simon B, Kather H. Gastroenterology 1978 74, 722–725
121. Singh M, Webster PD. Gastroenterology 1978 74, 294–309
122. Sundler F, Alumets J, Häkanson R, Ingemansson S, Fahrenkrug J, Shaffalitzky de Muckadell O. Gastroenterology 1977 72, 1375–1377
123. Sundler F, Alumets J, Häkanson R, Fahrenkrug J, Schaffalitzky de Muckadell O. Histochemistry 1978 55, 173–176
124. Szecoboa J, Sandberg E, Effendíc S. Diabetelogia 1980 19, 137–142
125. Thulin L, Olsson P. Acta chir scand 1973 139, 681–697
126. Uddman R, Alumets J, Edvinsson L, Häkanson R, Sundler F. Gastroenterology 1978 75, 5–8
127. Uddman R, Fahrenkrug J, Malm L, Alumets J, Häkanson R, Sunder F. Acta physiol scand 1980 110, 31–38
128. Ungar G, Parrott JL. C r seanc Soc Biol 1936 122, 1052–1055
129. Von Euler US. In the Handbook of Physiology 1959, Sect 1, Vol I, eds J Field, HW Magoun, VE Hall, pp 215–238. American Physiological Society, Washington DC
130. Wharton J, Polak JM, Bryant MG, Van Noorden S, Bloom SR, Pearse AGE. Life Sci 1979 25, 273–380.
131. Wills JH. Amer J Physiol 1941 134, 441–449.

# Removal of the Ganglionated Plexuses from the Gut Wall: Advantages for Studies of the Enteric Nervous System

K. R. JESSEN
MRC Neuroimmunology Project, Dept of Zoology, University College London,
Gower Street, London WC1E 6BT, UK

Methods have been developed for removing the myenteric and submucous plexuses from the gut wall. This offers significant advantages for studies of the enteric nervous system, some of which are illustrated below.

Firstly, the plexuses can be maintained in culture as explants for many weeks, during which period, neurite outgrowth, glial and fibroblast proliferation and cellular interactions, follow a characteristic and predictable pattern. Both neurones and glial cells in these cultures retain, to a high degree, their in situ properties. The usefulness of these preparations for complementing in situ studies is described. In addition, the cultures make it possible to tackle new types of problems, which could not, or only with difficulty, be approached without an in vitro model. Two examples are discussed: a) the search for specific growth factors required for enteric neurons and glial cells in vivo; b) the studies of cell and tissue interactions required for histogenesis in the enteric nervous system.

Secondly, the ability to dissect the ganglionated plexuses from the gut wall, offers the simple advantage that biochemical measurements can be carried out without contamination by other cell types. This is illustrated in studies of putative GABAergic neurons in the myenteric plexus, including measurements of glutamic acid decarboxylase (GAD) activity in plexus homogenates and studies of GABA and homocarnosine synthesis in intact enteric neurons.

Thirdly, the freshly dissected plexuses offer unique advantages, when compared to other parts of the vertebrate peripheral or central nervous system, for investigation of cell surface molecules, increasingly believed to be of central importance in development, histogenesis and the establishment of specific connections, in the nervous system. Comparative studies are described on the cell surface chemistry of neurones and glial cells in the enteric nervous system, other divisions of the peripheral nervous system and brain. Evidence is presented for two, and possibly three, new neuronal subpopulations in the myenteric plexus, identified by the distribution of surface antigens defined by monoclonal antibodies.

*K. R. Jessen, MRC Neuroimmunology Project, Dept of Zoology, University College London, Gower Street, London WC1E 6BT, UK*

The enteric ganglia have, until recently, remained the only major part of the vertebrate nervous system which has not been available for study except as part of another tissue, in this case the connective and muscle tissue of the gut wall. As a result, some important lines of approach, long since commonplace in research on other divisions of the nervous system, could only be applied to the enteric nervous system with difficulty. The most notable examples are biochemical measurements of nervous tissue uncontaminated by other cells, and tissue culture studies, both of which have played central roles in studies on other autonomic and sensory ganglia, peripheral nerves and the central nervous system.

We have recently developed methods for removing the major components of the enteric nervous system, the ganglionated myenteric and submucous plexuses, from the gut wall, thus freeing them from the connective tissue and muscle that surrounds them in vivo (20). I will discuss below some of the uses for this preparation. They fall into three broad classes: tissue culture studies; direct biochemical measurements of enteric nervous tissue, illustrated by studies on α-amino butyric acid (GABA) as an enteric neurotransmitter; and investigations of the cell surface chemistry of enteric neurons and glial cells.

## 1) TISSUE CULTURE STUDIES

### a) *Behaviour of enteric plexuses in culture*

Following incubation of pieces of gut wall in a solution of enzymes such as collagenase, elastase or hyaluronidase, for 2–4 hours, the myenteric and submucous plexuses can be dissected free from other tissues of the gut wall, under the dissecting microscope. We have applied this method, with appropriate modifications, to several gut areas of guinea pigs, rats, rabbits and

chicks, of various ages from newborn to a few weeks.

For culturing, the plexuses are explanted on glass coverslips, which are then mounted in modified Rose chambers and kept at 37°C. These chambers provide optimum optical conditions for light microscopical studies of outgrowth pattern and development of the plexuses, which can be maintained in this manner for many weeks. The growth pattern and cellular interactions have been most closely studied in case of the myenteric plexus from the guinea pig taenia coli (19, 20). Since a detailed account of these observations will be given elsewhere, they will only be described briefly below.

The characteristic organisation of the plexuses into compact ganglia separated by short nerves, breaks down during the first few days in culture. The enteric glial cells play a major role in this process. During the first 2–3 days in culture, they migrate out from the plexus onto the glass coverslip as flat cells carrying extensive, thin, mem-

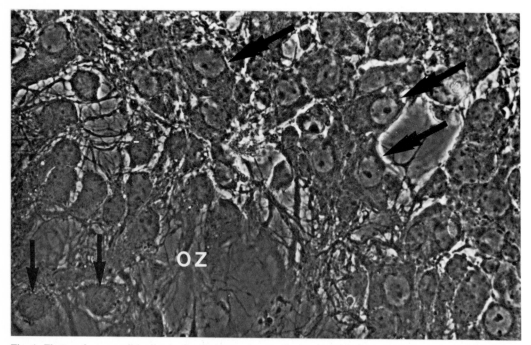

Fig. 1. Flattened nerve cell bodies in the explant area, near its border with the outgrowth zone which occupies the bottom left hand corner of the picture. Big arrows: examples of neurones; small arrows: glial nuclei in the outgrowth zone; OZ: outgrowth zone. Myenteric plexus from the guinea pig taenia coli, 7 days in culture; ×695.

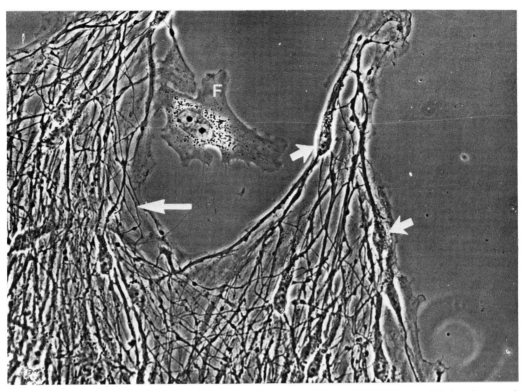

Fig. 2. Arrowhead-shaped glial cell sheet at the edge of the outgrowth zone. The continuous glial sheet is covered by a dense meshwork of neurites. Small arrows: examples of glial nuclei; big arrow: neurites; I: fibroblasts. Myenteric plexus from the guinea pig taenia coli, 4 days in culture ×512. (From 20 with permission.)

branous expansions, filling in the holes in the plexus-meshwork and forming the initial outgrowth around the explant.

After about one week in culture, the explant has developed into an unbroken monolayer of clearly visible neuronal cell bodies and associated glial cells, with a loose, irregular mesh of neuronal and glial processes interweaving between them (Fig. 1). Surrounding this area lies an extensive outgrowth zone: the neurons have by this time grown long processes which radiate from the explant in all directions, lying on top of a continuous sheet of flat, proliferating glial cells (Fig. 2). Inevitably, the terminals of the nerve fibers which innervate the plexus from external sources, are part of the original explant. These fibers degenerate during the first few days in culture, leaving only those nerve fibers that have regen-

erated from neurons intrinsic to the explanted plexus itself.

During the 2nd to 5th week in culture, the organization described above changes radically. The loose monolayer of neurons and glial cells gradually disappears as these cells rearrange into many small and compact aggregates (Fig. 3). Investigations of these aggregates by electron microscopy, show them to consist of neurons, glial cells and areas of neuropil where many synapses can be seen, the overall appearance being very similar to that seen in the enteric ganglia in situ (1). The aggregates are interconnected by thick bundles of neurites and are usually surrounded by connective tissue cells. Those cells originate from a few fibroblasts, that adhere to the plexuses when explanted and proliferate rapidly during the culture period. The arrangement

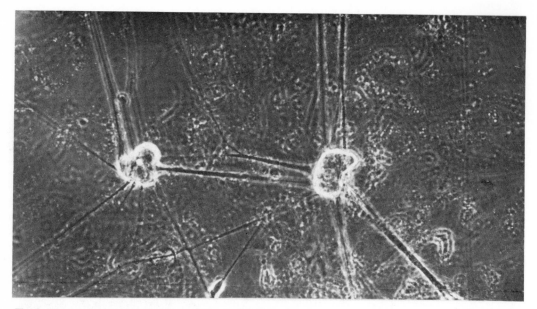

Fig. 3. Two compact aggregates of neurons and glial cells, which are connected by thick neurite bundles. Several other neurite bundles connecting these aggregates to other similar ones lying outside the field, can also be seen. A layer of fibroblasts, which is out of focus in this picture, lies under the neuronal elements. Myenteric plexus from the guineal pig taenia coli. 21 days in culture; ×270.

of neurons, glial cells and connective tissue described here, which is achieved after a minimum of 1 week in culture, shows clear similarities to the relationship between these tissue elements in vivo.

b) *Retention of neuronal and glial differentiation in culture*

In evaluating the present culture system as an in vitro model of enteric nervous tissue, it is important to assess to what extent the cells retain in culture the various features that characterize them in situ. We have used morphological, enzyme-histochemical, immunohistochemical and autoradiographic methods to compare a number of neuronal and glial properties in culture with those observed in situ (25).

These studies show, that the cultured neurones maintain their characteristically wide diversity in gross-morphology, and at the ultrastructural level both the neurons and glial cells exhibit the general features found in in situ studies. As in situ, most or all of the neurons contain histochemically demonstrable acetylcholinesterase and mono-amine oxidase activities, while neuronal subpopulations continue to synthesize and accumulate the neuropeptides VIP, substance-P and enkephalin, again mirroring observations made in situ (27, 36). Even some of the smallest neuronal subgroups found in the guinea pig myenteric plexus in situ, such as VIP immunoreactive neurons in the small intestine (9), catecholamine fluorescent neurons in the proximal colon (12) and neurons possessing high affinity uptake sites for $^3$H-GABA (23) in the taemia coli, are represented in cultured plexuses from these gut areas.

While no evidence has so far been found for qualitative changes in transmitter metabolism during maintenance in culture for periods of up to 2 weeks, the question of transmitter shift (6, 33) in these cultures has only been addressed to a limited extent. It has, however, been found, that when neurons are maintained in explants, rather than as dissociated cells, the resistance to such changes increases with increased developmental maturity of the ganglia, when taken into culture. Thus the labile period does not seem to exceed the 3rd postnatal week in explants of rat sympathetic ganglia (28). This observation tends to argue against transmitter shift occurring in enteric neurones obtained from newborn guinea pigs, since they, unlike the rat, are born at a very advanced stage of development.

Immunohistochemical studies using monoclonal antibodies have shown that the neuronal surface antigens 38/D7 and TR-2, found on enteric neurons in situ, are also synthesized and expressed in the cell membrane of these cells in culture (22). Similarly the glial surface antigen RAN-1 and the intracellular glial proteins glial fibrillary acidic protein (GFAP) and glutamine synthetase, are all demonstrable with immunohistochemical methods in enteric glial cells in culture as well as in situ (21, 22). In preliminary electrophysiological studies, using intracellular recordings, neurons have been found with AH-, or Type I-like and S-, or Type II-like characteristics as found in situ. Some spontaneously active neurons have been detected and there is evidence for the existence of polysynaptic pathways in mature cultures (16, 20).

All of these observations show a considerable similarity of individual neurons and glial cells in culture, to that found in these cells in situ. Electron microscopical studies on the aggregate formation, which takes place during the 2nd to 5th week in culture, indicate further, that cellular and tissue relationships develop in these cultures, that at least in histology and ultrastructure, closely resemble the organization of the enteric nervous system in situ.

c) *Studies combining the use of cultured plexuses with in situ experiments*

Cultures of the guinea pig myenteric and submucous plexuses have already proved of considerable use in complementing and extending in situ investigations of the enteric nervous system. The greatly improved visual resolution achieved in culture, was invaluable for the unambiguous identification of the enteric glial cells, rather than other tissue elements, as the sites of GFAP and glutamine synthetase immunoreactivity, in stud-

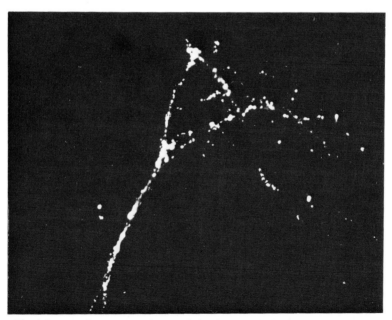

Fig. 4. Immunofluorescence micrograph showing enkephalin-like immuno-reactivity in a thick fiber bundle, which can be seen branching into smaller bundles or single fibers. Myenteric plexus from the guinea pig taenia coli, 10 days in culture; ×457. (From 27 with permission.)

ies which provided the first evidence of a biochemical similarity between enteric glial cells and the astrocytic glial cells of the central nervous system (21, 22). The easy visualization of individual neurons, glial and connective tissue cells in the cultures, was also essential for clearly establishing the cellular distribution of autoradiographically demonstrable high affinity uptake sites for $^3$H-GABA in enteric nervous tissue, discussed in more detail in Section II (23).

In a study of the sources of the various peptide containing nerve fibers, found in the guinea pig gastrointestinal tract, cultures of the myenteric and submucous plexuses from various gut areas where employed (27). Immunostaining of nerve fibers in the cultures, with antisera to VIP, substance-P and enkephalin (Fig. 4), revealed the type of peptide fiber originating in each of the plexuses, since all the nerve fibers present in such cultures emanate from neurons intrinsic to the explanted plexus itself. In combination with in situ studies on normally innervated and extrinsically denervated caecum, these experiments also provided evidence for a substance-P containing pathway running from the myenteric to the submucous plexus, and for a VIP containing pathway, running from the submucous to the myenteric plexus (24).

In addition, the cultured plexuses are in some instances the only preparation in which the molecular nature of cell surfaces of enteric neurons and glia can be investigated, as discussed in Section III.

d) *New directions in research on the enteric nervous system by use of the cultured plexuses*

In addition to expanding and complementing in situ studies of the type described above, the culture preparations make it possible to ask new types of question about the enteric nervous system, which would be difficult to approach without an in vitro model. I will mention here some examples of such studies, although experimental work along these lines is still only in preliminary stages.

The cultures provide an ideal system for quantitative assays, in the search for specific growth factors required by enteric neurons and glial cells

in vivo. The importance of such molecules for normal development and maintenance of neurons is most clearly illustrated in the extensive work on nerve growth factor (NGF), which supports the survival of sympathetic and sensory neurons (for recent review see 38). Further indication of the complexity and significance of neuronal growth factors comes from more recent experiments in tissue culture, on developmentally regulated growth factor requirements of neurons from dorsal root sensory ganglia, and from studies on two different components influencing respectively the choline acetyltransferase activity and growth rate of parasympathetic neurons in culture (2, 31). By analogy with work carried out on these systems, neuronal survival, axon elongation and biochemical measurements of enzyme or transmitter levels in the enteric cultures, can all be used to analyse the effects of soluble factors, secreted by enteric glial cells and connective tissue, gut smooth muscle cells and other sources. It seems likely, that a search for growth and trophic factors for enteric neurons will be fruitful, the enteric nervous system being the only major division of the peripheral nervous system where evidence regarding such substances has not yet been sought.

The problem of how the cells of the nervous system interact, forming specific and area dependent histological patterns, has been the subject of extensive experimentation in the central nervous system (15, 30, 37). Histogenetic processes in the peripheral nervous system, which have been much less studied, deal almost exclusively with the histogenesis of the peripheral nerve (e.g. 5, 7). The histological organization of the enteric nervous system is of particular interest for several reasons (13). It is distinctly different from that of all other peripheral nervous tissue, and shows clear similarities with central nervous tissue in its compactness, existence of large areas of synaptic neuropil and the exclusion of connective tissue. The overall organization is complex, since it consists of an extensive network of ganglia and nerves, i.e. the interconnecting strands, both the size and shape of the ganglia, and the length and orientation of the interconnecting strands varying in a specific manner between the different areas of the gut. Further, this structure is subject to an unusual mechanical stress, being situated between the two main muscle layers of the gut wall. The culture preparations of the myenteric plexus from the guinea pig taenia coli, should provide an excellent model for studies on the cell and tissue interactions involved in both histogenesis and maintenance, in enteric nervous tissue. As described in Section IA above, these cultures provide the opportunity to study a complex process of cell migration and recognition, leading to the formation of a cellular arrangement, which is histotypic to enteric nervous tissue, both in the relationship of the nervous tissue cells i.e. neurons and glia, to each other, and in their relationship to connective tissue. Furthermore, the reverse process can also be studied, i.e. the disintegration and subsequent merging of the compact ganglia into a rather loose monolayer of neurons and glia, which takes place during the first few days in culture. Both of these processes can be interfered with experimentally. Monoclonal antibodies, raised against extracellular antigens of enteric neural and connective tissue cells, can be used to analyse their cell surface chemistry and to block specific cell-cell interactions, based on the action of surface molecules. Alternatively, certain tissue components can be added to, or subtracted from the cultures. In this regard the role of the enteric connective tissue is of special interest. There is evidence that connective tissue elements are necessary to trigger normal interactions between Schwann cells and autonomic axons (5) and observations on the development of the myenteric plexus in culture suggest the possibility of a similar role for enteric connective tissue (26).

## 2) AUTORADIOGRAPHIC AND BIO-CHEMICAL STUDIES ON GABA AS AN ENTERIC NEUROTRANSMITTER

The ability to dissect the ganglionated plexuses from the gut wall, offers the simple advantage that biochemical measurements can be carried out without contamination by other tissues. Below I will illustrate this, in the context of studies carried out on putative GABAergic neurons in the myenteric plexus (18, 23).

GABA is a major neurotransmitter in the vertebrate brain and spinal cord. Although it is also employed by nerves in the invertebrate periphery, there has until recently been no evidence for the presence of GABAergic neurons in the vertebrate peripheral nervous system, and it has become accepted that in vertebrates, they are restricted to the central nervous system only (17, 32, 35). Through the vast amount of work devoted to GABA as a neurotransmitter during the last 20 years or so, it has emerged that GABAergic neurones possess two properties, which unambiguously distinguish them from all other neurons, although both may be present in lower quantities in some non-neuronal cells. These characteristics are the presence of the enzyme that synthesizes GABA from glutamic acid, glutamic acid decarboxylase (GAD), and the presence in the neuronal cell membrane of high affinity uptake sites for GABA (17, 32, 35). Autoradiography is a convenient way of revealing high affinity uptake sites. The cells that possess these sites rapidly accumulate radioactive GABA, when incubated in very low concentration for short periods of time, and as a result become selectively labelled with autoradiographic grains. This method is now widely used for the unequivocal identification of GABAergic neurons, either following in vivo injection of $^3$H-GABA or by incubation of tissue sections, cell suspensions or neurons maintained in tissue culture in $^3$H-GABA (17, 32, 35).

In autoradiographic studies of $^3$H-GABA uptake in cultures of the myenteric plexus from the guinea pig taenia coli, it was found that some neurones in the cultures became selectively and heavily labelled with autoradiographic grains, following incubations in $2 \times 10^{-8}$M $^3$H-GABA for 20 min at 20°C (Fig. 5) (23). This uptake was unaffected by β-alanine which preferentially blocks glial GABA uptake sites, while it was abolished by cis-1,3 aminocyclohexane carboxylic acid (ACHC), an inhibitor of neuronal GABA uptake. Electron microscopic autoradiography of $^3$H-GABA uptake in the myenteric plexus in situ, confirmed the existence of high affinity GABA uptake sites in a small population of myenteric neurons.

In the light of all available knowledge con-

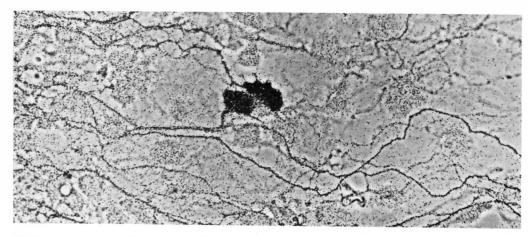

Fig. 5. Autoradiograph of the myenteric plexus from the guinea pig taenia coli, maintained in culture for 10 days before incubation with ³H-GABA. Two heavily labelled neurons and their processes can be seen. Note other labelled processes as well as light labelling concentrated over the nuclear areas of glial cells, which form a continuous sheet underneath the neurons. ×626. (From 23 with permission.)

cerning the distribution of high affinity GABA uptake sites on neurons, both in vertebrates and invertebrates, these observations already constituted very strong evidence for the presence of GABAergic neurons in the myenteric ganglia. This idea was pursued, both by showing that the taenia coli, containing the myenteric plexus, contains 3–4 times more endogenous GABA that a control tissue, and also by using the myenteric plexus, freshly dissected from the gut wall, for two types of experiment (18, 23). Firstly, the presence of GAD activity was demonstrated in homogenates of the dissected plexus. Secondly, the ability of the enteric neurons to synthesize and accumulate ³H-GABA was tested by incubating the plexus, without homogenizing, in ³H-glutamic acid, the immediate precursor to GABA in neuronal GABA synthesis. It was found that the plexus accumulated about 3.3 times more newly synthesized ³H-GABA than did sympathetic ganglia, where there is no evidnece for GABAergic neurons and where GABA synthesis presumably takes place in glial cells only (17). Slices of cerebellum, a tissue rich in GABAergic neurons (35), accumulated about 2 times more newly formed ³H-GABA than did the myenteric plexus. Unexpectedly, the myenteric plexus also syn-

thesized and accumulated considerable amounts of ³H-homocarnosine in this assay. Homocarnosine is a dipeptide, made from GABA and histidine (for refs see 23). Its presence or synthesis in the peripheral nervous system has not been reported before, while homocarnosine is found in the brain, with a heterogenous distribution which does not parallel that of GABA. Homocarnosine possesses some potent central actions and it has been suggested that it may be a central neurotransmitter. The results obtained in these studies indicate that the formation of homocarnosine is not a feature of glial GABA synthesis, since it was not made by the glial cells of the sympathetic ganglia. Further, its accumulation is not a general corollary of GABA synthesis by GABAergic neurons in this type of assay, since it was not found in the GABA neurons of the cerebellum slices.

In summary, these biochemical studies lend support to the strong autoradiographic evidence for the presence of a population of GABAergic neurons in the myenteric plexus. In addition, they have revealed that homocarnosine, a putative neurotransmitter in the brain, can also be synthesised and accumulated by enteric nervous tissue.

## 3) IMMUNOHISTOCHEMICAL STUDIES OF CELL SURFACE MOLECULES

### a) *General considerations*

Cell surface molecules have long been thought to perform a major role in the specific intercellular communication, involved in processes such as development, histogenesis and the establishment of appropriate synaptic connections. Recently, great advances have been made in the study of cell surface molecules in the nervous system, by the introduction of antibodies for analysing the cell surface chemistry of neurons and glia (4). The value and promise of this line of research has been greatly enhanced by the advent of techniques for producing monoclonal antibodies, allowing antibodies to particular cell types or subpopulations thereof, to be selected at will, form immunizations with heterogenous cell populations, carrying a multitude of different antigens (29, 40). This approach is of great potential value for studies involving cell identification and cell type purification in culture, and for investigations of intercellular communication by blockade of specific surface molecules. This type of experiment is also providing fresh insights into the heterogeneity of neurons and glial cells, revealing new subclasses of both cell types, the significance of which is at present not understood.

### b) *Methodological advantages in using the enteric plexuses for studies of cell surface antigens in the vertebrate nervous system*

The localization of cell surface antigen in tissue sections has proved difficult for technical reasons, although in some instances, presumably where the antigen is present in very high concentrations, this has been successfully accomplished (e.g. 10). It has been found that studies of this type are more easily carried out on intact cells, maintained in tissue culture, where large areas of the cell surface are exposed and accessible to antibodies (34, 39). It is, however, clear that the use of cultured cells has several drawbacks in this context. These are especially obvious when attempts are made to reveal the significance of novel neuronal subgroups, defined by the sharing of common surface antigens. In culture, all information

about such subgroups which might derive from the distribution of the cells within the nervous system in question and from their position relative to other identified cells or subgroups is lost. The normal synaptic connections of the cells are ruptured, thereby limiting the information obtainable by the use of electrophysiological methods, in conjunction with immunostaining. Further, the expression of both surface antigens and intracellular molecules, such as peptides, transmitters or transmitter related enzymes can change during maintenance in culture. Thus separate experiments may be needed to ascertain that a relationship between extra- and intracellular features found in culture, also was valid in situ.

Preliminary experiments using the monoclonal antibodies TR-2, A2B5 and A-4 indicate, that the freshly dissected myenteric plexus provides a very attractive preparation for the study of neuronal surface antigens in the vertebrate nervous system. While overcoming the objections raised against the use of cultures and discussed above, these preparations possess the essential advantage of cultured cells, because the neurons and glia are arranged in a semi-monolayer, with extensive surface areas exposed to the surrounding solution. The dissection procedure appears to play an essential part in loosening the normally compact tissue organization and providing access for antibodies, since immunostaining of surface antigens in stretch or whole-mount preparations of the myenteric plexus has so far yielded much poorer results. For technical reasons, therefore, the dissected plexuses appear to possess important advantages, when compared to all other parts of the vertebrate nervous system, for the immunohistochemical localization of cell surface molecules. The availability of the cultured plexuses provide additional versatility, since the cultures sometimes allow a more satisfactory visualization of antigens, already detected in the freshly dissected preparation; this appears to apply especially to glial surface antigens. Comparative studies on antigen expression in situ, i.e. in the freshly dissected plexuses, to that of the same cells maintained in culture, also offers the possibility of analysing the factors that control the expression of particular surface antigens.

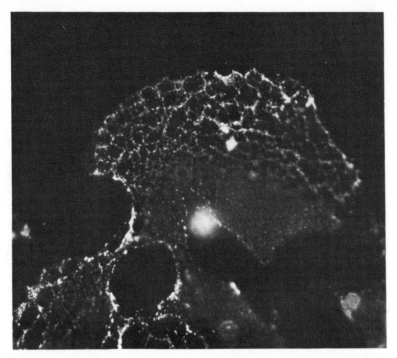

Fig. 6. Immunofluorescence micrograph showing the surface antigen RAN-1 on an enteric glial cell maintained in culture. One flat cell and parts of two others, can be seen, all exhibiting typical speckled surface fluorescence. Myenteric plexus from the rat colon, 7 days in culture; ×842.

In addition to these methodological considerations, the enteric nervous system may be a particularly rewarding model for studies on the significance of neuronal cell surface heterogeneity. It is composed of a large number of neuronal subpopulations, defined by differences in gross morphology, ultrastructure, transmitter and peptide content, electro-physiological properties and the type of function carried out. By combining the appropriate methods for detecting these subdivisions, with immunolabelling of surface molecules, this system should allow detailed studies to be made on relationships between defined neuronal surface antigens and a variety of other extra and intracellular neuronal features.

c) *Surface characteristics of glial cells and neurons in the rat myenteric plexus*

The glial cells of the enteric nervous system show similarities with the astrocytic glial cells of the central nervous system in a number of gross- and fine-structural features, as well as in their structural relationship with neuronal cell bodies and processes (13). We investigated whether these morphological and histological similarities between the two types of glial cells were reflected in their cell surface chemistry, by studying two surface antigens, RAN-1 and RAN-2 (22). RAN-1 is present on peripheral glial cells such as satellite cells and Schwann cells, but not on astrocytes, while RAN-2 is found on astrocytes but is not expressed by satellite or Schwann cells (3, 11). It was found, that the enteric glial cells were similar to other peripheral glial cells, but dissimilar to astrocytes, in that they expressed RAN-1, while RAN-2 was only detectable in very low quantities (Fig. 6). In an extension of this study to intracellular glial proteins we found on the other hand, that enteric glial cells and astrocytes share at least two intracellular proteins, neither of which are found in satellite cells nor in most Schwann cells. These are the intermediate filament constituent glial fibrillary acidic protein (GFAP), and the enzyme glutamine synthetase, until recently thought to be specifically present in astrocytes only (21, 22).

In an analogous comparison of the cell surface of enteric neurons to that of other peripheral neurons on the one hand, and central neurons on the other, it was found that the enteric neurons resembled other peripheral neurons, in that they expressed the antigen 38/D7, which is absent from all central neurons. Studies on enteric neurons in culture showed further, that the surface antigen A4, present on all central neurons, but absent from peripheral sympathetic and sensory neurons, is also absent from cultured enteric neurons (8). We are currently investigating the interesting possibility, that in spite of its absence on cultured cells A4 may in situ be expressed by a subpopulation of enteric neurons. An additional similarity between the cell membrane of enteric and other peripheral neurons, is the presence of the antigen TR-2 on a subdivision of both enteric neurons and neurons from other peripheral ganglia, while this antigen has so far not been found on any central neurons (22). A further example of surface heterogeneity among enteric neurons, is provided by the distribution of the neuronal antigen A2B5 (10). Preliminary studies indicate that this antigen is present in high levels on some enteric neurons, while being absent from others.

Taken together, these studies show that so far, the cells of the enteric nervous system share extracellular cell surface characteristics with cells from other divisions of the peripheral nervous system, rather than with cells from the central nervous system. While this is of interest in light of the common histological arrangement and neuroglia interrelationship in the enteric and central nervous systems, these similarities may be related to common embryological origin of enteric and other peripheral neurons and glia. On the other hand, two intracellular proteins, GFAP and glutamine synthetase, normally associated with astrocytic glial cells in the central nervous system, are also made by the enteric glial cells in the peripheral nervous system, perhaps reflecting the functional similarities of these cells to astrocytes.

## ACKNOWLEDGEMENT

The author is the recipient of a Senior Research Fellowship from the Mental Health Foundation.

## REFERENCES

1. Baluk P, Jessen KR, Saffrey MJ, Burnstock G, 1981. In preparation
2. Barde YA, Edgar D, Thoenen H. Proc Nat Acad Sci 1980, 77, 1199–1203
3. Bartlett PF, Noble MD, Pruss RM, Raff MC, Rattrey S, Williams CA. Brain Res 1981 204, 339–352.
4. J. Brockes (ed) 1981. In Immunological Markers for Neural Cells. Plenum Press, New York. In press
5. Bunge RP, Bunge MB. J Cell Biol 1978, 78, 943–950
6. Bunge R, Johnston M, Ross CD. Sci 1978 199, 1409–1416
7. Bunge MB, Williams AK, Wood PM, Uitto J, Jeffrey JJ. J Cell Biol 1980 84, 184–202.
8. Cohen J, Selvendran Y. Nature 1981 291, 421–423
9. Costa M, Furness JB, Butta R, Said SI. Neurosci 1980 5, 587–596.
10. Eisenbarth GS, Walsh FS, Nirenberg M. Proc Natl Acad Sci USA 1979 76, 4913–4917
11. Fields KL, Gosling C, Megson M, Stern PL. Proc Nat Acad Sci USA 1975 72, 1286–1300
12. Furness JB, Costa M. Physiol Rev 1974 69, 1–52
13. Gabella G. Intern Rev Cytol 1979 59, 129–193
14. Gabella G. Neurosci 1981 6, 425–436
15. Garber BB 1977. In Cell Tissue and Organ Cultures in Neurobiology, pp 516–537 (eds S Fedoroff and L Hertz). Academic Press
16. Hanani M, Baluk P, Burnstock G. J Auton Nerv Syst 1981. In press
17. Iversen LL, Kelly JS. Biochem Pharmacol 1975 24, 933–938
18. Jessen KR. Molecular and Cellular Biochem 1981 38, 69–76
19. Jessen KR, Burnstock G. 1981. Trends in Autonom Pharmacol. In press
20. Jessen KR, McConnel JD, Purves, RD, Burnstock G, Chamley-Campbell J. Brain Res 1978 152, 573–579
21. Jessen KR, Mirsky R. Nature Lond 1980 286, 736–737
22. Jessen KR, Mrisky R. Neurosci Letters 1981
23. Jessen KR, Mirsky R, Dennison ME, Burnstock G. Nature Lond 1979 281, 71–74
24. Jessen KR, Polak JM, Van Noorden S, Bloom SR, Burnstock G. Nature 1980 283, 391–393
25. Jessen KR, Saffrey MJ, Baluk P, Burnstock G. 1981. In preparation
26. Jessen KR, Saffrey MJ, Burnstock G. 1981. In preparation
27. Jessen KR, Saffrey MJ, Van Noorden S, Bloom SR, Polak JM, Burnstock G. Neurosci 1980 5, 1717–1735
28. Johnston MF, Ross CD, Bunge RP. J Cell Biol 1980 84, 692–704
29. Kohler G, Milstein C. Nature 1975 256, 495–497

30. Moscona AA. Exp Cell Res 1961 22, 455–475
31. Nishi R, Berg DK. J Neurosci 1981 1, 505–513
32. Nistri A, Constanti A. Prog Neurobiol 1979 13, 117–235
33. Patterson PH. Ann Rev Neurosci 1978 1, 1–17
34. Raff MC, Fields KL, Hakomori S, Mirsky R, Pruss RM, Winter J. Brain Res 1979 174, 283–308
35. Roberts E, Chase TN, Tower DB. (eds) 1976, GABA in Nervous System Function. Raven Press, New York
36. Schultzberg M, Hökfelt T, Nilson G, Terenius L, Rehfeld, JF, Brown M, Elde R, Goldstein M, Said S. Neurosci 1980 5, 689–744.
37. Seeds NW, Haffke SC, Krystosek A. 1980. In Tissue Culture in Neurobiology (eds E Giacobini, A Vernadakis, A. Shahar), pp 145–154. Raven Press, New York
38. Thoenen H, Barde YA. Physiol Rev 1980 60, 1284–1312
39. Vulliamy T, Rattray S, Mirsky R. Nature 1981 291, 418–420
40. Zipser B, McKay R. Nature 1981 289, 549–554.

# The Neuropathology of Pseudo-obstruction of the Intestine

B. SMITH
St. Bartholomew's Hospital, London EC1, UK

Destruction of the myenteric plexus impairs ongoing peristalsis and produces dilatation of the gut lumen with thickening of the gut wall.

Achalasia of the cardia, hypertrophic pyloric stenosis and non-Hirschsprung megacolon are well-known examples of damage to the bowel nerve supply.

There are many causes, some of which are unknown, but the common ones can be divided into three groups.

Congenital developmental failure may be total and incompatible with life, or less severe, in which case resection may be possible. Acquired inflammatory damage, other than Chagas' disease, can occur anywhere in the gut. Autonomic neuropathy may involve either the neurons or the Schwann cells. The former is often due to drugs because the autonomic ganglia are outside the blood-brain barrier. The latter is frequently associated with metabolic disease, such as diabetes mellitus.

*B Smith, St. Bartholomew's Hospital, London EC1, UK*

The clinical syndrome of intestinal obstruction without any organic impediment to the passage of food, has come to be known as intestinal pseudo-obstruction. If the colon only is involved it may present as non-Hirschsprung megacolon. It is due to the loss of neurological control of normal on-going peristalsis.

The smooth muscle of the bowel wall has an intrinsic rhythmicity, and will contract in the absence of a nerve supply. This segmentation is only partly organised and although some progress of the bolus may occur, in time the abdomen gets more and more distended, and the patient more and more constipated. Pain is, as a rule, not a feature. An important finding at laparotomy is considerable thickening of the bowel wall as a result of smooth muscle hypertrophy and possibly hyperplasia. It is a true enteromegaly in contrast to other conditions in which the bowel is dilated but the wall is thin. This thickening is much greater than that seen proximal to an organic destruction and can readily be recognised by an experienced surgeon at laparotomy. It may have two causes. One is that, as the bolus does not move adequately, the bowel becomes over-stretched; stretch of smooth muscle is a stimulus to hypertrophy. The other is that, in contrast to skeletal muscle, the overall effect of the innervation is to suppress contraction as has been shown physiologically in the guinea-pig by Wood (5). Denervated smooth muscle overworks.

The effect of the nervous control of the bowel muscle is to organise peristalsis and to some extent to control its rate. The intrinsic innervation of the alimentary canal, which controls movement, consists of the myenteric plexus. The submucous plexus has a different function. The myenteric plexus contains ganglia connected to one another by nerve trunks lying between the muscle coats. These ganglia have two types of neurons, distinguished by their affinity for silver. The argyrophil cells stain darkly and have a number of well-stained processes. Many autonomic nerve cells are multi-axonal in contrast to those of the central nervous system which have only one axon (Fig. 1). Bipolar and monopolar forms are also seen but whether the different morphology denotes a different function is not known. The processes of these cells, together with some extrinsic axons, form the nerve trunks of the plexus. They terminate on other nerve cells, both argyrophil and argyrophobe, sometimes branching many times so that one nerve cell communicates with many others. They do not appear to supply any branches to the muscle fibres. The argyrophobe cells may stain a very light brown with silver and sometimes cannot be seen at all in the normal. No processes can be seen on silver staining but using other methods, such as cholinesterase, some can be seen supplying the muscle fibres of the bowel wall. It is probable that many fibres cannot be seen at the light microscopical level, and the tracing of fibres for long distances at the ultrastructural level is difficult.

The nerve trunks of the plexus are made up of the axons of the intrinsic argyrophil cells together with extrinsic nerve fibres. Sympathetic fibres enter the plexus along the blood vessels, and sympathetic endings can be demonstrated around the neurons. These are visible with catecholamine fluorescence and under the electron microscope. However no noradrenergic nerve cells have every been seen in the plexus. Parasympathetic fibres derived from the vagus or the sacral outflow also enter the plexus and end on intrinsic nerve cells. It is probable that all these endings are on argyrophil cells in man but it is very difficult to be certain.

In man the vagus below the diaphragm is a small nerve, and most of it is unmyelinated. It would seem impossible for it to control directly the whole length of the alimentary canal as well as the rest of the abdominal viscera. It probably ends on a number of nerve cells, called "mother" cells by Bayliss and Starling (1) and these may pass the message on via other argyrophil cells to the argyrophobe cells and thus to the muscle. The vagus thus exerts some over-riding control over the speed of peristalsis. This peristalsis is the result of selective inhibition of segmentation in front of the bolus by the argyrophil cells so that it tends to progress in an anal direction.

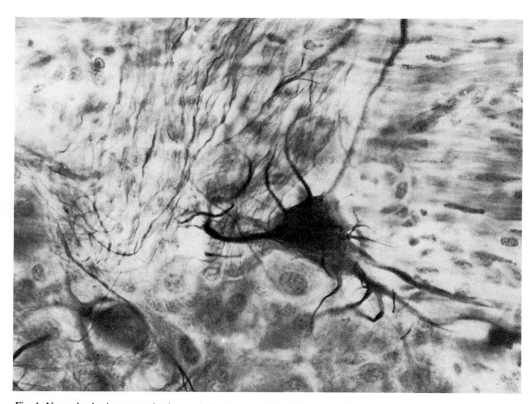

Fig. 1. Normal colonic myenteric plexus. A single argyrophil cell is shown with a number of well-stained processes. Also in the ganglion rather shadowy non-argyrophil neurons can be seen with very pale cytoplasm and no stainable processes. (× 750)

The impairment of normal peristalsis may be due to the absence or destruction of all myenteric neurones, or it may be due to selective damage to the argyrophil cells leaving the rest intact. In this case paraffin sections will appear normal. The effect of vagotomy in man is slight except at the pylorus. It is noteworthy that some parts of the intestine are much more affected by denervation than others. In these parts the proportion of nerve cells which are argyrophil is much higher and the innervation is more important. These areas are the cardia, the pylorus and the colon. Patients with Chagas' disease often have myenteric destruction affecting the entire bowel but they usually complain of dysphagia and constipation. It is also true, as in other autonomic diseases that the damage to the argyrophil cells has to be virtually total before significant symptoms arise, partial damage having little effect. This may perhaps be qualified in the case of the elderly, when their constipation may be a combination of some atrophy of the muscle together with some fall-out of nerve cells, both the result of wear and tear. Another feature of note is the ability of the autonomic nervous system to repair itself, or find a way round an obstruction. The temporary effect of surgical sympathectomy exemplifies this well. Following an intestinal resection the plexus is completely divided. This has no clinical effect, and the portion of gut has actually to be reversed before there is any hold-up in peristalsis.

If pseudo-obstruction occurs in the colon the clinical effect is constipation. If it occurs in the small intestine the main clinical effect may be a blind loop syndrome because of bacterial infestation of the stagnant bowel contents. In the pylorus, hypertrophic pyloric stenosis and at the cardia, dysphagia are obvious results.

In order to demonstrate lesions histologically, it is necessary to see as much plexus as possible.

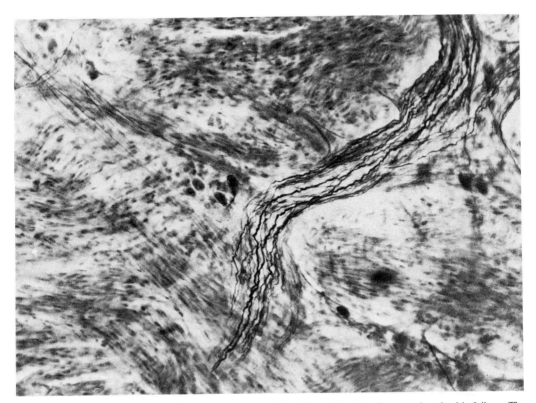

Fig. 2. Myenteric plexus from the small intestine of a child of 7 months dying from total peristaltic failure. The extrinsic trunks are normal and well formed but do not appear to communicate at all with the ganglia which contains neurons without processes. (× 375)

Frozen sections measuring 50 μm in thickness are cut parallel to it. Sections cut transverse to the bowel, even if frozen are not very helpful, and paraffin sections are usually non-contributory. Full thickness rectal biopsy does not contain enough plexus for diagnosis except in Hirschsprung's disease. Damage to the myenteric plexus may be due to many causes, some of which are unknown. Frequently seen nowadays is the effect of drugs with an anti-cholinergic component such as tranquillizers and anti-depressants. There is a condition known as mental hospital megacolon, which seems to be due to large doses of phenothiazines being given for long periods. After some time the condition becomes irreversible, as is tardive dyskinesia, from the same cause. It is not always realised that if the constipation is due to the effect of drugs on nerve cells, purgatives which act on nerve cells will be ineffective. If the argyrophil cells are not functioning attempts to drive either nerve cells or the muscle directly will only increase segmentation and not aid on-going peristalsis.

Known organic causes of myenteric plexus damage can be divided into three types, congenital, inflammatory and those associated with an autonomic neuropathy.

Congenital failure of myenteric plexus development may be total. In these cases oral feeding can never be established and life expectancy is limited. In many cases survival is very short and the diagnosis missed. There are different types of this failure. The commonest is associated with a short mal-rotated intestine and pyloric stenosis (4). Histologically there are no argyrophil cells and the ganglia contain pale-staining neurons without any processes. The extrinsic trunks can be seen, but there are no endings in the ganglia, presumably because there are no dendrites available (Fig. 2). This particular condition has been shown to be familial (2). There are other similar conditions in which ganglia contain far too many nuclei, probably neuronal. In all mammals at birth there is normal deletion of nerve cells in the brain and probably elsewhere too, as nature provides more than are necessary. In this particular condition this deletion does not occur in the plexus and the findings may be useful in a small

biopsy in which only one or two ganglia are present. There is another rare condition in which the ganglia themselves seem to be absent and presumably migration of neuroblasts from the cord has not occurred.

Another variety of developmental failure occurs which is not so devastating. The children are constipated from birth but the condition usually gets worse as they get older. They seem to come to resection in their late teens or early twenties. Pathologically there is usually some thickening of the bowel wall and dilation of the lumen but this is not very severe. Histologically, a few relatively normal argyrophil cells are seen, but some are obviously distorted and numbers are grossly reduced. Most of the cells within the ganglia have distended pale brown cytoplasm and a slightly eccentric nucleus. This nucleus contains no nucleolus but otherwise may be similar to, although rather darker than, a normal neuronal nucleus. Other examples may show a rather spindle-shaped or rectangular nucleus giving the cell a very similar appearance to that of the Opalski cell in the brain (Fig. 3). This latter is thought to be a degenerative form and it is possible that the condition is not a congenital deficiency but a gradual fall-out of cells, which for some reason or other, cannot maintain a normal existence. It is thus a type of autonomic motor neurone disease. In most patients with this condition the pathology appears to be confined to the colon and they do well following resection and ileo-rectal anastomosis. More long term clinical follow-up is needed to confirm this. Lesser operations such as sigmoid resection or anal sphincter procedures do not seem to be adequate and a further surgery later seems to be the rule.

Inflammatory damage to the myenteric plexus is well exemplified by Chagas' disease. This is due to infection by *Trypanosoma cruzi* which has a specific affinity for the heart and the myenteric plexus. There are 7,000,000 cases of Chagas' disease in South America, many of whom need surgery. Comparatively few of them get it, and there is a vast pool of misery and ill-health as a result of this disease.

There is a condition in Western Europe and North America which also appears to have an

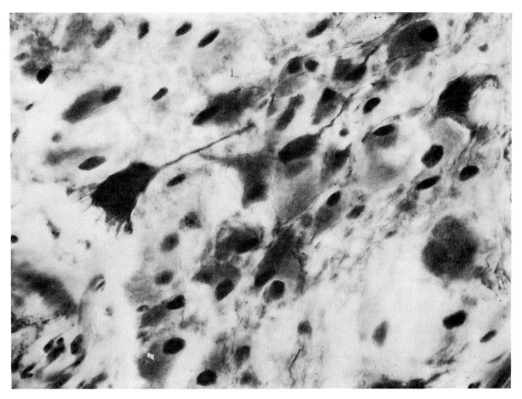

Fig. 3. A myenteric ganglion from a patient with congenital disease of the plexus. The nerve cells have abnormal spindle shaped nuclei and distended pale cytoplasm. One argyrophil cell is seen with an abnormal configuration. (× 750)

inflammatory lesion of the plexus, usually in the colon, although achalasia of the cardia is probably a similar condition. There is also a type of adult hypertrophic pyloric stenosis of the same nature.

Pathologically the wall of the colon is thick and the lumen large, the haustrae having almost disappeared. Histologically, there may be a trace of an inflammatory reaction but it has usually gone by the time surgery is performed and one is just looking at a scar. This is also frequently true to Chagas' disease and achalasia of the cardia. Normal argyrophil cells are absent, the few remaining are grossly distorted with swollen clubbed processes. Many intrinsic axons are also lost, and as a result there is marked hyperplasia of the Schwann cells. This is similar to the bands of Büngner seen in skeletal muscle after axons have been lost. Provided the affected bowel can be resected the prognosis is good. Very rarely it affects so much small intestine that resection is impractical and little can be done.

Autonomic neuropathy can be due to disease of the autonomic neuron or disease of the Schwann cell which supports the axon. The autonomic nerve cells, like those of the posterior root ganglia are outside the blood-brain barrier. They are not protected from neurotoxins in the circulation. These include particularly, drugs used in cancer chemotherapy, such as Daunorubicin and Vincristine.

Degenerative changes in autonomic neurons have come to be called the Shy-Drager syndrome. It is probable that it affects most nerve cells in peripheral ganglia, both sympathetic and parasympathetic, but the clinical effects of sympathetic loss, mainly postural hypotension, predominate. Constipation does occur and the occasional case actually presents with megacolon. Histolog-

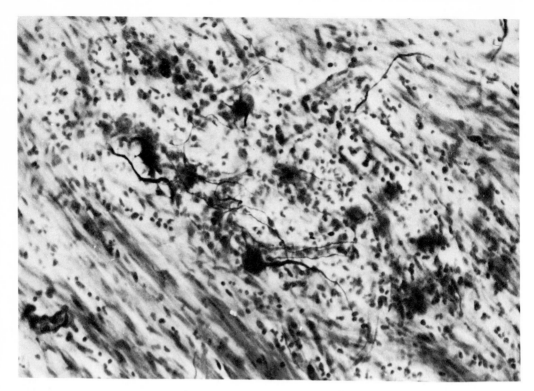

Fig. 4. A myenteric ganglion from a patient dying from carcinoma of bronchus. The ganglion is invaded by lymphocytes and there is severe neuronal damage. (× 375)

ically the nerve cells show a vacuolar change similar to that described in nerve cells in the sympathetic chain by Shy and Drager (3).

Pathology of the Schwann cells is common in many metabolic conditions such as diabetes mellitus or myxoedema, and is found in some types of collagen disease. It may also be a toxic or immunological manifestation. In the somatic sensory nervous system where it presents as a peripheral neuropathy the pathology consists of segmental demyelination as the segment of myelin between two nodes of Ranvier related to one Schwann cell is lost: the myenteric plexus and most of the extrinsic fibres are unmyelinated. The pathology consists of swellings and apparent discontinuities of the axons again related to a single Schwann cell. It is probable that, like segmental demyelination, this condition is reversible. If the myenteric plexus is examined in severe diabetes mellitus neurological pathology is nearly always

found although clinical symptoms such as dysphagia are very rare. Constipation often occurs but is ignored. The changes are most obvious in the extrinsic nerves particularly the vagus. Diabetic diarrhoea is probably due to this vagal lesion and is thus the same as post-vagotomy diarrhoea. In the ganglia the nerve cells themselves may be unremarkable but there are obvious irregularities and boutons terminaux of the endings on those nerve cells.

A rare but interesting cause of myenteric damage is as part of the neuropathy associated with malignant disease. The pathology of the myenteric ganglia is the same as that of the posterior root ganglia. It consists of infiltration with inflammatory cells, mainly lymphocytes, and destruction of the nerve cells (Fig. 4). Thus yet another clinical presentation of carcinoma of the bronchus may be megacolon.

In the upper alimentary tract the clinical and

radiological diagnosis of pseudo-obstruction is straight forward. Differentiating functional and organic constipation may be difficult. Many drugs are constipants and purgative addicts are still occasionally seen. The fact that organic disease responds poorly to anthraquinone purgatives may be useful, although this may have to be done under hospital supervision. Certainly, in the older age groups, the sort of pathology described here is rare except for obvious metabolic conditions.

Surgeons are often very reluctant to embark on a procedure which is not without risk, on patients with constipation. However, many patients who have had ileo-rectal anastomosis do very well, provided the disease is confined to the colon. It is perhaps unfair to condemn young patients to a life of enemas, and given the choice, most would willingly accept the risk.

REFERENCES

1. Bayliss WM, Starling EH. J Physiol 1900, 26, 107–118
2. Royer P, Ricour C, Nihoul-Fekete C, Pellerin D. Arch Franc Pe'd 1974, 31, 223–229
3. Shy M, Drager GA. Arch Neurol 1960, 2, 511–516
4. Tanner MS, Smith B, Lloyd JK. Arch Dis Childn 1976, 51, 837–841
5. Wood JD. Phys Rev 1975, 55, 307–324

# Ultrastructural Changes in the Gut Autonomic Nervous System Following Laxative Abuse and in Other Conditions

J. F. RIEMANN & H. SCHMIDT

Dept of Internal Medicine, University of Erlangen-Nuernberg, Erlangen, FRG

Electronmicroscopical studies have been carried out on colonic biopsies from patients with long-term laxative abuse, amyloidosis, diabetic autonomic neuropathy or chronic inflammatory bowel disease. The results of these investigations indicate that submucosal nerve fibres are damaged to an extent dependent upon the intensity of the toxic agent. The main pathological features range from distension or ballooning of axons, reduction of nerve-specific cell structures and increase in lysosomes to a total degeneration of whole nerve fibres. While the degenerative process is uniform, differentiation between disease states can be made on the basis of specific additional lesions such as the presence of typical amyloid fibrils, diabetic microangiopathy or the inflammatory process in inflammatory bowel disease. No changes were found in Whipple's disease or gluten-sensitive enteropathy. It is concluded that the structural alterations may provide a morphological explanation for the disturbances in gut motility, as an intact intramural nervous system is a necessary prerequisite for the regular coordination of normal peristalsis.

*Dr. J. F. Riemann & Dr. H. Schmidt, Department of Internal Medicine, University of Erlangen-Nuernberg, Krankenhausstrasse 12, D-8520 Erlangen, FRG*

The existence in the intestinal tract of contraction mechanisms which are independent of the central nervous system, has been recognised for several decades. Bayliss & Starling (5) showed that the peristaltic contractions of the intestine are true coordinated reflexes, which are triggered by mechanical stimulation of the intestine and are transmitted via local neural mechanisms in the myenteric plexus. In the following years innumerable investigations have dealt with the morphology, physiology, biochemistry and pathology of the enteric nervous system, and these are discussed in detail in the accompanying chapters. The classification of the enteric nervous system as a third, independent branch of the autonomic nervous system dated back to Langley (38).

There appears to be only a minor degree of influence of the central nervous stystem on enteric neurons as there are considerably more neurons extending throughout the intestine than there are pre-ganglionic nerve fibres from the central nervous system (26). This phenomenon emphasises the physiological independence of the enteric nervous system. Intestinal motility is controlled by muscular, neural and neurohumoral mechanisms and the enteric nervous system serves as a coordinator within this complex (9).

Anatomically the intramural nervous system is composed of two connected nerve plexuses. The submucous plexus is directly connected to the myenteric plexus via innumerable fascicles, forming a uniform network (13, 56, 60). Each network of nerves is made up of bundles of axons with accumulations of ganglion cells at the nodes. Synaptic connections exist between these cells and the sympathetic and parasympathetic nervous systems, particularly the vagus nerves.

Apart from the local ganglia, additional elements include the axons with accompanying Schwann cells and the nerve terminals (28, 37). The neurosecretory vesicles are aggregated in the terminal area and these can be differentiated according to morphological, biochemical and fluorescence-optical criteria. The vesicles are usually classified as cholinergic, noradrenergic, serotonergic, purinergic or peptidergic (2, 10, 11, 32).

The non-differentiated release of neurotransmitters is demonstrated by the fact that the electrically coupled muscle cells are exclusively excited by the release of transmitters from the gap between the myenteric plexus and the muscle cell (4, 17, 27). Acetylcholine constitutes the transmitter of most of the pre-ganglionic and sacral nerve fibres which reach the gastrointestinal tract. These cholinergic pre-ganglionic fibres innervate excitatory as well as inhibitory enteric ganglion cells (50). Cholinergic neurons are essential for the propulsive molitity. They can be inhibited by either muscarinic or nicotinic blockers (24). The secretory vesicles found within cholinergic fibres are small spheres with a mean diameter of 50 nm.

In contrast with these cholinergic fibres, the adrenergic nerves are distinguished by populations of small granular vesicles. Stimulation of sympathetic nerves relaxes the intestine. There are anatomical suggestions for the existence of noradrenergic axo-axonic synapses in the myenteric plexus. Their distribution, particularly in the periphery, explains an axo-axonal interaction and most likely constitutes the morphological representation of the reciprocal adrenergic-cholinergic axo-axonal synapse of the gastrointestinal tract (70).

Other types of vesicles have been classified as being "p-type". These appear to be serotonergic, purinergic or peptidergic. The term p-type vesicles includes those which contain a number of different neuropeptides, which probably act as neurotransmitters (8, 10). These "p-type" vesicles are large and granular.

## Laxative abuse

During the past few years, the side effects of drugs and the consequences of drug abuse have increasingly attracted the attention of physicians (7, 15, 16). Within this field, the abuse of laxatives represents a frequently occurring phenomenon and problem (54).

Investigations of the gut intramural nerves, using the electron microscope, have yielded accurate information on their morphology and have helped in the interpretation of the pathogenesis of disorders of this system (37, 39, 62). Changes resulting from the abuse of laxatives were initially described on the basis of histological investigations (63–65), which are widely quoted in reviews on the side effects of laxatives. Reports of ultrastructural findings in this condition consist so far of isolated observations (67), or those results published by our group (51, 54, 55). In 1968 B. Smith (64) first demonstrated histologically, that abuse of laxatives containing anthraquinones, over a period of several years, results in remarkable pathological changes in the colon. These changes take the form of gross loss of intrinsic innervation, an atrophy of the smooth muscle and melanosis coli. In advanced cases, also designated as "cathartic colon", the colon is an inert tube, without active function and the ultimate treatment is compulsory colectomy. However, such terminal cases are rare and intermediate cases of intestinal damage by laxatives are much more important and may frequently be overlooked during diagnosis.

Our own investigations have established that the submucous plexus can be taken as being representative of the intramural nervous system where damage caused by laxatives has occurred (51, 54, 55). An additional advantage of studying this plexus is that it is easily accessible via an endoscopic biopsy (39). The most important finding in the enteric nervous system, from the point of view of the clinical symptoms of persistent constipation and/or diarrhoea, concerns the nerve fibres and the terminal formations (Fig. 1 and 2). The degenerative process manifests predominantly as an oedematous distension or ballooning of individual axons, which can extend to total lysis of the axo-plasma. This dissolution is accompanied by a loss of specific structural elements, such as neuro-tubuli and neuro-secretory granules, sometimes leaving the axon content completely homogenous. A simultaneous rise in the number of lysosomes (Fig. 3) indicates the

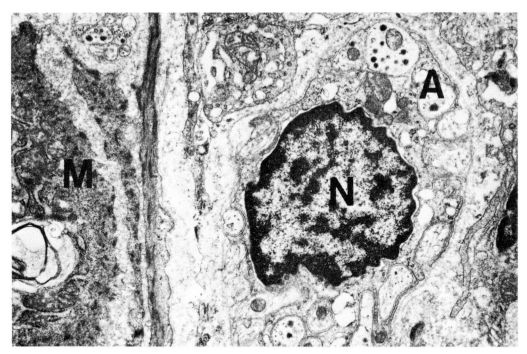

Fig. 1. Electron micrograph showing a cross section through a normal nerve, located in the submucosa of the large bowel. A = Axon, N = Nucleus, M = Muscle cell. Magnification: ×15,053.

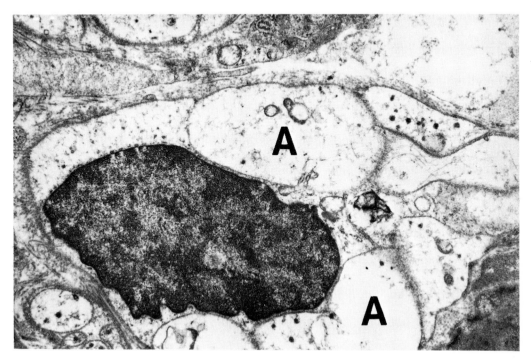

Fig. 2. Cross section of a degenerated nerve with ballooned axons (A). Long term laxative abuse. Magnification: ×12,230.

Table I. Distribution of neurosecretory granules and lysosomes per 100 μm² axonal area

| Patient groups | Vesicles | | | Lysosomes |
| --- | --- | --- | --- | --- |
| | Cholinergic | Adrenergic | Purinergic or peptidergic | |
| Normals, no. = 10 | 205 ± 73 | 500 ± 137 | 73 ± 34 | 10 ± 6 |
| Irritable bowel syndrome, no. = 10 | 371 ± 96* | 586 ± 142† | 73 ± 31† | 17 ± 9† |
| Laxative abuse, no. = 35 | 87 ± 35* | 265 ± 103* | 23 ± 9* | 34 ± 16* |

* P < 0.01 compared with normals.
† Not significant compared with normals.

inclusion of degenerated cells via such processes as auto-digestion. In extreme cases, complete bundles of nerves are subject to toxic degeneration. Obviously the transmission in the periphery is severely disturbed, as a result of the reduction in all populations of synaptic vesicles and the loss of the specific conductive system of neurotransmitters (Table I). The morphometric results also prove quantitatively that there is an increase in the axonal cross sections and areas, caused by the

sometimes considerable oedematous distension (Fig. 4). Similar changes are found throughout the entire colon but there is a general tendency for the damage to decrease towards the serosa.

Experimental investigations, involving chemical destruction of the ganglia and cutting of nerve fibres (34, 36, 37, 48) indicate that the degenerative changes are not necessarily specific for laxatives only. Damage to the intramural nervous system has also been reported for other sub-

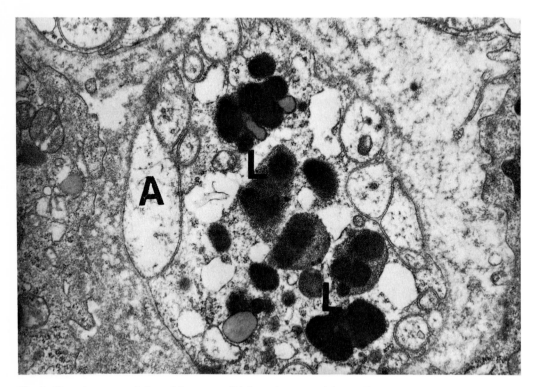

Fig. 3. Excessive accumulation of lysosomes (L) in a degenerated nerve fibre. Laxative abuse. A = Axon. Magnification: ×18,816.

DISTRIBUTION OF AXON-DIAMETERS IN %

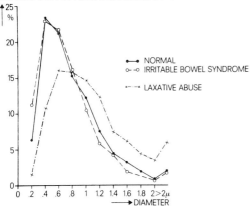

Fig. 4. Distribution of axon diameters, expressed as a percentage of the total measured. A significant difference (p < 0.01) between normals and patients with laxative abuse. No difference between normals and patients with iritiable bowel syndrome but with no purgative abuse.

stances, for example cytotoxic agents such as vinblastine sulphate (63). Spurious inflated axons are seen as signs of wear in healthy persons with unimpaired intestines and these increase in intensity with age. These defects however never assume the extent of the lesions caused by the toxic effects of laxatives. Quite obviously the changes described are not specific for a single group of laxatives irritating the mucosa. The changes mentioned are also observed for example after the use of diphenolic laxatives. If pigment of a melanin type is found in the macrophages (Fig. 5), there can be no doubt as to the diagnosis.

Long standing laxative abuse, extending over several years, results in motor and probably also sensory dysfunction of the colon. The morphological evidence for this damage is seen as the qualitative reduction of components of the intramural nervous system, transmitting excitation. The laxatives irritating the mucosa stimulate the

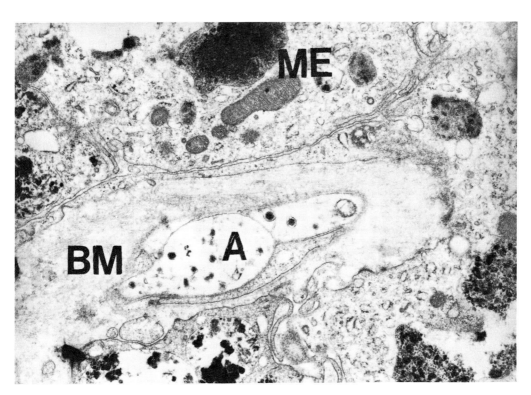

Fig. 5. Degenerated nerve fibre with ballooned axons (A), disintegrated basement membrane (BM), surrounded by melanin-laden macrophages (ME). Magnification: ×18,816.

intramural ganglia directly. The ensuing toxic degenerative damage to the submucous plexus proceeds in a centripetal direction. In specimens obtained during surgery, we were able to demonstrate that the myenteric plexus is likewise negatively affected.

These degenerative changes, the extent of which depends on the length of time the abuse was maintained and on the daily dose of laxatives, may result in serious impairment of the coordinated peristalsis of the gut. They provide evidence that initial functional disorders of the intestinal transport mechanism may develop into an organic change, forming an acquired hypoganglionosis as a consequence of laxative abuse. While this deterioriation is not numerical, it is quantitative and consists of lesions of the gut autonomic nervous system.

## Amyloidosis

Amyloidosis is a rare disease which is related to disturbed protein metabolism. Extracellular deposits of hyaline substances can be found in pericollagenous and perireticular tissues (69). In the gastrointestinal tract, a clear association can be seen with collagenous fibres in the perivascular tissue, muscularis mucosae, submucous tissue and nerve plexuses (53, 59). Amyloidosis presents with a variety of gastrointestinal symptoms (44, 45), the most important of which are diarrhoea and constipation (12, 40). Participation of the digestive tract can almost always be demonstrated in this disease (29, 30). Electron microscopy has shown that the amyloid fibrillae have a characteristic structure (14). The different amyloid proteins show a peculiar beta folded leaf structure (21), which, with other features, provides an explanation for the characteristic reaction to different dyes. Motility disorders can be due to muscular, as well as to neural or neurovascular damage (23). Where there is an extensive infiltration of the bowel muscles, a mechanical obstruction of muscle contractility can usually be described. The result of this is often an atrophy of the muscle cells, due to mechanical pressure,

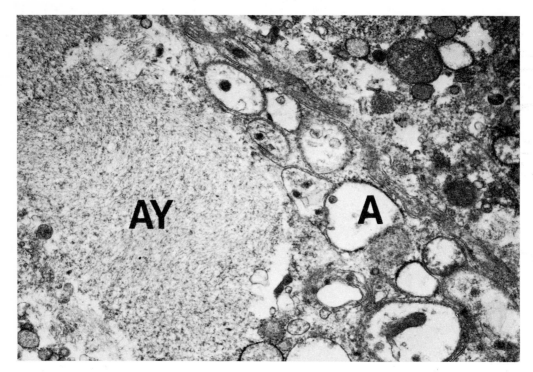

Fig. 6. Degenerated nerve with ballooned axons (A), infiltrated by amyloid deposits (AY). Magnification: ×18,816.

as well as impairment of the individual nexuses, which are dissociated by interposition of amyloid (53).

Far more important, however, is the neuropathy of the extrinsic and intrinsic gut nervous system (3, 25, 46). By means of fluoresence histochemistry it was demonstrated that, in visceral amyloidotic neuropathy, a depletion of catecholamines in the intramural nervous system occurs (57). Ultrastructural studies show that there is significant damage to the intrinsic nervous system in intestinal amyloidosis (41, 53, 58). As in laxative abuse, ballooning of the axons can be seen in parts of the nerve fibres (Fig. 6). Moreover, a significant reduction can be found in the neurosecretory granules, which play a decisive role in storing the neurotransmitters. The nerve plexuses are surrounded by a massive amyloidotic wall (Fig. 7).

These fibrillae can be seen encircling the nerve fibres like plates of armour. Thus disorders of the intestinal motility in this condition may be explained by the fact that there is a barrier surrounding partly normal axons which prevents the diffusion of transmitter substances from the axons to the reacting organs (59).

*Diabetes*

Autonomic neuropathy is a common complication of diabetes (31, 33, 66). It has been well known for many years that parts of the autonomic nervous system can be affected; this fact however is not often taken into consideration in clinical diagnosis (43). In 1956 Berge & Sprague (6) reported that a diabetic diarrhoea exists which can probably be traced back to lesions of the autonomic nervous system, but that no pathological findings had been found. Katz & Spiro (35), too, postulated, in 1966, an autonomic neuropathy, but did not find any correlation between the pathology and anatomy.

As other diabetic complications, for example

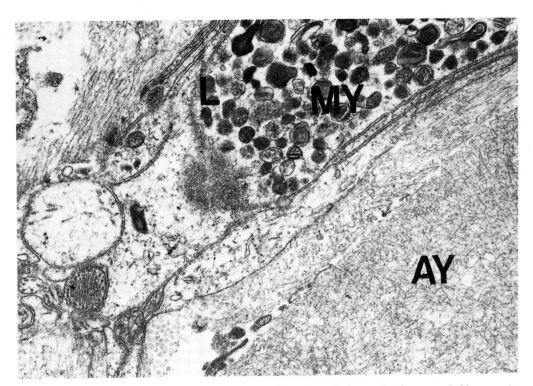

Fig. 7. Terminal part of a nerve fibre, rich in lysosomes (L) and myelin figures (MY), surrounded by excessive amyloid deposits (AY). Magnification: ×25,520.

retinopathy, are more dangerous, relatively little attention has been paid to autonomic neuropathy (33). Autonomic neuropathy manifests itself as a disturbance of the different bowel functions (42), the most important of which is constipation. Some workers feel that metabolic disorders like increased incorporation of glucose, fructose and sorbitol, quantitative changes in myelin composition and synthesis as well as Schwann-cell dysfunction are prime factors. On the other hand, others have suggested that segmental demyelinisation and axonal degeneration play an important role as morphological disorders. These investigations were carried out almost exclusively on autopsy specimens and they are rather controversial. Up to now it has not been possible to confirm or to disprove the involvement of the intramural nervous system of the intestinal tract. From the clinical point of view, diabetic enteropathy is a well known phenomenon. The clinical picture is dominated by spasmodic episodes of profuse diarrhoea, which are often painless, mostly nocturnal and connected with incontinence. Clinical investigations made by our group have shown that, indeed, there is a morphological correlation with clinical symptoms (52). Surprisingly, as in laxative abuse, we have found marked degenerative changes. The main signs here too, are the axons, which are swollen and lucent with a reduction of specific structural elements such as synaptic vesicles, neurotransmitters, neurotubules and neurofilaments (Fig. 8).

In diabetic enteropathy too, the degenerative process involves all parts of the nervous system, from the terminal region up to the ganglion cells, and ranges from oedema to complete lysis of the cellular compartments. Unlike laxative abuse, where degeneration is decreased towards the serosa, there is a uniform level of degeneration over all regions of the gut wall. Microangiopathy,

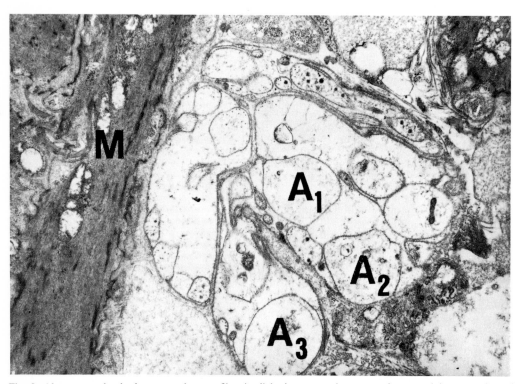

Fig. 8. Almost completely degenerated nerve fibre in diabetic autonomic neuropathy, containing a number of swollen axons ($A_1$–$A_3$) with diminished numbers of neurotubules and neurofilaments. M = Muscle cell. Magnification: ×10,765.

which is also pathognomonic in diabetes, can even be seen in the capillaries of the gut wall (Fig. 9).

The microangiopathy, which is an accompanying phenomenon, indicates a trophic disturbance which may possibly play an important role in the pathogenesis of the nerve lesions. In this case too, the functional mechanism of coordinated motility is badly hampered. In patients without any clinical symptoms of autonomic diabetic neuropathy, no similar changes could be detected.

*Chronic inflammatory bowel disease (IBD)*

The clinical symptoms of inflammatory bowel disease demonstrate that, in this disorder too, an impairment of the autonomic nervous system should be expected. In 1943 Storsteen, Kernohan & Bargen (68) observed a significant increase in the number of ganglion cells in ulcerative colitis. The same results have been obtained in regional enteritis (1, 18, 71). These findings were interpreted as overreactivity of the gut and were thus judged as a secondary phenomenon. Investigation of experimental gut stenosis has shown that, in a time period of 60 days, no changes in the gut nervous system occurred proximal to the stenosis (22). For this reason, the changes described are probably dependent upon the relatively long duration of the stenotic lesion. Electron microscopical studies of Van der Zypen (72) and Oka-

moto, Kakutani, Iwasaki, Namba & Ueda (47) have shown, for the first time, that in ulcerative colitis nerve damage occurs in inflamed areas of gut. These findings have been confirmed by other groups (19, 20, 61). It was recently reported that the intramural nervous system is involved in the inflammatory process, regardless of whether the tissue sample was removed from inflamed or normal parts of the gut (20). There have also been a report that especially in Crohn's disease there are significant changes in the peptide-containing nerve terminals (8).

The results of extensive ultrastructural studies made by our group of surgical specimens of the colon, as well as the ileum, in Crohn's disease are in accordance with these reports. We have found significant changes in all parts of the affected gut. In addition to a distinct hyperplasia of the nerves, all the ganglion cells showed marked signs of degeneration, mainly dilatation of endoplasmic reticulum, destruction of mitochondria and deposits of lipofuschin granules. In the nerve bundles (Fig. 12) there was a focal, massive dilatation of single axons, the content of which seemed to be completely homogenous. Similar changes could also be demonstrated in the terminal parts of nerves. These signs of degeneration were apparent only in regions with inflammatory changes. In areas free of inflammation, expecially

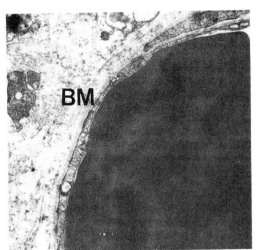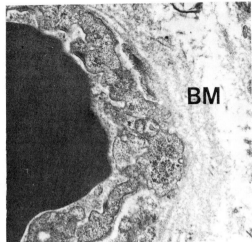

Fig. 9. Comparison between a normal (left) and diabetic capillary basement membrane. Submucosa, large bowel. Note the thickened and split basement membrane (BM) on the right. Magnification: ×13,520.

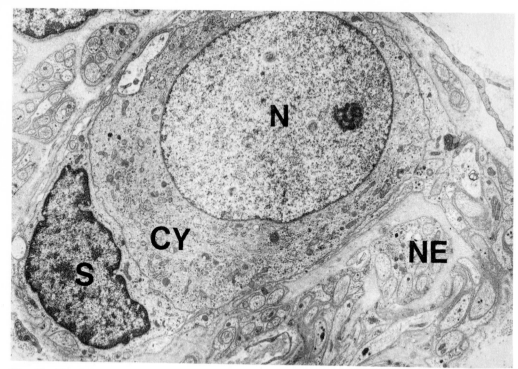

Fig. 10. Fine structure of a hypertrophied ganglion cell from the submucous plexus in Crohn's disease. N = Nucleus, CY = Cytoplasm, NE = Nerve, S = Schwann cell. Magnification: ×7,160.

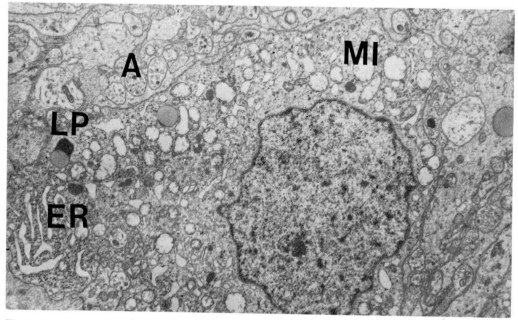

Fig. 11. Focal degeneration of a ganglion cell of the submucous plexus, with dilated endoplasmic reticulum (ER), swollen mitochondria (MI) and lipofushin granules (LP). A = Normal axons. Magnification: ×7,526.

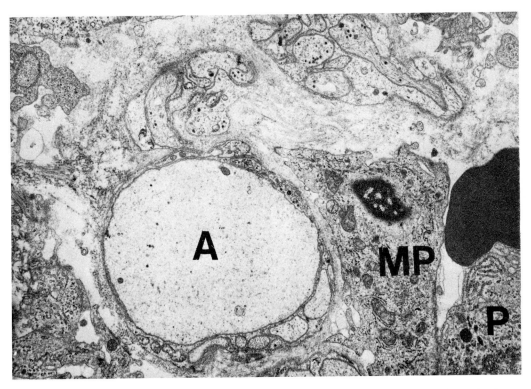

Fig. 12. Massively dilated, homogeneous axon (A) in Crohn's disease, surrounded by macrophages (MP) and plasma cells (P). Magnification: ×7,903.

proximal to stenoses, only a hyperplasia of nervous elements could be found.

### Whipple's disease

Whipple's disease is characterised by a distinct aggregation of so-called SPC-cells, in which the typical Whipple bacteria or their derivative products are condensed. In addition, these bacteria may be found in capillary basement membranes, in endothelial cells of lymph vessels and, occasionally, in the cytoplasm of Schwann wells (49). Toxic-degenerative changes of the autonomic nervous system have not been previously described in this condition. Studies made by our group on 5 patients with Whipple's disease did not reveal any lesions of the gut nerves. Intact nerve fibres were usually found, sometimes surrounded by SPC-cells but free of bacteria (Fig. 13).

### Gluten-sensitive enteropathy (Coeliac disease)

Gluten-sensitive enteropathy is characterised morphologically by variable atrophy of the villi as well as submucosal infiltration with lymphocytes and plasma cells. This can result in a malabsorption syndrome. This disease, which is caused by a nutritional allergy does not appear to affect the autonomic nervous system as degenerative changes do not occur more frequently than in normals. Our investigations on 14 patients with this syndrome did not show any damage to nervous elements of the submucosal gut layer. Nerve bundles were surrounded by plasma cells, but their fine structure was normal in appearance (Fig. 14).

In summary, it may be concluded that the gut intramural nervous system reacts in a uniform manner, irrespective of the nature of the primary damaging agent. The reaction consists of swelling

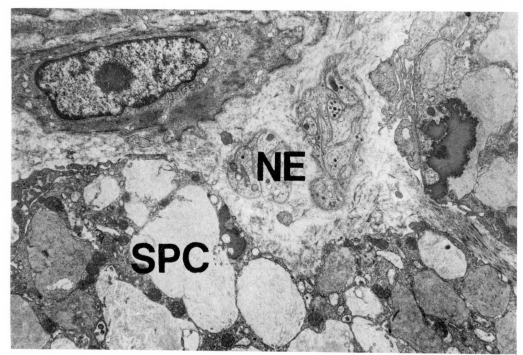

Fig. 13. Normal nerves (NE) in a case of Whipple's disease: Note the impressive SPC-cells. Magnification: ×7,526.

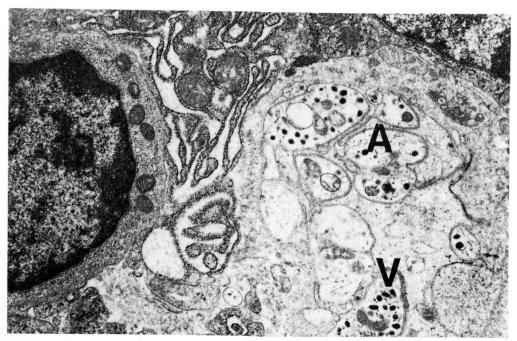

Fig. 14. Normal nerve fibre in gluten-sensitive enteropathy, surrounded by plasma cells. A = Axons, V = Varicosities. Magnification: ×12,800.

and ballooning of axons, reduction of specific nervous elements up to total degeneration of whole nerves. The loss of substance and therefore the loss of function explains the clinical symptoms, which are fairly similar in each clinical entity, and manifest as motility disorders of varying severity.

## ACKNOWLEDGEMENT

Thanks are due to Mrs. A. Schmidt for expert technical assistance.

## REFERENCES

1. Antonius JI, Gump FE, Lattes R, Lepore M. Gastroenterology 1960, 38, 889–907
2. Baumgarten HG, Holstein AF, Owman Ch. Zeit Zellforsch Mikros Anat 1970, 6, 376–397
3. Battle WM, Rubin M, Cohen S. Snape Jr, WJ. New Engl J Med 1979, 301, 24–25
4. Barr L, Berger W, Dewey MM. J Gen Physiol 1968, 51, 347–368
5. Bayliss WM, Starling EH. J Physiol (Lond) 1899, 24, 99–143
6. Berge KG, Sprague RG, Bennett WA. Diabetes 1956, 4, 289–294
7. Binder HJ, Donowitz M. Gastroenterology 1975, 69, 1001–1005
8. Bishop AE, Polak JM, Bryant MG, Bloom SR, Hamilton S. Gastroenterology 1980, 79, 853–860
9. Bortoff A. Ann Rev Physiol 1972, 24, 261–290
10. Burnstock G, Iwayama T, Progr Brain Res 1971, 34, 389–404
11. Burnstock G. Pharmacol Rev 1972, 24, 509–581
12. Carrizosa J, Lin KY, Myerson RM. Am J of Gastroenterol 1973, 59 541–546
13. Cavazzana P, Borsetto PL. Acta Anat 1948, 5, 17–23
14. Cohen AS, Calkins E. Nature 1959, 183, 1202–1203
15. Cooke WT. Clinics in Gastroenterology 1977, 3, 659–673
16. Cummings JH. Gut 1974, 15, 758–766
17. Daniel EE, Daniel VP, Duchon G. J Membr Biol 1976, 28, 207–239
18. Davis DR, Dockerty MB, Mayo CW. Surgery Gynecology & Obstetrics 1955, 101, 208–216
19. Dvorak AM, Dickersin GR. Human Pathology 1980, 11, 561–571
20. Dvorak AM, Osage JE, Monahan RA, Dickersin GR. Human Pathology 1980, 11, 620–634
21. Eanes EC, Glenner GG. J Histochem Cytochem 1968, 16, 673–678
22. Earlam RJ. Gut 1971, 12, 393–398
23. Ek BO, Holmlund DEW, Sjödin J-G, Steen LE. Am J Gastroenterology 1978, 70, 365–370
24. Feldberg W. J Physiol (Lond) 1951, 113, 483–585
25. French JM, Hall G, Smith Th. Am J of Medicine 1965, 39, 277–284
26. Furness JB, Costa M. Ergeb Physiol 1979, 19, 676–681
27. Gabella G, Blundell, D. J Cell Biol 1979, 82, 239–247
28. Gershon MD, Erde St M. Gastroenterology 1981, 80, 1571–1594
29. Gilat T, Revach M, Sohar E. Gut 1969, 10, 98–104
30. Gilat T, Spiro HM. Am J Dig Dis 1968, 13, 619–633
31. Hensley GT, Soergel KH. Arch Path 1968, 85, 587–597
32. Hokfelt T. pp 424–443 in Burnstock G, Gershon MD, Hokflet T, Iversen LL, Kosterlitz HW, Szurszweski TH. (eds). MIT Press, Cambridge 1979
33. Hosking DJ, Bennett T, Hampton JF. Diabetes 1978, 27, 1043–1054
34. Jabonero V. Acta neuroveg (Wien) 1965, 27/4, 496–518
35. Katz, LA, Spiro HM, New Engl J of Medicine 1966, 275, 1350–1360
36. Knoche H, Terwort H. Z f Zellforsch 1973, 141, 181–189
37. Knoche H, Addicks K. pp 1–142 in Sturm A, Birkmayer W. (eds). Fischer Verlag, Stuttgart 1976
38. Langley IN. J Physiol 1922, 56, 39–54
39. Lassmann G. Virchows Arch A Path Anat Histol 1975, 365, 257–261
40. Legge DA, Wollaeger EE, Carlson HC. Gut 1970 11 764–767
41. Low PA, Walsh JC, Huang CY, McLeod JG. Brain 1975, 98, 341–356
42. Malins JM, Mayne N, Diabetes 1969, 18, 858–866
43. Mencer Martin M. The Lancet 1, 1953, 560–565
44. Monteiro JG. Am J of Gastroenterology 1973, 60, 47–59
45. Monteiro JG. Gut 1968, 9, 353–354
46. Nordborg C, Kristensson K, Olsson Y, Sourander, P. Acta Neurol Scandinav 1973, 49, 31–38
47. Okamoto, E, Kakutani T, Iwasaki T, Namba M, Ueda T. Med J of Osaka Univ 1964, 15, 85–106
48. Otto HF. Zbl allg Path 1972, 115, 445–452
49. Otto HF. Morbus Whipple Georg Thieme Verlag: Stuttgart 1975
50. Paton WDM, Vizi ES, Zar MA. J Physiol (Lond) 1971, 215, 819–848
51. Riemann JF, Zimmermann W, Gastroenterology 1978, 74, 1085
52. Riemann JF, Schmidt H, Zimmermann W. Diabetes 1979, Suppl., 28, 408
53. Riemann JF, Schmidt H, Liendl I. Fortschr Med 1981 (in press)
54. Riemann JF, Schmidt H, Zimmermann W. Scand J Gastroent 1980, 15, 761–768
55. Riemann, JF, Schmidt H. Coloprotology 1980, 2, 348–353
56. Rhodin JAG. A Text and Atlas, New York—Oxford University Press, London-Toronto 1974
57. Rubenstein AE, Yahr, MD, Mytillneou C, Bajaj K. Mt Sinai J Med 1978, 45, 782–789
58. Schmidt H, Frühmorgen P, Riemann JF, Becker V. Endoscopy 1981, 4, 181–183
59. Schmidt H, Riemann JF. Leber Magen Darm 1981, 11, 105–111
60. Schofield GC. Brain 1960, 83, 490–514

61. Siemers PT, Dobbins WO. Surgery Gynecology & Obstetrics 1974, 138, 39–42
62. Schuffler MD, Bird ThD, Sumi SM, Cook A. Gastroenterology 1978, 75, 889–898
63. Smith B. J Neurol Neurosurg Psychiatr 1967, 30, 506–510
64. Smith B. Gut 1968, 9, 139–143
65. Smith B. Dis Col & Rect 1973, 16, 455–458
66. Smith B. J of Neurology Neurosurgery and Psychiatry 1974, 37, 1151–1154
67. Steer H, Colin-Jones DG. J Path 1975, 115, 199–205
68. Storsteen KA, Kernohan JW, Bargen JA. Surgery Gynecology and Obstetrics 1953, 97, 335–343
69. Sohar E, Merker H-J, Missmahl HP, Gafni J, Heller H. J Path Bact 1967, 94, 89–93
70. Vanhoutte PM. Fed Proc 1977, 36, 2444–2449
71. Van Patter WN, Bargen JA, Dockerty MC, Feldmann WH, Mayo CW, Wangh JM. Gastroenterology 1954, 26 347–351
72. Van der Zypen E. Dtsch Z Nervenheilk 1965, 187, 787–836

# Clinical Aspects of Autonomic Nerve Dysfunction of the Gut

S. COHEN, M.D.
University of Pennsylvania School of Medicine, Philadelphia, Pennsylvania, USA

Autonomic dysfunction leads to a variety of clinical disorders involving all parts of the gut. These neural disorders are distinct from the four other recognised categories of disorders involving myogenic function, myoelectric activity, hormonal regulation and abnormal humoral factors. Criteria for establishing that a disorder has a neurogenic aetiology vary in different diseases. Absence of a neural mediated response with intact muscle function has been the major criterion used in most studies. Neural mediated responses of peristalsis, sphincteric relaxation and intestinal contraction following distension or feeding are the major parameters of assessment. Abnormalities in neural function have been demonstrated in achalasia, symptomatic diffuse oesophageal spasm, diabetes mellitus, amyloidosis, scleroderma and chronic idiopathic intestinal pseudoobstruction. The anatomical site and type of gut neurological disorder varies in each condition. Morphological studies have been helpful in demonstrating specific intranuclear inclusion bodies in some pseudoobstruction patients, and vagal and ganglionic lesions in achalasia. Intact muscle and myoelectric function as well as normal responsiveness to drugs acting directly upon muscle may be established by morphological study. Advancement in basic technology should provide a rewarding area for future study of the pathogenesis and treatment of the gut neurological disorders.

*S. Cohen, M.D., Gastrointestinal Section of the Dept of Medicine, Hospital of the University of Pennsylvania, 3400 Spruce Street, Philadelphia, Pennsylvania 19104, USA*

Despite considerable knowledge concerning the normal physiology of the autonomic innervation to the gut, the clinical disorders of neural function are less well understood. In most clinical conditions, the pathophysiology of the disorder has not been clearly determined. Studies in man have been limited, and are mostly descriptive in character. Careful histological, physiological, or biochemical studies of isolated tissue are rare. Despite these limitations, major areas of clinical importance have been defined. The purpose of this presentation is threefold: First, to provide a rational classification of the gastrointestinal motor disorders; second, to discuss several selected disorders in gut neural function; and third, to describe possible approaches to further study of these disorders. The discussion will be limited to the gastrointestinal motility disorders due to neurological dysfunction of smooth muscle in man since this area is of major clinical importance.

## Classification of the gastrointestinal neuromuscular disorders

In Table I, the gastrointestinal motor disorders are classified into five major categories. In each category a brief definition of the specific classification is given, with a list of clinical conditions that may be considered in each group. This classification into specific categories stresses the particular component of the neuromuscular apparatus that is impaired in each disease. I have categorised these entities, but realise that reclassification or subclassification may be required in the future.

Table I. Classification of gastrointestinal neuromuscular disorders

I. Disorders of gut innervation: Diminished responsiveness to indirect acting stimuli such as distension, feeding or certain drugs acting upon nerves.
   A. Achalasia
   B. Symptomatic diffuse oesophageal spasm
   C. Diabetes mellitus
   D. Schleroderma (early)
   E. Amyloidosis
   F. Chronic idiopathic intestinal pseudo-obstruction
   G. Hirshprung's disease
II. Disorders of smooth muscle contractility: Diminished muscle contractility in response to direct stimulation.
   A. Primary visceral myopathy
   B. Scleroderma (late)
   C. Ulcerative colitis
III. Disorders of myoelectric activity: Abnormal frequency or pattern of muscle contraction due to an abnormal slow wave rhythm.
   A. Irritable bowel syndrome
   B. Tachygastria
IV. Disorders due to an abnormal humoral substance either in the gut lumen or in the circulation: An increase or decrease in gut motility related to the presence of some endogenous or an exogenous humoral substance that acts on either nerve or gut.
   A. Bacterial toxins
   B. Prostaglandins
   C. Bile salts
   D. Laxatives
V. Disorders in hormonal regulation: An alteration in gut motility due to either an increased or decreased amount of circulating hormone or an altered gut sensitivity to a hormone.
   A. Lower oesophageal sphincter incompetence
   B. Achalasia
   C. Symptomatic diffuse oesophageal spasm
   D. Irritable bowel syndrome
   E. Bilary dyskinesia

Classification of a given clinical condition is based on all available data including morphology, in vitro tissue studies and animal studies. In some cases, the evidence is indirect.

The decision that a gastrointestinal motor disorder is due to impaired innervation is based upon several observations. Firstly, the abnormality in function in man is clearly a derangement in a neural mediated response as determined in an animal or in man (9, 19, 20, 40, 41). An actual creation of a chronic animal model of that disease following nerve destruction has been rare (16, 21). Secondly, a neural disease may be defined by specific morphological abnormalities in the autonomic nerves or ganglia as seen in achalasia or Hirshprung's disease (6, 8, 9, 16, 32). Thirdly, evidence of intact muscle should be demonstrated by either morphological criteria or normal contractile responses to agents acting directly upon the muscle membrane, or by the demonstration of intact slow wave activity (1–3, 10, 11, 14, 17, 34, 35). Fourthly, a neural disorder may be suggested by demonstrating an abnormality in the gut response to indirect acting stimuli (distension, feeding, or drugs acting upon nerves or ganglia) despite an intact response to direct acting agents (drugs or hormones) stimulating muscle directly (1–3, 10, 14, 35). Thus, concluding that a clinical disorder in man is due to an abnormality in autonomic neural function is based on a variety of evidence. Obviously, the more criteria that have been fulfilled, the stronger is that conclusion.

The other categories of the neuromuscular disorders are defined by direct evidence. In the disorders of muscle function, morphological evidence of muscle disease by either vacuolar degeneration or fibrosis with atrophy is seen in primary visceral myopathy and late scleroderma, respectively (13, 28–30, 38). In irritable bowel syndrome and tachygastria, abnormal slow wave frequencies have been recorded in the colon and stomach, respectively (33, 36, 37). In the disorders due to a humoral substance, the findings have been mainly in animal models. In an ileal loop model, bacterial toxins of cholera, E. coli and shigella as well as several strains of salmonella have been shown to induce a unique pattern of action potential complexes (5, 24, 25, 42). This disorder has been shown to be prostaglandin mediated through cholinergic pathways (24). This disorder is thus due to an exogenous toxin, but requires neural pathways for its expression.

Abnormalities in hormonal control of gut motility have been controversial since the physiological effect of these hormones on motility is still uncertain (9, 10). The most relevant findings in man concern the disorders of altered muscle sensitivity to the hormones due to denervation. A denervated structure has an altered responsiveness to a stimulus (39). This law of denervation supersensitivity indicates that the altered responsiveness of the denervated structure may be non-specific, giving increased activity to agents that are not the usual transmitter substances. In several disorders in man, altered smooth muscle responsiveness to several hormones has been described. These changes have been noted for the lower oesophageal sphincter in achalasia and the oesophageal body in diffuse oesophageal spasm (12, 15). In both disorders, an increased responsiveness to gastrin has been reported. Although altered sensitivity to the hormone is present, the role of this supersensitivity to gastrin in the pathogenesis of the clinical disorder is not clear. However, these findings do indicate that autonomic nerve dysfunction may lead to altered hormonal responses in vivo. These changes may or may not be related to the pathophysiology of the clinical condition.

*Achalasia and symptomatic diffuse oesophageal spasm*

The classical clinical features of achalasia are dysphagia, regurgitation of retained food and chest pain. The oesophagus shows aperistalsis, lower oesophageal sphincter hypertension and failure of the sphincter to relax completely (16, 17, 41). The evidence that achalasia is a neural disorder is strong. I will examine the evidence using the criteria outlined above as a framework.

There has been supposition that damage to the vagi, the dorsal vagal nucleus in the brain stem and the ganglia in the oesophageal wall accounted for the disorders in peristaltic and sphincter function in this disease (6–8, 9, 16, 17, 32, 41). How-

ever, the actual role of the vagal system was unclear since it was assumed to be a parasympathetic nerve releasing acetylcholine, the latter increasing sphincter pressure. In recent years, experimental data in the opossum and in the cat clarify the role of the vagi on oesophageal function (19, 20, 22, 27, 40). Section or cooling of both vagi fails to alter lower oesophageal sphincter pressure, but does cause aperistalsis and impaired sphincter relaxation. The vagi induce sphincter relaxation during swallowing or direct electrical vagal stimulation (19, 27). The neurotransmitter is not cholinergic but is rather a purine nucleotide or vasoactive intestinal peptide (20, 40). Impairment of both vagi are required to alter peristalsis or sphincter relaxation (19, 22, 27). Destruction of a single vagus has no effect. The impairment of vagal function must be high in the thorax since lower thoracic levels of vagal nerve section have no effect on sphincter function (22). It would seem that the oesophagus is innervated proximally by the vagus, with distal function being controlled by intramural pathways. Thus, an acute bilateral preganglionic interruption causes changes similar to achalasia (aperistalsis and impaired sphincter relaxation) but not sphincter hypertension or tertiary oesophageal contractions. Several chronic models of achalasia in animals were produced by bilateral cervical vagotomy, destruction of the dorsal vagal nuclei or neural destruction, using a toxin. The actual production of sphincter hypertension in these chronic animal models is unclear since the method of recording pressure was imprecise in these earlier studies (7, 16).

In achalasia, muscle morphology is normal but lesions have been observed in the vagi, dorsal vagal nucleus, the brain stem and in the oesophageal intra-mural ganglia (6, 16, 41). Further

Table II. Summary of myoelectric findings in proposed neural disorders of the colon

|  | CIIP* | Scleroderma | Diabetes | Amyloidosis |
|---|---|---|---|---|
| Slow wave activity | Intact | Intact | Intact | Intact |
| Response to a meal | Absent | Absent | Diminished | Diminished |
| Cholinergic stimulation | Normal | Normal (early) Decreased (late) | Normal | Normal |

* Neural form of disease.

evidence for intact muscle is obtained from studies showing intact responses to direct acting muscle agonists. Therefore, achalasia fulfills each of the criteria, indicating a true autonomic neural dysfunction.

The evidence that symptomatic diffuse oeso-phageal spasm is also a neural disorder is less well established, but supported by considerable indi-rect evidence (7, 9, 16, 41). Firstly, several of the manometric features of diffuse oesophageal spasm are similar to those seen in achalasia (8, 41). In animals, partially denervated by vagal cooling, peristaltic and sphincter relaxation can be impaired selectively, similar to that seen in some patients with diffuse oesophageal spasm (27). Secondly, neural pathology but not muscle changes have been prominent in this disorder (7, 8). Thirdly, muscle response to directly acting agonists is intact (8, 15). Fourthly, in some patients more classical features of achalasia may evolve following documented evidence of diffuse oesophageal spasm (8, 9, 41). The oesophageal motor disorders of achalasia and diffuse oeso-phageal spasm plus other variants variously called dyschalasia, unclassified motor disorders, and hypertensive lower oesophageal sphincter appear to represent a spectrum of disorders (8, 9, 41). The degree of vagal nerve dysfunction most likely determines the manometric and clinical picture.

An interesting aspect of these oesophageal motor disorders is that patients with these dis-orders do not have more widespread evidence of vagal nerve dysfunction. Some patients with achalasia have been shown to have evidence of vagal nerve dysfunction based on a negative acid secretory response to insulin-induced hypo-glycemia (16). A proximal vagal or brain stem lesion, as reported in achalasia, would be expected to alter other aspects of gut motor func-tion similar to those observed in the more gener-alised disorders such as diabetes mellitus or intes-tinal pseudoobstruction (6, 16). A more distal oesophageal neural lesion would be suggested by the absence of more widespread symptoms.

*Chronic idiopathic intestinal pseudoobstruction*

Chronic idiopathic pseudoobstruction (CIIP) exists in at least two forms, a neural disorder and

a myopathic disorder (28–31, 35). The myopathic disorder is known as primary hollow visceral myopathy and is characterised by vacuolar degeneration of gut smooth muscle (29, 30). The neuropathic variety has been studied in our lab-oratory and will be discussed in detail (35).

CIIP is a chronic disorder which manifests itself by episodes of intestinal dilation simulating true organic obstruction. In most cases, multiple operations have been performed to relieve a nonexistent obstruction. The small intestine is dilated in all cases and the colon is dilated in most cases. The oesophagus shows features of achalasia by radiographic examination.

In some cases with CIIP, characteristic neu-ronal lesions are seen. Intramural ganglia contain filamentous inclusion bodies (29). The inclusion bodies are not characteristic of any known viral lesion. These neuronal changes are not seen in patients with primary visceral myopathy.

The evidence of widespread gut neural dys-function is quite convincing. In the oesophagus, there is usually aperistalsis and impaired lower oesophageal sphincter relaxation similar to that seen in achalasia (31, 35). The sphincter pressure is usually not elevated and most patients, there-fore, do not have dysphagia. In the small intestine and colon, slow waves generated within the smooth muscle remain intact. The small bowel responds poorly to distension and the colon responds poorly to a meal (23, 35). Both responses are neural mediated. The small and large intestine responded normally with increased spike and motor activity to direct stimulation with a cholinesterase inhibitor (23, 35). In one patient, anal sphincter relaxation was impaired. Thus, in this serious, often fatal, clinical condition, mor-phological and physiological evidence of wide-spread neural dysfunction with intact muscle activity is present. Attempts at therapeutic stimu-lation of the smooth muscle by direct agonists (bethanechol or metaclopramide) have not been successful. Simple pharmacological stimulation of the muscle does not indicate a restoration of normal integrated gut function.

*Diabetes mellitus*

In patients with long-standing, insulin-dependent diabetes mellitus, gut involvement is not uncommon. Available evidence suggests that this is a visceral neuropathy similar to the peripheral neuropathy in this disease. However, the correlation between the two forms of neuropathy in any given patient may be poor. Although gastroparesis may be the clinical manifestation of diabetes mellitus that is most troublesome to manage, the most common gastrointestinal complaint in patients with this disease is constipation (2). We studied colonic function in patients with insulin-dependent diabetes mellitus.

The colonic myoelectric and motor activity was measured in patients with mild and severe constipation. In all patients with diabetes, colonic slow wave activity was intact, suggesting preserved smooth muscle function. The spike activity of the colon in response to a 1,000 calorie meal was markedly diminished in patients with severe constipation and only minimally reduced in patients with mild constipation as compared to normals. The colonic spike and motor responses to direct muscle stimulation using 10 mg or 20 mg of metaclopramide were normal (2). These findings suggest that intact muscle was present despite abnormal neural responses. Similar conclusions were drawn by other investigators studying the mechanism of diabetic gastroparesis. Whether the site of the neural defect is in the afferent or efferent limb is not clear.

In diabetes mellitus, the oesophagus shows nonspecific motor changes with many simultaneous and non-peristaltic contractions. The lower oesophageal sphincter pressure and relaxation are normal. Oesophageal symptoms are rare despite the presence of peristaltic abnormalities in many patients with diabetes mellitus.

*Progressive systemic sclerosis*

Progressive systemic sclerosis (PSS) or scleroderma is a systemic disorder that may affect all portions of the luminal gastrointestinal tract (3, 10, 11, 13, 14, 28, 38). Most postmortem studies in PSS emphasise the prominent smooth muscle fibrosis and atrophy (13, 28). However, considerable evidence has been presented to indicate that some of the early gastrointestinal motility changes in this disease are related to

neural dysfunction rather than muscle destruction. The initial evidence was presented in a correlative study between oesophageal motility changes before death and postmortem morphological examination of the oesophagus (38). In this study, it was demonstrated by manometry that areas of diminished oesophageal peristalsis were present in portions of the oesophagus with normal muscle. It was suggested that cholinergic nerve dysfunction may be related in some way to the sympathetic hypertonicity causing the Raynaud's phenomenon. Raynaud's phenomenon is closely correlated with gut dysfunction in this disease (10, 11). This supposition was further supported by a yet unconfirmed study showing that intra-arterial sympathetic blockade with reserpine restored normal oesophageal function (43).

In studies performed in our laboratory on the oesophagus, small intestine and colon, considerable pharmacological and physiological data were obtained to support the contention that an early neurological dysfunction precedes the later changes of smooth muscle atrophy and fibrosis. These studies demonstrate two phases of the illness affecting the gut (3, 10, 11). Early in the disease, all evidence indicates intact myogenic function with impaired neurological response (3, 10, 11, 14). The muscle of the oesophagus, small intestine and colon respond normally to direct stimulation with various agonists such as methacholine, metaclopramide or cholecystokinin. Also, the small intestine and colon generate normal slow wave activity (3, 14). Despite normal myogenic responses to direct-acting agonists, the small intestine fails to respond to distension and the colon fails to respond to a meal (3, 14). Late in the disease, the same organs lose their response to direct agonists as well, indicating the stage of muscle damage and fibrosis. Gut dysfunction is present in both stages, but the serious sequelae occur at the later stage of the disease. Oesophagitis and stricture of the oesophagus, small intestinal dilation with bacterial overgrowth, steatorrhea, and colonic widemouth diverticula are more common at the second stage of the disease (3, 10, 11, 13, 14).

Evidence of neural lesions by histological examination is lacking in this disease (13, 38).

However, it is well established that many sympathetic or catecholamine-containing nerves terminate on Auerbach's ganglia and act by inhibiting ganglionic release of acetylcholine (4, 26). A functional neural disorder may then be hypothesied in which sympathetic inhibiton of ganglionic acetylcholine release causes widespread gut dysfunction preceding the stage of muscle destruction. This hypothesis would explain the close correlation of Raynaud's phenomenon and gut dysfunction, and would also explain the absence of actual neural destruction. The early gut dysfunction in scleroderma may be reversible but has been demonstrated in only one study (43).

## CONCLUSIONS

It is apparent from this discussion that further study of the neuromuscular disorders of the gut is needed. The evidence supporting that specific disease of the gut are due to neural dysfunction is based in many cases on less than optimal information. To delineate the pathophysiology, the aetiology and possible therapy, a multifacted approach will be required. Firstly, it is important that basic research describing the functions of the gut and its innervation be continued on a high level. It is only possible to implicate a specific neural disorder if one knows the functions of that nervous system. Secondly, studies in man should be continued at multiple levels. Clinical studies as described above are necessary to determine the nature of the disorder, its motor and myoelectric patterns. These studies should be supplemented by morphological investigation and, most importantly, in vitro studies of smooth muscle from these patients. Animal models of disease should be sought when possible. Available techniques of electron microscopy, sucrose gap recording, force velocity recordings, electrical recordings and smooth muscle organ culture can all be applied to the study of disease in man. A large body of available technology has not yet been applied to the study of the neuromuscular disorders in man.

## REFERENCES

1. Battle WM, Rubin MR, Cohen S, Snape WJ Jr. New Engl J Med 1979, 301, 24–26
2. Battle WM, Snape WJ Jr, Alavi A, Cohen S, Braunstein S. Gastroenterology 1980, 79, 1217–1221
3. Battle WM, Snape, WJ Jr, Wright S, Sullivan M, Cohen S, Myers A, Tuthill R. Ann Intern Med 1981, 94, 749–752
4. Beani L, Bianchi C, Crena A. Br J Pharmacol 1969, 36, 1–12
5. Burns TW, Mathias JR, Carlson GM. Am J Physiol 1978, 4, E311–E315
6. Cassella RR, Brown AL, Sayre GP, Ellis FH. Ann Surg 1964, 160, 474–487
7. Cassella RR, Ellis FH, Brown AL. JAMA 1965, 191, 379–382
8. Castell DO. Arch Intern Med 1976, 136, 571–579
9. Cohen S. New Engl J Med 1979, 301, 184–192
10. Cohen S, Fisher R, Lipschutz W, Schumacher R. J Clin Invest 1972, 51, 2663–2668
11. Cohen S, Laufer I, Snape WJ Jr, Shiau YF, Levine G, Jiminez S. Gastroenterology 1980, 79, 155–166
12. Cohen S, Lipshutz W, Hughes W. J Clin Invest 1971, 50, 1241–1247
13. D'Angelo WW, Fries JF, Mori AT. Am J Med 1969, 46, 428–440
14. DiMarino AJ, Carlson G, Myers A, Cohen S. New Engl J Med 1973, 289, 1220–1223
15. Eckardt V, Weigand H. Gut 1974, 15, 706–709
16. Ellis FH, Olsen AM. Achalasia of the Esophagus. Major Problems in Clinical Surgery. WB Saunders Co, Philadelphia 1969
17. Fisher R, Cohen S. Annual Rev Med 1975, 26, 373–390
18. Fisher R, Cohen S. Gastroenterology 1976, 5, 29–47
19. Goyal RK, Rattan S. J Clin Invest 1975, 55, 1119–1126
20. Goyal RK, Said SI, Rattan S. Nature 1980, 288, 378–380
21. Higgs B, Kerr FW, Ellis FH Jr, J Thorac Cardiov Surg 1965, 50, 613–625
22. Kravitz J, Snape WJ Jr, Cohen S. Am J Physiol 1978, 234, E359–E364
23. Lewis TD, Daniel EE, Sarna SK, Waterfall WE, Marzio L. Gastroenterology 1978, 74, 107–111
24. Mathias JR, Carlson GM, Bertiger G, Cohen S. Am J Physiol 1977, 235, E529–E534
25. Mathias JR, Carlson GM, DiMarino AJ, Cohen S. J Clin Invest 1976, 58, 91–96
26. Paton WO, Vizi ES. Br J Pharmacol 1969, 35, 10–18
27. Ryan JP, Snape WJ Jr, Cohen S. Am J Physiol 1977, 232, E159–E164
28. Schuffler MD, Beegle RG. Gastroenterology 1979, 77, 664–671
29. Schuffler MD, Bird TD, Sumi SM. Gastroenterology 1978, 75, 889–896
30. Schuffler MD, Lowe MC, Bill AH. Gastroenterology 1977, 73, 327–332
31. Schuffler MD, Pope CE. Gastroenterology 1976, 70, 677–682
32. Smith B. Gut, 1970, 11, 388–391

33. Snape WJ Jr, Carlson G, Matarazzo S, Cohen S. Gastroenerology 1977, 72, 383–387
34. Snape WJ Jr, Wright SH, Cohen S, Battle WM. Gastroenterology 1979, 77, 1235–1240
35. Sullivan MA, Snape WJ Jr, Matarazzo SA, Petrokubi R, Jeffries G, Cohen S. New Engl J Med 1977, 297, 233–238
36. Taylor I, Darby C, Hammond P. Gut, 1978, 19, 923–929
37. Telander RL, Morgan KG, Kreulen DL, Schmalz PF, Kelly KA, Szurszewski JH. Gastroenterology 1978, 75, 497–501
38. Treacy WL, Baggenstoss AH, Slocumb CH, Code C. Ann Intern Med 1963, 59, 351–356
39. Trendelenburg V. Pharmacol Rev 1966, 18, 629–656
40. Tuch AF, Cohen S. J clin Invest 1973, 52, 14–20
41. Vantrappen G, Janssens H, Hellemans J. Gastroenterology 1979, 76, 450–457
42. Weisberg P, Carlson G, Cohen A. Gastroenterology 1978, 74, 47–51
43. Willerson JT, Thompson RH, Hookman P, Heidt J, Decker JL. Ann Intern Med 1970, 72, 17–23

# Studies of Autonomic Nerves in the Gut—Past, Present and Future

G. BURNSTOCK
Dept. of Anatomy and Centre for Neuroscience, University College London,
Gower Street, London WC1E 6BT, UK

The findings of the last few years, reviewed today, present some new insights into the complexity of integrative nervous activity in the gut. However, it is imperative that we increase our understanding of these basic neurological mechanisms if we are to have any chance of understanding and treating abnormalities in these mechanisms that occur in various gastrointestinal diseases.

*G. Burnstock, Dept. of Anatomy and Centre for Neuroscience, University College London, Gower Street, London WC1E 6BT, UK*

We have heard today some exciting new discoveries about the innervation of the gut and the extraordinary number of putative neurotransmitters. In summary, I would like first to briefly put these new findings into historical perspective and secondly to present for discussion what I think are some of the crucial questions that we now face, most of which have been raised during the day.

## HISTORICAL BACKGROUND

Classically the non-sphincteric smooth muscle of the gut was considered to be controlled by antagonistic parasympathetic cholinergic excitatory nerves and sympathetic adrenergic inhibitory nerves (23)-

In the early 1960's transient hyperpolarisations were recorded in intestinal smooth muscle cells during stimulation of intramural nerves in the presence of atropine and guanethidine (11). These hyperpolarisations were unaffected by sympathectomy, but abolished by tetrodoxin; thus they represented inhibitory junction potentials, and the presence of non-adrenergic, non-cholinergic inhibitory nerves was established in the smooth muscle of the muscularis externa of the gut (4).

Extensive investigations were carried out to discover the transmitter in these non-adrenergic inhibitory nerves in the gut. A number of criteria need to be satisfied to establish a substance as a neurotransmitter. These include: synthesis and storage in nerve terminals; release by a $Ca^{++}$-dependent mechanism; mimicry of the neurogenic response by receptor occupation; inactivation by ectoenzymes and/or neuronal uptake; modification of response by drugs in a comparable manner to that of the neurogenic response. Somewhat surprisingly a purine nucleotide, probably adenosine 5-triphosphate (ATP), best satisfied the criteria listed above from a wide variety of biologically active substances examined; these nerves were consequently termed 'purinergic' (4). Since that time, a considerable body of evidence has grown in support of this hypotheses (7, 8).

Between 1975 and 1977, important new findings suggested that, in addition to intramural purinergic inhibitory nerves supplying smooth muscle, there may be further non-adrenergic, non-cholinergic transmitters present in other nerve types in the gut, including interneurones, sensory nerves and nerves supplying mucosal epithelial secretory cells, sphincteric muscles and blood vessels; this work has been summarised in a monograph by Burnstock, Hökfelt, Gershon, Inversen, Kosterlitz & Szurszewsky (12). Immunohistochemical methods for localising biologically active polypeptides have revealed autonomic nerves containing enkephalin, substance P, vasoactive

POSSIBLE ROLES OF NON-ADRENERGIC, NON-CHOLINERGIC NEUROTRANSMITTERS IN GUT

| PUTATIVE TRANSMITTERS | INTERNEURONES | | NERVES TO SMOOTH MUSCLE | | | VASO-DILATOR NERVES | NERVES TO MUCOSAL SECRETORY CELLS | SENSORY NERVES | NERVES MODULATING RELEASE OF: | |
|---|---|---|---|---|---|---|---|---|---|---|
| | | | NON-SPHINCTERIC | | SPHINCTERIC | | | | | |
| | EXCITATORY | INHIBITORY | EXCITATORY | INHIBITORY | | | | | ACh | NA |
| ATP | − | − | ? | + | ? | ? | ? | − | +↓ | +↓ |
| 5-HT | + | ? | ? | − | − | − | ? | − | +↓ | − |
| DOPAMINE | − | ? | − | ? | ? | ? | − | − | − | +↓ |
| GABA | ? | − | − | − | − | − | − | − | ?↓ | ?↓ |
| ENKEPHALIN | − | + | − | − | − | − | − | − | +↓ | ?↓ |
| SOMATOSTATIN | ? | ? | − | − | − | − | ? | ? | ?↓ | − |
| VIP | ? | − | − | ? | + | + | + | − | ?↑ | − |
| SUBSTANCE-P | + | − | + | − | ? | ? | − | + | ?↓ | ?↓ |
| BRADYKININ | − | − | − | ? | − | ? | − | − | − | − |
| NEUROTENSIN | ? | − | − | − | − | − | ? | − | ?↑ | − |
| GASTRIN/CCK | − | − | ? | − | − | ? | − | − | ?↑ | − |

$\left.\begin{array}{l}\text{BOMBESIN} \\ \text{ANGIOTENSIN} \\ \text{ACTH} \\ \text{PANCREATIC POLYPEPTIDE (PP)}\end{array}\right\}$    LITTLE KNOWN

Fig. 1.

intestinal polypeptide (VIP), neurontensin, somatostatin, and more recently, bombesin and gastrin/cholecystokinin (CCK). In addition to polypeptides, there is growing evidence largely on the basis of autoradiographic and electrophysiological studies, that 5-hydroxytryptamine (5-HT) or a related indoleamine may be a transmitter in some autonomic nerves in the gastrointestinal tract (see 17), and recent evidence from our own laboratory suggests that GABA may be a transmitter in some myenteric neurones (21). Pharmacological experiments have also led to the suggestions that dopamine and bradykinin are autonomic transmitters (see 12).

## CURRENT PROBLEMS

### 1) Ultrastructural identification of neurotransmitters

Electronmicroscopic studies have revealed about eight morphologically distinct nerve profiles (largely in terms of predominant vesicle types) in the gastrointestinal tract (1, 13, 15).

Attempts to relate these profile types to the various putative neurotransmitters have been largely unsuccessful to date (see (9)—Vol. 1 of this series), and the question is complicated by the growing evidence that different transmitters may co-exist within the same nerve terminals (see 5, 18).

Preparative procedures will need to be developed that give high quality electronmicrographs of nerve profiles following the application of specific cytochemical reactions for putative transmitters and associated enzymes, before this problem can be resolved.

### 2) The localisation, roles and interactions of different enteric nerve types

The combination of surgical experiments, designed to work out the projections of enteric neurones containing different substances, and pharmacology, have allowed some speculations to be made about the effector sites for different nerve types (10, 14).

Figure 1 summarises the current situation as I

see it, the shaded squares indicating those roles best supported by existing data (8, 10, 12, 14, 16, 17, 19, 26). Thus, there is growing evidence for: 5-HT in excitatory interneurones; enkephalin in inhibitory interneurones; ATP in intrinsic non-adrenergic inhibitory nerves to smooth muscle; substance P in non-cholinergic excitatory nerves to smooth muscle and perhaps some sensory nerves; VIP in vasodilator nerves and nerves supplying mucosal secretory cells and perhaps some sphincters. In addition, several substances including ATP, 5-HT, dopamine and enkephalin are known to modulate release of acetylcholine and noradrenaline and there is evidence suggestive of axoaxonic interactions.

The culture methods recently developed in our laboratory for growing myenteric and submucous plexuses have much to offer to help distinguish the various roles and interactions on non-adrenergic, non-cholinergic transmitters (20, 21). First, the neurones are denervated of fibres arising from neurones in the other ganglionated enteric plexus as well as of both extrinsic parasympathetic and sympathetic nerve connexions. Secondly, the nerve cells are easy to penetrate with micro-electrodes because the glial and satellite cells migrate away from the surface. They can then be recognised by their membrane characteristics and their responses to ionophoretic application of putative transmitters, and they can be identified morphologically following injection with horseradish peroxidase (HRP). Thirdly, they provide convenient monolayer preparations for immunohistochemical, autoradiographical and ultrastructural analysis.

### 3) Neurochemical differentiation of transmitters

The question of the factor or factors that determine the time and direction of differentiation of neurotransmitters is of considerable interest. All cells contain the genetic machinery to produce all transmitters, but normally they are programmed to utilize one or perhaps a few substances as chemical messengers. Considerable progress has been made in recent years in understanding the neurochemical differentiation of sympathetic nerves into adrenergic or cholinergic forms (3, 6, 25), but much less is known of the factors

controlling differentiation of the different neurone types in the gut.

Both the ingenious in vivo system of Le Douarin and her colleagues (see 24) and the in vitro system described by my colleague Kristjan Jessen at this meeting (20, 22) seem to offer opportunities to further our understanding of this problem.

### 4) Central control mechanisms

There is a need to extend our knowledge of the autonomic centres in the central nervous system that modulate the intramural reflex activity of the gut (see 2), as well as the roles of both classical afferent nerve fibres supplying the gut with their cell bodies in the dorsal root ganglia, and the special intramural sensory neurons within the gut wall.

### REFERENCES

1. Baumgarten HG, Holstein AF, Owman CH. Z. Zellforsch 1970, 106, 376–397
2. Brooks FP, Evers PW (eds), Nerves and the Gut. Charles B Slack Inc, New Jersey 1977
3. Bunge R, Johnson M, Ross CD. Science 1978, 199, 1409–1416
4. Burnstock G. Pharmacol Rev 1972, 24, 509–581
5. Burnstock G. Neuroscience 1976, 1, 239–248
6. Burnstock G. Prog. Neurobiol 1978, 11, 205–222
7. Burnstock G. pp 3–32 in Baer HP, Drummond GI (eds), Physiological and Regulatory Functions of Adenosine and Adenine Nucleotides. Raven Press, New York 1979
8. Burnstock G. J Physiol (Lond) 1981, 313, 1–35
9. Burnstock G. Scand J Gastroent 1981, 16, Suppl 70, 1–9
10. Burnstock G. in Cytochemical Methods in Neuroanatomy. Alan Liss, New York 1981, in press
11. Burnstock G, Campbell G, Bennett M, Holman ME. Int J Neuropharmacol 1964, 3, 163–166
12. Burnstock G, Hökfelt T, Gershon MD, Iversen LL, Kosterlitz HW, Szurszewski JH. Neurosciences Res Prog Bull 1979, 17, (3), MIT Press, Boston
13. Cook RD, Burstock G. I Neuronal elements J Neurocytol 1976, 5, 171–194
14. Furness JB, Costa M. Neuroscience 1980, 5, 1–20
15. Gabella G. J Anat 1972, 111, 69–97
16. Gabella G. pp 197–241 in Physiology of the Gastrointestinal Tract. Johnson LR (ed), Raven Press, New York 1981
17. Gershon MD. Ann Rev Neurosci 1981, 5, 1–20
18. Hökfelt T, Lundberg JM, Schultzberg M, Johnsson O, Skirboll L, Änggard A, Fredholm B, Hamberger B, Pernow B, Rehfeld J, Goldstein M. Proc Roy Soc Lond B 1980, 210, 63–77
19. Hökfelt T, Johansson O, Ljungdahl A, Lundberg

JM, Schultzberg M. Nature (Lond) 1980, 284, 515–521

20. Jessen KR, McConnell JD, Purves RD, Burstock G, Chamley-Campbell J. Brain Res 1978, 152, 573–579
21. Jessen KR, Mirsky R, Dennison M, Burstock G. Nature (Lond) 1979, 281, 71–74
22. Jessen KR, Saffrey MJ, Van Noorden S, Bloom SR, Polak JM, Burnstock G. Neuroscience 1980, 5, 1717–1735
23. Langley JN. The Autonomic Nervous System Part I W Heffer Cambridge 1981
24. Le Douarin N. pp 19–46 in Elliot K, Lawrenson G (eds), Development of the Autonomic Nervous System, Ciba Foundation Symposium 83. Pitman Medical, London 1981
25. Patterson PH. Ann Rev Neurosci 1978, 1, 1–17
26. Polak JM, Bloom SR. Invest Cell Path 1978, 1, 301–326

# Adaptation
## Pathophysiology of Intestinal Response to Disease

# Introduction

## "L'intelligence, c'est l'adaptation"

C. C. BOOTH
Clinical Research Centre, Watford Road, Harrow, Middx. HA1 3UJ, England

The ability to absorb substances from the external environment is vital to living organisms. In primitive unicellular organisms it is this ability, together with the capacity for cell division, that differentiates living matter from the inanimate.

In mammals the absorption of nutrients has become specifically the function of the small intestine, and it is on the adequate function of this organ that growth, development, intellectual activity and reproductive performance depends. There is in addition an important relationship between nutrient intake and absorption. Even if absorptive capacity may be seriously compromised, overall absorption may be sufficient to maintain the integrity of the organism if the nutrient intake is sufficiently high. Conversely, there are situations in which nutrient intake may be severely limited. Under such circumstances, absorptive capacity may be markedly enhanced.

This capacity to adapt to external circumstances is clearly fundamental to living organisms. Without adaptation, no species develops and it is the failure to adapt that leads to the elimination of the species. It is therefore not surprising that the intestine, which represents the most intimate interface between the *milieux extérieur* and *intérieur*, has a remarkable capacity to adapt to environmental changes. Adaptation, or changes in intestinal structure and function, occurs in response to three main situations—changes in the diet, changes in the structure of the intestine as a result of surgical intervention or disease, or changes in hormonal status.

Dietary change may include hyperalimentation and hyperphagia, semistarvation or starvation, and may involve either selected nutrients or the entire caloric intake. Hyperalimentation may result both in increase in villous size of the small intestine and increase in intestinal function. Conversely, total starvation, or the deprivation of a segment of intestine from the nutrients in the luminal contents, may result in intestinal atrophy and reduction in absorptive function. Perhaps the most interesting response to dietary change is that produced by semistarvation, either in terms of total calories, or as a result of selective restriction of nutrient intake. In iron deficiency or when there is a lower calcium intake, for example, the intestine adapts by markedly increasing its absorption and this response occurs without significant morphological change. It would perhaps be expected that in the total absence of the substrate requiring absorption the mechanism for that absorption may be reduced. It is of immensely greater interest that the mere reduction in substrate results in an increase in absorptive capacity. The precise mechanism, however, whereby a reduction in substrate results in an increased capacity of the mechanism for absorption of that substrate is at present uncertain but it should not be beyond the ingenuity of modern research techniques to elucidate these events.

Surgical interference with the small intestine has provided a model for the study of adaptive changes since the middle of the nineteenth century. Both resection and bypass operations have been carried out and enlarged villi have been particularly seen to develop following partial resection of the small intestine. Subsequent work using models of intestinal resection in parabiotic animals, or in those in whom a cross circulation was created, have suggested that the adaptive responses, which involve increase in villous height, could be due to hormonal mechanisms. Theoretically, however, such a hypothesis is unattractive. When surface membranes are partially removed in other areas of the body's integument there is normally no adaptive hypertrophic response in other areas. In the dermis, for example, the removal of a section of skin does not enhance cell turnover or production rate anywhere else than locally at the site of the lesion and the same is true for both stomach and colon. It would therefore be curiously unique if removal of sections of small intestine alone resulted in villous hyperplasia. It was the work of the Hammersmith group that first showed that there was probably a response to something other than resection going on after partial resection of the small intestine (1). In the first place, it was demonstrated that the jejunal response following ileal resection was markedly less than the ileal response after jejunal resection. Subsequent studies showed that even when there was no resection but the ileum was simply transposed to the position of the jejunum and the jejunum to that of the ileum, the same degree of ileal hyperplasia would occur (2). This led to the proposal that in fact it was the caloric value of luminal contents reaching the transposed ileum that was important in producing the adaptive response, comparable to that occurring in hyperalimentation or hyperphagia in experimental animals. The term 'topical nutrition' was used to describe this phenomenon, which was thought to be predominantly independent of hormonal influences.

Nevertheless, it had been clear for a long time that hormonal influences could produce changes in small intestinal function (3). Both thyroid hormone and cortisone influence intestinal function, and there is evidence to suggest an effect of insulin. Pregnancy and lactation are also situations where it has been suggested that hormones may influence both structure and function of the intestine (4). Whether growth hormone produces intestinal hyperplasia has not hitherto been clearly established. It was a piece of clinical serendipity that necessitated a radical rethink of the Hammersmith position. A patient was referred to the Gastroenterology Department at Hammersmith Hospital for investigation of a curious illness associated with hair loss, skin rash, oedema, abdominal distension and obstinate constipation. The patient was ultimately shown to have a tumour of the kidney producing the gut type of glucagon, and jejunal biopsy showed that the villi were markedly hypertrophic. The villi returned to normal following successful removal

of the tumour (5). Enteroglucagon has not yet been shown to have direct trophic effects on the small intestinal mucosa but it seems likely that regulatory peptides may influence intestinal growth and changes in circulating peptides may be related to the adaptive response that occurs both after resection of the intestine and in coeliac disease, a condition in which the ileum adapts to the severe malabsorption in the jejunum. The explosion of our knowledge of the gut hormones has resulted in an enormous expansion of our knowledge in this field even if it has not yet enhanced our comprehension of adaptive phenomena.

This Symposium provides a valuable forum for the interchange of ideas between those involved in the whole field of intestinal adaptation. There are to be sections on morphology and function, together with discussion of mechanisms of regulation, as well as of clinical situations where adaptive responses are important.

Whether there is anyone at this Symposium who can tell me how it is that a villus whose cells turn over every two to three days throughout life remains precisely the same length and size throughout the whole of a life span of three score years and ten I do not know. One of the most important things we have to understand, however, in studying how villi undergo morphological changes during adaptation, is what determines mitosis in the cells of the crypts of Lieberkühn. If you remove a villus tip, do you get a burst of mitosis in the crypts associated with that villus? All our current notions of cell turnover suggest that you should. But if this is so, what is it about the removal or damage to cells at the tip of a villus that encourages mitosis of cells in the crypt far beneath its base?

## REFERENCES

1. Booth CC, Evans KT, Menzies T, Street DF. Brit J Surg 1959, 46, 403–410
2. Dowling RH, Booth CC. Clin Sci 1967, 32, 139–149
3. Levin RJ. J Endocrinol 1969, 45, 315–348
4. Fell BF, Campell RM. In Intestinal Adaptation, Schattauer Verlag, Stuttgart-New York, 1974, pp 227–237
5. Gleeson MH, Bloom SR, Polak JM, Henry K, Dowling RH. Gut 1971, 12, 773–782

# The Experimental Analysis of Changes in Proliferative and Morphological Status in Studies on the Intestine

N. A. WRIGHT
Department of Histopathology, Royal Postgraduate Medical School,
Hammersmith Hospital, Ducane Road, LondonW12 0HS, U.K.

Two of the mainstays of the study of intestinal adaptation are morphological and cell kinetic methods; however, an analysis of many current techniques for the assessment of intestinal proliferation and morphological status reveals that few methods are robust enough to withstand critical examination. It is essential that investigators in this field think critically about what to measure before investing time and effort in complex experiments which need such morphokinetic end points. This article sets out briefly a methodology which appears to offer most in accuracy and precision and to be suitable for critical morphokinetic analysis in intestinal adaptation.

*N. A. Wright, Dept. of Histopathology, Royal Postgraduate Medical School, Hammersmith Hospital, Ducane Road, London W12 0HS, U.K.*

In recent years there has been a remarkable increase in interest in the study of the mechanisms and phenomena of intestinal adaptation, and essential to such studies is the assessment of proliferative and morphological changes by which this adaptation can be detected. One of the most prominent features of intestinal adaptation after resection is an increase in the rate of crypt cell production and an increase in the size of the component parts of the intestinal mucosa, namely the crypts and the villi. Consequently many investigators have concentrated on measuring the results of this change without giving a great deal of thought to the measurements which ought to be made. On the other hand, cell kinetics and morphometric measurements can be difficult. It is especially hard for investigators, who need to maintain a wide appreciation of intestinal adaptation, not only from the viewpoint of morphology and cell proliferation, but also from the functional aspect, to choose the most appropriate measurements from among the many available. There is no point in performing highly sophisticated adaptation experiments if the results used to assess the induced changes are inappropriate or cannot withstand critical scrutiny. This paper looks briefly at the available methods and attempts to analyse their strengths and weaknesses and,

finally, a methodology, which appears to withstand critical evaluation, is proposed for the simultaneous assessment of proliferative and morphological status in the intestine.

## METHODS FOR THE ASSESSMENT OF SMALL INTESTINAL MORPHOLOGY

The small intestine has a complex three-dimensional configuration and, consequently, presents many problems in the study of its quantitative morphology. Investigators often want to correlate structure with function and, in this respect, the most important part of the epithelium is the villus, which houses functional cells. Thus, investigators often wish to know the size of the villus cell population and also the number of cells in the crypt. Such information is important when studying intestinal growth after resection (12) or after putative trophic hormone action (11, 16).

The size of the villus or crypt population is a difficult parameter to measure with accuracy and precision and so most investigators have relied upon an indirect estimator, in the unproven hope that it is equivalent to the epithelial cell population size. There are two types of measurements which have been frequently used; firstly morphometric measurements, usually made in sections, and secondly, estimation of the total or mucosal DNA content of the intestine. In the first instance, measurements made in sections have included the height of the villus (15, 21) or the number of cells in vertical, well orientated villus sections, sometimes dignified by the term 'the villus row count' (7, 18). It is usually assumed that these measurements reflect the number of cells present on the villus. It is implicit in such an assumption that all villi are the same shape, do not change their shape during the experimental manoeuvre and possibly, if all villi were finger shaped, this hope might be vindicated. Unfortunately, both rodent and human villi are notoriously variable in shape, not only changing between normal and experimental conditions, but also varying in shape with position in the intestine. In addition to this problem, there are technical factors such as bending or distortion of the villus during sectioning, the fact that the lamina propria of the villus contains smooth muscle fully capable of contracting and, additionally, the bias inherent in counting nuclei in microtome sections (4).

Perhaps the only way of showing what these measurements mean is by checking them against an absolute measurement of the villus cell population size, in both normal and abnormal conditions. This has in fact been done, in both animals (2, 23, 25) and man (9, 29). The method used consists of bulk staining of the intestinal tissue with the Feulgen technique, followed by micro-

dissection and counting of epithelial cells in carefully squashed villi and crypts. Table I shows the standard errors of the mean villus cell population. These values are small compared with the mean values at each site. Moreover, the standard deviation of individual sample measurements (Table I) obtained from replicate counts on the same villus, is small compared to the within animal variation. Additionally, in animals kept under standardised conditions there are no significant between animal variations. Consequently, this method does allow absolute values to be obtained with considerable precision.

It is a convenient fact that, in both rat and mouse small intestine, there is a proximodistal linear gradient in the villus size from duodenum to terminal ileum and use can be made of this in comparing the size of the villus population with the various morphometric measurements in the control, normal animal. In abnormal states, the morphometric measurements can be compared with villus population size in abnormally shaped villi, seen in the intestine undergoing regeneration after cytotoxic drug treatment. The appropriate method of comparison is by linear regression with least squares approximation. Table II shows the sample correlation coefficients for both groups. In normal villi, villus height and row count are highly correlated with the villus population and this correlation can be improved upon by product estimators, by combining a length with a width

Table I. Sample standard errors of measurements of the mean villus cell population compared with the sample error measurements of individual villus cell populations for control animals.

| | Position/Animal† | 1 | 2 | 3 | 4 | 5 |
|---|---|---|---|---|---|---|
| Sample standard errors of mean villus population* | A | 350.1 | 183.2 | 236.4 | 218.1 | 75.5 |
| | B | 568.2 | 338.5 | 192.7 | 157.0 | 61.4 |
| | C | 489.4 | 286.1 | 215.2 | 230.8 | 75.8 |
| Sample error measurement: standard deviation of villus cell populations‡ | A | 164.2 | 93.6 | 39.6 | 78.7 | 28.0 |
| | B | 173.6 | 158.7 | 48.0 | 31.8 | 26.1 |
| | C | 122.9 | 103.6 | 55.3 | 32.9 | 14.5 |

* Obtained from measurements of the villus cell population in a sample of 10 villi from each site per animal.
† These refer to bowel positions: 1, 0%; 2, 25%; 3, 50%; 4, 75%; 5, 100%.
‡ Obtained from 5 replicate counts on the same villus squash.

Table II. Sample correlations of measured morphometric variables with the villus cell population in the mouse small intestine.

| Number | Variable | Sample correlations Control | Experimental (ara-C treated) |
|---|---|---|---|
| 1 | Position | 0.984 | |
| 2 | Row count | 0.836 | 0.653 |
| 3 | Height | 0.843 | 0.619 |
| 4 | Core height | 0.840 | 0.616 |
| 5 | Maximum width | 0.422 | 0.501 |
| 6 | Maximum core width | 0.142 | 0.0716 |
| 7 | Basal width | 0.762 | 0.554 |
| 8 | Basal core width | 0.166 | 0.151 |
| 9 | Basal column count | 0.845 | 0.0819 |
| 10 | (max and min) basal diameter | 0.700 | 0.315 |
| 11 | (max and min) core diameter | 0.660 | 0.422 |
| 12 | Height and max width | 0.927 | 0.579 |
| 13 | Height and basal width | 0.846 | 0.656 |
| 14 | Height and basal count | 0.962 | 0.0587 |
| 15 | Height (max and min) core diameter | 0.888 | 0.459 |
| 16 | Row count and max width | 0.961 | 0.299 |
| 17 | Row count and basal width | 0.950 | 0.560 |
| 18 | Row count and basal count | 0.942 | 0.706 |
| 19 | Core height and basal width | 0.934 | 0.609 |
| 20 | Core height and max width | 0.947 | 0.646 |
| 21 | Core height and basal count | 0.961 | 0.734 |
| 22 | Core height and (mas and min) core diam. | 0.910 | 0.292 |
| 23 | Height (max and min) basal diameter | 0.957 | 0.572 |

parameter. However, in abnormally shaped villi, correlation coefficients are smaller and analysis of variance on the linear regression shows significant departure from linearity. In most instances, the slopes of the line differ between the two groups. It would appear that, in experimental material, the use of morphometric estimators of the villus cell population cannot be recommended where there is variation in villus shape. In human villi, results are disparate; Zucoloto et al. (29), analysing both normally shaped villi and abnormally shaped villi in gluten challenged coeliac patients, found that comparison of cell population and villus height revealed no correlation. However, Ferguson et al. (9) have claimed a good correlation between the height of human villi measured in microdissected specimens and the villus population. Further work is evidently needed in this sphere, but it should be emphasised that those workers who do use linear measurements should show that such measurements are meaningful before drawing conclusions from them.

The second measurement is that of DNA content. In this method the total amount of DNA in a bowel segment or the DNA in mucosal scrapings from a defined length of bowel (11, 16, 22) is measured and used as an estimate of the cell mass.

The essential parameter is the amount of epithelial DNA, but these crude estimates will include the not inconsiderable amounts of DNA present in lymphoid cells in the lamina propria. Therefore, it is assumed that the lymphoid cell populations are not different in experimental and control groups. However, it is well known that disordered bowel function and/or flora initiated by experimental manoeuvres, could well modify the numbers of lymphoid cells. Again, for accurate work, this method should be modified by following the procedure of Altmann (3), in which the total amount of DNA was measured and the amount of epithelial DNA was estimated by multiplying the DNA content by the fraction of tissue sections occupied by epithelial cells. However, most workers do not bother with this step, which has yet to be checked against absolute measurements.

## PROLIFERATIVE STATUS

What is usually required from a measurement of proliferative status? The majority of people want to know if the rate of cell proliferation is increased or decreased by any experimental or clinical manoeuvre. This is a very simple question to state, but extremely difficult to answer (2). It is germane to the argument to enquire as to what defines the rate of cell production in the intestine. Fig. 1 shows the various parameters which must be appreciated before all the different facets of cell production in any proliferative unit in the gastrointestinal tract can be understood. The three factors which together make up the cell production rate (in the small intestine this would be the crypt cell production rate) are *the cell cycle time* (the duration of the cell cycle or the interval between two successive divisions of a proliferating cell), *the growth fraction,* (that portion of the cell population which is devoted to proliferation) and the *cell population size,* (the number of cells in the proliferative unit, which in the small intestine is the crypt). The crypt cell production rate could be increased by a reduction in the cell cycle time (i.e. an increase in the rate at which cells traverse the cell cycle), an increase in the growth fraction (or relative number of proliferating cells) and thirdly by an increase in the number of cells in the crypt. There are experimental and clinical situations where all of these changes occur to both

increase and decrease the crypt cell production rate (2).

However, in the small intestine, this is only half the argument. Unfortunately, the final arbiter of cell proliferation is not even the crypt cell production rate, since, because of the complex three-dimensional structure, it is known that villi receive cells from several crypts, i.e. there is a crypt:villus ratio in excess of one. In the jejenum of rat, mouse and man, the crypt villus ratio is 30 to 1, 11 to 1 and 6 to 1 respectively (2). Consequently, in order to know the number of cells moving into the functional compartment (the net villus influx) the product of the crypt cell production rate and the crypt:villus ratio would have to be taken. Omission of such a measurement could lead to a serious anomaly if an experimental or clinical manoeuvre led to changes in the crypt:villus ratio.

These considerations may seem self evident but it is interesting to note the various short cuts that investigators have tried to use to measure the rate of cell production in the intestine. Few workers in fact measure the crypt cell production rate or net villus influx (but see Clarke (6)), and again, investigators have relied upon indirect measurements. These include *the incorporation of tritiated thymidine into DNA.* This has been widely used as a measurement of DNA synthesis in the gut (11) and, of course, is readily and rapidly measured by liquid scintillation counting. It is usual to express the amount of incorporated tritiated thymidine as the specific activity of extracted DNA, although some workers do express the measurement as radioactivity per mg wet weight or per mg of protein (17), although this could incur further inaccuracies because of changes in cell number. However, it has become increasingly apparent over recent years that there are large numbers of actual and potential errors associated with this technique, which have been aptly summarised by Maurer (2, 13, 14), and there are numerous assumptions that must be made before this measurement becomes a definitive proliferative parameter. Thus, it is necessary to assume that there is no change in a) the activity of either thymidine kinase or thymidine synthetase, b) the size of the endogenous thymidine pool, caused

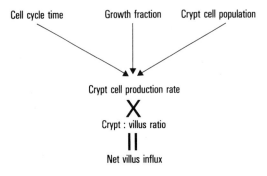

Fig. 1. The components of the crypt cell production rate and net villus influx in the intestine.

by the experimental manoeuvre, and c) the uptake of precursor and transport of thymidine across the cell membrane. Numerous other *caveats* are necessary with this method (13). In fact, the amount of work required to make this a definitive measurement, i.e. measurement of all the above variables, would make the technique extremely tedious. There is the additional problem that the scintillation counting of whole blocks of tissue can be criticised because there are numerous other cell populations in the intestine apart from the target epithelial cell production, particularly the lymphoid infiltrate in the lamina propria, which contains cells fully capable of dividing and incorporating tritiated thymidine (6). This objection can, in fact, be overcome by measuring tritiated thymidine incorporation into whole, microdissected crypts (19), but the *caveats* listed above will still apply. Consequently, this technique does not have a great deal of future as a definitive measurement of crypt cell production.

Other measurements which have been used include the mitotic and flash thymidine labelling indices, which give the proportion of cells undergoing mitosis and DNA synthesis, respectively. These measurements have the distinct advantage that the counts are confined to the epithelial component of the intestine, but the limitations of these methods include the fact that these are state parameters, merely reflecting the fraction of cells in mitosis and DNA synthesis and changes in the duration of the phases would also alter the index. There are also problems in counting cells in tissue sections (4); the factors which affect thymidine availability and incorporation could also modify the labelling index.

Of course, measurement of the three parameters which are the components of the crypt cell production rate could provide a definitive estimator of cell proliferation. However, measurement of the cell cycle time by the fraction of labelled mitoses method is a very time consuming procedure; in the small intestine this will take at least 16 hours. It is thus remarkably time dependent and not suitable for detecting rapid changes in proliferative rate. There are several other assumptions implicit in this method, not all of which can be assumed to be operative in the

small intestine in experimental circumstances (2), and besides, the method is very expensive in terms of counting procedure, autoradiography, exposure time and animal number. At the same time, the growth fraction would have to be measured, either from the fraction of labelled mitoses curve (1) or from the distribution of labelled cells in autoradiographs of the crypt. In addition to this, these measurements also require a measurement of crypt cell population, which would necessitate microdissection and squashing and the counting of component crypt cells. All of this would make the series of measurements, i.e. cell cycle time, growth fraction and crypt population, extremely cumbersome and really inappropriate for routine use.

Some investigators have measured the migration rate of labelled cells in the villus and have proposed this as a suitable estimator of the rate of cell proliferation. Unfortunately, the migration rate (more properly called the transit rate) on the villus is not only proportional to the transit time, but also to the size of the villus population. If the migration rate was the sole parameter for comparing proliferative rates between two experimental groups, it would be necessary to assume that the size of the villus population was unchanged between the two groups, or to measure it. In this respect, measurements of the transit time in the villus population are also very much time dependent, and, in point of fact, it is very difficult to obtain an estimate of the mean or median transit time through the villus epithelium (26).

Still other investigators have relied on the measurement of the rate of mucosal cell exfoliation into the lumen, as evidenced by the amount of DNA lost into the lumen which can be measured in bowel perfusates (8). This method has been used mainly in man but it has been adapted for use in animals (10). However, exfoliated cells are trapped in the mucus overlying the villus tips and, consequently, the number of cells removed is proportional to the perfusion pressure (6).

In addition, there is the distinct probability that some of the cells will be non-epithelial in nature. In fact, Croft et al. (8) showed that some 15%

of cells are non-epithelial and, of course, experimental manoeuvres could change this proportion.

## A PROPOSED METHODOLOGY

In the assessment of proliferative status, the measurement of a rate parameter has intrinsic attractiveness. Rate measurements are available at several points in the cell cycle and perhaps the most appropriate measurement is the birth rate or rate of production of new cells. The most readily available method is the metaphase arrest, or stathmokinetic, technique in which the ability of certain drugs, such as vincristine, to arrest cells in metaphase is used to measure the rate of entry of cells into mitosis. Since each mitosis results in the net production of one cell, the rate of entry into mitosis reflects the birth rate of new cells. The metaphase arrest method has found wide usage in the gut, mainly in histological sections (27), but, as is evident from Fig. 1, a better denominator would be the proliferative unit, i.e. the number of cells produced per crypt per hour. Since the birth rate summarises the growth fraction and the cell cycle time when it is expressed on a *per crypt* basis, as the crypt cell production rate, this will compensate for cell population changes (see Fig. 1). Measurement of crypt cell production rate can be achieved by combining the metaphase arrest method with microdissection (5, 26). There are several advantages of this method; a) the method gives the crypt cell production rate; the crypt:villus ratio can be measured on the same material, allowing the net villus influx to be calculated, which would detect any three-dimensional changes; b) the precision of the crypt cell production rate estimate is definable in terms of the confidence interval of the slope of the regression line (see Tables III and IV), and it is readily comparable with other experimental groups; c) there are no hidden errors from the use of sectioned material; d) measurements are completed over a period of $2\frac{1}{2}/3$ hours, allowing ephemeral responses to be monitored; e) the method is economical in terms of animals and counting time, adequate precision being achieved by counting 10 crypts per reading; f) the method can be used in man (28); g) the method compares well with the apparently more sophisticated tritiated thymidine autoradiographic methods. Table IV shows that estimates of birth rate obtained used the two methods of measuring the crypt cell production rate are in good agreement.

There are of course, several practical points to bear in mind (24). These include the use of the optimal dosage of the agent, which in rats and mice is 1 mg per kg of body weight for the small intestine, the avoidance of any delay period before metaphase arrest is complete, proof of linearity of metaphase correction by taking serial readings over the experimental period and avoidance of metaphase degeneration, since a prolonged experimental period invites degeneration and loss of arrested metaphases, with consequent underestimation of the crypt cell production rate. In the mouse gut this appears to begin after $2\frac{1}{2}$ hours (1) and thus the experimental period should not be longer than 2/3 hours. Finally, the

Table III. A comparison between birth rate ($K_B$) in the intestine as measured by the metaphase arrest method and by tritiated thymidine ($^3$HTdR)

| | | cells/1000 cells/hr | |
| Tissue | Kinetic state | metaphase arrest $K_B$ | $^3$HTdR $K_B$ |
|---|---|---|---|
| mouse jejunum | normal | 52 | 49 |
| mouse jejunum | 15 hr after ara-C | 73 | 83 |
| rat jejunum | normal | 72 | 55 |
| rat jejunum | 90 hr starvation | 38 | 38 |
| rat jejunum | 15 hr after hydroxyurea | 63 | 62 |
| mouse ascending colon | normal | 26 | 19 |
| mouse transverse colon | normal | 13 | 14 |
| mouse descending colon | normal | 16 | 16 |
| mouse rectum | normal | 18 | 20 |

Table IV. Crypt Cell Production Rates (CCPR) as measured by different methods

| Rat | CCPR (cells/crypt/hr) |
|---|---|
| (i) metaphase arrest method | 35 |
| (ii) $K_B = I_m/t_m \cdot N_p$ | 32.4 |
| (iii) $K_B = I_p/T_c \cdot N_c$ | 35.6 |
| (iv) double labelling (Clarke 1971) | 32 |

| Mouse | |
|---|---|
| (i) metaphase arrest method | 13.7 |
| (ii) $K_B = I_m/t_m \cdot N_p$ | 14.5 |
| (iii) $K_B = I_p/T_c \cdot N_c$ | 13.8 |

$K_B$ = birth rate; $I_m$ = mitotic index; $t_m$ = mitotic duration; $N_p$ = number of proliferative cells; $I_p$ = growth fraction; $T_c$ = cell cycle time; $N_c$ = total crypt cell number.

correct line for the data should be fitted. Since in this instance the whole crypt is being considered and the age distribution is rectangular (20), routine regression analysis with least squares approximation is appropriate.

It is evident that, when used correctly, this method fits the requirements of a suitable procedure for the assessment of proliferative status of the intestine. Combined with the measurement of the crypt:villus ratio, the influx onto the villus can be assessed with both accuracy and precision. It possesses few if any of the numerous deficiencies of indirect methods and would appear to be the method of choice for use in the assessment of proliferative status in the field of intestinal adaptation.

At the same time, using the microdissection method, it would be possible to measure the numbers of cells in the various compartments, i.e. the crypts and villi in the small intestine. In this respect, it should perhaps be emphasised that measurements such as villus length or row count cannot be used even to provide data of relative worth, unless it is shown that, in the relevant experimental situation, these measurements do correlate with the number of cells per villus. If villus shape varies, they are unlikely to.

## CONCLUSIONS

Even within the environs of this brief review, it is evident that there are numerous methods available for the assessment of morphological and proliferative status. Few of these methods with-

stand even superficial examination and it is considered very important that investigators think carefully before employing them in the assessment of these important aspects. The bottom line of this message is that, if inappropriate measurements are used, then often elegant experiments cannot yield robust conclusions and will have to be done again.

## REFERENCES

1. Aherne WA, Camplejohn RS, Wright NA. An introduction to cell population kinetics. Edward Arnold, 1977
2. Al-Mukhtar MY, Polak JM, Bloom SR, Wright NA. In 'Intestinal Adaptation' ed. Dowling H, Robinson W, 1982
3. Altmann GG. Am J Anat 1971, 132, 167–178
4. Clarke RM. J Roy Microscop Soc 1968, 88, 189–196
5. Clarke RM. Cell Tissue Kinet 1971, 4, 263–271
6. Clarke RM. Digestion 1973, 8, 161–175
7. Clarke RM. MD Thesis, Cambridge University 1975
8. Croft DN, Loehry CA, Taylor CFN, Cole J. Lancet, ii, 1968, 70–73
9. Ferguson A, Sutherland A, MacDonald TT, Allan F. J Clin Path 1977, 30, 1008–1073
10. Goldsmith DPJ. Digestion, 1973, 8, 130–141
11. Johnson LR, Guthrie PD. Gastroenterol 1974, 67, 453–459
12. McDermott FD. Gastroenterol 1976, 70, 707–711
13. Maurer HR. Cell Tissue Kinet 1981, 14, 111–120
14. Maurer HR, Laerum OD. In 'Chalones', ed. Houck JC, pp 331–349, North Holland, 1976
15. Menge H, Grafe M, Lorenz-Meyer H, Reiken EO. Gut 1975, 16, 468–472
16. Oscarson JEA, Veen HP, Williamson RCN, Ross JS, Malt RA. Gastroenterol 1977, 72, 890–895
17. Ryan GP, Dudrick SJ, Copeland EM, Johnson LR. Gastroenterol 1979, 27, 658–663
18. Sato F, Muramatsur S, Tsuchi S et al. Cell Tissue Kinet 1972, 5, 227–235

19. Sharp JG, Lipscomb HL, Cullen GE et al. In 'Cell Proliferation in the Gastrointestinal Tract', ed. Appleton DR, Sunter JP, Watson AJ pp. 66–88. Pitman Medical 1980.

20. Steel GG. Growth kinetics of tumours 1971, OUP

21. Tutton PJM. Control of epithelial cell proliferation in the small intestine—the villus longistat. J Anat 1978, 128, 68.

22. Williamson RCN, Bauer FLR, Ross P, Malt RA. Gastroenterol 1978, 74, 16–23

23. Wright NA. In 'Cell Proliferation in the Gastrointestinal Tract' ed. Appleton DR, Sunter JP, Watson AJ. pp 3–21. Pitman Medical 1980

24. Wright NA, Appleton DR. Cell Tissue Kinet 1980, 13, 643–662

25. Wright NA, Carter J, Irwin M. Cell Tissue Res 1982, (submitted)

26. Wright NA, Irwin M. Cell and Tissue Kinetics 1982, (In press)

27. Wright NA, Morley AR, Appleton DR. Cell Tissue Kinet 1972, 5, 521–534

28. Wright NA, Watson AJ, Morley AR et al. Gut 1973, 14, 603–606

29. Zucoloto S, Wright NA, Bramble M, Record C. Gut 1979, 20, 921

# Proliferative and Morphological Adaptation of the Intestine to Experimental Resection

W. R. HANSON
Department of Therapeutic Radiology;
Joint Appointment: Department of Dermatology,
Rush University, Presbyterian-St. Luke's Medical Centre,
Chicago, Illinois 60612, U.S.A.

The proliferative and morphological adaptation of the residual intestine following resection is briefly reviewed. Within days after a partial intestinal resection, the number of crypt cells increases. There is a proportional increase in the number of proliferative cells, thus there is no change in the growth fraction. Villus height and morphological complexity increases, particularly in the ileum. The thickness of the muscularis mucosae increases, most likely through an increase in cellularity. The size of the adaptive response is dependent on the amount of tissue removed.

The possibility of an adaptive change in the number and proliferative characteristics of rat intestinal stem cells was investigated using the microcolony assay (38). Regenerative foci of mucosal epithelium were quantitated as a function of $^{137}$Cs $\gamma$ ray irradiation in control or 30 days after a 60% resection of the combined jejunum and ileum. Hydroxyurea, (HU), an S phase cytotoxic agent was given to one group of control and one group of resected rats five minutes before a single dose of radiation. HU had little effect on control jejunum or ileum, however, HU reduced the clonogenic cell survival by over tenfold in resected animals which implies a post-resection change in the intestinal stem cell age distribution. The radiation dose-survival curve of clonogenic cells was shifted to the right after resection compared to control values. These results suggest that an increase in intestinal stem cell number and a shift in the proliferative characteristics (from slowly to rapidly cycling) occur as an adaptive response to intestinal resection.

*Dr. Wayne R. Hanson, Director, Research Section, Department of Therapeutic Radiology, Rush-Presbyterian-St. Luke's Medical Centre, 1753 West Congress Parkway, Chicago, Illinois, 60612, U.S.A.*

## INTRODUCTION

Partial small bowel resections are required for a variety of pathological conditions such as volvulus, strangulated hernia, coeliac disease (18, 30) and radiation-induced fibrosis and stenosis after abdominal treatment for cancer (25). Intestinal resection is well tolerated in man due to the reserve functional capacity of the residual intestine and to the adaptive response which quickly increases functional capability. Many experimental perturbations of the intestinal cell renewal system such as irradiation (5, 6) or the administration of cytotoxic drugs (7, 12, 31) cause transient mucosal changes, however, intestinal resection produces a permanent alteration which is considered a true adaptive or compensatory response (3, 4, 19, 26, 34, 35). The proliferative and morphological alterations that occur in the residual intestine to partial resection have been widely studied mainly in rats using a variety of assays generally applicable to the study of cytokinetics of any tissue. However, the proliferative and morphological arrangement of the intestinal mucosa offers certain problems and challenges along with some advantages in the assessment of normal cytodynamics and the alterations that occur following partial resection of the small intestine.

In spite of the variety of techniques employed to study the phenomena of adaptation and the problems associated with each assay (See Wright, this symposium), there is general agreement.

## Crypt adaptation

Bizzozero (2) suggested in 1892 that cells produced in the crypt of Lieberkühn migrate towards the tips of villi to replace cells shed into the intestinal lumen. The details of this cell renewal process have been constantly refined as new biomedical techniques have become available. The introduction of the concept of the cell cycle (17) and autoradiographic techniques to determine cell cycle time (27) led to a refinement of the investigation of intestinal crypt cell production. One current concept of the epithelial cell renewal process is that a stem cell, perhaps a pluripotent cell analogous to the bone marrow colony forming unit—spleen or CFU-S (24), gives rise to an amplification division cell which is rapidly proliferating. A cell in this compartment may go through three or four divisions and reach about two-thirds of the way up the crypt before it differentiates beyond the capacity to proliferate under normal conditions and enters the non-dividing functional compartment as migration continues toward the tips of the villi.

The average cell cycle time of crypt epithelial cells in the amplification or proliferative compartment is about 11.5 hours in control or sham resected rats as measured by the per cent tritiated thymidine ($^3$HTdR) labeled mitosis method (13). Following partial resection, the cell cycle time is slightly but consistently reduced, mainly by a reduction in the S phase time of the cell cycle (13, 21). This alteration occurs both proximal and distal to the site of anastomosis. Although the reduction in cell cycle time is slight, the increase in total crypt cellularity and size of the proliferative compartment is great. These permanent increases, unrelated to surgical trauma began between two and four days post-resection (Figs. 1 and 2). The increase in crypt cellularity was complete by about 12 days post-resection but the size of the increase depended on the amount of tissue removed (14). In general, a small resection elicited a small but permanent response whereas a large resection produced a much larger change. In fact, the increase in crypt cellularity was nearly linear as the degree of resection increased. The number of S phase cells, which is representative of the proliferative compartment (since the

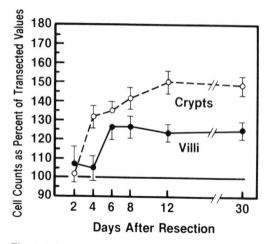

Fig. 1. Jejunal epithelial cell counts in crypts and villi at increasing times after a 70% resection expressed as a percentage of transected values. The 100% value for crypts = 36 cells ± 1.4 (1 S.E.M.). The 100% value for villi = 79 cells ± 4.8 (1 S.E.M.).

change in the cell cycle is slight after resection) increased proportionally, hence, there was no change in the per cent of labeled cells per crypt or the labeling index, no matter how much tissue was resected (14). Since the S phase time is about half the total cell cycle time, the number of labeled cells represents about half the crypt growth fraction, therefore, the crypt growth fraction is

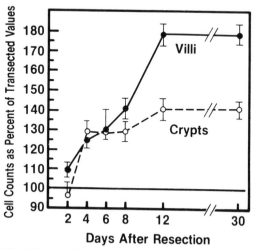

Fig. 2. Ileal epithelial cell counts in crypts and villi at increasing times after a 70% resection expressed as a percentage of transected values. The 100% crypt value = 33 cells ± 1.1 (1 S.E.M.) and the 100% value for villi = 45 cells ± 3.1 (1 S.E.M.).

unaltered by resection. The per cent mitotic index or number of mitotic figures per number of cells in the crypt section increased slightly, perhaps due to the slight decrease in total generation time of the proliferative cells. The measurements of total cells and labeled cells per crypt column (two-dimensional representations of complex three-dimensional changes) have been confirmed with appropriate three-dimensional techniques; for example, whole crypts have been microdissected (37) from control and resected rats killed one hour after a single injection or pulse label of $^3$HTdR. These crypts have been squashed to count the total number of cells per crypt. The results confirmed the increase in total cellularity after resection estimated by the measurement of cells per crypt column. From the same crypt squashes, autoradiographs confirmed not only the increase in the proliferative compartment, but also confirmed that the increase is proportional to the change in total cellularity, therefore, no change in the labeling index or crypt growth fraction occurred after partial resection. Changes in the proliferative compartment of microdissected crypts from control or resected animals were also measured by liquid scintillation counting of the amount of radioactive tritium expressed as the number of disintegrations per minute (DMP) per

crypt. However, to insure that a measured change in the radioactivity per crypt was not a result of a change in the incorporation of $^3$HTdR into individual S phase cells, the DPM per crypt was divided by the number of labeled cells per crypt squash autoradiograph to determine the DPM per labeled nuclei in both control and resected rats. There was no difference between the two and the DPM per crypt is therefore an accurate measure of the size of the proliferative compartment in crypts from both control or resected animals. The DMP per crypt increased in a step-wise fashion as the amount of resection was increased (Fig. 3). Further, the DPM per mg of dried intestinal tissue was obtained by liquid scintillation counting along with the total mg of small intestine tissue by weighing it directly. Using the following relationships first used by Hagemann (8) to estimate the total number of intestinal crypts in mice, the number of crypts per residual rat intestine was estimated for control and resected rats:

$$\frac{DPM}{mg \text{ of intestinal dry weight}} \times \frac{Crypts}{DPM} = \frac{\dfrac{Crypts}{}}{mg \text{ of intestinal dry weight}}$$

By measuring the total dry weight of the various areas of the residual intestine, for instance, the duodenum or jejunum + ileum, the total number of crypts in each area was calculated after increasing percentages of resection compared to values that would be expected if no increase in crypt number occurred. For example, if the partial resection was 50% of the combined jejunum and ileum, 50% fewer crypts would be expected in the residual jejunum and ileum if there were no change in intestinal crypt number in response to resection. However, duodenal crypt number would be expected to remain the same since none of this tissue was removed. Estimates of the number of crypts per duodenum did not change from control values of about $5 \times 10^5$ even after 80% partial resection whereas the number of crypts in the combined jejunum and ileum decreased by the same percentage as the per cent resection. Therefore, 30 days after a 50% resection of the combined jejunum and ileum, the crypt number

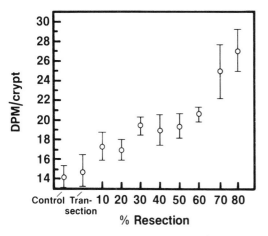

Fig. 3. Disintegrations per minute (DPM) per crypt microdissected from the mid-duodenum 30 days after no surgery (control), transection, or resection of increasing amounts of jejunum and ileum. Tissue was sampled 1 hour after the intravenous administration of tritiated thymidine.

was estimated at $2.4 \times 10^6$ crypts or about half the control value of $4.4 \times 10^6$ crypts.

To summarize the hyperplastic response of the residual intestinal crypts to partial resection; there is a rapid and permanent increases in total crypt cellularity, both proximal and distal to the anastomosis. The size of the increase is dependant on the amount of tissue removed. There is a proportional increase in the proliferative compartment, thus the growth fraction is unchanged no matter how much tissue is removed. The increase in crypt cellularity appears to reach a maximum by about day 12 post-resection (15) and remains in the new steady state apparently permanently. There is a slight decrease in the S phase of the cell cycle with a slight increase in the mitotic index. The frequency of labeled cells within the crypt measured as a function of cell position (crypt labeling profile) reflected only the change in the sizes of the crypt and the proliferative compartment. When the crypt profiles from resected rats were corrected for the size of the crypt and the size of the proliferative compartment, they were similar to control crypt profiles (14). The hyperplastic response of each crypt is independent of its position in the small intestine. The total number of crypts in each segment of intestine does not change in response to resection, thus the total number of crypts in the residual intestine is reduced by the same degree as the amount of resection.

## Villus adaptation

Contrary to the similarity of crypts from the duodenum or ileum, the normal morphology of villi depends on the location (1, 3, 4). Low power scanning electron micrographs of the luminal side of intestinal mucosa (Fig. 4) reflect the proximal (panel a)—distal (panel d) villus height gradient as do villus column cell counts from tissue sections (15). Column counts of the number of villus epithelial cells gradually fall from about 85 in the rat jejunum to about 40 in the lower ileum. This villus height gradient is maintained in isographs of fetal mouse duodenum compared to fetal ileum when sampled at various post-natal ages. The cephalad-caudal size gradient is also maintained

in germ-free mice (22) and rats (10). However, when the duodenal papilla was transplanted to the distal ileum, the ileal villi were transformed into jejunal-like villi (1). Furthermore, when a distal ileal segment with its own intact nerve and blood supply was inserted into the proximal jejunum, the ileal villi became similar to those in the surrounding jejunum (32). These results suggest both an inherent and an environmentally controlled morphology and point to the complexity of control mechanism. Intestinal resection in adult rats caused an increase in the size and height of villi but the amount of increase was dependent on the location as well as on the degree of resection (14). As in the crypts, a small resection elicited a small but rapid increase in epithelial cellularity and a large resection produced a large change. The increase in villus cellularity occurred rapidly after resection as measured by two-dimensional column counts or by three-dimensional villus squashes to count total villus cellularity and was complete by about day 12 post-resection (Figs. 1 and 2). It can be noted that there appears to be a delay in the response of the jejunal villi after resection compared to the crypt response (Fig. 1) however, in the ileum, both crypts and villi increase in size at nearly the same time, at least within the measurement limits of these experiments, (Fig. 2). The change was much greater in the ileum after resection than in the jejunum and obliterated the size gradient. The villus change was similar to the results obtained when an ileal segment was transposed to the jejunum (32). Low power scanning electron micrographs of jejunal villi (Fig. 4, panel e), compared to ileal villi, (panel h) 30 days after 60% mid small intestinal resection show great similarity in size and shape along with height.

When a segment of jejunum or ileum was removed from continuity and made into a Thiry-Vella fistula (16), the villi underwent atrophy as shown in Fig. 4, panels b and c. However, the fistulae of both the jejunal (panel f) and ileal (panel g) tissue responded to a 60% resection of the in situ intestine. The villi of the jejunal fistula in particular took on the appearance of the villi in the post-resection jejunum in continuity. These results, confirmed by Williamson & Bauer (36)

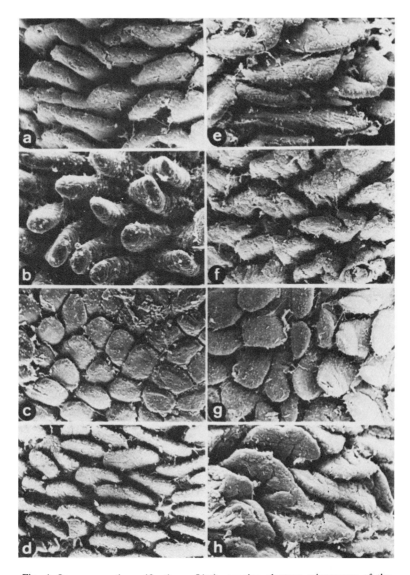

Fig. 4. Low power (magnification = 54×) scanning electron microscopy of the luminal surface of the small intestine: (a) normal jejunum, (b) jejunal fistula, (c) ileal fistula, (d) normal ileum, (e) jejunum after 60% resection (f) jejunal fistula after 60% resection (g) ileal fistula after 60% resection and (h) ileum after 60% resection. Tissues were sampled 30 days after surgery. (Reprinted from Hanson et al., Cell and Tissue Kinet (1977) 10, pp 543–555. (Courtesy Blackwell Publishing Co London.)

suggested a systemic factor in the adaptive response.

*Non-epithelial adaptation*

Most experimental attention has been given to the cell kinetics and morphology of the epithelial lining of the intestine, but what was described in the early literature as tissue hypertrophy as a response to resection was not only due to hyperplasia of crypts and villi but also hyperplasia of the muscle layers. The increased longitudinal and circular muscle thickness was likewise dependent on the amount of tissue removed. Direct measurements of cellularity were not made, but there was an impression that cellularity was increased and there was an increase in the number of rarely seen ³H labeled smooth muscle cells in tissue from resected animals killed one hour after a pulse label of ³HTdR (14).

One would assume that the elements of the lamina propria increase along with the size of the villi, but this aspect of intestinal adaptation has not received the appropriate attention due mainly to the difficulties of quantitative endpoints.

*Crypt stem cell adaptation*

There are many aspects of intestinal proliferative adaptation which have not been widely explored. One such area of interest in our laboratory is the adaptive response of the intestinal stem cell; the progenitor of the mucosal epithelium. Morphologically, the stem cell zone is toward the base of the crypt. Electron microscopy reveals characteristics within these cells ascribed to stem cells in general such as a scarcity of organelles and an abundance of free ribosomes (20). However, the normal proliferative characteristics of these cells and their role in the cell renewal process is not well understood. There is some evidence that crypt stem cells are few in number and proliferate slowly (11, 12, 29), characteristics that mask the stem cell population

from study by conventionally used cytokinetic methods (11). One indirect method of investigation is the microcolony assay described by Withers & Elkind (38). Intestinal stem cells that survive a large dose of radiation and maintain reproductive integrity form small regenerative foci of epithelium in the intestinal mucosa. Animals are killed about 4 days following whole body irradiation and after routine histology procedures, the number of microcolonies are counted per intestinal cross-section and plotted as a semi-log function of irradiation dose. The resulting dose-survival curve has a wide shoulder region followed by an exponential region. The basic assumptions attendant to this assay are 1) each microcolony comes from a single surviving stem cell (or clonogenic cell) and; 2) clonogenic cell survival is independent from the survival of other clonogenic cells, assumptions which are reasonable but difficult to test.

Using the indirect microcolony assay, the effect of intestinal resection on the proliferative characteristics of intestinal stem cells was investigated.

## MATERIALS AND METHODS

Male Charles Rivers CD rats, (Portage stock) weighing about 300 g were anesthetized with Sodium Pentabarbitol (40 mg/kg). Following a

Table I. Schedule of single ¹³⁷Csγ doses to indirectly assay the radiosensitivity and proliferative characteristics of rat intestinal stem cells before and after resection

| Irradiation Dose (Gy)† ¹³⁷Csγ | Control (no surgery) | Control +HU†† | Transection | 60% Resection | 60% Resection +HU |
|---|---|---|---|---|---|
| 0.0 | 4* | | | 4 | |
| 10.0 | 3 | | | | |
| 10.5 | 4 | | | | |
| 11.0 | 4 | 4 | 4 | | |
| 11.5 | 4 | | | 4 | |
| 12.0 | 4 | | 4 | 4 | 4 |
| 12.5 | 4 | | | 4 | |
| 13.0 | 4 | | | 4 | |
| 14.0 | 4 | | | 4 | |
| 15.0 | | | | 4 | |
| 16.0 | | | | 4 | |

† 1 Gray is an equivalent dose of radiation to 100 rad.
†† Hydroxyurea (0.5 mg/g body wt) was given within 5 min before the animals were irradiated.
* Number of animals at each dose of radiation.

midline laparotomy, 60% of the mid-portion of the combined jejunum and ileum was resected and the residual 20 cm of jejunum was anastomized to the 20 cm of ileum with 6–0 silk. A small cylinder of soluble gel-foam was inserted into the intestinal lumen and positioned perpendicular to the suture line at the time of intestinal closure to insure intestinal lumen continuity. The intestine was kept moist with warm saline throughout the procedure to prevent later adhesions. In a second group of animals, transections were performed by dividing the intestine midway between the ligament of Treitz and the cecum. The anastomosis of the two ends was performed as described for the resection group. The peritoneum and abdominal muscle layers were closed with 3–0 silk suture and the skin was closed with wound clips in both resected and transected rats. A third group of rats had no surgery.

About 30 days after transection or resection, animals of these two groups along with the third group (no surgery) were irradiated whole body with single doses of $^{137}$Cs gamma ($\gamma$) rays using the schedule in Table I.

Hydroxyurea (HU, 200 mg/average 400 g rat) an S phase specific cytotoxic agent (12, 28) was given to one group of 4 control animals and one group of 4 resected animals immediately before irradiation. Any clonogenic cells which were in the S phase of the cell cycle would be killed by the HU and the shoulder of the clonogenic survival curve would be reduced. If, however, there are few or no clonogenic cells in DNA synthesis, clonogenic cell survival at the selected radiation dose levels should be the same as without HU. By comparing the effect of HU on the clonogenic survival in control and resected animals a qualitative estimate of a shift in the stem cell age distribution due to resection was assayed. Jejunal and ileal tissue was taken from 4 unirradiated control and 4 resected rats and the number of crypts was counted per cross-section. Three and a half days after irradiation, rats were killed and proximal jejunum and distal ileum was sampled, fixed in alcohol, formalin and acetic acid (AFA) and processed for histology in such a way that cross-sections were obtained. The number of microcolonies in a minimum of 6 cross-sections

of tissue was counted and plotted on a semi-log scale versus irradiation dose.

## RESULTS

The surgical procedures were well tolerated; 2 transected and 1 resected animal died within 4 post-operative days. New animals were added in their place.

The number of crypts per intestinal cross-section in control animals was about 140 for both jejunum and ileum. In spite of the increased intestinal diameter after resection, the number of crypts per cross-section was unchanged at 140 in both jejunum and ileum, therefore, no correction factor was applied to the number of microcolonies per circumference and a direct comparison of clonogenic dose-survival curves was possible.

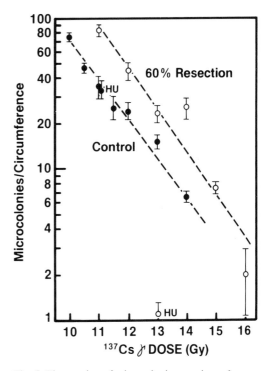

Fig. 5. The number of microcolonies per circumference of intestine versus dose of $^{137}$Cs$\gamma$ ray irradiation in control *jejunum* (●) or 30 days after 60% resection of the jejunum + ileum (○). The control single dose survival when HU was given 5 min before irradiation is shown (● HU) along with the single dose survival after HU in resected animals (○ HU). Mean ± S.E.M.

The radiation, dose-survival curves for the jejunum of resected compared to control rats is shown in Fig. 5. The control curve has a $D_0$ of about 1.67 Gy. The $D_0$ is defined as the radiation dose required to reduce clonogenic survival by 37% on the exponential portion of the curve. The clonogenic survival in the jejunum of animals having intestinal transections was the same as in control (no surgery) animals at the selected radiation doses (Table I). These values are not shown. The $D_0$ of the jejunal clonogenic cell survival curve was not greatly altered in resected animals (Fig. 5) however, the curve is shifted to the right. Hydroxyurea (HU) had little effect on the clonogenic cell survival in control animals (Fig. 5) however, HU reduced clonogenic survival by at least tenfold in resected animals.

Clonogenic cell survival in the ileum of control rats was greater than in control jejunum especially at lower doses of irradiation (Fig. 6). The control ileal $D_0$ appears to be lower (about 1.4 Gy) compared to the control jejunum, however, the scatter of the data does not allow a precise determination of the shoulder. It is clear, though, that the survival curve in the ileum is shifted to the right after resection and the $D_0$ remains about the same. HU had little effect on the single dose control survival, however, there was a greater than tenfold effect on the single dose cell survival after resection (Fig. 6).

## DISCUSSION

The permanent proliferative and morphological adaptation of the residual intestine to partial resection is multifaceted and complex. Along with the adaptive change briefly reviewed in the introduction, the results of the experiments outline in this report suggest that the number and proliferative characteristics of the intestinal stem cells are altered after resection.

The actual number of stem cells or clonogenic cells per crypt in the normal intestine is unknown and controversial. Analysis of split-dose or multi-fraction radiation survival curves gives a wide range of estimates from less than 20 (11, 12, 26) to over 150 (9, 23, 33) clonogenic cells per crypt. The higher estimates must include the rapidly proliferating amplification division cells. However, in experiments in which mice were given HU (12), high specific activity $^3$HTdR or prolonged colcemid treatment (11) to selectively kill the rapidly cycling crypt cells, results did not show any shift in the clonogenic dose-survival curve to the left. These results suggest that the rapidly cycling crypt cells are not clonogenic.

There has been no resolution to the apparent discrepancy of stem cell estimates given by multifraction radiation studies compared to deductions from observations of the effect of cytotoxic drugs and the stem cell number remains a mystery. However, a more precise estimate of stem cell number is needed not only to better understand the normal intestinal cell renewal process, but to assess alterations in intestinal disease processes and the potential cytotoxicity of a treatment to the dose-limiting intestinal tissue.

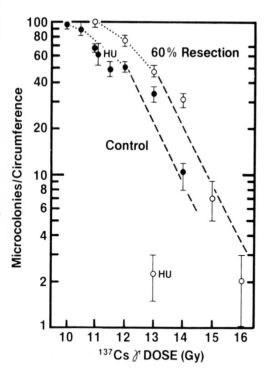

Fig. 6. The number of microcolonies per circumference of intestine versus dose of $^{137}$Cs$\gamma$ ray irradiation in control *ileum* (●) or 30 days after 60% resection of jejunum + ileum (○). The control single dose survival when HU was given 5 min before irradiation is shown (● HU) along with single dose survival after HU in resected animals (○ HU). Mean ± S.E.M.

In the experiments reported here, hydroxy-urea, specifically cytotoxic to S phase cells, had little effect on the single dose clonogenic cell survival in control jejunal or ileal tissue (Figs. 5 and 6). These results imply that in these rats, few clonogenic cells were in the S phase of the cell cycle during the time of drug availability. As in similar experiments with mice using cytotoxic drugs including HU (12), the conclusion can be reached that in the normal rat intestine, crypt stem cells are few in number and slowly proliferating. This conclusion assumes that cells toward the top of crypts which are differentiated beyond the capacity to proliferate normally, are not clonogenic after injury and although this assumption has not been tested, it does not seem likely that these cells would be clonogenic if the less differentiated rapidly dividing cells are not. By the process of elimination then, the conclusion of a few slowly dividing $G_1$ or $G_0$ stem cells per crypt can be reached.

After intestinal resection, the effect of HU was considerably different than in controls. HU reduced the single dose clonogenic cell survival by greater than tenfold in both the residual jejunum (Fig. 5) and ileum (Fig. 6). The number of clonogenic cells in S phase of the cell cycle was greatly increased after resection apparently though a shift in the cell age distribution of clonogenic cells from a slowly cycling or perhaps predominantly $G_0$ state to a rapidly cycling state.

Along with the apparent shift in the cell age distribution of stem cells after resection, there appears to be an increase in stem cell number per crypt. The clonogenic cell survival curve of the control ileum is higher than in the jejunum (Figs. 5 and 6). A slightly greater number of stem cells per ileal crypt compared to jejunal crypt could account for the difference in the control curves. Thirty days after a 60% resection, the radiation dose survival curve is shifted to the right of the control curves in both residual jejunum (Fig. 5) and ileum (Fig. 6). The shift in the survival curve is mainly through an increase in the shoulder which suggests an increase in clonogenic cell number per crypt.

It should be emphasized that these measurements are indirect, however, direct assays such as per cent labeling index, mitotic index, direct microscopic cell counts or cell sorting data cannot discriminate stem cells from other proliferating crypt cells. Even though the measurements are indirect, it appears that the number of crypt stem cells are increased after resection and that their proliferative characteristics are changed from a slowly cycling state to a more rapidly cycling state. These alterations reduce the radiosensitivity of intestinal tissue but greatly increase the tissues' sensitivity to phase specific cytotoxic drugs. Consideration of these stem cell alterations and the subsequent response of the intestine to radiation or chemotherapy should be given when a candidate for treatment has had a prior intestinal resection.

## ACKNOWLEDGEMENTS

The excellent technical assistance of Ms. Yoonyee Choi and Mr. Wayne Kickels is greatly appreciated along with the typing of the manuscript by Ms. Sandra Bates. The work was supported by the Rush Cancer Center and the Rankin Memorial Fund.

## REFERENCES

1. Altmann GG, Leblond CP. Am J Anat 1970, 127, pp 15–36
2. Bizzozero G. Arch F Mikr Anat 1892, p 325
3. Booth CC, Evans KT, Menzies T. Br J Surg 1959, 46 pp 403–410
4. Dowling RH, Booth CC. Clin Sci 1967, 32, pp 139–149
5. Galjaard H, Bootsma D. Exp Cell Res 1969, 58, pp 79–88
6. Galjaard H, Van der Meer-Fieggen W, Giesen J. Expl Cell Res 1972, 197–109
7. Hagemann RF, Lesher S. In Drugs and the Cell Cycle, Academic Press 1973, pp 195–217
8. Hagemann RF, Lesher S. Radiat Res 1971, pp 159–167
9. Hagemann RF, Sigdestad CP, Lesher S. Radiat Res 1971, 46, pp 533–546
10. Hanson WR, Fry RJM, Balish E. Second International Conference on Intestinal Adaptation, May, 1981, Falk Symposium No 30 (in press)
11. Hanson WR, Fry RJM, Sallese AR. Cell Tissue Kinet 1979, 12, pp 569–580
12. Hanson WR, Henninger DL, Fry RJM. Int J Rad Onc Biol Phys 1979, 5, pp 1685–1689
13. Hanson WR, Osborne JW. Gastroenterology 1971, 60, pp 1087–1097

14. Hanson WR, Osborne JW, Sharp JG. Gastroenterology 1977, 72, pp 692–700
15. Hanson WR, Osborne JW, Sharpe JG. Gastroenterology 1977, 72, pp 701–705
16. Hanson WR, Rijke RPC, Plaisier HM, Van Ewijk, Osborne JW. Cell Tissue Kinet 1977, 10, pp 543–555
17. Howard A, Pelc, SR. Heredity (Suppl) 1953, 6, p 261
18. Jackson WPU. pp 243. In Jones FA (ed). Modern Trends in Gastroenterology, 2nd Ed Paul B Hoeber, Inc, New York, 1958
19. Johnson LR, Copeland, EM Dudrick SS, et al, Gastroenterology 1975, 68, pp 1177–1183
20. Leblond CP, Cheng H. pp 7–31 in Cairnie, AB, Lala PK, Osmond DG (eds). Stem Cells of Renewing Cell Populations. Academic Press, New York, 1976
21. Loran MR, Althuausen RL. J Biophys, Biochem. Cytol 1960, 7, pp 667–672
22. MacDonald TT, Ferguson A. Second International Conference on Intestinal Adaptation May, 1981, Falk Symposium No 30 (in press)
23. Masuda K, Withers HR, Mason KA, Clen KY. Radiat Res 1977, 69, pp 65–75
24. McCulloch EA, and Till JE. Radiat Res 1964, 22, p 383
25. Nussbaum H, Kagan AR, Wollin M, Rao A, Hintz B, Gilbert H, Chan P, Winkley J, Kwan D. Cancer Clin Trials 1981, 4, pp 295–299
26. Nygaard K. Acta Chir Scand 1967, 133, pp 233–248
27. Painter RB, Drew RM. Lab Invest 1959, 8, p 278
28. Philips FS, Sternberg SS, Schwartz HS, Cronin AP, Sodergren JE, Vidal PM. Cancer Res 1967, 27 pp 61–74
29. Potten CS, Hendry JH. Int J Radiat Biol 1975, 27, pp 413–424
30. Pullen JM. Proc Roy Soc Med 1959, 52, pp 31–37
31. Quastler H, Sherman FG. Exp Cell Res 1959, 17, p 420
32. Rijke RPC, Hanson WR, Plaiseir HM. Cell Tissue Kinet, 1977, 10, pp 399–406
33. Thames HD, Withers HR, Mason KA, Reid BO. Int J Rad Onc Biol Phys 1981, 7 pp 1591–1597
34. Tilson MD, Wright HK. Surgery 1970, 67, pp 687–693
35. Weser E, Hernandez MH. Gastroenterology 1971, 60, pp 69–75
36. Williamson RC, Bauer FL. Br J Surg 1978, 10 pp 736–739
37. Wimber DE, Quastler H, Stein OL, Wimber DR. J Biophys Biochem Cytol 1960, 8, pp 327–331
38. Withers HR, Elkind MM. Int J Rad Biol 1970, 17, pp 261–267

# Intestinal Adaptation: Factors that Influence Morphology

R. C. N. WILLIAMSON
University Department of Surgery, Bristol Royal Infirmary, U.K.

The lining of the intestinal tract is constantly renewed in a brisk but orderly fashion. Further acceleration of cell renewal is elicited by various stimuli, notably surgical shortening of the intestine and hyperphagia, which lead to prompt but persistent increases in mucosal mass. Progressive hypoplasia ensues when the small and large bowel are deprived of their normal contents, either by fasting (with or without parenteral nutrition) or by exclusion from intestinal continuity. All atrophic changes are reversed by refeeding or restoration of the normal anatomical disposition. Intestine responds to mucosal damage by regeneration from the crypts. Pancreatobiliary secretions mediate some of the tropic effects of chyme; systemic influences, both neurovascular and humoral, also play a part in the adaptive response of the gut.

*Professor R. C. N. Williamson, M.A., M.B., M.Chir., F.R.C.S., Department of Surgery, Bristol Royal Infirmary, Bristol BS2 8HW.*

## INTRODUCTION

'. . . (body) tissues may be divided into three groups. First, one in which they continue to multiply throughout the life of the individual; to this class belong . . . epithelial coverings and their glandular prolongations, etc. These are tissues with transient elements (*elementi labili*).'
Giulio Bizzozero, Professor of General Pathology, Turin (1894) (6).

Intestinal epithelium is a prime example of an *elementum labilis*. Indeed, its enormously rapid cell turnover must impose a considerable demand on the body's resources. For reasons unknown the lining of the small and large bowel is replaced every 2–8 days in rodents and man (114). Despite the continual flux of cells from crypt base to luminal surface, the overall mass of intestinal mucosa remains remarkably constant in healthy adult animals. Equilibrium must therefore exist between cell birth in the crypts of Lieberkühn and cell loss into the lumen of the bowel.

The normal intrinsic control of cell renewal is presumably facilitated by the fact that the 3 main indigenous cell types (columnar, mucous, endocrine) differentiate from a common precursor in the stem cell compartment before migrating onto the villus (11); in the small bowel alone a fourth type, the Paneth cell, remains at the base of the crypt throughout its longer life-span (10). The pericryptal sheath of mesenchyme also undergoes renewal and may migrate in synchrony with the crypt epithelium in rabbits, if not in rats (61, 80, 81). The pattern of mucosal recovery from cytotoxic damage by transient ischaemia or low-dose irradiation suggests a local feedback device, by which cell proliferation in the crypts is regulated by the number of mature cells on the villi (85, 86). But the adaptive response to disease or injury is governed by a number of powerful extrinsic factors acting by either the luminal or the systemic route (115, 125).

From the original studies of Senn (94) in 1888 and Flint (24) in 1912 until recent years, nearly all that was known about intestinal adaptation had been learned from animal experimentation. A tangential benefit of intestinal bypass surgery for obesity has been to supplement this animal data with an increasing amount of evidence about

Table I. Principal agents affecting intestinal morphology

| Agent | Hyperplasia | Hypoplasia |
|---|---|---|
| 1. Resection/bypass* <br> Surgical transposition | Residual functioning bowel <br> Ileum transplanted proximally ⎫ <br> Ileum distal to PBD ⎭ | Defunctioned segments <br> ⎰ ?Jejunum transplanted distally <br> ⎱ — |
| 2. Food intake | Refeeding, hyperphagia | Fasting, TPN |
| 3. Mucosal damage | Recovery phase <br> Bacterial infection <br> Coeliac disease, ulcerative colitis <br> Chemical carcinogens | Irradiation, cytotoxics, ischaemia <br> Germ-free state <br> — <br> — |
| 4. Miscellaneous | Tropic hormones <br> Diabetes, lactation, hypothermia | Antitropic hormones <br> Sympathectomy |

* of small intestine or large intestine
PBD = pancreatobiliary diversion, TPN = total parenteral nutrition

adaptation in man. No major differences between species have yet been established. Structural adaptation is primarily a mucosal phenomenon, though the muscular coat of the intestine can probably hypertrophy or atrophy in response to certain stimuli. Generally much less is known about large-bowel adaptation than about corresponding events in the jejunum and ileum. The principal agents that affect intestinal morphology are listed in Table I and considered individually below.

## 1.   POSTOPERATIVE ADAPTATION

### A.   *Partial enterectomy*

No stronger stimulus to compensatory growth of the small bowel has yet emerged than loss of functioning tissue. The villi that remain after partial resection soon become hyperplastic: increased mucosal mass is detectable within 48 hours (34, 76, 122). About a week after 30–50% proximal small-bowel resection, contents of RNA and DNA in ileal mucosa reach a peak around 175% of preoperative values (117, 118). Unlike the modest and ephemeral response to transection and resuture of the bowel (122), post-resectional hyperplasia persists for at least 3–6 months and probably indefinitely (112, 120).

Enteric growth is achieved by increased segmental weight, with luminal dilatation and mural thickening. Elongation of the residual small bowel may follow massive resection in animals and man

(75, 90, 126), but could not be confirmed after 60% distal enterectomy in rats (124). Although adaptation develops on either side of a resected segment, it is always maximal downstream, and the degree of hyperplasia reflects the length of bowel excised (35, 116, 117).

The stomach and colon share in the compensatory response to partial enterectomy. Major resections of jejunum and ileum in rats, dogs or monkeys give rise to increased acid output (9, 69, 113) and parietal-cell hyperplasia (93, 127). Though often transient, gastric hypersecretion can exacerbate the symptoms of short-bowel syndrome in man (110, 128); it is accompanied by hypergastrinaemia (101, 113), and abolished by antrectomy (33). Adaptive growth of the caecum and proximal colon might be anticipated after ileal resection and does indeed take place in rats (74, 124). Some colonic hyperplasia even follows jejunal resection, but this early response diminishes after the ileum has become fully adapted (118, 120).

### B.   *Ileojejunal transposition*

Despite their overall structural similiarity, jejunum and ileum have rather different functions, which are reflected in different brush-border enzymes and a progressive decrease in mucosal mass from pylorus to ileocaecal valve (3). Ingested nutrients are almost completely absorbed before reaching the mid small bowel, so that ileal chyme is relatively devoid of energy (14). When conjugated with fluorescein, plant lectins that bind to specific sugar residues will normally label the jejunum but not the ileum (25). The ileum possesses 2 functions: it has specific transport mechanisms for absorbing vitamin $B_{12}$ and bile salts, and it provides a functional reserve which may sometimes help to prevent malabsorption of fat in particular.

Distal enteric mucosa responds to proximal transposition as it does to proximal resection; in each case it becomes exposed to chyme that is rich in nutrients. Ileal segments transposed to the jejunum soon become hyperplastic, and their villi grow to resemble those of the adjacent jejunal epithelium (31, 65, 84). Furthermore, after 8 weeks the adapting ileum can be labelled with fluorescein-conjugated lectins (25). By contrast, jejunal segments transposed to the ileum appear to retain their normal complement of sugar residues and may not even undergo hypoplasia (114).

## C.   *Enteric bypass*

If luminal nutrition were all that controlled adaptation, excision and exclusion of the jejunum could be expected to produce the same amount of distal hyperplasia. In practice minor differences exist, at least in rats. The early response of the ileum is greater after resection than bypass, though the ultimate effect is the same, and resection alone causes colonic hyperplasia (29, 75, 118). The large bowel can respond to enteric bypass of sufficient extent, however; our preliminary findings suggest that crypt cell production rate in the transverse and descending colon is more than doubled 30 weeks after 85% jejunoileal bypass (7).

Bypassed small bowel undergoes severe hypoplasia, whether self-emptying blind loops are examined or Thiry-Vella fistulae (27, 29, 63, 118). Jejunum is particularly susceptible to defunction

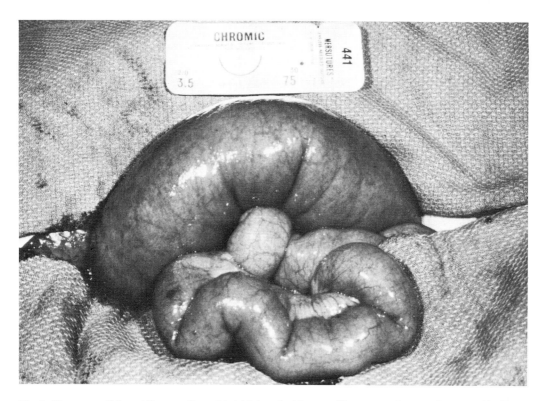

Fig. 1. Human small bowel 3 years after subtotal jejunoileal bypass. The contrast between hypertrophic (functioning) and atrophic (defunctioned) jejunum is apparent. The patient was a 23-year-old woman successfully treated for morbid obesity. Because of intractable diarrhoea intestinal continuity was restored, and gastric bypass was performed.

atrophy: already reduced at 2 days, mucosal contents of nucleic acids fall to 60% of normal by 1 month, although continuing cell proliferation is indicated by unaltered thymidine incorporation (expressed as DNA specific activity) (118). Ileum is unaccustomed to high nutrient loads, and its mucosal integrity is relatively well preserved during total exclusion from the nutrient stream (36, 117). The absorptive power of bypassed small bowel diminishes pari passu with the progressive hypoplasia (29, 63), despite the suggestion that individual enterocytes have greater functional maturity (66). All atrophic changes are promptly reversed by restoration of intestinal continuity (63).

Adaptation to enteric bypass for obesity in man has been studied radiographically and through biopsies obtained either at repeat laparotomy or by the peroral route. The findings are very similar to those in experimental animals (45, 114). The hypertrophic bowel in continuity is strikingly different from the atrophic defunctioned loops (Fig. 1). The functioning remnants are dilated and elongated; their villi are taller throughout, though deeper crypts are confined to the ileum (16, 21, 42). A fourfold increase in absorptive surface area develops during the first 2 years and correlates with the plateau in weight loss (26); nevertheless, changes in body weight seem to be independent of adaptation (83). Basal acid output and circulating levels of gastrin may be increased (as after massive resection), but peptic ulceration is not a common problem (4, 114). The defunctioned loop of small bowel probably undergoes some villous hypoplasia (114).

### D. *Pancreatobiliary diversion*

Besides food, pancreatobiliary secretions help to maintain normal mucosal mass and modulate adaptive changes in the shortened gut. Some post-resectional hyperplasia can occur in rats after ligation of the pancreatobiliary duct, but the response is blunted (95). As a corollary, diverting these secretions into the ileum enhances the compensatory response to jejunectomy (111). Pancreatobiliary diversion to mid small bowel without concomitant resection produces intense ileal hyperplasia persisting for 30 weeks, as well as a

smaller and shorter colonic response (118, 121). Stimulation of pancreatobiliary secretions could readily explain the ability of a combined infusion of cholecystokinin and secretin to reverse the intestinal hypoplasia seen in fasting dogs (40). Bile and pancreatic juice are independently tropic to the ileum (28, 119). Since they are just as effective when rats are given an elemental diet, their effect is independent of any improved digestion of foodstuffs increasing the availability of luminal nutrients (28, 111).

There is conflicting evidence regarding events in the jejunum deprived of pancreatobiliary secretions. Marked hyperplasia has recently been described (67), but we and others have found no evidence of such a response, rather a tendency towards hypoplasia (28, 118). These and other unresolved questions are no longer academic, now that biliopancreatic bypass has been introduced as a treatment for morbid obesity (91, 92).

### E. *Colectomy*

The major function of the colon is to reabsorb most of the daily load of water (1500 ml), sodium (200 mmol) and chloride (100 mmol) that traverses its luminal surface (82, 129). After removal of the colon in man, the ileum appears to adapt. The reduction in ileostomy effluent that usually occurs during the first few weeks correlates with the increased villous height detectable in the terminal ileum (41, 130). Likewise, subtotal colectomy provokes compensatory ileal hyperplasia in rats, though the response is relatively slow to develop (8, 60, 131). The rectum may share in this compensatory response (78). Rats certainly tolerate ileoproctostomy much better than ileostomy, but each operation appears to increase mitotic index and villous height throughout the small bowel and expecially in the ileum (129). Some ileal growth occurs after lesser colectomies, including local excision of the caecum and right hemicolectomy (60, 89, 123).

Adaptive changes are less pronounced in the shortened colon itself, unlike the vigorous response of the small bowel to partial enterectomy. We have observed modest hyperplasia in the right colon 8 months after caecal resection or left hemicolectomy in rats (123). Conversely, others have found marked hyperplasia of the left colon 3 months after right hemicolectomy (60). The colonic response to partial colectomy may be limited by the presence of an intact distal small bowel. Perhaps ileal adaptation can compensate in part for loss of colon, since caecectomy has little effect on the residual large bowel unless accompanied by resection of the terminal ileum (89). Nevertheless, a recent study of faecal losses in postoperative patients attributed a greater importance to the extent of colectomy than that of ileectomy in the pathogenesis of diarrhoea (68).

F.  *Colostomy*

After defunctioning proximal colostomy in rats, the changes in the distal colon mimic those observed in bypassed loops of small bowel. The amounts of protein, RNA and DNA are reduced (in similar proportions) by a third at 1 week and by a half at 1 month (103). Presumably this hypoplasia reflects the loss of mechanical stimulus that follows faecal diversion, rather in the same way that a paralysed limb will atrophy from disuse.

Closure of the transverse colostomy is followed by a burst of proliferative activity in the crypts, which restores distal colonic mass precisely and completely within 7 days (103). Although creation of the colostomy has no demonstrable effect on the proximal colon, its closure is followed by transitory growth of this segment. We have not observed in the colon any evidence of the short-lived hyperplasia shown by the small bowel in response to transection and resuture (103, 122). The temporary diarrhoea that may ensue after colostomy closure in man has been attributed to the loss of absorptive surface area in the defunctioned bowel (104).

2.  THE DOMINANT ROLE OF FOOD

A.  *Starvation*

The small bowel is ideally placed to receive nourishment directly from the nutrients it absorbs for the rest of the body. It is therefore not surprising that enteric epithelium is extraordinarily sensitive to the withdrawal of oral food, being more adversely affected than any other organ in the body (50). After 6 days of complete starvation in rats, the total weight of small bowel and its mucosal mass were approximately halved, while body weight was only reduced by a third (98). Dietary restriction rapidly reduces the number of proliferating enterocytes, prolongs the cell cycle and delays cell migration (1, 32, 39, 51). As in bowel excluded from the nutrient steam, individual villous cells become hypermature (13). As in bypass also, the jejunum undergoes greater atrophy than the ileum (2). Hypoplasia is promptly reversed by refeeding (1, 2).

Fasting has a remarkably severe effect on the large bowel as well, with similar lengthening of the cell cycle, notably the $G_1$ and S phases (32). Not only sugar and protein are required to reverse these effects, but also an adequate supply of dietary salt (99). In contrast to the small bowel, mechanical distension preserves the integrity of colonic mucosa (15, 87, 100).

B.  *Parenteral nutrition*

Intravenous alimentation is quite unable to prevent the intestinal atrophy that occurs with fasting. Parenterally-nourished rats and rabbits develop hypoplasia of the small intestine (especially jejunum) and large intestine, but not of any other organs except the pancreas and gastric fundus (19, 49, 52, 87). Moreover, total parenteral nutrition abolishes post-resectional hyperplasia in rats and dogs (20, 53, 72). By contrast, liquid elemental diets given by mouth permit relatively normal adaptation of the small bowel to resection or bypass (22, 105), although they do not prevent colonic atrophy (44, 71, 87).

Food has direct and indirect effects on the gut, since its absence alters the release of other tropic factors. Besides causing pancreatic hyposecretion, parenteral nutrition changes the gastrointestinal hormone profile (30, 49). Defunctioned small bowel undergoes further hypoplasia during starvation or intravenous feeding (12, 17), and ileal infusions of nutrients cause jejunal hyperplasia (97).

C.  *Hyperphagia*

Villous hypertrophy occurs in several different models of experimental hyperphagia, including intermittent starvation, hypothalamic lesions, tube feeding, high-lactose diets and insulin injections (114). Hyperphagia is also a feature of certain other conditions associated with increased small-bowel growth, such as lactation, hyperthyroidism, hypothermia, diabetes mellitus and intestinal resection; but pair feeding and other experiments suggest that humoral factors contribute to adaptation in these cases (114). In man, adaptation to subtotal jejunoileal bypass develops in spite of reduced oral intake (4), and the early response of rat small bowel to partial resection is independent of hyperphagia (64).

## 3.   MUCOSAL DISEASE AND INJURY

Agents that damage the intestinal epithelium without causing the death of the host lead to increased epithelial-cell proliferation during the recovery phase (18, 114). In chronic injury states, such as coeliac disease and ulcerative colitis, superficial 'atrophy' coexists with intense hyperplasia in the crypts. Indeed, the persistent acceleration in cell renewal (18, 132) presumably underlies the increased risk of malignant change in these hyperproliferative conditions. Enhanced ileal absorption in coeliac disease (96) and gastric hypersecretion in Crohn's disease (23) suggest some adaptation by healthy gut to segmental disease.

Both irradiation and cytotoxic drugs inhibit mitotic activity in the crypts of animals and man; the subsequent burst of proliferative activity repopulates the villus with immature enterocytes (86, 102). Other agents that perturb intestinal cytokinetics are alcohol, uraemia and deficiency of folic acid and vitamin $B_{12}$ (114). Bacteria exert a physiological role in maintaining normal cell turnover; germ-free animals have a hypoplastic mucosa, and microbial infection stimulates crypt-cell proliferation (5, 114).

Intestinal epithelium exhibits a triphasic response to specific chemical carcinogens like azoxymethane and dimethylhydrazine. Healing of the initial cytotoxic injury is followed in a few weeks by increased cell proliferation leading to hyperplasia and ultimately to neoplastic transformation (120). The abnormal appearance of replicating cells in the upper third of the colonic crypts and the subsequent accumulation of these cells are features of the preneoplastic epithelium both in rodents receiving dimethylhydrazine and in patients with familial polyposis coli (56, 58). Besides suggesting a common process of transformation in spontaneous and induced neoplasms, these subtle kinetic changes offer the possibility of screening for malignant change in high-risk individuals (57).

## 4.   SYSTEMIC       INFLUENCES       ON ADAPTATION

### A.   *Neurovascular*

Villous cells are preferentially damaged by temporary intestinal ischaemia (85), and increased blood flow precedes (but clearly need not cause) post-resectional adaptation (106). Nevertheless noradrenaline, a vasoconstrictor, increases intestinal cell proliferation, and this effect is reversed by $\alpha$-adrenergic blockade; adrenaline inhibits proliferation, and this effect is reversed by $\beta$-adrenergic blockade (108).

The intestinal mucosa has a rich autonomic innervation; electrical stimulation of mesenteric nerves and cholinergic drugs both stimulate mitosis, whereas sympathectomy is inhibitory (107). The enteric hypoplasia that first follows truncal vagotomy may result from reduced mucosal blood flow and is reversed by splachnicectomy (79); later, mucosal integrity is restored by increased crypt-cell proliferation (55).

### B.   *Hormonal*

A humoral contribution to the control of intestinal adaptation is supported by inadequacies in the theory of luminal nutrition plus the development of post-resectional hyperplasia in sequestered bowel, i.e. in Thiry-Vella fistulae or cross-circulated parabionts (117, 122, 125). Subordinate enterotropic hormones comprise the anterior pituitary hormones and those produced by their target organs, viz thyroxine, testosterone and corticosteroids (115). Muller & Dowling (73) have now convincingly shown that prolactin does not have any tropic role in the intestine and is not responsible for the hyperplasia of lactation.

The stimulatory effect of saliva on intestinal cell renewal probably depends upon its high content of epidermal growth factor (54). Somatostatin, vasoactive intestinal polypeptide and perhaps secretin appear to have antitropic effects (37, 47, 115).

A tropic role throughout the gastrointestinal tract has been postulated for *gastrin* (46, 47, 48). Much of the supporting evidence comes from experiments involving exogenous administration of pentagastrin to fasted animals, but several studies have failed to confirm any tropic action beyond the ligament of Treitz in fed animals (59, 62, 70). Alterations in endogenous gastrin levels were without obvious effect on the intestinal response to short-term starvation or jejunal resection (77). It therefore seems unlikely that gastrin has a physiological role in jejunoileal adaptation (109, 115).

*Enteroglucagon* remains the strongest candidate for the label of 'enterotropin' (115). Increased circulating levels coexist with intestinal hyperplasia in lactation, hypothermia, enterectomy and enteric bypass (38, 43, 88). The major distribution of enteroglucagon in man lies in the lower ileum and colon (88), which provides an explanation for the fact that adaptation to proximal enterectomy exceeds that observed after distal enterectomy. (For details see paper by Bloom & Polak, this symposium).

## CONCLUSIONS

Loss of functioning tissue and absence of normal chyme or faeces are the principal agents affecting the morphology of the intestine. Luminal nutrients maintain the small-bowel epithelium and luminal bulk maintains the large-bowel epithelium. Further, the stomach, pancreas and intestine itself depend upon tropic hormones secreted in response to meals. Within the small bowel, the greater sensitivity of jejunum than ileum to starvation and bypass is consistent with the normal aboral gradients of both mucosal mass and nutrient concentrations within the small bowel. Colonic adaptation is broadly similar to enteric adaptation, except that partial resection

may provoke a lesser response in the presence of an intact small bowel.

Further developments of clinical relevance are likely to be in 3 areas: the identification of enterotropic hormones and their possible therapeutic use in the short-bowel syndrome, the optimal means of nutritional support during the period of intense adaptation to surgical stress, and the precise relationship between hyperplasia and neoplasia of the intestinal tract.

## ACKNOWLEDGEMENTS

Some of the original work described in this review has been supported by generous grants from the Cancer Research Campaign and the South Western Regional Health Authority, United Kingdom.

## REFERENCES

1. Aldewachi HS, Wright NA, Appleton DR, Watson AJ. J. Anat 1975, 119, 105–121
2. Altmann GG. Am J Anat 1972, 133 391–400
3. Altmann GG, Enesco M. Am J Anat 1967, 121, 319–336
4. Barry RE, Barisch J, Bray GA, Sperling MA, Morin RJ, Benfield J. Am J Clin Nutr 1977, 30, 32–42
5. Barthold SW. Cancer Res 1981, 41, 2616–2620
6. Bizzozero G. Br Med J 1894, 1 728–732
7. Bristol JB, Williamson RCN. Br J Surg 1982, in press
8. Buchholtz TW, Malamud D, Ross JS, Malt RA. Surgery 1976, 80, 601–607
9. Caridis DT, Roberts M, Smith G. Surgery 1969, 65, 292–297
10. Cheng H. Am J Anat 1974, 141, 521–536
11. Cheng H, Leblond CP. Am J Anat 1974, 141, 537–562
12. Clarke RM. Clin Sci Mol Med 1976, 50, 139–144
13. Dowling RH. Br Med Bull 1967, 23, 275–278
14. Dowling RH, Booth CC. Clin Sci 1967, 32, 139–149
15. Dowling RH, Riecken EO, Laws JW, Booth CC. Clin Sci 1967, 32, 1–9
16. Dudrick SJ, Daly JM, Castro G, Akhtar M. Ann Surg 1977, 185, 642–648
17. Dworkin LD, Levine GM, Farber NJ, Spector MH. Gastroenterology 1976, 71, 626–630
18. Eastwood GL. Gastroenterology 1977, 72, 962–975
19. Eastwood GL. Surgery 1977 82, 613–620
20. Feldman EJ, Dowling RH, McNaughton J, Peters TJ. Gastroenterology 1976, 70, 712–719
21. Fenyö G, Backman L, Hallberg D. Acta Chir Scand 1976, 142, 154–159

22. Fenyö G, Hallberg D. Acta Chir Scand 1976, 142, 270–274
23. Fielding JF, Cooke WT, Williams JA. Lancet 1971, 1, 1106–1107
24. Flint JM. Bull Johns Hopkins Hosp 1912, 23, 127–144
25. Freeman HJ, Etzler ME, Garrido AB, Kim YS. Gastroenterology 1978, 75, 1066–1072
26. Friedman HI, Chandler JG, Peck CC, Nemeth TJ, Odum SK. Surg Gynecol Obstet 1978, 146, 757–767
27. Garrido AB Jr, Freeman HJ, Kim YS. Dig Dis Sci 1981, 26, 107–112
28. Gélinas, MD, Morin CL. Can J Physiol. Pharmacol 1980, 58, 1117–1123
29. Gleeson MH, Cullen J, Dowling RH. Clin Sci 1972, 43, 731–742
30. Greenberg GR, Wolman SL, Christofides ND, Bloom SR, Jeejeebhoy KN. Gastroenterology 1981, 80, 988–993
31. Grönqvist B, Engström B, Grimelius L. Acta Chir Scand 1975, 141, 208–217
32. Hagemann RF, Stragand JJ. Cell Tissue Kinet 1977, 10, 3–14
33. Hall AW, Moossa AR, Wood RAB, Block GE, Skinner DB. Ann Surg 1977, 186, 83–87
34. Hanson WR, Osborne JW, Sharpe JG. Gastroenterology 1977, 72, 692–700
35. Hanson WR, Osborne JW, Sharpe JG. Gastroenterology 1977, 72, 701–705
36. Hanson WR, Rijke RPC, Plaisier HM, van Ewijk W, Osborne JW. Cell Tissue Kinet 1977, 10, 543–555
37. Holmes SJK, Moossa AR. Br J Surg 1981, 68, 819–820
38. Holst JJ, Sørensen TIA, Andersen AN, Stadil F, Andersen B, Lauritsen KB, Klein HC. Scand J Gastroenterol 1979, 14, 205–207
39. Hopper AF, Rose PM, Wannemacher RW. J Cell Biol 1972, 53, 225–230
40. Hughes CA, Bates T, Dowling RH. Gastroenterology 1978, 75, 34–41
41. Hultén L, Holm C, Kewenter J. Acta Chir Scand 1971, 137, 689–691
42. Iversen BM, Schjønsby H, Skagen DW, Solhaug JH. Eur J Clin Invest 1976, 6, 355–360
43. Jacobs LR, Polak J, Bloom SR, Dowling RH. Clin Sci Mol Med 1976, 50, 14P–15P
44. Janne P, Carpentier Y, Willems G. Dig Dis 1977, 22, 808–812
45. Joffe SN. Gut 1981, 22, 242–254
46. Johnson LR. Gastroenterology 1976, 70, 278–288
47. Johnson LR. Gastroenterology 1977, 72, 788–792
48. Johnson LR. World J Surg 1979, 3, 477–487
49. Johnson LR, Copeland EM, Dudrick SJ, Lichtenberger LM, Castro GA. Gastroenterology 1975, 68, 1177–1183
50. Ju JS, Nasset ES. J Nutr 1959, 633–645
51. Koga A, Kimura S. J Nutr Sci Vitaminol 1979, 25, 265–267
52. Levine GM, Deren JJ, Steiger E, Zinno R. Gastroenterology 1974, 67, 975–982
53. Levine GM, Deren JJ, Yezdimir E. Dig Dis 1976, 21, 542–546
54. Li AKC, Schattenkerk ME, Huffman RG, Ross JS, Malt RA. Clin Res 1980, 28 483A
55. Liavåg I, Vaage S. Scand J Gastroenterol 1972, 7, 23–27
56. Lipkin M. Cancer 1974, 34, 878–888
57. Lipkin M. Cancer 1975, 36, 2319–2324
58. Lipkin M and Deschner E. Cancer Res 1976, 36, 2665–2668
59. Mak KM, Chang WWL. Gastroenterology 1976, 71, 1117–1120
60. Masesa PC, Forrester JM. Gut 1977, 18, 37–44
61. Maskens AP, Rahier JR, Meersseman FP, Dujardin-Loits RM, Haot JG. Gut 1979, 20, 775–779
62. Mayston PD, Barrowman JA, Dowling RH. Digestion 1975, 12, 78–84
63. Menge H, Bloch R, Schaumlöffel E, Riecken EO. pp 61–67, in Dowling RH, Riecken EO (eds), Intestinal Adaptation, Schattauer Verlag, Stuttgart, 1974
64. Menge H, Gräfe M, Lorenz-Meyer H, Riecken EO. Gut 1975, 16, 468–472
65. Menge H, Robinson JWL. Acta Hepato-Gastroenterol 1978, 25, 150–154
66. Menge H, Robinson JWL, Schroeder P. J Physiol 1978, 280, 33–34P
67. Miazza BM, Levan H, Vaja S, Dowling RH. Gut 1980, 21, A917
68. Mitchell JE, Breuer RI, Zuckerman L, Berlin J, Schilli R, Dunn JK. Dig Dis Sci 1980, 25, 33–41
69. Moossa AR, Hall AW, Skinner DB, Winans CS. Surgery 1976, 80, 208–213
70. Morin CL, Ling V. Gastroenterology 1978, 75, 224–229
71. Morin CL, Ling V, Bourassa D. Dig Dis Sci 1980, 25, 123–128
72. Morin CL, Ling V, Caillie M van. Paediat Res 1978, 12, 268–271
73. Muller E, Dowling RH. Gut 1981, 22, 558–565
74. Nundy S, Malamud D, Obertop H, Sczerban J, Malt RA. Gastroenterology 1977, 72, 263–266
75. Nygaard, K. Acta Chir Scand 1967, 133, 233–248
76. Obertop H, Nundy S, Malamud D, Malt RA. Gastroenterology 1977, 72, 267–270
77. Oscarson JEA, Veen HF, Williamson RCN, Ross JS, Malt RA. Gastroenterology 1977, 72, 890–895
78. Owen RJ, Lyttle JA. Gut 1979, 20, 444
79. Padula RT, Noble PH, Camishion RC. Surg Forum 1967, 18, 317–319
80. Parker FG, Barnes EN, Kaye GI. Gastroenterology 1974, 67, 607–621
81. Pascal RR, Kaye GI, Lane N. Gastroenterology 1968, 54, 835–851
82. Phillips SF, Giller J. J Lab Clin Med 1973, 81, 733–746
83. Pilkington TRE, Gazet J-C, Ang L, Kalucy RS, Crisp AH, Day S. Br Med J 1976 1, 1504–1505
84. Rijke RPC, Hanson WR, Plaisier HM. Cell Tissue Kinet 1977, 10, 399–406
85. Rijke RPC, Hanson WR, Plaisier HM, Osborne JW. Gastroenterology 1976, 71, 786–792
86. Rijke RPC, Plaisier H, Hoogeveen AT, Lamerton LF, Galjaard H. Cell Tissue Kinet 1975, 8, 441–453

87. Ryan GP, Dudrick SJ, Copeland EM, Johnson LR. Gastroenterology 1979, 77, 658–663
88. Sagor GR, Almukhtar MYT, Ghatei MA, Wright NA, Bloom SR. Br J Surg 1982, 69, 14–18
89. Scarpello JHB, Cary BA, Sladen GE. Clin Sci Mol Med 1978, 54, 241–249
90. Schleflan M, Galli SJ, Perrotto J, Fischer JE. Surg Gynecol Obstet 1976, 143, 757–762
91. Scopinaro N, Gianetta E, Civalleri D, Bonalumi U, Bachi V. Br J Surg 1979, 66, 613–617
92. Scopinaro N, Gianetta E, Civalleri D, Bonalumi U, Bachi V. Br J Surg 1979 66, 618–620
93. Seelig LL Jr, Winborn WB, Weser E. Gastroenterology 1977, 72, 421–428
94. Senn N. Ann Surg 1888, 7, 99–115
95. Shellito PC, Peterson Dahl E, Terpstra OT, Malt RA. Proc Soc Exp Biol Med 1978, 158, 101–104
96. Silk DBA, Kumar PJ, Webb JPW, Lane AE, Clark ML, Dawson AM. Gut 1975, 16, 261–267
97. Spector MH, Levine GM, Deren JJ. Gastroenterology 1977, 72, 706–710
98. Steiner M, Bourges HR, Freedman LS, Gray SJ. Am J Physiol 1968, 215, 75–77
99. Stragand JJ, Hagemann RF. Am J Clin Nutr 1977, 3, 918–923
100. Stragand JJ, Hagemann RF. Am J Physiol 1977, 233, E208–E211
101. Straus E, Gerson CD, Yalow RS. Gastroenterology, 1974, 66, 175–180
102. Taminiau JAJM, Gall DG, Hamilton JR. Gut 1980, 21, 486–492
103. Terpstra OT, Peterson-Dahl E, Williamson RCN, Ross JS, Malt RA. Gastroenterology 1981, 81, 475–480
104. Tilson MD, Fellner BJ, Wright HK. Am J Surg 1976, 131, 94–97
105. Touloukian RJ, Mitruka B, Hoyle C. Surgery 1971, 69, 637–645
106. Touloukian RJ, Spencer RP. Ann Surg 1972, 175, 320–325
107. Tutton PJM. Med Biol 1977, 55, 201–208
108. Tutton, PJM, Helme RD. Cell Tissue Kinet 1974, 7, 125–136
109. Weser E. Gastroenterology 1978, 75, 323–324
110. Weser E, Fletcher JT, Urban E. Gastroenterology 1979, 77, 572–579
111. Weser E, Heller R, Tawil T. Gastroenterology 1977, 73, 524–529
112. Weser E, Tawil T. Gastroenterology 1976, 71, 412–415
113. Wickbom G, Landor JH, Bushkin FL, McGuigan JE. Gastroenterology 1975, 69, 448–452
114. Williamson RCN. N Engl J Med 1978, 298, 1393–1402
115. Williamson RCN. N Engl J Med 1978, 298, 1444–1450
116. Williamson RCN. Ann Roy Coll Surg Engl 1979, 61, 341–348
117. Williamson RCN, Bauer FLR. Br J Surg 1978, 65, 736–739
118. Williamson RCN, Bauer RLR, Ross JS and Malt RA. Gastroenterology 1978, 74, 16–23
119. Williamson RCN, Bauer FLR, Ross JS, Malt RA. Surgery 1978, 83, 570–576
120. Williamson RCN, Bauer FLR, Ross JS, Oscarson JEA, Malt RA. Cancer Res 1978, 38, 3212–3217
121. Williamson RCN, Bauer FLR, Ross JS, Watkins JB, Malt RA. Gastroenterology 1979, 76, 1386–1392
122. Williamson RCN, Buchholtz TW, Malt RA. Gastroenterology 1978, 75, 249–254
123. Williamson RCN, Davies PW, Bristol JB, Wells M. Gut 1982, in press
124. Williamson RCN, Lyndon PJ, Tudway AJC. Br J Cancer 1980, 42, 85–94
125. Williamson RCN, Malt RA, pp 230–243, in Appleton DR, Sunter JP, Watson AJ (eds), Cell Proliferation in the Gastrointestinal Tract, Pitman Medical, Tunbridge Wells, 1980
126. Wilmore DW, Dudrick SJ, Daly JM, Vars HM. Surg Gynecol Obstet 1971, 132, 673–680
127. Winborn WB, Seelig LL, Nakayama H, Weser E. Gastroenterology 1974, 66, 384–395
128. Windsor CWO, Fejfar J, Woodward DAK. Gut 1969, 10, 779–786
129. Woo ZH, Nygaard K. Scand J Gastroent 1978, 13, 903–910
130. Wright HK, Cleveland JC, Tilson MD, Herskovic T. Am J Surg 1969, 117, 242–245
131. Wright HK, Poskitt T, Cleveland JC, Herskovic T. J Surg Res 1969, 9, 301–304
132. Wright NA, Watson A, Morley A, Appleton D, Marks J, Douglas A. Gut 1973, 14, 603–606

# Assessing small intestinal function in Health and Disease in vivo and in vitro

R. J. LEVIN
Department of Physiology, University of Sheffield,
Sheffield S10 2TN, Yorkshire, U.K.

Diet, dysfunction and disease induce primary and secondary changes in intestinal structure and function. The major techniques used to assess such changes in human and animal intestinal absorption and secretion in situ, in vivo and in vitro are reviewed concisely but critically and the problems of normalisation of the data explored. Exploitation of the various electrical potential differences generated by and across the intestinal epithelium allows the kinetic characterisation of the electrogenic glucose absorption mechanism, the measurement of functional lactase activity, the assessment of the thickness of the unstirred layer, the estimation of intestinal ionic (diffusive) permeability and the recording of electrogenic secretion coupled with motility changes in the jejunum, in situ, of conscious man in health and disease. The use of animal intestine has allowed direct and indirect evidence of multiple hexose carriers to be obtained and a new technique allowing corrected kinetic parameters of $K_m$ and $J_m$ to be estimated in vivo. Application of the technique to experimental conditions will allow a better assessment of the adaptive capabilities of the enterocytes absorptive functions.

*R. J. Levin, Department of Physiology, University of Sheffield, Western Bank, Sheffield S10 2TN, Yorkshire, U.K.*

## INTRODUCTION

*The intestine as a living barrier*

The brief for this article was to review techniques used to assess changes in small intestinal function. If the small intestine were simply the 'tube lined with cells' of the textbooks where the chyme is transported along or across, the task would be relatively easy. The small intestine cannot however, be so described, for it is a true living barrier adapting its structure and functions to the changed circumstances imposed upon it. The population of enterocytes undertaking absorption and secretion is in a dynamic state, constantly being shed and renewed by mitosis. The enterocytes moreover are unique in that they have two sources of nutrition. During the interdigestive state they obtain their nutriments, like other cells, from the interstitial fluid via the blood but during the digestive phase they receive a considerable supply from the normal food intake, the proteinaceous secretions of the gastro-intestinal tract and from the exfoliated, degenerating enterocytes. This 'luminal nutrition' (72) of the enterocytes profoundly influences their number (116, 141, 142) and functions. Apart from diet, changes in the population dynamics can also be induced by dysfunction and disease. The triad can alter intestinal function not only by direct or primary actions on the enterocytes but also by indirect, secondary effects on the systems that subserve the intestine and the processing of its nutrient supplies. The secondary effects may often be very marked and can swamp the sometimes more modest primary changes. In order to simplify the complexity of the secondary actions, they can be separated into two schemes, one focussing on their influence on crypt-villous dynamics (Fig. 1) the other on the control mechanisms affecting absorption and secretion (Fig. 2).

Diet, dysfunction and disease by affecting appetite and food intake alter the nutrient and bulk supply to the bowel (Fig. 1). A review of the many conditions where nutrition influences human gastro-intestinal function has been published (46). The changes of motility, intestinal flora, bile and pancreatic secretions, enzymic breakdown of nutrients and the absorption of their hydrolysis products influence the production and loss of cells at the crypt and villous top extrusion zones respectively. The absorbed nutrients by affecting intestinal blood and lymph flows, the endocrine/paracrine/neural control of the gut by direct local effects or through mediation via hypothalamic 'appestats' and the differentiation of enterocytes as they progress up the villi can decrease or increase the enterocyte numbers and even their degree of maturation. The new population will possess a changed absorptive/secretory capacity which may be expressed on a per cell or on an organ basis. To emphasise the intimate relationships between systems, a further analysis is presented schematically in Fig. 2. The focus here is on the absorption and secretion of ions and fluid by the intestine, the net balance between these leading to elimination by excretion.

Absorption is influenced not only by gastric

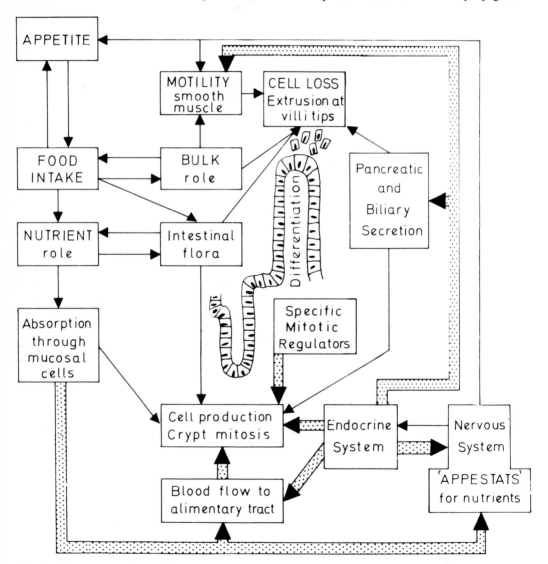

Fig. 1. Diagrammatic schema of the complex interactions influencing crypt-villous dynamics modified from Levin (72). The shaded bars represent blood or tissue fluid pathways.

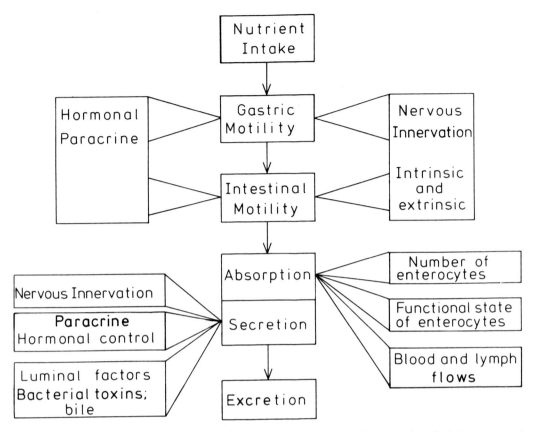

Fig. 2. Diagrammatic schema of the control mechanisms and other factors influencing intestinal absorption and secretion of ions and fluid.

and intestinal motility but also by the functional state of the enterocytes and the ability of the lymph and blood flow to clear transferred substances away from their contraluminal membranes. Gastric motility controls the amount of nutrients delivered to the small bowel for hydrolysis and absorption. Small bowel motility affects absorptive efficacy because it mixes and moves the luminal contents, preventing the development of localised high concentrations of hydrolysis products and reducing diffusion barriers, i.e. the unstirred layers. The propulsive motility governs the transit of chyme through the intestine and thus to a large extent controls the residence or contact time that the mucosa has with the luminal contents. Changes in these times can increase or reduce the ability of the intestine to absorb efficiently. Experimental increases in transit rate of

the small bowel reduce its capacity to absorb (58, 83). The fibre content of the diet acting as a bulking agent plays a role in influencing absorption because it can speed the passage of bowel contents and thus reduce absorption. The small bowel becomes less efficient as the fibre content of diet is increased (135).

The net amount of fluid and ions absorbed will obviously be related to the amounts secreted by the small intestine. Such secretion is thought to arise mainly from the crypt regions and is influenced not only by nervous, paracrine and hormonal control but also by luminal factors such as bacterial toxins and bile (9, 82). Alterations in any of these factors can lead to pathophysiological changes in the intestinal handling of fluid and electrolytes. Ignored for many years, the secretory mechanisms of the intestine have recently

Table I. The major in vivo and in vitro techniques used to study small intestinal absorptive/secretive functions in humans and animals

| In vivo techniques | | In vitro preparations | | |
| Human | Animal | isolated intact intestine | intact epithelia | disrupted epithelia |
| --- | --- | --- | --- | --- |
| *Tolerance tests*<br>Serial plasma/urine levels after ingestion | *Gastric intubation*<br>(with or without markers) | *Continuous circulation*<br>i) luminal and serosal fluids | everted sacs<br>rings | isolated villi<br>isolated enterocytes |
| *Breath tests*<br>Production of $H_2$ or $C^{14}$ labelled $CO_2$ from ingested substrates | *Intestinal loops*<br>Acute—static (tied off) or circulated.<br>Chronic—Thiry—Vella | ii) luminal but no serosal fluid | sheets<br>strips | brush border vesicles<br>basolateral vesicles |
| *Balance studies*<br>Whole alimentary tract absorption.<br>Input/output measured often with non-absorbable markers | *Balance studies*<br>Whole alimentary tract absorption.<br>Input/output measured often with non-absorbable markers | *Segmental luminal flow* | biopsy | enterocyte mitochondria |
| *Isolated loops*<br>Acute/chronic preparations | *Sampling systemic/body fluids using special surgical preparations*<br>Collecting portal, mesenteric blood or lymph.<br>Blood vessel perfusion | *Perfusion blood vessels* | | |
| *Intubation methods*<br>Single, double or triple lumen tubes (with or without occluding balloon(s)) Sample liquid test meals segmental luminal perfusion (with or without non-absorbable markers). | *Transintestinal p.d.*<br>Transfer p.d. kinetics; Osmotic and diffusion p.d. | | | |
| *Transintestinal p.d.*<br>Transfer p.d. kinetics; secretory, osmotic and diffusion p.d. | | | | |

become fashionable to study and much investigative work has been undertaken (28, 56, 118). Unfortunately, the multiplicity of factors affecting the intestine will not only influence its functions per se but will also influence specific methods designed to assess such functions, especially if they are carried out in the in vivo or in situ condition. Two examples should suffice, if a solute is fed to an animal or human, gastric emptying, intestinal motility and transit will obviously affect the rate at which the substance is absorbed. In vitro experiments, where the intestine is removed from such influences and studied out of the body, would seem unaffected by such effects. However, if the intestine has been removed from the alimentary tract of a human or animal that has previously been exposed to a changed dietary, hormonal or a diseased condition, the enterocytes removed will still have been affected by the indirect or secondary actions of the condition as well as the primary actions. The technique chosen to investigate the adaptive changes of the intestine will often play a decisive role in their interpretation as either primary or secondary changes.

*Techniques to assess intestinal function*

A large number of techniques have been developed and a vocabulary of terms and parameters created to characterise and quantify solute and fluid movements across the small intestine in vitro, in vivo and in situ. Because many articles and reviews have been published containing much critical discussion about the various techniques (25, 49, 70, 72, 75, 100, 105, 124, 126, 127, 128, 131, 132, 144), repetition would be wasteful of space and time. The general survey of techniques to follow, biased to human studies, will merely list the major methods with brief comments. More detailed discussion will be reserved for newer methods not described in the above reviews and for the techniques that exploit the electrical activity generated by the enterocytes as an index of intestinal function.

*In vitro methods*

The variety of in vitro techniques, listed in Table I, is extensive. It starts from the preparation that allowed the clear-cut demonstration of active transport of amino acids and sugars—the much-used, classic everted sac of rodent small intestine first prepared at Sheffield (145) with its modifications (19). There is a range of preparations that use whole isolated intestine whose mucosa and serosa are bathed with oxygenated buffers circulated continuously (32) or whose serosa is bathed only in a moist, oxygen/carbon dioxide allowing the collection of transferred fluid and solutes undiluted by any buffer solution (130). An innovation has been the use of segmented flow, where the buffer circulated through the intestinal lumen is interrupted by bubbles of the aerating gas mixture. It is claimed to yield better preparations (30) but it does make recording of electrical activity across the gut wall technically difficult.

Greater control over the serosal milieu of enterocytes is achieved by perfusing the blood vessels of the isolated intestine (31). This technique has also been used when the intestine is left in situ (see section on in vivo techniques in animals).

Intestinal sheets prepared from animal ilea (122) and jejuna (37) and human ilea (39, 40) and jejuna (8) have been clamped as a membrane between two chambers allowing electrical measurements of potential difference (p.d.) short-circuit current (SCC) and tissue conductance. These parameters, together with isotopic flux measurements of the solute and fluid movements across the tissue, are essential to characterise the mechanisms involved in the transfer processes of absorption and secretion. More detailed analysis of the electrical activity across the individual membranes of the enterocyte has been accomplished by the use of micro-electrodes (2, 75). Rings (1), strips of intestine (60) and isolated villi (18) have been employed for uptake studies but have become less popular. In humans, biopsy samples can be taken from normal and diseased intestine for direct in vitro measurement of uptake or enzyme studies (12, 26, 84, 94, 117), for assessing changes in the kinetics of uptake (136), for assessing accumulation of nutrients into enterocytes by autoradiography (137) or for experiments during or after growing biopsy material in tissue culture (78, 139).

Isolated enterocytes prepared from animal intestine have become a useful preparation in the hands of some investigators expecially for exploring in detail the energetics of entry and exit mechanisms of the enterocyte for sugars and amino acids (61, 62). Sealed vesicles obtained from the brush border membranes of animal (93) and human enterocytes (79) and from their basolateral membranes (92) can now be manufactured with a high degree of purification using sophisticated techniques of separation. Recently controlled-pore glass bead column chromatography (99) has been claimed to produce quickly a more homogenous size of vesicle with better transporting properties than those previously manufactured by laborious and time-consuming repeated ultracentrifugation (79) or free-flow electrophoresis (92). One of the great advantages of the vesicles is that they allow discrete analysis of events that take place at the brush border or basolateral membranes of the enterocyte. They have become tools for the analysis of epithelial transport and were the key to confirming the detailed electrogenic mechanism of Na-dependent active translocation of hexoses and amino acids across the brush border membrane. Vesicles could be made that transported hexoses and amino acids against their concentration difference when the only possible energy source was either a $Na^+$ concentration gradient or an electrical potential difference (51). The vesicles have also been used to study the kinetics of glucose transfer (52), to distinguish between different models for cotransport (53) and to examine possible changes in the movement of neutral amino acids across the brush border membrane in different dietary conditions (42, 50). Some workers attempted to study the transfer mechanisms of brush borders not only at the phenomenological level but also at the molecular level by extracting possible carrier complexes with detergent and inserting them into liposomes (vesicles made from plant phospholipids) to assess their properties and compare them with vesicles made from brush borders (17). Even mitochondria have been prepared from enterocytes to study their properties during the life span of the cells (64).

Early attempts at localising amino acids and hexoses transferred into enterocytes in vitro utilised autoradiography in frozen sections (65). A development of this technique uses glutaraldehyde to fix the amino acids inside the enterocytes. With automatic scanning of the density of the autoradiographs the method promises to be useful in analysing the acquisition of transfer functions by the enterocytes as they move up from crypt to villus and mature (63). This appears to be one of the few techniques that can tackle this problem. To conclude this section, the development of in vitro methodology has been the major factor in allowing rigorous analysis of the transport processes at the levels of the membrane, the cell and when the cells are coupled together as an epithelium (Fig. 4). The methods possess the obvious advantage of fine experimental control of many variables allowing specific transfer/secretory mechanisms to be isolated and studied. Apart from some technical problems (adequate oxygenation of tissue, choice of correct buffer pH for incubation, provision of correct metabolisable substrates), the main disadvantages of in vitro methods lie in their obvious lack of blood and lymph flows, systems that can play a substantial role in normal fluid (41) and solute absorption, in the disruption of normal motility patterns and of hormonal and nervous control. Tearing the intestine from the body upsets the neural balance, an important aspect when studying secretory phenomena. Because of these factors studies of intestinal function in vivo, or better in situ, must of need be the 'final court of inquiry' (70).

*In vivo methods*

A brief listing of the major techniques available for the task of measuring function in vivo and in situ is given in Table I. By far the greatest number of studies on human intestine have employed these techniques. Details can be found either in the general reviews of methods previously quoted (70, 100, 131, 132, 144) or in those especially dealing with human studies (25, 49, 124, 126, 127). The appropriate choice depends on the question to be answered and the level of analysis desired. Methods used to assess malabsorption for diagnostic purposes will clearly not need to be as rigorous as those in experiments attempting to elucidate the mechanisms of enter-ocyte function. Developments in the clinical evaluation of bowel function, however, are often the stimulus for more exacting studies in the laboratory while physiological techniques occasionally become incorporated into clinical assessment.

### In vivo techniques in humans

The ingestion of a test substance either by mouth or by tube and the serial measurements of their appearance in the blood or urine (Tolerance tests) are much-used clinical tests of the efficacy of absorptive function of the small bowel. Their great weakness is that the body fluid levels are the result not only of absorption processes per se but also of gastrointestinal motility and hepatic and renal function. These can be controlled for to some extent by comparing the oral load with that given intravenously but then the effects of the oral load in releasing or affecting the secretion of the numerous gastrointestinal hormones (104) is bypassed and the two experimental conditions are not exactly equivalent. A current non-invasive development of the technique is the sampling of excretory products in the breath created by the ingestion of specific substrates (45, 95). Fats and carbohydrates labelled with $^{14}C$ have been employed as substrates for the production by the intestine (and its bacteria) of labelled $^{14}CO_2$ (13, 120). Hydrogen has also been used as it is generated exclusively by gut bacteria acting on dietary carbohydrates. Various forms of sugar malabsorption, especially of lactose, have been detected by this approach (86). In the most recent development the breath is analysed for hydrogen by a sensitive electrochemical detector (14).

The simple principle behind balance studies, that absorption is equated to the difference between oral ingestion and faecal excretion, is often confounded in practice by complications of metabolism, completeness and regularity of bowel evacuation and of the necessity for the daily collection of stools. The advent of non-absorbed markers has made the technique more useful but while the method has traditionally been used clinically to assess fat and nitrogen absorp-tion, it is really only suited to the study of substances excreted without modification, viz calcium, iron and $B_{12}$ (128). The serial measurement of whole body retention of a substance labelled with radioactivity is a variant of the balance study. It is only applicable to substances retained by the body in an unmodified form for prolonged periods (128).

Only rarely can absorption be measured, (as it is often done in animals) from acute isolated loops of intestine in anaesthetised man (4, 80) undergoing an abdominal operation or from chronic, surgically prepared loops (54). The latter suffer from the lack of 'luminal nutrition' and their enterocyte population may be abnormal (72, 116, 141, 142).

By far the most important techniques used to assess human intestinal absorptive/secretive function in situ are the various intubation methods. Since the introduction of a long rubber intestinal tube with a balloon by Miller and Abbott (87) in 1934, many types have been developed and rubber has been superceded by fine plastic tubing. These can even be passed along the whole length of the gut allowing any region to be studied (10). The major difficulty of the complete recovery of any unabsorbed material infused down the tubes (in order to assess the absorptive function) was overcome by the introduction of inert, non-absorbed markers. The most satisfactory and reliable for human work appears to be polyethylene glycol (PEG) which can be obtained labelled with $^{14}C$ or $^3H$ (69, 146) greatly facilitating its estimation. The tubes have been used to aspirate intestinal contents after feeding liquid test meals containing the non-absorbable marker and fats, carbohydrates, proteins, peptides and free amino acids (11, 96, 97, 123). This type of experiment gives information about the site and the amount of net absorption. The most popular approach however, has been the steady-state perfusion of an intestinal segment. Three types of tube are used i) the simple double lumen, ii) the triple lumen with a mixing segment and iii) the triple lumen with occluding balloon. Much discussion and criticism about the validity of techniques i and ii exist (34, 49, 124, 126, 127, 128, 133), the general agreement is that the use of an occluding balloon with aspiration above the balloon prevents refluxing of the perfused solution and its contamination from upper gastrointestinal endogenous secretions and is preferable if kinetic studies are contemplated (90). Balloons however, are not too well tolerated by conscious subjects and if tight control of the infusion solution entering the test segment is not essential (as it is for kinetic studies) then technique ii) with the mixing segment is satisfactory.

### In vivo techniques in animals

The investigation of intestinal absorption in animals allows, obviously, the employment of a greater variety of techniques (Table I). The classic early studies using gastric intubation of the material and then killing of the animal to see how much has been absorbed (15) are now little used because of the concentrated solutions fed and the complicating effects of gastric emptying and intestinal motility (114). Balance studies have, on the whole, been used more in the context of nutritional assessment than for defining mechanisms (5, 125). A great number of studies have been undertaken using intestinal loops either of the acute type in anaethetised animals where a specific segment of intestine is isolated by ligatures at cephalic and arboral ends. The solute under study is injected into the lumen and absorption allowed to take place (static loop) (59) or (dynamic loop) the material is circulated through the cannulated lumen (with or without non-absorbable markers) by hydrostatic pressure (134), gas lift (57) or peristaltic pump (16, 115). Static loops, with their lack of stirring or mixing, can create conditions where the absorption of the solute becomes rate limited by its diffusion from the bulk phase, this leads to difficulties in interpreting results obtained from animals whose intestines have different absorbing capacities (74). Dynamic loops do not usually suffer from this difficulty and lend themselves to kinetic studies where serial measures of absorption can be made and even the electrical p.d. generated by the processes measured (21). Circulating fluid containing air bubbles ('segmented flow') through rat intestine in vivo has been used to greatly increase luminal mixing (147). When tried in chicken intestine in vivo, the intestinal perfusate became extremely cloudy indicating discharge of material from the gut wall.

Two intriguing in vivo preparations have been published but neither has been embraced by other workers. The first is unique in that it not only allows the electrical p.d. across the rat intestine to be measured in vivo but also its short-circuit current and resistance (98). The current, of course, is not claimed by the authors to be identical with that measured under in vitro conditions but is purported to be related to ion transfer. The second preparation cannulates segments of jejunum and ileum independently in a rat under anaesthesia. After surgery, the animal is placed in a restraining cage and the loops used for kinetic absorption experiments, one hour after recovery from the anaesthesia, for up to 5 hours by circulating hexose and PEG as a marker (7). The absorption data (in the conscious rat) were calculated per length of intestine (after sacrificing the animal) but special measurements also allowed it to be calculated per enterocyte. It is not known if perfusing jejunum and ileum simultaneously with sugar solutions in conscious animals affects the absorptive functions of either segment but recently it has been claimed that ileal perfusion significantly modified jejunal hexose absorption in anaesthetised rats (24).

Mention should be made of the preparations where the blood supply of the intestine is cannulated in vivo and is perfused with buffers or blood allowing control of the serosal milieu. It has been much used with intestine from amphibians (102, 103) and can be used in the more exacting mammalian preparation (55).

Special surgical techniques can be undertaken in animals allowing the creation of Thiry-Vella loops of intestine and the sampling of portal and mesenteric blood or lymph (100, 131). Using these highly specialised methods, absorption can be studied especially in conscious animals. While essential for answering specific questions (viz. how much fat enters the lymphatic route as compared with the portal route, what type of products enter the blood from the absorption of proteins etc), the surgical techniques need skill, the animals need excellent post-operative care and the experiments need generous funding for they are usually expensive! The use of the electrical activity generated by the movement of ions across human and animal intestine to assess intestinal function in vivo, as previously mentioned, will be discussed in a later section.

*The normalisation of absorption data—which base to use?*

The limitations of the methods used to assess intestinal function in vivo are important in relation to the interpretations placed on the data obtained. A significant problem exists when attempting to make comparisons between conditions that change not only intestinal function but also intestinal morphology. A large literature has grown up over the years as to the choice of base upon which to calculate or normalise absorption data (7, 22, 70, 73, 89). This choice can be critical as different bases for calculation can change the interpretation placed on the initial measurements. Absorption, for example, may be found to be decreased from normal when measured per segment of intestine. However, if related to the actual number of enterocytes present, it may then be actually greater than normal! This type of confusion is always possible and depends upon the focus of the study—is the experimenter trying to discover how each enterocyte adapts to the condition or is he only trying to learn the nutritional implication of the change. In a study of the maximum absorptive capacities of the jejunum and ileum for two amino acids, distinct differences were observed if the absorptive function was calculated on a mucosal surface area basis (an index of the enterocyte number) and on a regional, segmental basis (89). One criticism of the attempts used to calculate or normalise absorption data, even that based per enterocyte (7), is that they all assume that the whole of the villus or all the enterocytes in the mucosa are undertaking the transfer. Studies undertaken in

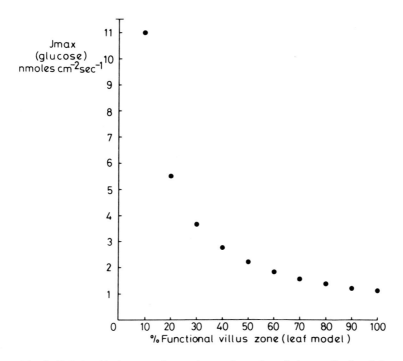

Fig. 3. Relationship between the maximum absorption of glucose ($J_{max}$) and the percentage area of the villus assumed to be undertaking the transfer (% functional villus zone assuming a leaf shaped villus model). (When the total area of the villus is transferring the % functional zone = 100, when the upper third is transferring the % functional zone = 30). From Mitchell & Levin (88).

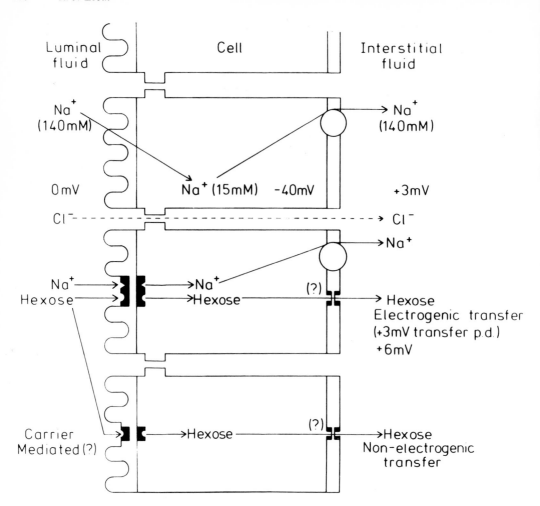

Fig. 4. Enterocytes of the small intestinal epithelium illustrating the concepts of linking the extracellular/intracellular Na$^+$ gradient (upper enterocyte) with hexose active transfer through the agency of co-transfer mediated by the Na$^+$-hexose carrier at the brush border membrane and the outward directed Na$^+$ pump at the basolateral membrane (middle enterocyte). The enterocyte interior is approximately 40 mV negative to the luminal fluid (assuming the potential here is 0). In the interdigestive phase the basal potential difference (p.d.) across the epithelium is approximately 3 mV (interstitial fluid or serosa positive to the luminal fluid) which increases to 6 mV, on addition of an hexose to the luminal fluid. The electrogenic hexose transfer creates a hexose transfer p.d. of +3 mV. A non-electrogenic path for hexose absorption, probably carrier mediated, is also present in the brush border membrane. Exit of the hexose is thought to be via a carrier process at the basolateral membrane. The tight junctions between cells and the intercellular channels represent the major shunt pathway for passive ion movement, in this case exemplified by Cl$^-$ movement. The diagram is a composite made from a variety of experimental data given in the review by Levin (75).

vitro have indicated that the best intracellular accumulation of amino acids and sugar is at the top third of the hamster villus (65) while apparent similar results have been observed more recently with rabbit intestine in vitro (129). Conditions *in vitro* are very different from those in vivo where

the possibility of villous motility (pumping up and down) exists (67) but against this is the close packing of villi reducing the anatomic surface area accessible to luminal solutes. The effects of calculating the maximum absorptive capacity ($J_{max}$) in vivo for glucose absorption over different percentages of functional villus zones have been explored by Mitchell & Levin (88) and are shown in Fig. 3. The absorption calculated over the whole villus (% functional zone = 100) appears to be approximately ⅓ to ¼ less than if it was assumed the absorption took place over the top third (% functional zone = 30%). This approach will allow any absorption calculated per whole villous area to be corrected to any fraction deemed to be the functional zone in vivo.

The problem of the base upon which to calculate absorption has usually been ignored in human studies where absorption in vivo can be related only to the assumed length of intestine perfused, in reality the measured distance between the inlet and outlet ports of the intubaton tube. In human intubation studies, the intestine can concertina over the tube (33) and thus make the actual area performing the absorption much different from the assumed one. The length of segment perfused can be critical in experiments designed to illustrate certain aspects of intestinal transfer (124). Relating the decrease in glucose absorbed (in children with monosaccharide intolerance) with the change in the calculated absorptive surface has been attempted in a recent

study (66). This type of approach offers promise for future studies in humans but it does necessitate both biopsy and intubation.

*Electrical potentials across the small intestine—exploitation to assess intestinal functions in vivo*

Movements of ions across the small intestinal epithelium in vitro and in vivo produce measurable electrical potential differences (p.d.) (2, 6, 75). The types and mechanisms involved in their generation are listed in Table II. A model of the epithelium featuring certain mechanistic aspects of the electrical activity is shown in Fig. 4.

*The potential difference in the interdigestive phase in vivo and intestinal secretion*

During the interdigestive phase in vivo, most measurements have recorded a variable, but small, electrical potential difference (p.d.) of a few millivolts (normal polarity lumen negative to the blood side) (6, 75, 119). A recent updating (43) of an older human study (44) has claimed, however, a much higher and stable value of 12 mV. No specific name has ever been given to the potential; basal or endogenous p.d. is perhaps most appropriate. Although always measured

Table II. Electrical potential differences (p.d.) recorded across the human/animal small intestinal epithelium

| Transintestinal electrical potential difference (p.d.) | Probable mechanism of generation |
| --- | --- |
| Basal or endogenous | Complex generation-sum of secretory p.d., electrogenic $Na^+$ transfer (lumen to blood) and diffusion p.d.'s. Normal polarity lumen negative to blood. |
| Secretory | Change in transintestinal p.d. (lumen becoming more negative) due to electrogenic secretion of anion ($Cl^-$ or $HCO_3^-$) blood-to-lumen. Under neural influences. |
| Transfer (amino acid/hexose) | Increase in endogenous p.d. (serosa becoming more positive) on addition of actively transferred hexose/amino acid to luminal fluid due mainly to increased electrogenic $Na^+$ entry and transfer (Fig. 4). |
| Diffusion | Change in transintestinal p.d. due to differential movements of cations/anions across the tight junctions (paracellular pathway) and enterocyte membranes (Fig. 4). |
| Osmotic | Change in transintestinal p.d. induced by ion/fluid movements due to hypertonic osmotic loads |

Table III. Characteristics of pressure waves (using categorisation of Foulk et al. (36)) and associated fluctuations of endogenous potential differences observed in jejuna of conscious human subjects (from 113)

| Pressure wave | PD fluctuation | Amplitude (mV) | Peak-to-peak delay (secs) | Duration (secs) |
|---|---|---|---|---|
| Type III | Spike | $0.51 \pm 0.1$ | 0 | $5 \pm 1$ |
|  | wave | $3.1 \pm 0.1$ | $45 \pm 3$ | $120 \pm 3$ |
| Type III with basic rhythm superimposed |  | $7.8 \pm 0.4$ | — | $452 \pm 48$ |

during 'basal' small bowel activity, its generation is complex and probably represents the algebraic sum of electrogenic secretion (blood to lumen; (20, 43), electrogenic $Na^+$ transfer (lumen to blood) and difffusion p.d.'s across the enterocytes membranes (Table II). While the basal p.d. is important as the physiological driving force for $K^+$ movement (38), its variation in anaesthetised animals and in vitro did not appear initially to be useful in delineating changes in absorptive and secretive functions (71). Recent studies in conscious man and dog, however, recorded considerable spontaneous changes in the basal p.d. of up to 10 mV. These correlated temporally with specific patterns of small intestinal motility measured by simultaneous pressure recordings (113). A summary of the pressure waves and characteristics of the p.d. fluctuations is given in Table III.

Typical recordings showing some of these features are shown in Fig. 5. Both the fluctuations in the p.d. and the motility were suppressed after injection of the anticholinergic drug propantheline bromide (Probanthine, 30 mg intramuscularly); luminal pilocarpine stimulated the p.d. but not the motility. The conclusion from these experiments and others in the literature was that the major cause of the spontaneous, large electrical change in the endogenous p.d. correlated with motility was intestinal electrogenic ion secretion (Table III) modulated by cholinergic mechanisms. Interestingly in patients with coeliac disease, where intestinal secretion is enhanced (35), the amplitude of the p.d. with Type III wave ($5.1 \pm 0.3$ mV, Mean $\pm$ S.E. n = 77, 6 patients) was highly significantly greater than in normal controls ($2.3 \pm 0.2$, n = 80, 7 subjects). Whether this is due to a genuinely enhanced electrogenic secretion or to changes in intestinal resistance (71) inferred from the greater diffusional resistance of the sprue intestine to solutes (112) is not yet clear. Further studies on the relationships between motility and the transintestinal endogenous p.d. discovered previously clearly demonstrated that in normal subjects, the phases of the migrating motor complex (MMC) are associated with characteristic patterns and amplitudes of the transintestinal p.d. (107). These are shown in Table IV. The phases of the MMC had previously

Table IV. Characteristics of the basal (interdigestive) transintestinal p.d. with the phases of the migrating myoelectric complex (MMC) obtained from 3 jejunal sites in 9 young healthy subjects (from 107)

| Phases of MMC | Quiescent | Intermittent activity | Regular |
|---|---|---|---|
| Contractions/min | 2 | 5–8 | 8 |
| Transintestinal p.d. characteristics | Flat, little change | irregular small fluctuations (peaks) | single large peak |
| Amplitude p.d. (mV) Mean $\pm$ S.E.M. | $1.3 \pm 0.3$ | $2.7 \pm 0.5$ | $5.3 \pm 0.5$ |

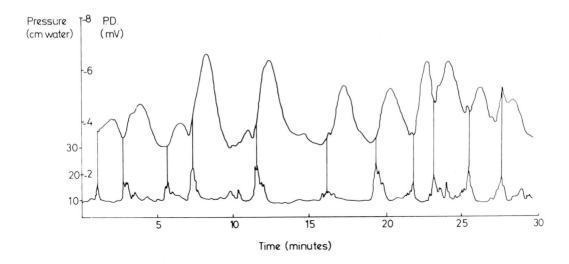

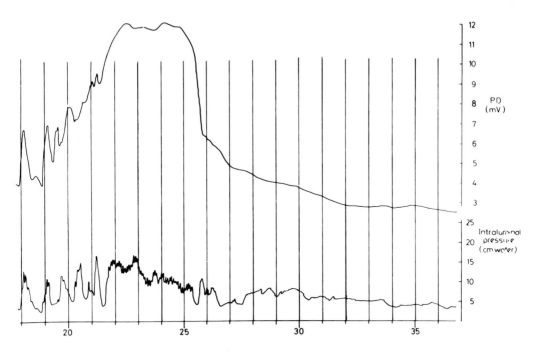

Fig. 5. Recordings of intraluminal pressure and the transintestinal p.d. in two conscious subjects. In the upper record lines have been drawn from the peaks of the pressure waves to emphasis their association with large delayed p.d. waves. Lower record shows the type III wave with basal rythm superimposed and the corresponding large increase in p.d. (numbers represent minutes), both activities then fall to basal levels. This type of wave is characteristic of a migrating myoelectric complex. See text for details. (From Read et al, 113).

only been associated with fluctuations in gastric and pancreatic secretion (140). It now appears that as the MMC progresses down the alimentary canal, it activates not only secretion in the stomach and pancreas but also in the small intestine. Confirmation of this intestinal secretory behaviour obviously requires chemical/isotopic measurements using intubation and perfusion. Unfortunately, the present techniques need long perfusion periods to demonstrate net ion movements and are not suitable to reveal the changes in anion movement during the brief passage (in minutes) of the MMC wave so easily revealed by the on-line electrical and pressure recordings. Combined p.d. and pressure monitoring, however, could well provide new insights into electrogenic secretion in healthy and dysfunctional intestine.

*The intestinal 'unstirred layer' and its effects*

Solid surfaces create a stationary layer of adherent fluid when immersed in a moving fluid. Many experiments, especially those using animal intestine in vitro have demonstrated clearly that this layer adhering to the mucosal surface of the intestine provides a significant barrier to the diffusive movement of solutes being transferred by mechanisms in the brush border membrane. This is especially so in the intestine in situ. While fluid in the bulk phase can be mixed, the flow closer to the mucosal surface becomes increasingly more laminar and slower until the final stationary layer at the fluid/membrane interface itself. These fluid lamellae (together with the mucus and glycocalyx) constitute the in vivo 'unstirred layer'. It has crucially important consequences on the kinetics of active and passive transfer across the intestine, causing underestimation of the passive permeability coefficient and over-estimation of affinity parameters of carriers (the Km of carrier kinetics). A recent review gives all the relevant references (75). The unstirred layer creates experimental difficulties when trying to characterise the type of absorption kinetics in vivo. Slow rates of luminal perfusion will always yield diffusion limited rates of solute movement and the kinetics will become indistinguishable from those of diffusion even if a saturable, active transfer carrier

mechanism is present (29). This is the probable reason for the recent surprising report that the absorption of glucose in vivo was a linear rather than a curvilinear function of glucose concentration (68).

The relationship between the thickness of the unstirred layer (d cm), the 'actual' Km of the carrier site (mM), the measured or 'apparent' Km of the carrier site (mM), the maximum transporting capacity of the site of mechanism $J_{max}$ ($\mu$moles/cm$^2$/sec) and the free diffusion coefficient of the solute under study D (cm$^2$/sec) has been formulated (101) into the simplified but useful equation

$$\text{'Apparent' Km} = \text{'Actual' Km} + J_{max}\frac{d}{D}$$

While clearly showing the effects of changes in $J_{max}$ and d, the unstirred layer, in obscuring the 'actual' Km, the equation, for practical purposes, is not too easy to employ with data obtained in vivo and other formulations have to be used (75, 109). The equation, however, emphasises that in any experimental condition or diseased state, changes in the unstirred layer thickness, with or without changes in the $J_{max}$, will cause artificial changes in the 'apparent' Km possibly unrelated to any real change in the affinity (or 'actual' Km) of the carrier. Thus a study of the changes in the unstirred layer thickness in various conditions became essential for a better understanding of the real changes in intestinal absorption mechanisms. The measurement of the functional unstirred layer thickness under in vivo conditions was first attempted in anaesthetised rats using the time course of the development of an osmotic potential (Table II) induced by a mannitol load (21). Subsequently, the same technique has been applied uniquely to studies in human jejunum in situ in conscious healthy subjects and in patients with active and controlled coeliac disease and functional and pathological diarrhoea (109). Pro-Banthine was given to create conditions favourable to the recording technique (the equivalent of anaesthesia in the rat study). The various measures of the functional unstirred layer so obtained are listed in Table V. In healthy subjects, the functional unstirred layer was of similar thickness

Table V. Functional thickness of jejunal unstirred layer and values (mean ± S.E.M.) of the kinetic parameters characterising the electrogenic component of glucose absorption in healthy controls and patients with intestinal pathology or dysfunction. Numbers in brackets represent number of subjects (from Read et al. (109))

| | Functional unstirred layer thickness (μm) | Apparent Km (mM) | $PD_{max}$ (mV) |
|---|---|---|---|
| Controls (healthy) | 632 ± 24 (7) | 36 ± 6 | 7.6 ± 0.6 |
| Active coeliac | 442 ± 23 (9) | 11 ± 1 | 6.8 ± 0.7 |
| Treated coeliac | 585 ± 26 (7) | 31 ± 5 | 10.6 ± 0.9 |
| Functional diarrhoea | 557 ± 34 (5) | 36 ± 9 | 9.2 ± 1.15 |
| Pathological diarrhoea | 416 ± 16 (9) | 12 ± 2 | 7.6 ± 0.6 |

to the height (500–600 μm) of a human villus. During active coeliac disease, the thickness decreased significantly but was restored after removal of gluten during treatment. The thickness of the layer in the pathological diarrhoea group was significantly less than the healthy controls unlike that of the functional group. The possible consequences of these changes in unstirred layer thickness on the kinetics of absorption of glucose in coeliac disease have been reported and interpreted by computer simulation (75, 108, 109) and will be briefly discussed in the next section.

*Kinetic parameters characterising electrogenic glucose absorption and coeliac disease*

Animal experiments showed that the glucose transfer p.d.'s (Table II and Fig. 4) measured in vivo and used as an index of glucose absorption allowed the kinetic characterisation of the electrogenic glucose transfer mechanism in jejunal enterocytes (21). Apparent Km's obtained electrically matched those obtained in fed (21) and in fasted rats (22) by chemical estimation after correction of the total chemical absorption for the non-electrogenic linear component (Fig. 4). The presence of this linear component of hexose absorption in vivo has been independently confirmed in rat (91) and although clearly present in many kinetic studies published previously, its effects on the kinetics had been overlooked (3, 21 for references). It is probably mediated by a carrier with a very high Km only blocked by high concentrations of phloridzin, the specific hexose carrier inhibitor (75).

Application of the technique to measure the kinetics of electrogenic glucose absorption in conscious man using the glucose transfer p.d. generated by increasing concentrations of luminally infused glucose (111) was accomplished by creating a stable electrical recording system between the luminal electrode, (the infusion electrolyte) and a saline-filled plastic cannula inserted subcutaneously in the forearm and using propantheline bromide (Pro-Banthine, i.m.) to abolish the spontaneous fluctuations in the basal p.d. and motility (113). Continuous aspiration from the infusion site increased the sensitivity of the method, the stability of the recordings and prevented pooling of the infusions (109). Although technically difficult, it was possible in a few healthy subjects to measure simultaneously the amount of glucose absorbed, using a double lumen perfusion technique (47), and the electrical p.d. generated (108). The results obtained are shown in Fig. 5. Interestingly, the glucose transfer p.d. has a curvilinear relation with the amount of glucose absorbed, a result compatible with the dual mechanism of glucose absorption discussed previously for rat, i.e. an electrogenic and a non-electrogenic route. The electrogenic route saturates but the non-electrogenic component has a capacity and a greater proportion of glucose goes via this route as the infused concentration of glucose is increased. This causes the curvilinear nature of the relationship, a maximum transfer p.d. is generated but glucose transfer still increases.

The kinetics of electrogenic glucose absorption was studied (109) in healthy controls and in patients with active coeliac disease, treated coeliac disease, functional diarrhoea and pathological

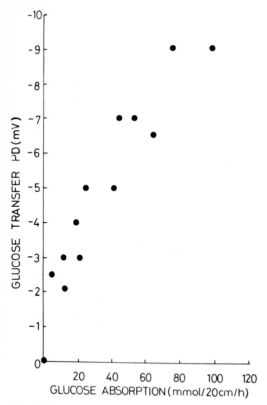

Fig. 6. Relation between the glucose transfer p.d. and the amount of glucose absorbed, measured simultaneously in the jejunum of conscious, healthy subjects. See text for details. Modified from Read (108).

diarrhoea (Table V). The 'apparent' Km for electrogenic glucose absorption was much reduced in active coeliacs compared with healthy controls but it returned to normal values after 6 months on a gluten-free diet (treated coeliacs). The values for the maximum P.D. generated (P.D. max) were not significantly different. Patients with functional diarrhoea (of unknown aetiology) had normal 'apparent' Km's but those with pathological diarrhoea (of known aetiology) had significantly reduced 'apparent' Km's. The reduction in 'apparent' Km could be interpreted as an increase in the affinity of the transfer mechanism (carrier?) for glucose. It will be recalled, however, that changes in 'apparent' Km can occur due to changes in the unstirred layer and maximum transfer capacity while the actual Km could remain unchanged. A computer simulation allowed an exploration of the possible relation-

ships between changes in the unstirred layer thickness, $J_{max}$ and 'apparent' Km and the possible combinations of 'actual' Km and $J_{max}$ that interact through the unstirred layer yielding the experimental observed values of 'apparent' Km for the control and active coeliac conditions (109). This is the first intestinal disease state to be so analysed.

It was clear that the difference in 'apparent' Km between controls and active coeliacs could not be explained by the changes in the unstirred layer thickness (previously measured by an electrical method). If the published values for glucose absorption kinetics in coeliacs (48, 121) are analysed it is clear that the $J_{max}$ in coeliacs is only a fraction of that in health. This reduced $J_{max}$ acting through the reduced unstirred layer will produce the artificial change in 'apparent' Km. The decreased $J_{max}$ could be caused solely by the loss of enterocytes that occurs in the diseased state and need not reflect any change in the transport characteristics of the remaining enterocytes.

A preliminary study in fasting man has reported that the 'apparent' Km for electrogenic glucose absorption ($16 \pm 2$ mM, Mean $\pm$ S.E.M.) was increased significantly by repeated perfusions of glucose or sucrose (106) a result remarkably similar to that obtained in fed and fasted animals by electrical (21, 22, 23) and chemical methods (77).

The advantages of the electrical method of assessing kinetics in man are its speed (approximately 1 hour to construct a concentration/transfer p.d. curve), low concentrations of glucose can be used, unstirred layer thickness and diffusion p.d.'s can also be assessed with little extra time, computer simulation can be applied and it can be adapted for electrogenic amino acid transfer. Its major disadvantage is that it characterises only the electrogenic component of intestinal transfer and thus does not give any information about the total absorptive capacity of the intestinal segment.

*Electrical technique for estimating functional lactase activity in situ*

Although tolerance tests are available for the clinical determination of hypolactasia, they do not provide a direct estimate of functional lactase activity for they utilise glucose levels in the blood and as argued in the previous sections, these are influenced by many other systems. Breath tests suffer from similar problems. Even estimation of lactase in biopsy material will not necessarily reveal functional lactase activity because of the differences of lactase activity between intact cells and homogenates (148). Attempts to correlate the absorption of hexose from lactose hydrolysis in patients with lactase deficiency with the lactase activity have been unsuccessful although the hexose absorbed was reduced (81). The failure was probably due to the great difficulty in measuring low rates of hexose absorption by intubation studies. Because of these problems, the development of a new method for assessing functional lactase activity in situ in conscious man by electrical techniques was undertaken. Because lactose per se does not yield a transfer p.d. but its hydrolysis products do, the magnitude of the transfer p.d. created by lactose infusion into the human jejunum could be used as an index of functional lactase activity in situ. The obvious difficulty of different intestines giving rise to different hexose transfer p.d.'s due to non-specific changes (resistance, active transfer changes etc) was overcome by the simple expedient of measuring the glucose transfer p.d. in the same subject by infusion of a glucose load and then using the ratio of the $\frac{\text{lactose p.d.}}{\text{glucose p.d.}}$ as the index of lactase activity (110). This ratio when plotted against the lactase activity measured in jejunal biopsies from the same subjects clearly distinguished those patients with a lactase deficiency (biopsy lactase < 4 lactase units). There was a highly significant linear reaction between the ratio and the lactase activity. Higher normal levels of lactase activity (biopsy activity > 4 lactase units) did not show any evidence of correlation with the potential ratio. Thus, unlike other lactase assessments, the electrical technique can provide a specific index of functional lactase activity of the jejunal mucosa in situ. The efficacy of the technique has been independently confirmed (106). The method offers the possibility of investigating changes in lactase activity in various diseased states and experimental conditions.

*Multiple transport systems for hexoses—the isocarrier concept*

Although the level of dietary sugar is known to influence absorption of sugars, the complexities of the mechanisms involved were not realised until specific sugars were fed to fasting animals and then their effects on the various transfer mechanisms for these sugars were tested (23). The feeding of glucose, galactose and $\alpha$-methyl glucoside produced differential effects in the kinetic parameters characterising the transport mechanisms for the various sugars. This was interpreted as strong evidence for the possession by enterocytes of more than a single carrier for hexose transport. There is now a convincing body of direct and indirect evidence that intestinal sugar transfer is mediated by multiple carriers (23, 74, 138). Unfortunately, there is not enough information to define their physiological roles. It may be that the multiple hexose carriers are isocarriers of glucose—in analogy to isozymes (multiple forms of the same enzyme with highly similar qualitative but different quantitative properties). They may be involved in the facultative responses of the enterocytes to changes in dietary intake—especially of sugars. Multiple carriers can obviously cause complications in the kinetic analysis of hexose transfer mechanisms if glucalogues (artificial analogues of hexose) are used to characterise the kinetics rather than glucose and galactose—the dietary sugars. In an animal model none of the three glucalogues employed exactly characterised the changes in glucose and galactose kinetics (138). The possible source of error in using glucalogues to characterise transfer in human biopsy material from patients has been emphasised (23). At present, no study has set out to explore the specific presence of multiple hexose carriers in human intestine but in the rare condition of glucose/galactose malabsorption, patients show a residual glucose absorption (85).

*Using corrected kinetic parameters of in vivo absorption to assess intestinal responses to dietary changes*

A technique has been developed (76, 77) that allows, in animals, the best estimates of the kinetic

Table VI. Flow chart for the estimation of 'real' $K_m$ and $J_{max}$ for the in vivo absorption of hexoses and amino acids (Levin & Mitchell (76, 77))

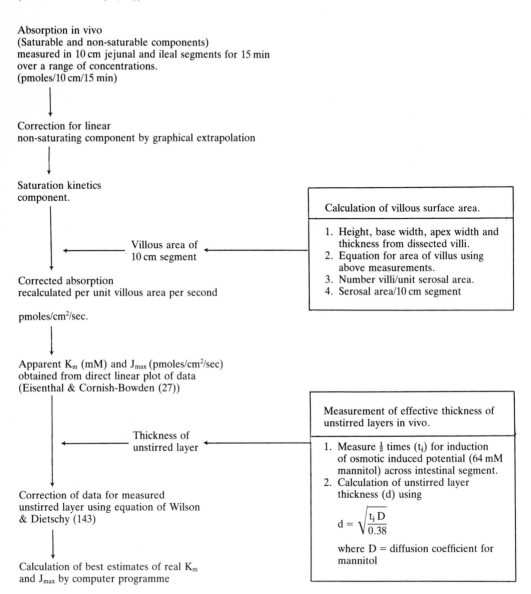

Absorption in vivo
(Saturable and non-saturable components)
measured in 10 cm jejunal and ileal segments for 15 min
over a range of concentrations.
(pmoles/10 cm/15 min)

Correction for linear
non-saturating component by graphical extrapolation

Saturation kinetics
component.

Villous area of
10 cm segment

Calculation of villous surface area.

1. Height, base width, apex width and thickness from dissected villi.
2. Equation for area of villus using above measurements.
3. Number villi/unit serosal area.
4. Serosal area/10 cm segment

Corrected absorption
recalculated per unit villous area per second

pmoles/cm²/sec.

Apparent $K_m$ (mM) and $J_{max}$ (pmoles/cm²/sec)
obtained from direct linear plot of data
(Eisenthal & Cornish-Bowden (27))

Thickness of
unstirred layer

Measurement of effective thickness of unstirred layers in vivo.

1. Measure $\frac{1}{2}$ times ($t_\frac{1}{2}$) for induction of osmotic induced potential (64 mM mannitol) across intestinal segment.
2. Calculation of unstirred layer thickness (d) using

$$d = \sqrt{\frac{t_\frac{1}{2}\, D}{0.38}}$$

where D = diffusion coefficient for mannitol

Correction of data for measured
unstirred layer using equation of Wilson
& Dietschy (143)

Calculation of best estimates of real $K_m$
and $J_{max}$ by computer programme

parameters Km and $J_{max}$ to be obtained under in vivo conditions from the 'apparent' values. These best estimates have been designated 'real' Km's to distinguish them from the 'apparent' and 'actual' Km. The various steps of the method are shown in the flow chart in Table VI. When animals were fasted, significant changes in the 'real' Km's and $J_{max}$'s for five different amino acids and for glucose and galactose were observed (77). The responses could be classified into six different combinations of change in the Km and $J_{max}$ (theoretically nine such combinations exist). The observations reveal that fasting induces highly specific adaptations of intestinal transfer processes for hexose and amino acids. Application of the technique to other experimental situations will allow a better understanding of the adaptive capabilities of the enterocyte's absorptive functions.

## ACKNOWLEDGEMENTS

Acknowledgement is given to the Agricultural Research Council for research support.

## REFERENCES

1. Agar WT, Hird FJR, Sidhu GS. Biochim Biophys Acta 1954, 14, 80–84.
2. Armstrong WMcD. pp 45–65 in Csaky TZ (ed). Intestinal Absorption and Malabsorption, Raven Press, New York, 1975
3. Atkins GL, Gardner MLG. Biochim Biophys Acta 1977, 468, 127–145
4. Atwell JD, Duthie HL. Gastroenterology 1964, 46, 16–22
5. Aubert JP, Bronner F, Richelle LJ. J Clin Invest 1963, 42, 885–891
6. Barry RJC. Brit Med Bull 1967, 23, 266–269
7. Batt RM, Peters TJ. Clin Sci Mol Med 1976, 50, 499–509
8. Binder H. Gastroenterology 1974, 67, 231–236
9. Binder HJ. pp 159–178, in Field M, Fordtran JS, Schultz, SG (eds). Secretory Diarrhea. American Physiological Society, Bethesda, USA, 1980
10. Blankenhorn DH, Hirsch J, Ahrens EH. Proc Soc Exp Biol Med 1955, 88, 356–362
11. Borgstrom D, Dahlqvist A, Lundh G, Sjovall J. J Clin Invest 1957, 36 1521–1536
12. Brice RS, Owen EE, Taylor MP. Gastroenterology 1965, 48, 584–592
13. Burrows PJ, Fleming JS, Garnett ES, Ackery DN, Colin-Jones DG, Bamforth J. Gut 1974, 15, 147–150
14. Corbett CL, Thomas S, Read NW, Hobson N, Bergman I, Holdsworth CD. Gut 1981, 22, 836–840
15. Cori CF. J Biol Chem 1925, 66, 691–715
16. Cramer CF, Dueck J. Am J. Physiol 1962, 202, 161–164
17. Crane RK, Malathi P, Preiser H. Biochim Biophys Res Comm 1976, 71, 1010–1016
18. Crane RK, Mandelstam P. Biochim biophys Acta 1960, 45, 460–476
19. Crane RK, Wilson TH. J Appl Physiol 1958, 12, 145–146
20. Davis GR, Santa Ana CA, Morawski S, Fordtran JS. J Clin Invest 1980, 66, 1326–1333
21. Debnam ES, Levin RJ. J Physiol 1975, 246, 181–196
22. Debnam ES, Levin RJ. J Physiol 1975, 252, 681–700
23. Debnam ES, Levin RJ. Gut 1976, 17, 92–99
24. Debnam ES. J Physiol 1982, Proc Physiological Society, in press
25. Duthie HL. Brit Med Bull 1967, 23, 213–216
26. Eggermont E, Loeb H. Lancet 1966, ii, 343–344
27. Eisenthal R, Cornish-Bowden A. Biochem J 1974, 139, 715–720
28. Field M, Fordtran JS, Schultz SG. Secretory Diarrhea. American Physiological Society, Bethesda, USA, 1980
29. Fisher RB, pp 339–353 in Dickens F, Neil E (eds). Oxygen in the Animal Organism, Pergamon Press, 1964
30. Fisher RB, Gardner MLG. J Physiol, 1974, 241, 211–234
31. Fisher RB, Gardner MLG. J Physiol, 1974, 241, 235–260
32. Fisher RB, Parsons DS. J Physiol 1949, 110, 36–46
33. Fordtran JS. Gastroenterology 1966, 51, 1089–1093
34. Fordtran JS. Gastroenterology 1969, 56, 987–989
35. Fordtran JS, Rector FC, Locklear TW, Ewton MS. J Clin Invest 1967, 46, 287–298
36. Foulk WT, Code CF, Morlock GG, Bargen J. Gastroenterology 1954, 26, 601–611
37. Fromm D. Am J Physiol 1973, 224, 110–116
38. Gilman A, Koelle E, Ritchie JM. Nature 1963, 197, 1210–1211
39. Gradey GF, McGaffey, Moore EW, Chalmers EW. Gastroenterology 1966, 50, 883
40. Gradey GF, Madoff MA, Duhamel RC, Moore EW, Chalmers TC. Gastroenterology 1967, 53, 737–744
41. Granger DN, Taylor AF. Am J Physiol 1978, 235, E429–E436
42. Groseclose R, Hopfer U. Membrane Biochem 1978, 2, 135–148
43. Gustke RF, McCormick P, Ruppin H, Soergel KH, Whalen GE, Wood CM. J Physiol 1981, 321, 571–582
44. Gustke RF, Whalen GE, Geenen JE, Soergel KH. Gastroenterology 1967, 52, 1134 (Abstract)
45. Hepner GW. Gastroenterology, 1974, 67, 1250–1256
46. Herman RH. pp 105–140 in Hughes RE (ed). Human Nutrition—a comprehensive treatise Vol 4, Nutrition—Metabolic and Clinical Applications, Plenum Press, New York, 1979
47. Holdsworth CD, Dawson AM. Clin Sci 1964, 27, 371–379
48. Holdsworth CD, Dawson AM. Gut 1965, 6, 387–391
49. Holdsworth CD, Sladen GE. pp 338–397 in Duthie HL, Wormsley KG (eds). Scientific Basis of Gastroenterology, Churchill–Livingstone, Edinburgh, 1979
50. Hopfer U. Proc Nat Acad Sci 1975, 72, 2027–2031
51. Hopfer U. Am J Physiol 1977, 233 (6) E445–E449
52. Hopfer U. J Supramol Struct 1977, 7, 1–13
53. Hopfer U. Fed Proc 1981, 40, 2480–2485
54. Jackson WPU. Clin Sci 1952, 11, 209–216
55. Jacobs P, Bothwell TH, Charlton RW. Am J Physiol 1966, 210, 694–700
56. Janowitz HD, Sachar DB. Frontiers of knowledge in the Diarrheal Diseases, Projects in Health, Inc, Upper Montclair, New Jersey, 1979

57. Jervis EL, Johnson FR, Sheff MF, Smyth DH. J Physiol 1956, 134, 675–688
58. Kendall MJ. Brit Med J 1973, 2, 179
59. Kershaw TG, Neame KD, Wiseman G. J Physiol 1960, 152, 182–190
60. Kimberg DV, Schachter D, Schenker H. Am J Physiol 1961, 200, 1256–1262
61. Kimmich GA. pp 51–115 in Korn E (ed). Methods in Membrane Biology, Plenum Press, New York, 1975
62. Kimmich GA. Fed Proc 1981, 40, 2474–2479
63. King IS, Sepúlveda FV, Smith MW. J Physiol 1981, 319, 355–368
64. Kinnula VL, Hassinen IE. Acta Physiol Scand 1981, 112, 387–393
65. Kinter WB, Wilson TH. J Cell Biol 1965, 25, 19–39
66. Klish WJ, Udall JN, Rodriguez JT, Singer DB, Nichols BL. J Pediatrics 1978, 72, 566–571
67. Kokas E. Pflügers Arch für Physiol 1932, 229, 486–489
68. Kotler DP, Levine GM, Shiau Y. Am J Physiol 1981, 240, G432–G436
69. Krag E, Krag B, Lenz K. Scand J Gastroenterol 1975, 10, 105–108
70. Levin RJ. Brit Med Bull 1967, 23, 209–212
71. Levin RJ. Gut 1969, 10, 868–870
72. Levin RJ. J Endocr 1969, 45 315–348
73. Levin RJ. Life Sciences 1970, 9, 61–68
74. Levin RJ. pp 63–116 in Boorman KN, Freeman BM. Digestion in the Fowl, British Poultry Science Ltd, Edinburgh 1976
75. Levin RJ pp 308–337 in Duthie HL, Wormsley KG (eds). Scientific Basis of Gastroenterology Churchill Livingstone, Edinburgh, 1979
76. Levin RJ, Mitchell MA, J Physiol 1979, 295, 20–21P
77. Levin RJ, Mitchell M, in Robinson JWL, Dowling RH, Riecken EO (eds). Mechanisms of Intestinal Adaptation, MTP Press Ltd, Lancaster, 1982
78. Lichtenberger LA, Lechago J, Miller TA. Gastroenterology 1979, 77, 1291–1300
79. Lucke H, Berner W, Menge H, Murer H. Pflügers Arch 1978, 373, 243–248
80. McColl I. Proc Roy Soc Med 1971, 64, 1026–1028
81. McMichael HB, Webb J, Dawson AM. Brit Med J 1966, 2, 1037–1041
82. Makhlouf GM. Gastroenterology 1974, 67, 159–184
83. Manninen V, Melin J, Apajalahti A, Karesoja M. Lancet 1973, 1, 398–399
84. Meeuwisse G, Dahlquist A. Acta Paediatr Scand 1968, 57, 273–280
85. Meeuwisse GW, Kerstin M. Acta Paediat Scand, 1969, 188 (Suppl) 1–24
86. Metz G, Jenkins DJA, Peters TJ, Newman A, Blendis LM. Lancet 1975, 1, 1155–1157
87. Miller TG, Abbott WO. Am J Med Sci 1934, 187, 595–599
88. Mitchell MA, Levin RJ, in preparation
89. Mitchell MA, Levin RJ. Experientia 1981, 37, 265–266
90. Modigliani R, Bernier JJ. Gut 1971, 184–193

91. Murakami E, Saito M, Suda M. Experientia 1977, 33, 1469–1470
92. Murer H, Hopfer U, Kinne-Saffran E, Kinne E. Biochim Biophys Acta 1974, 345, 170–179
93. Murer H, Kinne R. J Membrane Biol 1980, 55, 81–95
94. Newcomer AD, McGill DB. Gastroenterology 1966, 51, 481–488
95. Newman A. Gut 1974, 15, 308–323
96. Nixon SE, Mawer GE. Br J Nutr 1970, 24, 227–240
97. Nixon SE, Mawer GE. Br J Nutr 1970, 24, 241–258
98. Noble HM, Matty AJ. J Endocrinol 1971, 49, 377–386
99. Ohsawa K, Kano A, Hoshi T. Life Science 1979, 24, 669–678
100. Parsons DS. pp 1177–1216 in Code CF (ed). Handbook of Physiology Vol 3, Section 6, American Physiological Society, Washington DC, 1968
101. Parsons DS. pp 407–430 in Robinson JWL (ed). Intestinal Ion Transport MTP Press Ltd, England, 1976
102. Parsons DS, Pritchard JS. J Physiol 1968, 198, 405–434
103. Parsons DS, Sanderson IR. J Physiol 1980, 309, 447–460
104. Polak J, Bloom S. pp 71–111 in Duthie HL, Wormsley KG (eds). Scientific Basis of Gastroenterology Churchill Livingstone, Edinburgh, 1979
105. Quastel JH. pp 273–286 in Quastel JH (ed). Methods in Medical Research, Vol 9, Year Book Medical Publishers, Chicago 1961
106. Rask-Madsen J, Gudmand-Høyer E, Krag E. Scand J Gastroent 1976, 11, (Supplement 38) 46 Abstract
107. Read NW. pp 299–306 in Christensen J (ed). Gastrointestinal Motility, Raven Press, New York, 1980
108. Read NW. pp 45–52 in Ruppin H, Domschke W, Soergel H (eds). Diarrhea in Disorders of Intestinal Transport, Georg Thieme Verlag, Stuttgart and New York, 1981
109. Read NW, Barber DC, Levin RJ, Holdsworth CD. Gut 1977, 18, 865–876
110. Read NW, Davies RJ, Holdsworth CD, Levin RJ. Gut 1977, 18, 640–643
111. Read NW, Holdsworth CD, Levin RJ. Lancet 1974, 2, 624–627
112. Read NW, Levin RJ, Holdsworth CD. Gut 1976, 17, 444–449
113. Read NW, Smallwood RH, Levin RJ, Holdsworth CD, Brown BH. Gut 1977, 18, 141–157
114. Reynell PC, Spray GH. J Physiol 1956, 134, 531–537
115. Rider AK, Schedl HP, Nokes G, Shining S. J Gen Physiol 1967, 50, 1171–1182
116. Riecken EO, Menge H. Acta Hepato-Gastroenterol 1977, 24, 389–399
117. Rosensweig NS, Stifel FB, Herman RH. Biochim Biophys Acta 1968, 170, 228–234
118. Ruppin H, Domschke W, Soergel KH. Diarrhea in Disorders of Intestinal Transport, Georg Thieme Verlag, Stuttgart, 1981

119. Sachar DB, Taylor JO, Saha JR, Phillips R. Gastroenterology 1969, 56, 512–521
120. Sasaki Y, Iio M, Kameda H, Ueda H, Aoyagi T, Christopher NL, Bayless TM, Wagner HN. J Lab Clin Med 1970, 76, 824–835
121. Schedl HP, Clifton JA. J Clin Invest 1961, 40, 1079–1080
122. Schultz S, Zalusky R. J Gen Physiol 1964, 47, 1043–1059
123. Silk DBA, Chung YC, Berger KL, Conley K, Beigler M, Sliesenger MH, Spiller GA, Kim YS. Gut 1979, 20, 291–299
124. Silk DBA, Dawson AM. pp 151–204 in Crane RK (ed). International Review of Physiology Gastrointestinal Physiology 111 Vol 19. University Park Press, Baltimore, 1979
125. Skoryna SC, Waldron-Edward D (eds). Intestinal absorption of metal ions, trace elements and radionuclides, Pergamon Press, Oxford, 1971
126. Sladen GE. Gut 1968, 9, 624–628
127. Sladen GE, Dawson AM. Gut 1968, 9, 530–535
128. Sladen GE. pp 1–49 in McColl I, Sladen GE (eds). Intestinal Absorption in Man Academic Press, London 1975
129. Smith MW. Experientia 1981, 37, 868–870
130. Smyth DH, Taylor CB. J Physiol 1957, 136, 632–648
131. Smyth DH. pp 260–272 in Quastel JH (ed). Methods in Medical Research, Vol 9, Year Book Medical Publishers, Chicago, 1961
132. Smyth DH. pp 241–283 in Smyth DH (ed). Biomembranes, Intestinal Absorption Vol 4A, Plenum Press, New York, 1974.
133. Soergel KH. Gut 1969, 10, 601–602
134. Sols A, Ponz F. Revta esp Fisiol 1947, 3, 207–211
135. Southgate DAT, Durnin JVGA. Brit J Nutrition 1970, 24, 517–535
136. Steiner M, Bourges HR, Farrish GCM, Koss JR, Gray SJ. Am J Med Sci 1969, 257, 234–241
137. Stirling CE, Schneider AJ, Wong MD, Kinter WB. J Clin Invest 1972, 51 438–451
138. Syme G, Levin RJ. Brit J Nutr 1980, 43, 435–443
139. Trier JS. pp 365–384 in Harris CC, Trump BF, Stoner GD (eds). Methods in Cell Biology, Vol 21B, Academic Press Inc, New York, 1980
140. VanTrappen G, Peeters TL, Janssens J. Gastroenterology 1979, 76, 1264
141. Williamson RCN. New Eng J Med 1978, 298, 1393–1402
142. Williamson RCN. New Engl J Med 1978, 298, 1444–1450
143. Wilson FA, Dietschy JM. Biochim Biophys Acta 1974, 363, 112–126
144. Wilson TH. Intestinal Absorption, WB Saunders, Philadelphia, 1962
145. Wilson TH, Wiseman G. J Physiol 1954, 123, 116–125
146. Wingate DL, Sandberg RJ, Phillips SF. Gut 1972, 13, 812–815
147. Winne D. Naunyn-Schmiedeberg's Arch Pharmacol 1978, 304, 175–181
148. Zoppi G, Hadorn B, Gitzelman R, Kistler H, Prader A. Gastroenterology 1966, 50, 557–561

# Small Bowel Adaptation and its Regulation

R. H. DOWLING
Gastroenterology Unit, Dept. of Medicine, Guy's Hospital & Medical School,
London, SE1 9RT, U.K.

Since the subject of intestinal adaptation was last reviewed (16, 20, 97), there have been relatively few major advances but many useful minor additions and extensions which have helped to consolidate our knowledge of the field. The aim of this chapter is to summarise the results of a series of experiments which build up to our present state of knowledge. In doing so, the results of relatively old studies carried out some 15 years ago are briefly reviewed since they provide an essential background for, our current work. However the article concentrates mainly on the new developments and in discussing these, areas of doubt and controversy are emphasised.

*R. H. Dowling, Gastroenterology Unit, Dept. of Medicine, Guy's Hospital & Medical School, London SE1 9RT, U.K.*

## BACKGROUND

Our interest in intestinal adaptation started with studies of the residual intestine following small bowel resection and bypass. We began by asking questions such as: Does the intestinal remnant undergo adaptive changes in mucosal structure and function to compensate for loss of the resected segment? If so, are there regional differences in the adaptive response? Does the functional adaptation affect the absorption of all nutrients? Following ileectomy, for example, can the jejunum 'acquire' the specialised active transport functions of the terminal ileum for intrinsic factor-bound vitamin $B_{12}$ and conjugated bile acids? How soon after resection do the adaptive changes develop? And most important of all, what is the mechanism for these changes?

We now know the answers to some, but not all, of these questions and as often happens in the world of biological research, the story is not quite so simple as it first appeared. It is clear that no one unifying hypothesis can explain all the phenomena of intestinal adaptation which have so far been described.

### Classification of different types of intestinal adaptation

*Type I and Type II responses.* With few exceptions (see below) the small bowel mucosa seems

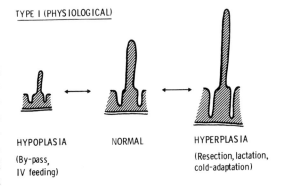

TYPE I (PHYSIOLOGICAL)

HYPOPLASIA (By-pass, IV feeding)   NORMAL   HYPERPLASIA (Resection, lactation, cold-adaptation)

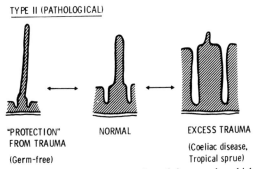

TYPE II (PATHOLOGICAL)

"PROTECTION" FROM TRAUMA (Germ-free)   NORMAL   EXCESS TRAUMA (Coeliac disease, Tropical sprue)

Fig. 1. Schematic representation of the ways by which the small bowel adapts. The Type I (physiological) response is considered by the author to be most common and important adaptive mechanism. The Type II (pathological) response is more correctly a repair process in response to trauma (or the lack of it). Examples are given of the experimental models in which these two types of responses are seen.

to undergo only two major types of adaptive response (Fig. 1)—a Type I or physiological response with adaptive hyper- or hypo-plasia (and corresponding changes in segmental digestive/absorptive function) and a Type II or pathological response which is really a repair process in response to mucosal injury (or conversely, to the lack of 'trauma' as happens, for example, in 'germ-free' animals) with secondary changes in absorptive function.

In the opinion of the author, Type II changes are completely different from the adaptive hyperplasia or hypoplasia seen in 'true' adaptation. The short or absent villi and tall 'hyper-regenerative' crypts (Type II changes) of coeliac disease, tropical sprue, radiation injury, ischaemia, immune-mediated mucosal damage, experimental self-filling blind loops and mucosal injury induced by luminal perfusion or instillation of noxious agents, such as lactic acid or formalin, have little or nothing in common with the Type I adaptive response to resection, bypass, hyperphagia, pregnancy and lactation, hypophysectomy, pancreatico-biliary diversion or to hormonal stimuli such as the effects of excess CCK or hyperenteroglucagonaemia—examples of Type I responses all of which are discussed below. For this reason, the present chapter is confined mainly to the classical Type I or physiological responses. In these responses, the increases or decreases in segmental digestive/absorptive function are secondary to the changes in mucosal surface area resulting from intestinal dilatation and villus hyperplasia (or narrowing and villus hypoplasia) and to the associated changes in the function of individual enterocytes which occur when crypt cell production and epithelial cell migration rates change.

*Exceptions to the Type I and Type II responses.* As mentioned before, there are only a few exceptions to the generalisation that adaptive changes in small bowel function are mainly due to changes in absorptive surface. Occasionally, however, functional adaptation may occur without corresponding changes in mucosal structure. This happens, for example, as a result of feeding high bulk diets (24), after cortico-steroid treatment (6) and during pregnancy (when vitamin $B_{12}$ absorption

increases (85)). This implies, of course, that since the absorptive surface, the size of the villi and the number of epithelial cells do not change, the function of the individual enterocytes must increase. As discussed later, the function of individual cells also changes with the more conventional Type I adaptive hyperplasia and hypoplasia, but usually in a paradoxical sense. In other words, with hyperplasia there is more rapid cell migration and the villus becomes populated with relatively immature cells whose individual function *diminishes*. With hypoplasia and slow cell migration, the reverse is true: the villus becomes populated with hypermature cells and their individual absorptive potential tends to *increase* (22).

## THE PHENOMENA OF INTESTINAL ADAPTATION

The phenomena of a Type I response can best be considered by taking the example of the adaptive changes seen in the mucosa after small bowel resection and by attempting to answer the rhetorical questions which were posed in the introduction (see 'Background' above).

(i) *Does the residual intestine develop adaptive changes?*

Following small bowel resection, the residual intestine becomes dilated* and both crypt depth and villus height increase. The resultant increase in absorptive surface area/unit length of intestine is associated with enhanced segmental absorption of many 'substrates' (20, 21).

(ii) *Is there functional adaptation for the absorbance of all nutrients?*

The answer to this question seems to be yes—at least for those substances studied to date. For example, there is increased segmental absorption of water, electrolytes, mono-, di- and oligo-saccharides, amino acids, di- and oligo-peptides, and probably also of the water soluble vitamins. Assuming that adequate luminal bile

---

* Some investigators maintain that the intestinal remnant also elongates: most, however, (including the author) find that it does not.

acid concentrations are maintained, it seems likely that mono- and di-glycerides, fatty acids, the fat soluble vitamins and sterols such as cholesterol, are also hyperabsorbed. In other words, there is a non-specific increase in segmental absorption—that is, in the amount of 'substrate' absorbed/unit length intestine (usually, but not exclusively, measured as luminal disappearance of perfused or instilled substrates).

### (iii) *Are there local differences in the adaptive response?*

The adaptive response to jejunectomy is marked—with increases in the various indices of mucosal structure and function in the region of 70–100%, when compared to controls. In contrast, the changes in the jejunal remnant after ileectomy are modest with, at most, 20–30% increases in the markers of the adaptive response.

### (iv) *After ileal resection, does the jejunum 'acquire' specialised active transport functions of the distal small bowel?*

The answer here is probably no. There is no evidence that the jejunum can inherit the specialised transport functions of the ileum. However, the inherent properties of the ileal enterocytes for the active transport of intrinsic factor(IF)-bound $B_{12}$ and conjugated bile acids are retained by the ileum, irrespective of its anatomical site. For example, $B_{12}$ absorption remains unchanged following ileal transposition to a proximal small bowel site (25). In fact, when ileal hyperplasia is induced by proximal small bowel resection, as the number of enterocytes increase, so the number of hypothetical $B_{12}$-IF receptor or binding sites increase, with the result that not only segmental, but also overall, absorption increases (64, 65).

For most nutrients, the loss of absorptive surface produced by resection diminishes overall absorption to subnormal levels in the immediate post-operative period. Ultimately, however, the net effect of the segmental hyperfunction is to maintain overall absorption at normal or near normal levels. (Whether or not the patient is left with permanent malabsorption depends on the site and extent of the resection, the 'health' of the residual bowel and the magnitude of the

adaptive response). For IF-bound $B_{12}$ and conjugated bile acids, however, the net effect of jejunectomy is to 'trick' the ileum so that instead of restoring overall absorption from subnormal to normal, it induces supranormal absorption (64, 65, 78). This curiosity is probably of no clinical importance. In the case of vitamin $B_{12}$, the hyper-absorbed vitamin is likely to 'spill' into the urine. In the case of the bile acids, even though the passive diffusion component of jejunal bile acid absorption may be lost as a result of resection, the net gain as a result of the increased active transport expands the bile acid pool (at least in the rat (78)), but if this happens in man, again it is unlikely to be of any clinical significance.

### (v) *How quickly do the adaptive changes develop after resection?*

This probably varies from species to species. In the rat, the first demonstrable change is an increase in mucosal DNA synthesis—as judged by the incorporation of $^3H$ thymidine into DNA—which develops in 24–36 h after resection (75). The sequence of events is then likely to be a temporary imbalance between crypt cell production (which is increased) and villus tip cell loss (which initially, at least, may be normal) until villus hyperplasia is produced. Then, when the hyperplasia becomes established, a new steady state is reached in which crypt cell production again matches cell loss from the villus tips—albeit that both variables remain increased when compared to normal. This hyperplasia seems to develop over 1–2 weeks before it reaches its maximum: certainly it is fully established by one month (21).

There have been no systematic studies on the speed on onset of post-resectional hyperplasia in the dog or in man but indirect evidence suggests that it may take 1–2 months in the dog and possibly one year in man before adaptive changes become fully established. However, this latter conclusion is based on clinical observations of gradually diminishing stool frequency and the wet weight and fat content of faeces, with time. In theory, many 'compensatory' influences other

Table I. Summary of major and minor factors believed to promote intestinal adaptation.

| Major Influences | Minor Influences |
|---|---|
| Luminal nutrition.<br>Pancreatico-biliary secretions.<br>Hormonal factors. | Changes in mucosal blood flow.<br>Neural (including peptidergic) factors.<br>Changes in luminal and mucosal bacteria.<br>Other factors (eg. salivary epidermal<br>growth factor). |

than small bowel adaptation—such as modifications in gastric emptying, small and large bowel transit and in functional colonic adaptation (89)—could all play a role in this gradual and progressive amelioration.

**(vi) *What are the mechanisms for small bowel adaptation?***

Having documented the phenomena of adaptation, the emphasis appropriately, is now on studies of its mechanisms. Ten years ago, there were three major and several minor factors known to influence small bowel mucosal structure and function and thought to regulate the adaptive response (Table I).

In 1982, the three major influences of a decade ago—luminal nutrition, pancreaticobiliary secretions (PBS) and hormonal factors—still hold sway but as mentioned earlier, with accumulating evidence it is clear that the influences are complex and multiple. The relatively simple hypotheses of ten years ago have now become confused. It is to be hoped that a critical analysis of the evidence for and against the various factors will help to clarify the mechanisms once more.

## MECHANISMS OF INTESTINAL ADAPTATION

### LUMINAL NUTRITION: THE CASE FOR (Table II)

#### (i) *Jejunal resection*

Normally most of the ingested nutrients are absorbed in the proximal small bowel and little nutrition remains in the chyme reaching the ileum. Following jejunal resection, however, the ileum receives a richer than normal supply of luminal nutrition and shows marked adaptive mucosal hyperplasia.

Table II. Summary of the evidence in favour of luminal nutrition as a mechanism for intestinal adaptation

| Mucosal hyperplasia and/or segmental hyperfunction in association with absolute or relative increases in luminal nutrition. | | Mucosal hypoplasia and/or segmental hypofunction in association with absolute or relative decreases in luminal nutrition. | |
|---|---|---|---|
| Absolute | Relative | Absolute | Relative |
| Hyperphagia associated with:— | In the ileum after:— | In:— | After:—<br>Hypophysectomy<br>During:— |
| —Hypothalamic damage | —Jejunal resection | —Thiry-Vella by-pass loops | Starvation |
| —Dietary training | —Jejunal by-pass | —Self-emptying blind loops | —semi-starvation |
| —Hyperthyroidism | —Ileo-jejunal transposition | —Ileal urinary conduits | —intermittent starvation |
| —Pregnancy | —Pancreatico-biliary diversion | —During TPN | —protein-calorie malnutrition |
| —Lactation | During:— | | In the jejunum:— |
| —Experimental diabetes | Luminal infusion of hydrolysed | | ileo-jejunal transposition |
| —Exposure to low temperatures | nutrients into by-passed loops ('Vivonex') or during TPN | | |

This finding is compatible with the luminal nutrition theory but the evidence is indirect and many other factors could have influenced the results such as a drop in ileal luminal pH, the effect of salivary, gastric, pancreatico-biliary or duodenal secretions (although many of these, in turn, are also affected by ingested nutrients). More direct evidence that luminal nutrition plays a major role in the adaptive ileal response to jejunectomy came from studies in the dog. Feldman et al. (30) showed that in orally-fed animals, the ileum showed the expected villus hyperplasia. Conversely, in parenterally-fed dogs there was no such adaptive response; in fact, there was a slight and significant fall in villus height (30) comparable to that seen in parenterally fed animals with an intact small bowel (41, 44). Thus, the presence of luminal nutrition is essential for the expression of the ileal adaptive response to jejunal resection (30, 59).

### (ii) *Ileo-jejunal transposition*

When the positions of the ileum and jejunum are interchanged anatomically (by transposing, surgically, the lower half of the small intestine to lie immediately distal to the ligament of Treitz), even though there is no stimulus to mucosal growth because of loss of absorptive surface, the ileum again receives more luminal nutrition than usual and develops obvious hyperplastic changes (21). Conversely, the jejunum, now lying downstream and receiving its chyme after proximal (ileal) absorption, shows modest, but significant, hypoplasia (21).

It seems, therefore that when the ileum receives more luminal nutrition than normal it becomes hyperplastic. Conversely, when the jejunum becomes the deprived member of the intestinal community, it becomes hypoplastic, but because the degree of proximal ileal absorption is unknown after ileo-jejunal transposition, this is a poor model in which to study the effects of excluding luminal nutrients from the small bowel mucosa. A much better model is the use of a Thiry-Vella bypass.

### (iii) *Jejunal bypass*

As with jejunal resection, jejunal bypass stimulates mucosal hyperplasia in the ileum remaining in continuity. Conversely, the jejunum deprived of luminal nutrition (and also, it must be admitted, of pancreatico-biliary secretions) becomes hypoplastic with a narrower calibre, shorter villi, shallower crypts, slower cell migration, fewer cells (mucosal DNA)/unit length intestine, reduced segmental absorption and diminished enzyme activity/cm intestine, than normal (35). Similar changes occur in self-emptying blind loops (70). This pattern of response also seems to occur in man and the results of most (but not all) studies have shown that in patients undergoing jejuno-ileal bypass for obesity, the mucosa in the excluded intestine becomes hypoplastic while that in the intestine remaining in continuity shows adaptive hyperplasia (27, 32, 38, 47). These findings lend further support to the luminal nutrition hypothesis.

### (iv) *Starvation and semi-starvation*

The results of many studies show that when food intake is restricted (or even completely excluded), the intestinal mucosa becomes hypoplastic and shows diminished segmental absorptive function. Indeed, this is the major (but not the sole) reason for the mucosal hypoplasia and hypofunction seen after hypophysectomy (96). Removal of the pituitary results in a marked reduction in food intake. In control animals with an intact small bowel, when food intake is restricted to match that of the hypophysectomised animals, a comparable degree of mucosal hypoplasia develops.

Thus there is accumulating evidence that when luminal nutrition is increased, the intestinal mucosa becomes hyperplastic and when it is decreased, the reverse is true. But because starvation and semi-starvation invariably cause associated malnutrition, proof that the effects of these experiments on the gut are due to exclusion of topical nutrition, rather than to secondary malnutrition, are wanting. The advent of total parenteral nutrition (TPN), therefore, provided a valuable experimental model for extending this hypothesis.

### (v) *Exclusion of exogenous luminal nutrition during parenteral feeding*

Results of studies in animals (41, 44, 59) and

in man (26) have shown that when nutrition is maintained by parenteral feeding, but exogenous luminal nutrition completely excluded, the intestinal mucosa becomes hypoplastic and/or develops hypofunction. This effect is greater in the jejunum than in the ileum and is compatible with the idea that the well known proximal-to-distal gradient in mucosal mass is stimulated by the presence of a rich supply of ingested nutrients in the jejunum and a relatively poor supply (because of proximal absorption) in the ileum. During TPN, therefore, the jejunum 'suffers' the effects of luminal deprivation to a greater extent than the ileum and as a result, the normal gradient disappears (93).

### (vi) *Hyperphagia induced by exposure to low temperatures*

When rats are chronically exposed to low temperatures (6°C), they develop hyperphagia within a few days (40) and after about one month, the resultant increase in luminal nutrition is associated with mucosal hyperplasia and segmental hyperfunction (49). However, these adaptive changes are prevented when food intake is limited to match that taken by normothermic, normophagic controls.

This observation is again compatible with the concept that the increase in luminal nutrition is responsible for the adaptive mucosal growth in the hypothermic rats. However, the evidence again is indirect.

### (vii) *Stimulation of mucosal growth by luminal perfusion of nutrients*

At least three separate studies have shown that infusion or instilling of nutrients directly into the intestinal lumen stimulates mucosal growth—or more correctly, prevents the hypoplasia which would otherwise have been expected when exogenous nutrients are excluded from the intestinal lumen of Thiry-Vella or self-emptying bypass loops or in parenterally-fed animals. (There are, in fact, several different, although related, ways of studying this—prevention of hypoplasia; reversal of hypoplasia after it has become established and stimulation of mucosal growth over and above that seen in controls.)

Jacobs et al. (52) found that in the dog with two jejunal Thiry-Vella fistulae, although instilling of 0.15 M saline every day for 12 weeks prevented the villus hypoplasia of the empty loop, it did not prevent the hypofunction. However, by instilling a dilute isotonic solution of the elemental diet 'Vivonex', they not only prevented the hypoplasia which would otherwise have occurred but they actually stimulated villus hyperplasia. This then was our first *direct* evidence that luminal nutrients were important in maintaining normal mucosal growth. But which of the individual nutrients was responsible?

In similar studies, Menge, Riecken et al. (72, 73) and Clarke (15) showed that glucose, galactose and methionine partially prevented the hypoplasia and hypofunction of self-emptying blind loops. However this experimental model has its limitations. The isoperistaltic loops may not be completely self-emptying. It seems likely that some luminal nutrients may reflux into the most distal parts of the bypassed loops with the result that as one progresses from the most proximal portion of the 'excluded' loop near its occluded stump to its mid segment and distal portion near the end-to-side anastomosis, one may find hypoplasia, normoplasia and even hyperplasia.

In the opinion of the author, the most valuable studies of direct stimulation of mucosal growth by luminal nutrients came recently from Canada. Morin and colleagues (79) found that in jejunectomised rats, although luminal (intra-gastric) infusion of carbohydrate and protein partially prevented the intestinal mucosal hypoplasia of TPN, fat provided by far the most potent stimulus for intestinal mucosal growth. When only 20% of the total daily energy (calorie) requirement was infused intragastrically in the form of long-chain triglycerides (corn oil), the structure and function of the small bowel mucosa of parenterally-fed animals was maintained at levels comparable to those seen in rats given a complete solid diet by mouth.

Thus, there is overwhelming evidence that luminal nutrition is important for maintaining normal small bowel mucosal structure and function and for stimulating adaptive changes in many experimental situations. However, the *mechanism* whereby luminal nutrition exerts its trophic (or tropic) effect is unknown. Although there is evidence that the epithelial cells can directly utilise absorbed nutrients as they traverse the enterocytes, it would be naive to imagine that they work on a commission basis, extracting their 'percentage' like a handling agent. In theory, the luminal nutrients could stimulate the release of trophic peptides from the APUD cells in the intestine which, in turn, could act as classical systemic hormones or they could act locally as paracrine substances. Alternatively, they might stimulate biochemical and cell biological regulators of tissue growth such as the ornithine decarboxylase/diamine oxidase system (63). In theory, they could also trigger neurovascular changes with secondary (or even tertiary) changes in mucosal growth. Yet again, they could provoke the release of other enterotrophic stimuli such as the pancreatico-biliary secretions. It should be emphasised that any or all of these hypothetical mechanisms may be involved; they should not be considered mutually exclusive.

## LUMINAL NUTRITION: THE CASE AGAINST

As stated before, no one putative mechanism can account for all the phenomena of intestinal adaptation. The case against luminal nutrition is largely based on negative evidence, which is indirect and circumstantial, rather than on positive proof—for example:—

### (i) *Jejunal adaptation following ileal resection*

With few exceptions (71), most investigators find no increase in food intake after ileal resection, either in experimental animals or in man. That being the case, the jejunum still receives its load of ingested nutrients directly from the stomach and duodenum—as normal. There is, therefore, neither an absolute nor a relative increase in luminal nutrition to explain the admittedly modest adaptive mucosal hyperplasia seen in the jejunum after ileal resection.

### (ii) *Ileal adaptation following colonic resection*

Similarly, there is no change in food intake nor, as far as we know, in the amount of nutrition reaching the distal small bowel lumen, after colonic resection but again the ileum shows modest adaptive changes both in experimental animals (108) and in man (107).

In the opinion of the author, the evidence from these two experiments neither negates nor destroys the luminal nutrition hypothesis: it simply suggests that in these two models some other mechanism must be operating.

### (iii) *Parabiotic and cross-circulation studies*

The same is true of experiments in parabiotic and cross-circulated animals where resection in the 'donor' animal apparently provokes an adaptive response in the 'recipient' whose food intake (and presumably also luminal nutrition) remains normal. The results of these experiments suggest that some hormonal factor must have cross-circulated to stimulate the adaptive hyperplasia in the recipient (parabiont). One up for the hormonal theory but if we accept that several mechanisms may act in concert and that none is mutually exclusive, then again this evidence complements rather than excludes the topical nutrition story. Indeed, the effects of the two mechanisms may be additive—as happens, for example, when resection and bypass are combined.

### (iv) *Effect of resection on excluded loops of intestine*

The results of studies both in the rat (98, 106) and dog (29) have shown that after either a one- or two-stage operation, the degree of mucosal hypoplasia in the excluded intestinal segment is diminished by partial resection of the gut in continuity. In other words, the anticipated hypoplasia of the bypassed loop which receives no luminal nutrients (or indeed pancreatico-biliary secretions), may be partially prevented or even reversed by resection of, say, half of the 'functioning' intestine. These and other findings (see below) strengthen the undisputed case in favour of a hormonal factor. But they say no more than 'the luminal nutrition hypothesis cannot be the sole mechanism' and cannot account for all the results.

Table III. Summary of evidence for and against pancreatico-biliary secretions (PBS) as enterotrophic factors in intestinal adaptation

| For | Against |
|---|---|
| —Trophic effect of PBS diverted to self-emptying ileal loops<br>—Trophic effect of pre-harvested pancreatic juice on self-emptying intestinal loops<br>—Ileal adaptive changes following pancreatico-biliary diversion (PBD)<br>—Enhancing effect of PBD on ileal adaptation seen during hyperphagia induced by hypothermia<br>—Enhancing effect of PBD on ileal adaptation of jejunal resection<br>—Prevention of hypoplasia of TPN by IV secretin + CCK | Diversion of PBS away from jejunum by PBD leads to:—<br>—Preserved or exaggerated proximal-to-distal gradient in mucosal mass<br>—Jejunal hyperplasia:<br>　—in rats made hyperphagic by exposure to low temperatures<br>　—in normophagic controls<br>　—in TPN rats |

(v) *Onset of post-resectional hyperplasia before luminal nutrition restored*

Hanson and colleagues (39) found that the first evidence of adaptive hyperplasia in the residual intestine occurred *before* the animals had fully recovered their appetite after intestinal resection, when they were still being fed a glucose/salt liquid diet.

## PANCREATICO-BILIARY SECRETIONS (PBS): THE CASE FOR (Table III)

So far we have emphasised the importance of luminal nutrition to explain the phenomena of adaptation acknowledging, *en passant*, that it may mediate its effect through hormonal factors, that luminal or topical nutrition cannot explain all the results and that hormonal factors undoubtedly play a role. But we have accorded only brief and parenthetic mention to the trophic effect of the pancreatico-biliary secretions. It is possible that changes in luminal nutrition simply trigger the release of varying amounts of pancreatico-biliary secretions and that these secretions, rather than the ingested food itself, are responsible for the adaptive changes in the gut.

(i) *Diversion of pancreatico-biliary secretions to the ileum*

Some ten years ago Altmann and Leblond pub-lished the results of technically brilliant experiments which showed that when bile, and particularly pancreatic secretions, were diverted to self-emptying loops of ileum, they provoked clear cut increases in ileal villus size (2, 3). The authors concluded that PBS were trophic to the intestine and that since the jejunum normally receives these secretions first, the PBS were also responsible for the proximal-to-distal gradient in villus size and in small bowel mucosal mass. These results are not in question but their interpretation is. Their findings were crucial in that other investigators (including ourselves) were influenced by their results and seduced—at least initially— by their hypothesis.

(ii) *The potentiating effect of PBS in other models of intestinal adaptation*

(a) Hypothermia: In animals exposed to low temperatures, the resultant hyperphagia stimulates ileal as well as jejunal mucosal hyperplasia (49). If, in addition, the ileum is enriched in pancreatico-biliary secretions by diverting the bile and pancreatic secretions to the mid-point of the small intestine, the ileal adaptive response become further increased (50). The effect of pancreatico-biliary diversion (PBD) is achieved not by transposing the duodenum with its attendant pancreas and bile duct to the mid-point of the small intestine but by interposing the proximal half of the small bowel between the pylorus and duodenum. If one accepts that the initial hyperplasia was due to the increase in luminal nutrition (which seems reasonable since it is abolished by restricting food intake to normal levels), then the superadded hyperplasia seem attributable to the pancretico-biliary secretions.

(b) Resection: Independently, and about the same time, Weser et al. (102) did similar experiments in jejunectomised rats. They showed that the ileal hyperplasia induced by jejunal resection could be further increased, downstream from the PBS, after PBD to the mid-point of the intestinal remnant. This finding was subsequently confirmed in a similar experiment, by Williamson et al. (104)

### (iii) *Effect of CCK and secretin during parenteral feeding*

Although the intestinal mucosal hypoplasia of TPN could be due to the absence of luminal nutrition, it is known that during parenteral feeding, not only the intestine but also the pancreas becomes hypoplastic (46). If the pancreatic secretions are indeed trophic to the intestine (2) then in theory the associated pancreatic hyposecretion, rather than the absence of topical nutrition, might be responsible for the intestinal changes.

To test this hypothesis, Hughes et al. (41) compared intestinal mucosal structure and function in two groups of dogs—one with TPN alone and one with TPN plus daily stimulation of the pancreas with one unit each/kg BW of 'bioextracted' CCK and secretin (GIH laboratory, Karolinska Institute, Stockholm) given as bolus IV injections over the course of one hour—in an attempt to simulate the pancreatic secretory response to the dogs' one meal of the day. The CCK and secretin completely prevented the villus hypoplasia of TPN alone.

At first sight, the results of this experiment might suggest that PBS are indeed trophic to the intestine. However, the 'protective' effect of the two hormones (in preventing the hypoplasia of TPN) could equally well be due to a direct trophic effect of CCK alone, of secretin alone, or of a combination of the two hormones, acting directly

on the gut. To study this further, Hughes et al. (43) and Breuer et al. (13) went on to look at the effect of low (4 µg kg$^{-1}$ day$^{-1}$) and high (40 µg kg$^{-1}$ day$^{-1}$) doses of CCK-octapeptide (CCK-OP) alone and of secretin alone in orally- and parenterally-fed rats. They found that in the doses used, neither the CCK-OP alone nor the secretin alone had any effect on the gut.

This surprising negative result raised many questions. Was the CCK-OP inactive? Based on parallel studies of pancreatic structure and function (see below), the answer, emphatically, was no. In both the low and high doses, the CCK-OP stimulated marked pancreatic growth both in orally- and in parenterally-fed rats.

Was there a species difference in the intestinal adaptive response between the dog and the rat? And did the protocol for the IV infusion influence the results? (In the dog, the CCK and secretin were given as bolus IV injections over the course of one hour in an attempt to simulate the normal response of endogenous hormones to a meal: in the rat, the peptides were infused with the IV nutrients at a constant rate throughout the 24 h period). The answer to both these possible explanations is again probably no. Hughes et al. (42) went back to the Karolinska preparations of CCK and secretin and showed that in parenterally-fed rats, as in the dog, the combination of the two hormone preparations prevented the hypoplasia which would otherwise have developed—suggesting that neither species difference* nor variation in infusion protocol, influenced the results.

Does this mean that the enterotrophic property of cholecystokinin (if it exists) resides between amino acids 8 (the number of residues in the synthetic octapeptide) and 33 (the number of amino acids in one of the major circulating forms of CCK)? Could the trophic effect of the Karolinska preparation of CCK belong to a contaminant peptide and have nothing to do with the CCK itself? Do CCK and secretin have synergistic or additive enterotrophic effects which are not apparent with the individual peptides alone?

---

* It must be admitted, however, that there is controversy about intestinal adaptive responses in different species (86).

Alternatively, could the results of the dog experiments (which were based on only 6 animals) be wrong? The answer to all these questions is that we simply do not know. This is one of the many areas of unresolved controversy referred to in the introduction. There are, however, a few additional shreds (but no more than shreds) of evidence suggesting that both peptides may stimulate intestinal growth. Based on the observation by Hughes et al. (41) that CCK + secretin prevented the hypoplasia of TPN, Weser et al. (101) also studied the effect of CCK alone in parenterally-fed rats, and concluded that CCK probably was the trophic peptide in the hormonal mixture. These results and their interpretation are discussed later (see section on hormones).

Furthermore, in a preliminary communication, Johnson and Guthrie showed that secretin (55) stimulated an increased rate of $^3$H-thymidine incorporation into intestinal mucosal DNA. Whilst these observations are compatible with a trophic effect of the peptide on the gut, they certainly do not prove it. In the opinion of the author, if CCK and/or secretin have any trophic effect on the gut, it is likely to be modest and unworthy of the effort, time and expense which would be needed to prove the point.

Although this whole question has been discussed under the heading of pancreaticobiliary secretions, it is obvious that the effect of CCK and/or secretin could equally well have been discussed under the heading of hormonal factors (see below).

### (iv) *Effect of pre-harvested pancreatic juice on self-emptying and Thiry-Vella bypass loops*

The key experiment to prove a trophic effect of pancreatic secretions on the gut is the perfusion of pooled, pre-harvested pancreatic juice into isolated intestinal loops.

In the context of intestinal adaptation, this was first done by Altmann (2) who found that the secretions did indeed play a modest trophic role in the ileum. Of course, enzyme secretions provide a rich protein meal for the intestine and it was important, therefore, to compare the effect of pancreatic juice on the gut with that produced by the equivalent 'load' of amino acids. In

essence, the effect of the amino acids was analogous to the methionine used by Menge & Riecken (72) and of the protein used by Morin et al. (79) when studying the specific properties of different luminal nutrients. To extend Altmann's studies and the observation that CCK and secretin prevented the hypoplasia of TPN, Hughes et al. (45) also infused pre-harvested pancreatic juice into the intestine. And in an attempt to exclude any specific, heat-labile, trophic factor, they compared the effect of non-boiled and boiled pancreatic juice on the gut and found that both boiled and particularly unboiled juice increased mucosal mass in self-emptying jejunal loops.

### PANCREATICO-BILIARY SECRETIONS: THE CASE AGAINST (Table III)

From the analysis of the preceding sections, it is clear that mucosal growth in the 'underprivileged' ileum may be stimulated relatively easily by an absolute or relative increase in luminal nutrition and that the trophic effect of pancreatico-biliary secretions may well be due to the associated luminal protein load. However, this remains an area of controversy and in the case of ileum, the evidence in favour of PBS is relatively strong. The principal case against PBS, however, comes from studies of the jejunum after pancreatico-biliary diversion (PBD).

### *Pancreatico-biliary diversion* (PBD)

If PBS are trophic to the intestine, since the jejunum normally receives these secretions first, one could reasonably argue that (i) PBS are responsible for the proximal-to-distal gradient in absorptive surface area and (ii) that the jejunum deprived of these secretions should become hypoplastic. This hypothesis can be tested by PBD—as described above—see section on the evidence in favour of PBS. (It must be admitted that our original aim in using this model in hypothermic rats (50) was to study the jejunum deprived of them). Later, when we repeated the studies in normothermic animals (76), our aim was to establish a baseline of jejunal structure and function after PBD so that we could see whether or not intravenous CCK and/or secretin had a direct trophic effect on the intestine *independent* of pancreatico-biliary secretions. In fact, we have yet to carry out this experiment. The changes in jejunal and pancreatic structure and function were so striking that the means became an end. In its own right, PBD became a valuable new model for inducing adaptive changes and for studying their mechanisms.

Whatever the original motives for the experiments, the results of the PBD studies cast serious doubt on the Altmann hypotheses—or more correctly, on its corollary which suggests that jejunum deprived of PBS should become hypoplastic. In orally-fed rats maintained at low (6°C) (50) or normal (22°C) temperatures (76) and in parenterally-fed rats housed at room temperature (76), PBD stimulated marked jejunal *hyperplasia*. In fact, rather than abolishing the proximal-to-distal gradient in villus height, mucosal mass and absorptive surface, PBD had the opposite effect: if anything it accentuated the gradient. Indeed, based on the results of the PBD studies, one could reasonably argue that the PBS were actually anti-trophic to the jejunum and that diversion of the secretions away from the upper small bowel removed their inhibitory influence with a rebound increase in jejunal mucosal growth.

If one accepts that there are only 3 *major* factors promoting intestinal adaptation, then by a process of exclusion one could argue that since neither luminal nutrition nor PBS are necessary for the jejunal adaptive response to PBD, one is left with a humoral mechanism. The intestinal adaptive response to PBD occurred in TPN rats which, by definition, had no exogenous nutrients in their intestinal lumen. Furthermore, the jejunal adaptive changes developed in the absence of PBS. *Ergo*, if neither luminal nutrition nor pancreatico-biliary secretions can explain the jejunal adaptive phenomena, we are left with hormonal factors. This, and many other lines of evidence in favour of a humoral mechanism, are discussed below.

## HORMONAL FACTORS: THE CASE FOR (Table IV)

Many snippets of evidence in favour of hormonal factors have already emerged from our analysis of the mechanisms of intestinal adaptation—for example, the suspicion that hormonal mechanisms may explain the jejunal adaptation seen after

Table IV. Summary of the evidence in favour of hormonal factors as a mechanism for intestinal adaptation

| Direct | Indirect |
|---|---|
| —Parabiotic studies where resection in 'donor' rat stimulates increased cell turn-over or mucosal DNA synthesis in 'recipient'<br>—Increased intestinal weight in recipient after resection of intestine in 'donor' cross-circulated pig | —Hyperplasia and segmental hyperfunction in by-passed jejunum during lactation<br>—Jejunal hyperplasia after ileal resection<br>—Ileal hyperplasia after colonic resection<br>—Modification of hypoplasia in by-passed intestine by partial resection of small bowel remaining in continuity<br>—Villus hyperplasia associated with enteroglucagonoma<br>—Intestinal enlargement in mice after intra-peritoneal injections of EG tumour extracts<br>—Increased intestinal tissue and plasma levels of EG (and other peptides) in animal models of intestinal adaptation<br>—Increased fasting and post-prandial plasma EG levels in diseases where intestinal adaptation occurs. |

ileectomy or following PBD and the ileal adaptation which has been documented after colectomy. (See also 'Luminal Nutrition: The case against, the effect of CCK and secretin during TPN and the discussion of the PBD experiment'—above.)

Much of the evidence in favour of a hormonal role for intestinal adaptation is indirect (the parabiotic studies in rats (61, 105) and cross-circulation studies in pigs (57). However there have been many studies (both *in vitro* and *in vivo*) on the effect of individual hormones or regulatory peptides on small bowel mucosal growth such as gastrin, pentagastrin, CCK, secretin, growth hormone, pancreatic glucagon, thyroid hormone, cortico-steroids and enteroglucagon and other hypothalamic/anterior pituitary hormones.

### (i) The gastrin family of peptides (Table V)

For several years Johnson claimed that gastrin was of paramount importance in regulating intestinal mucosal growth and his eloquent and persuasive arguments were stated forcibly in many original articles and in comprehensive reviews (53, 54). However, most other investigators remained unconvinced and the results of several studies challenged the role of gastrin in the small bowel adaptive response (69, 80, 83). There was often a dissociation between serum gastrin levels and the intestinal adaptive response. Many investigators, for example, found no changes in fasting

Table V. Candidate peptides and hormones for the role of 'enterotrophin',

---

1. Hypothalamic/anterior pituitary hormones—
   ? Growth hormone
   ? ACTH
   ? TSH
2. Enteroglucagon (GLI or the gut glucagon family of peptides)
3. Placental lactogen (for adaptation in IF-bound vitamin $B_{12}$ absorption)
4. Corticosteroids—prednisolone
   —dexamethasone
5. Epidermal growth factor
6. Cholecystokinin (and its family of peptides)
7. Secretin
8. Gastrin (including pentagastrin and the family of gastrins)

---

or post-prandial serum gastrin levels after small bowel resection—despite obvious adaptive mucosal changes in the residual intestine. Furthermore, small bowel mucosal hyperplasia has not been recorded in the Zollinger-Ellison syndrome or in Addisonian pernicious anaemia where serum gastrin levels are markedly increased.

Last year, however, during the Second International Conference on Intestinal Adaptation (86), Johnson stressed that however important gastrin was in stimulating parietal cell growth in the stomach (which no one doubts) and mucosal growth in the duodenum, it had little or nothing to do with intestinal adaptation.

### (ii) Cholecystokinin and/or secretin

Given its structural similarity to gastrin and the fact that strong claims had been made in favour of gastrin as an enterotrophic hormone, it was not surprising that CCK (or more correctly the family of CCK peptides) should have been considered for the role of 'enterotrophin'. Some of the studies using bioextracted CCK or its synthetic octapeptide alone, or in combination with secretin, have already been discussed in the context of pancreatico-biliary secretions. Indeed, in many of these studies it is impossible to distinguish between the direct effect of CCK and/or secretin on the gut from an indirect effect mediated through the PBS. A group of investigators from Los Angeles, however, has looked at the effect of CCK alone and of secretin alone on the rate of $^3$H-thymidine incorporation into DNA of intestinal mucosa grown in culture. They found that a dose of 125 µg secretin $kg^{-1} BW^{-1}$ given 8 hourly for 10 days significantly increased the rate of DNA synthesis but it is a long step from this pharmacological approach *in vitro* to proving that such peptides have a trophic role on the intestinal mucosa *in vivo* or indeed that in physiological concentrations they have anything to do with the maintenance of normal small bowel mucosal structure and function.

Having found that low (4 µg) and high (40 µg $kg^{-1} day^{-1}$) doses of CCK-OP infused IV have no effect on intestinal mucosal structure and function but marked effects on the pancreas, we are forced to conclude that this pancreatico-trophic peptide does *not* affect the gut. Whether or not some of the other molecular forms of CCK have an effect on the intestine remains untested and unproven and it seems unlikely that one part of the 'big' CCK molecule should be trophic to the gut. If this argument is valid, we still have to explain why the combination of bioextracted CCK and secretin should prevent the intestinal mucosal hypoplasia of TPN. At present this problem has not been resolved.

### (iii) *Anterior pituitary/hypothalamic hormones*

In classical hormonal studies, the effect of the hormone on the target organ or tissue can be inferred by removing the appropriate endocrine gland. When the pituitary is removed, for example, the intestine, amongst many other tissues, develops marked hypoplastic changes (18, 84, 96). Furthermore, the intestinal mucosal hypoplasia of hypophysectomy can be prevented, at least in part, by replacing individual hormones such as growth hormone, ACTH and TSH (84). At first sight, these results might suggest that some of the anterior pituitary/hypothalamic hormones have a trophic effect on the gut. However, as already discussed (see section on 'Starvation and semi-starvation' under the heading, 'Luminal Nutrition: the evidence in favour'), in animals with an intact small intestine the effect of hypophysectomy on the gut is almost certainly due to the associated reduction in food intake: a comparable degree of hypoplasia and hypofunction developed in pair-fed rats (96). This was not the case for hypophysectomised rats with jejunal or ileal resection. After removing the pituitary, the intestinal remnants still showed adaptive responses to resection but the *degree* of adaptation was significantly less than that seen in pair-fed controls. This suggests, indirectly, that the anterior pituitary hormones modify the intestinal adaptive response to resection.

Which hormone? Again methods are available to answer this question and in theory, it would be possible to repeat the mono-hormonal replacement studies in hypophysectomised—enterectomised rats. To date, however, such studies have not been carried out.

### (iv) *Lactation*

During pregnancy (31) and particularly during lactation (14, 16, 28), several animal species develop hyperphagia and the resultant increase in luminal nutrition is associated with intestinal mucosal hyperplasia and segmental hyperfunction. Unlike the hyperphagia induced by hypothermia, however, these adaptive changes in the intestine are not completely prevented by restricting food intake to normal levels. More important, when Elias & Dowling (28) studied mucosal structure and function in Thiry-Vella by-passed jejunal loops from lactating rats, they found comparable adaptive changes to those seen in lactating animals with an intact intestine. Thus, for the first time, we saw striking adaptive changes in loops of intestine completely isolated from exogenous (or ingested) luminal nutrition and from pancreatico-biliary secretions. The loops still had mesenteric neuro-vascular pedicles, however, and although in theory several influences could have been responsible for the adaptive change in the excluded segment, given the striking hormonal changes in lactation, it seemed to us much more likely that endocrine influences had modified mucosal growth in the by-passed loops.

### (v) *Prolactin*

Based on the results of the previous experiment (showing adaptive mucosal hyperplasia and hyperfunction in by-passed jejunum of lactating rats (28)), the most obvious candidate to account for the intestinal changes seemed to be prolactin. To study this further, Muller et al. (81) used two models of experimental hyperprolactinaemia—perphenazine injections and pituitary transplantation (where the pituitary glands from donor rats were transplanted to lie, two on each side, beneath the renal capsules of the recipient). Having confirmed that these models did indeed induce hyperprolactinaemia, at least as judged by radio-immunoassay, we next had to show that the circulating prolactin was biologically active. This was done simply by weighing the mammary tissue and by histology of the breast which showed obvious and enormous hyperplasia in both experimental models (Fig. 2). Whilst these findings strongly suggest that immunoreactive prolactin

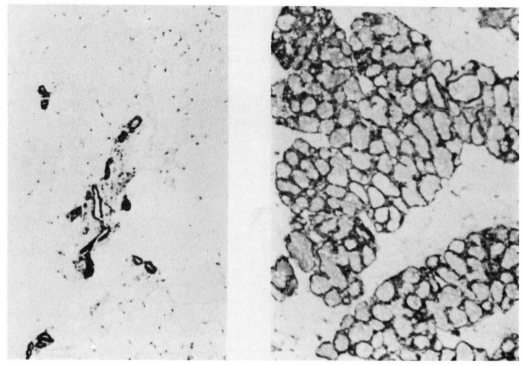

Fig. 2. Histological appearance of breast tissue from a virgin control rat (left) showing mainly ductular elements with surrounding adipose tissue, and from an animal with reduced hyperprolactinaemia (right) where there is obvious glandular enlargement—same magnification—(74).

is also biologically active, it must be admitted that many factors other than prolactin influence mammary growth. However, there was no such change in the intestine: measurements of villus height, crypt depth and of mucosal wet weight, protein and DNA per cm intestine, remained unchanged when compared with control values.

This was an important negative result since it showed clearly that prolactin was *not* trophic to the intestine (at least in these experimental models*) and that hyperprolactinaemia could *not* explain the adaptive changes seen in excluded jejunal segments of lactating rats.

If not prolactin, which hormone? A vital clue came from studies of a unique patient with an enteroglucagon secreting tumour of the kidney.

---

* In lactating rats, however, Mainoya (66) found that injections of the prolactin-secreting inhibitor, bromocriptin, partly prevented the increase in whole jejunal weight.

(vi) *The gut glucagon family of peptides*

(a) *The enteroglucagonoma case.* In 1971, Gleeson et al. (34) described a new clinical syndrome—that of changes in small bowel structure, motility and absorptive function in a patient with an enteroglucagon secreting tumour which arose in the right kidney. When the tumour was removed, the high circulating enteroglucagon levels returned to normal and the intestinal dilatation and marked villus hyperplasia disappeared. The following year Bloom (9) described biochemical, physiological and radioimmunoassay characteristics of the tumour showing that it contained gut-derived (enteroglucagon or gut glucagon like immunoreactivity) rather than pancreatic-derived glucagon. Furthermore, in unpublished studies, Gleeson & Dowling (36) went on to examine the effect in mice of intraperitoneal injections of simple saline extracts of the tumour. They found obvious macroscopic enlargement of the small bowel in the tumour injected animals which was

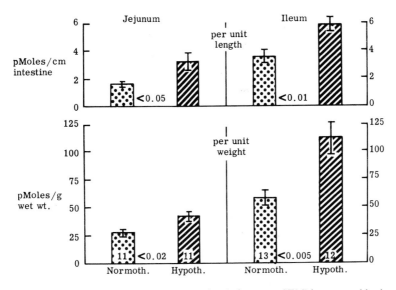

Fig. 3. Intestinal mucosal enteroglucagon levels (means ± SEM's) expressed both per unit length (upper panel) and per unit weight (lower panel) in normothermic control rats (stippled bars) and in rats maintained in a hypothermic environment of 6°C (lower panel) for 5 weeks (44). The hypothermic rats developed hyperphagia, increased luminal nutrition and both jejunal and ileal adaptive hyperplasia.

not seen in the saline injected controls. The experimental and clinical findings strongly suggested that enteroglucagon was trophic to the intestine—an observation which was tested subsequently in many experimental models of intestinal adaptation (see below).

When the clinical details of the enteroglucagonoma were first presented in public at the British Society of Gastroenterology in 1970, the audience included a medical registrar, Dr. Fiona Stevens, who was working with Professor Ciaran McCarthy in Galway. Shortly afterwards, during a routine endoscopy session, she noticed 'giant' duodenal villi and remembering Gleeson's presentation, she considered that the patient might have a similar enteroglucagon secreting tumour. This was subsequently confirmed (94) but the patients' relatives requested that he should undergo further investigations in the United States where he subsequently died. Unfortunately, the pancreatic tumour was not adequately characterised but it seems likely that he too had an enterotrophic, glucagon secreting tumour.

(b) *Tissue and plasma enteroglucagon in animal*

*models of adaptation*. Based on the clinical evidence from the enteroglucagonoma case, Jacobs et al. (48, 51) went on to measure fasting plasma, and intestinal mucosal tissue, concentrations of immunoreactive enteroglucagon and to study the immunofluorescent appearance of cryostat sections of small bowel mucosa in three experimental models of intestinal adaptation—resection, lactation and hyperphagia induced by hypothermia. Since the principle small bowel site for enteroglucagon synthesis is in the ileum, not surprisingly the greatest tissue concentrations of immunoreactive enteroglucagon were found in the distal half of the small bowel—both in controls and in the adaptation models. However, in all three experimental models, ileal mucosal enteroglucagon concentrations were increased not only when expressed/unit length (which might be expected with a non-specific increase in all epithelial cells—including the endocrine cells) but also when expressed unit weight mucosa (Fig. 3). This suggested that there must have been more EG secreting cells, larger cells, more actively synthesising cells or that the removal of EG from the cells was decreased. In fact, the results of the immunofluorescence studies suggested that many, if not all, these phenoma may be true: there were more cells and larger cells with more brightly fluorescing cytoplasms, than in the controls.

These findings, therefore, are compatible with the idea that enteroglucagon may be trophic to the intestine but they certainly do not prove it. Since then, however, there have been several more studies by Bloom, Wright and colleagues (1, 37) and from our own unit in collaboration with Bloom (74, 77) which confirm that in situations where adaptive mucosal hyperplasia develops in the intestine (particularly in the ileum), circulating enteroglucagon levels tend to rise. Indeed, Wright et al. have shown a strong correlation between crypt cell production rate (measured by vincristine metaphase arrest stathmokinetic techniques), and immunoreactive circulating enteroglucagon levels (1). (See also Bloom & Polak this symposium.)

The mechanism for the increased ileal tissue and for the increased fasting and post-prandial plasma EG levels is unknown but seems to be related again to absolute or relative increases in luminal nutrition.

(c) *Plasma enteroglucagon levels in man.* In a series of clinical studies, Bloom and colleagues have shown that in untreated coeliac disease (8) (which, being confined as it usually is, to the upper small bowel, causes proximal malabsorption with the result that the ileum is exposed to a richer than normal supply of luminal nutrition and in some cases, undergoes functional adaptation (65, 90, 91)), small bowel resection (11) or by-pass (10) and in the dumping syndrome (12) (where rapid small bowel transit delivers a relative increase in luminal stimuli to the ileum), the area under the integrated 4 h plasma EG concentration-time curve, increases markedly.

(d) *Mechanism for enteroglucagon release.* One of the main components of the luminal nutrients stimulating EG released is fat and it is tempting to speculate that Morin's exciting observation (79) showing the importance of luminal fat in maintaining mucosal growth in parenterally-fed rats, is due to the release of EG. (One could, with equal validity, also make a case for fat-stimulated CCK release.) These conjectures are amenable to testing and proof.

(e) *A 'priming' role for enteroglucagon in adaptation?* The results of recent studies in the rat suggest that increased circulating EG may play a role in intestinal adaptation (in this case the jejunal mucosal hyperplasia of pancreatico-biliary diversion), but is not needed to maintain it. In orally-fed rats studied 8 days after PBD, plasma EG levels were high and the intestinal mucosal hyperplasia had already become established. Three months after PBD, however, the degree of intestinal mucosal hyperplasia was unchanged but the plasma EG levels had returned to normal.

A more detailed 'kinetic' study of the speed of onset of jejunal mucosal hyperplasia after PBD, together with the demonstration of a rise and fall of plasma EG, would be necessary to consolidate this hypothesis. However EG is by no means the only candidate for a 'trigger mechanism' to initiate intestinal adaptation. Luk et al. (62, 63) have recently shown waxing and waning changes in the activity of ornithine decarboxylase, the first and rate-limiting enzyme in the polyamine biosynthesis pathway, which coincide with the onset and maintenance of the intestinal mucosal hyperplasia of lactation.

(f) *Conclusions about EG: the definitive proof.* Despite the strong circumstantial evidence, proof of a cause-and-effect relationship between EG and intestinal mucosal growth is wanting and until recently, definitive proof was impossible because the amino acid sequence of EG was unknown and the peptide had not been synthesised. Both these problems have now been overcome (97) and it remains to be seen whether or not synthetic gut glucagon will stimulate intestinal mucosal growth.

(vii) *Pancreatic glucagon*

The results of studies by Rudo, Rosenberg and colleagues from Chicago (87, 88) suggested that pancreatic glucagon might play a role in the intestinal adaptive changes of semi-starvation and experimental diabetes. It seems likely, however, that these findings are unrelated to studies with EG described above.

(viii) *Corticosteroids*

The results of two recent studies, one using

prednisolone (6) and the other using the gluco-corticoid, dexamethasone (56), deserve mention for separate and important reasons.

(a) Prednisolone: In previous studies (5, 7), Batt & Peters had studied the effect of chronic (4 weeks) administration of prednisolone in phar-macological doses, on small bowel mucosal struc-ture and function. However with short term (7 day) studies they found a 50% increase in the apparent $V_{max}$ for galactose absorption by indi-vidual enterocytes in the absence of changes in enteroblast (crypt cell) production or cell migration rates. As well as their scientific value (which is considerable), these studies are impor-tant in that they provide an example of functional adaptation without a corresponding change in absorptive surface. In fact, the authors presented evidence to show that prednisolone treatment increased the synthesis of jejunal brush border membrane proteins which, in turn, enhance the digestive/absorptive function of the organelle.

(b) Dexamethasone: The dexamethasone stud-ies are important in that they illustrate the result of a new 'tool' for studying adaptation—the use of jejunal mucosal explants from 6-day old rats cultured *in vitro* in the presence and absence of various candidate hormones to see if any were enterotrophic.

With this technique, Kedinger et al. (56) stud-ied the effect of epidermal growth factor, insulin, pentagastrin, thyroxine and dexamethasone on purified brush border enzyme activity. They con-cluded that in the doses used, dexamethasone alone induced sucrase and maltase (but not lactase and alkaline phosphatase) enzyme activity. The significance of these data is uncertain. They may represent induced maturation of neonatal intes-tine. Alternatively, the changes may be analogous to those described by Peters et al. (6) using prednisolone.

The technique of jejunal mucosal organ culture offers the advantage that the inevitably multiple variables present *in vivo*, can be controlled in the test tube. For example, the effect of luminal (and serosal) nutrition, luminal pH, digestive secre-tions, mucosal blood flow and neural factors can all be eliminated, or at least accurately manipu-lated. It suffers the disadvantage, however, of

being even further removed from normal physi-ology than in many of the experimental models described above, and of using dying tissue. In theory, however, the principle might be extended to organ culture of human jejunal biopsies with a different range and different doses of peptide hormones.

### (ix) *Epidermal growth factor*

Finally, in this long but necessarily incomplete list of potentially enterotrophic peptides, is epi-dermal growth factor (EGF). EGF, a chain of 53 amino acid residues, has been isolated from sal-ivary and duodenal glands. Konturek and col-leagues (17) showed that when given intraperi-toneally or intragastrically, chronic EGF administration stimulated increased DNA syn-thesis and also the weight and total DNA and RNA contents of the gastroduodenal mucosa and pancreas. It also stimulates ornithine decarboxyl-ase. Whether or not it affects other parts of the small bowel mucosa remains unknown.

In our long and detailed analysis of the ileal adaptation seen after jejunal resection, bypass, ileo-jejunal transposition and proximally con-fined coeliac disease, we have laboured the argu-ment that the ileum is exposed to a richer than normal supply of luminal nutrition. However we also conceded that in theory, some trophic factor in the salivary, gastric or duodenal secretions could have stimulated mucosal growth in the distal small bowel. Could EGF be that missing factor? As yet there is too little information by far to make such a conclusion and one should beware of the temptation of grasping at the latest and most fashionable straw. However studies with EGF are likely to prove a growing area in the adaptation field.

## HORMONAL FACTORS: THE CASE AGAINST

Few would doubt that hormonal factors are important in intestinal adaptation. Indeed they may be the final common pathway by which luminal stimuli affect intestinal mucosal growth. However there are some facts which are difficult to explain if one postulates a classical systemic hormonal effect. For example:—

### (i) *Small bowel by-pass*

If by-passed segments of intestine have an intact mesenteric blood supply, they should be stimulated by hormones in the systemic circulation. How then can we explain that the excluded loop becomes hypoplastic whilst the gut remaining in continuity—within the same abdominal cavity—becomes hyperplastic?

### (ii) *Effect of topical, prehydrolysed nutrients in bypassed intestinal loops*

In the double Thiry-Vella fistula model in the dog (52), if hormonal factors were operating, why should there be differences between the empty and perfused by-passed loops?

The answer to these rhetorical questions is unknown but may well be due to locally acting enterotrophic peptides—of the paracrine or even of the peptidergic or neuroendocrine type—areas of almost complete ignorance in the adaptation field.

It is quite conceivable, however, that the function of the brush borders at the apical portions of the APUD cells is to 'sense' luminal stimuli—whether nutrients or other trigger factors—which then release their secretory granules into the adjacent tissues thereby stimulating growth. It should be emphasised, perhaps, that at present this is speculation for which there is no experimental proof.

### (iii) *Studies of intestinal adaptation where a trophic effect of individual hormones has been denied*

This is not so much evidence against the role of humoral factors in intestinal adaptation as evidence that certain individual hormones or peptides cannot explain certain phenomena. The results of these studies with experimental hyperprolactinaemia (81), for example, the fact that pharmacological doses of pentagastrin did not seem to affect jejunal mucosal growth (69) and the fact that neither low nor high doses of CCK-OP stimulate mucosal hyperplasia (13, 43), does not really exclude the trophic effect of other peptides or exclude a hormonal mechanism in

other experimental models of intestinal adaptation.

In summary, one is hard pressed to make a case *against* the role of hormones in intestinal adaptation. Like luminal nutrition they cannot explain all the findings but in our present state of knowledge, the judgement is heavily in favour of humoral factors.

## OTHER POSSIBLE MECHANISMS FOR INTESTINAL ADAPTATION

Surprisingly little is known about changes in mucosal blood flow nor about the direct or indirect influence of neural factors on intestinal adaptation.

(a) Blood flow: From the macroscopic appearance of hyperplastic intestine (for example, the ileal remnant following jejunectomy), it is obvious that the segmental arteries and veins supplying the enlarged segment are much larger than normal. It seems likely that there is a corresponding increase in regional blood flow but if so, it is not known whether this antedates or postdates the onset of mucosal hyperplasia. Blood flow is notoriously difficult to measure, especially in small vessels and particularly when chronic measurements of blood flow over hours, days or even weeks are needed. Mechanical devices such as electromagnetic flow meter probes tend to distort the anatomy, and hence the blood flow, through small vessels. Dynamic exchange studies using marker gases such as argon or xenon cannot reliably distinguish between mucosal and seromuscular blood flow nor between villus and sub-villus mucosal blood flow because of intratissue shunting and problems such as countercurrent exchange within the villi. One possible exception is the use of rubidium and several years ago there were two brief reports by Touloukian & Spencer (99, 100) which suggested that blood flow was indeed increased in the enlarged residual bowel after resection and, based on studies carried out at only two time periods after enterectomy, that the increase in blood flow *preceded* the increase in tissue mass. These preliminary results badly need confirmation and extension. It is just conceivable that the mechanism whereby

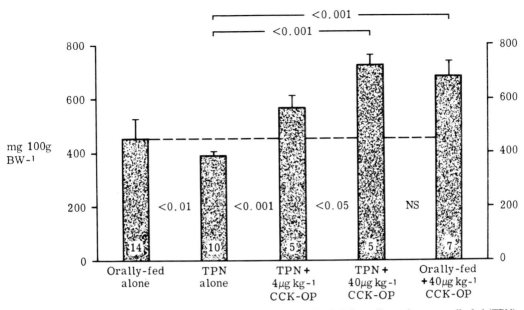

Fig. 4. Effect of CCK-OP on pancreatic wet weight, standardised/100 g BW in orally- and parenterally-fed (TPN) rats (38). The bars show mean values and the vertical lines, the SEM's. The numbers at the base of the bars are the numbers of the animals studied.

luminal nutrition and hormonal factors stimulate adaptive hyperplasia is by increasing blood flow in response to chemical, hormonal and neural stimuli.

(b) Neural factors: If little is known about the influence of blood flow, even less is known about the role of neural mechanisms. However the results of two recent studies shed a little light on this otherwise dark area of ignorance.

Laplace (58) studied the effect of cutting the afferent or sensory fibres of the vagus, on the adaptive response of the pig to partial small bowel resection. The sensory vagotomised animals ate and grew normally but 28 days after surgery there was no evidence of adaptive change in the resected plus 'deafferented' pigs but 37–60% increases in the weight/unit length of residual intestine in the non-vagotomised animals. The full significance of this new and important observation has yet to be established but may well be another link in the chain of evidence that nerves and hormones are intimately related. Although CCK is difficult to measure by radioimmunoassay, two recent reports have shown that the post-prandial rise in immunoreactive CCK and motilin and the contractile response of the gallbladder to a

test meal, are abolished by atropine (68, 95). Could it be that the mechanism for Laplace's observation is related to abolition of CCK release after cutting the vagal sensory fibres?

The sympathetic nervous system also influences intestinal mucosal growth: sympathectomy decreases the indices of cell proliferation and reduces mucosal mass. When Levine et al. (60) induced chemical sympathectomy (with 6-hydroxydopamine) in TPN rats, they accentuated the intestinal mucosal hypoplasia of IV feeding. However the mucosal 'atrophy' of sympathectomy was prevented by direct intragastric infusion of luminal nutrients.

## THE ENTERO-PANCREATIC TROPHIC AXIS

Although a relationship between the gut and the pancreas is already established with the entero-insular axis, the two organs seem to be related in another way—through an entero-pancreatic trophic axis. Thus, in classic physiological theory, the presence of food in the gut stimulates the release of CCK and secretin which then trigger the output of exocrine pancreatic secretions. With all the caveats discussed above (see 'Pancreatico-biliary secretions: the case against'), the exocrine secretions are thought to be trophic to the gut. In turn, it seems that for CCK, at least, the intestinal hormone not only stimulates enzyme secretion but also the growth of its target organ, the pancreas (Fig. 4). Whilst neither the low (4 µg) nor the high (40 µg kg$^{-1}$ day$^{-1}$) doses of CCK-OP were trophic to the intestine (13, 43), they were both markedly trophic to the pancreas (42). Indeed, in parenterally-fed rats, they not only prevented the pancreatic hypoplasia of TPN but actually stimulated pancreatic growth, over and above that seen in the orally-fed controls*. If there is indeed a balance between food-stimulated release of CCK from the gut and the maintenance of normal pancreatic structure and function, then the IV administration of 40 µg CCK-OP kg$^{-1}$ day$^{-1}$ must have swamped the physiological stimulus. The degree of pancreatic hyperplasia was comparable in orally- and parenterally-fed rats given the high-dose, CCK-octapeptide (42).

Surprisingly, pancreatic adaptation was also seen after pancreatico-biliary diversion (PBD). Only 8 days after PBD, pancreatic mass (wet weight, protein and DNA content) doubled (75). The mechanism for this extraordinary pancreatic growth is unknown but may be related to the mucosal hyperplasia in the transposed jejunum with secondary release of pancreatico-trophic CCK. When Miazza et al. (77) measured the circulating levels of gastrin, insulin, secretin, CCK, neurotensin and enteroglucagon, the only peptides to increase significantly after PBD were CCK and enteroglucagon. Since enteroglucagon is a strong candidate for the role of enterotrophin, might it not also be trophic to the pancreas? Apparently not: when PBD is achieved by interposing ileum rather than jejunum between the stomach and the duodenum, the ileal mucosa becomes markedly hyperplastic and plasma enteroglucagon levels increase markedly (to an even greater degree than occurs after jejunal

interposition) but the pancreas does not change in size.

While the hypothesis that pancreatic secretions influence the structure and function of the intestine, which in turn maintains the growth and regulates the secretion of the pancreas, is an attractive one, it should be emphasised that to date, the theory has not yet been proven. The weak link in the circular chain of argument is that pancreatic secretions have a specific trophic effect on the intestine—apart from contributing an endogenous protein-rich luminal stimulus to mucosal growth.

## CONCLUSION

The principle aim of this article has been to review the 'state-of-the-art' in small bowel adaptation. Compensatory changes in colonic mucosal structure and function have not been discussed and the relatively new topic of pancreatic adaptation has been mentioned only briefly.

Intestinal adaptation is a multidisciplinary field of interest to basic scientists (anatomists, biochemists, physiologists, cell biologists and cell kineticists), veterinarians, physicians and surgeons. For the clinician, however, the ultimate goal is to identify a trophic factor (or factors) which might have a therapeutic role in the treatment of patients with malabsorption and malnutrition secondary to extensive disease or resection of the small intestine. With long-term parenteral nutrition, these patients can be kept alive and well but this is a hugely expensive exercise and for all but the affluent few, the survival of these patients depends on the capacity of the residual intestinal system (not only the small bowel but also the pancreas, colon and perhaps even the stomach) to adapt. It remains to be seen whether or not we can improve on the spontaneous adaptive mechanisms which, arguably, are already working optimally in patients with the short bowel syndrome.

## ACKNOWLEDGEMENTS

The author wishes to thank the many colleagues, collaborators, and mentors (listed below in alphabetical order) who contributed to the studies

---

* The trophic effect of CCK (and of the structurally related gastrin family of peptides) on the pancreas have, of course, been studied many times before (4, 33, 67, 92).

described in this review. Thanks are also due to the Medical Research Council, the Wellcome Trust and to the Swiss National Fund, for financial support. Mrs. Suma Das kindly typed the script.

S. R. Bloom, C. C. Booth, R. Breuer, E. Elias, E. Feldman, M. H. Gleeson, D. Hatoff, C. A. Hughes, L. Hung, L. Jacobs, M. McKinnon, B. M. Miazza, H. Y. I. Mok, E. Müller, G. M. Murphy, T. J. Peters, J. Polak, B. Taylor.

## REFERENCES

1. Al-Mukhtar MYT, Sagor GR, Ghatei MA, Polak JM, Koopmans HS, Bloom SR, Wright NA. In 'Mechanisms of Intestinal Adaptation' ed. Robinson JWL, Dowling RH, Riecken EO. 1982, MTP Press Ltd., Lancaster, pp. 243–253
2. Altmann GG. Amer J Anat 1971, 132, 167–178
3. Altmann GG, Leblond CP. Amer J Anat 1971, 127, 15–36
4. Barrowman JA, Mayston PD. J Physiol (London) 1973, 238, 73
5. Batt RM, Peters TJ. Clin Sci Mol Med 1976, 50, 511–523
6. Batt RM, Peters TJ. Clin Sci Mol Med 1978, 55, 435–443
7. Batt RM, Wells G, Peters TJ. Clin Sci Mol Med 1978, 55, 435–443
8. Besterman HS, Bloom SR, Sarson DL, Blackburn AM, Johnston DI, Patel HR, Stewart JS, Modigliani R, Guerin S, Mallinson CN. Lancet 1978, i, 785–788
9. Bloom SR. Gut 1972 13, 520–523
10. Bloom SR. In 'Surgical Management of Obesity' ed. Maxwell JD, Gazet J-C, Pilkington TR. 1980, Academic Press, London, pp. 115–123
11. Bloom SR, Besterman HS, Adrian TE, Christofides ND, Sarson DL, Mallinson CN, Pero A, Modigliani R. Gastroenterology 1979, 76, 1101
12. Bloom SR, Royston CMS, Thompson JPS. Lancet 1972, 2, 789
13. Breuer RS, Hatoff DE, Hughes CA, Dowling RH. Gut 1979, 20, A911
14. Campbell RM, Fell BF. J Physiol 1964, 171, 90–97
15. Clarke RM. Digestion 1977, 15, 411–424
16. Craft IL. Clin Sci 1970, 38, 287–295
17. Dembinski A, Gregory H, Konturek SJ, Polanski M. In 'Mechanisms of Intestinal Adaptation' ed. Robinson JWL, Dowling RH, Riecken EO. 1982, MTP Press Ltd., Lancaster, pp. 281–284
18. Dorchester JEC, Haist RE. J Physiol 1953, 119, 226–273
19. Dowling RH. In 'Advanced Medicine 12' ed. Peters DK. Pitman Medical, London 1976, pp. 251–261
20. Dowling RH, Booth CC. Lancet 1966, ii, 146–147
21. Dowling RH, Booth CC. Clin Sci 1967, 32, 139–149
22. Dowling RH, Gleeson MH. Digestion 1973, 8, 176–190
23. Dowling RH, Riecken EO. 1974, 'Intestinal Adaptation', Schattauer Verlag, Stuttgart-New York
24. Dowling RH, Riecken EO, Laws JW, Booth CC. Clin Sci 1967, 32, 1–9
25. Drapanas T, Williams JS, McDonald JC, Heyden W, Bow T, Spencer RP. J Amer Med Asscn 1963, 184, 337–341
26. Ducker DA, Hughes CA. 1981, Personal communication
27. Dudrick SJ, Daly JM, Castro G, Mohamed Akhtar. Ann Surg 1977, 185, 642–648
28. Elias E, Dowling RH. Clin Sci Mol Med 1976, 51, 427–433
29. Feldman EJ, Carter D, Grossman MI. Gastroenterology 1978, 75, 1033
30. Feldman EJ, Dowling RH, McNaughton J, Peters TJ. Gastroenterology 1976, 70, 712–719
31. Fell BF, Smith KA, Campbell RM. J Path Bact 1963, 85, 179–188
32. Fenyö G, Backman L, Hallberg D. Acta Chir Scand 1976, 142, 154–159
33. Fölsch UR, Winckler K, Wormsley KG. Scand J Gastroenterol 1975, 13, 663
34. Gleeson MH, Bloom SR, Polak JM, Henry K, Dowling RH. Gut 1971, 12, 773–782
35. Gleeson MH, Cullen J, Dowling RH. Clin Sci 1972, 43, 731–742
36. Gleeson MH, Dowling RH. Unpublished observation
37. Gregor M, Bryant MG, Buchan AMJ, Bloom SR, Polak JM. Gut 1981, 21, A907
38. Grenier JF, Eloy MR, Jaeck D, Dauchel J. Chirurgie 1974, 100, 59–65
39. Hanson WR, Osborne JW, Sharp JG. Gastroenterology, 1977, 72, 701–705
40. Heroux O, Gridgeman NT. Canad J Biochem Physiol 1958, 36, 209–216
41. Hughes CA, Bates T, Dowling RH. Gastroenterology 1978, 75, 34–41
42. Hughes CA, Breuer RS, Ducker DA, Hatoff DE, Dowling RH. In 'Mechanisms of Intestinal Adaptation' ed. Robinson JWL, Dowling RH, Riecken EO. 1982, MTP Press Ltd., Lancaster, pp. 435–450
43. Hughes CA, Breuer RS, Hatoff DE, Ducker DA, Dowling RH. Europ J Clin Invest 1980, 10, 16
44. Hughes CA, Dowling RH. Clin Sci 1980, 59, 317–327
45. Hughes CA, Ducker DA, Warren IF, McNeish AS. Gut 1979, 20, A924–925
46. Hughes CA, Prince A, Dowling RH. Clin Sci 1980, 59, 329–336
47. Iversen BM, Schjønsby H, Skagen DW, Solhaug JH. Europ J Clin Invest 1976, 6, 355–360
48. Jacobs LR, Bloom SR, Dowling RH. Life Sciences 1981, 19, 2005–2007
49. Jacobs LR, Bloom SR, Harsoulis P, Dowling RH. Clin Sci 1975, 48, 13p
50. Jacobs LR, Dowling RH. Europ J Clin Invest 1975, 5, 203
51. Jacobs LR, Polak J, Bloom SR, Dowling RH. Clin Sci Mol Med 1976, 50, 14–15p
52. Jacobs LR, Taylor BR, Dowling RH. Clin Sci Mol Med 1975, 49, 26–27p

53. Johnson LR. Gastroenterology 1976, 70, 278–288
54. Johnson LR. Gastroenterology 1977, 72, 788–792
55. Johnson LR, Guthrie P. Gastroenterology 1976, 70, 59–65
56. Kedinger M, Simon PM, Raul F, Grenier JF, Haffen K. In 'Mechanisms of Intestinal Adaptation' ed. Robinson JWL, Dowling RH, Riecken EO. 1982, MTP Press Ltd., Lancaster, pp. 285–294
57. Laplace J-P. Digestion 1974, 10, 229
58. Laplace JP. In 'Mechanisms of Intestinal Adaptation' ed. Robinson JWL, Dowling RH, Riecken EO. 1982, MTP Press Ltd., Lancaster, pp. 321–331
59. Levine GM, Deren JJ, Yezdimir E. Amer J Dig Dis 1976, 21, 542–546
60. Levine GM, Kotler DP, Yezdimir EA. In 'Mechanisms of Intestinal Adaptation' ed. Robinson JWL, Dowling RH, Riecken EO. 1982, MTP Press Ltd., Lancaster, pp. 311–317
61. Loran MR, Carbone JV. In 'Gastrointestinal Radiation Injury' ed. Sullivan MF. 1968, Excerpta Medica, Amsterdam, pp. 127–139
62. Luk GD. Personal communication
63. Luk GD, Baylin SB. In 'Mechanisms of Intestinal Adaptation' ed. Robinson JWL, Dowling RH, Riecken EO. 1982, MTP Press Ltd., Lancaster, pp. 65–78
64. MacKinnon AM. Amer J dig Dis 1973, 18, 576–582
65. MacKinnon AM, Short MD, Elias E, Dowling RH. Amer J dig Dis 1975, 20, 835–840
66. Mainoya JR. Experientia 1978, 34, 1230–1231
67. Mainz DL, Black O, Webster PD. J Clin Invest 1973, 52, 2300–2304
68. Maton PN, Selden AC, Chadwick VS. Reg Pep 1981, 3, 76
69. Mayston PD, Barrowman JA, Dowling RH. Digestion 1975, 12, 78–84
70. Menge H, Bloch R, Schaumlöffel E, Riecken EO. Z Ges Exp Med. 1970, 153, 74–90
71. Menge H, Grafe M, Lorenz-Meyer H, Riecken EO. Gut 1975, 16, 468–472
72. Menge H, Muller K, Lorenz-Meyer H, Riecken EO. Virchows Arch Abt B Zellfach 1975, 18, 135–144
73. Menge H, Werner H, Lorenz-Meyer H, Riecken EO. Gut 1975, 16, 462–467
74. Miazza BM, Ghatei MA, Adrian TE, Bloom SR, Dowling RH. Reg Pep 1981, 3, 77
75. Miazza BM, Hung L, Vaja S, Dowling RH. In 'Mechanisms of Intestinal Adaptation' ed. Robinson JWL, Dowling RH, Riecken EO. 1982, MTP Press Ltd., Lancaster, pp. 481–490
76. Miazza BM, Levan H, Vaja S, Dowling RH. In 'Mechanisms of Intestinal Adaptation'. ed. Robinson JWL, Dowling RH, Riecken EO. 1982, MTP Press Ltd., Lancaster, pp. 467–477
77. Miazza B, Levan H, Ghatei M, Adrian T, Bloom S, Dowling H. Europ J Clin Invest 1982, 12, in press
78. Mok HYI, Perry PM, Dowling RH. Gut 1974, 15, 247–253
79. Morin CL, Grey VL, Carofalo C. In 'Mechanisms of Intestinal Adaptation' ed. Robinson JWL, Dowling RH, Riecken EO. 1982, MTP Press Ltd., Lancaster, pp. 175–184
80. Morin CL, Ling V. Gastroenterology 1978, 75, 224–229
81. Müller E, Dowling RH. Gut 1981, 22, 558–565
82. Obertop H, Nundy S, Malamud D, Malt RA. Gastroenterology 1977, 72, 267–270
83. Oscarson JEA, Veen HF, Williamson RCN, Ross JS, Malt RA. Gastroenterology 1977, 72, 890–895
84. Riecken EO, Menge H, Bloch R, Lorenz-Meyer H, Warm K, Ihloff M. In 'Intestinal Adaptation' ed. Dowling RH, Riecken EO. 1974, Schattauer Verlag, Stuttgart-New York, pp 239–247
85. Robertson JA, Gallagher ND. Gastroenterology 1979, 77, 511–517
86. Mechanisms of Intestinal Adaptation, ed. Robinson JWL, Dowling RH, Riecken EO. 1982, MTP Press Ltd., Lancaster
87. Rudo ND. Gastroenterology 1973, 64, 686, Abst
88. Rudo ND, Rosenberg IH. Proc Soc Exp biol Med 1973, 142, 521–525
89. Scarpello JHB, Carey BA, Sladen GE. Clin Sci 1978, 54, 241–249
90. Silk DBA, Kumar PJ, Webb JPW. Gut 1975, 16, 261–267
91. Schedl HP, Pierce CE, Rider A, Clifton JA. J Clin Invest 1968, 47, 417–425
92. Solomon TE, Petersen H, Elashoff J, Grossman MI. Am J Physiol 1978, 235, E714
93. Spector MH, Levine GM, Deren JJ. Gastroenterology 1977, 72, 706–710
94. Stevens FM, McCarthy C, Buchanan KD. Personal communication
95. Svenberg T, Christofides ND, Fitzpatrick ML, Bloom SR, Welbourn RB. Clin Sci 1981, 62, 20–21
96. Taylor B, Murphy GM, Dowling RH. Europ J Clin Invest 1979, 9, 115–127
97. Thim L, Moody AJ. Reg Pep 1981, 2, 139
98. Tilson MD, Wright HK. Surgery 1970, 67, 687–693
99. Toulokian RJ, Aghajanian GK, Roth RH. Ann Surg 1972, 176, 633–637
100. Toulokian RJ, Spencer RP. Ann Surg 1972, 175, 320–325
101. Weser E, Bell D, Tawil T. Dig Dis Sci 1981, 26, 409–416
102. Weser E, Heller R, Tawil T. Gastroenterology 1977, 73, 524–529
103. Williamson RCN. New Engl J Med 1978, 298, 1393–1402 and 1444–1450
104. Williamson RCN, Bauer FLR, Ross JS, Malt RA. Surgery 1978, 83, 570–576
105. Williamson RCN, Bucholtz TW, Malt RA. Gastroenterology 1978, 75, 249–254
106. Williamson RCN, Malt RA. In 'Mechanisms of Intestinal Adaptation' ed. Robinson JWL, Dowling RH, Riecken EO. 1982, MTP Press Ltd., Lancaster, pp. 215–224
107. Wright HK, Cleveland JC, Tilson MD, Herskovic T. Amer J Surg 1969, 117, 242–245
108. Wright HK, Poskett T, Cleveland JC, Herskovic TJ. Surg Res 1969, 9, 301–304

# Response of the Small Intestinal Mucosa to Oral Glucocorticoids

R. M. BATT & J. SCOTT*
Department of Veterinary Pathology, University of Liverpool, L69 3BX, U.K. and
*Department of Biochemistry and Biophysics, School of Medicine,
University of California, San Francisco, California 94143, U.S.A.

These studies explored the effects of oral pharmacological doses of glucocorticoids on the normal small intestine of the adult rat. Short-term (7 days) prednisolone had little effect on mucosal structure or cell kinetics but enhanced the maximum absorptive capacities of the jejunum and ileum for galactose. This was due to an increase in carrier-mediated transport in the individual enterocytes and not to a change in the cell population. Activities of brush border enzymes were elevated and turnover studies indicated an increased rate of synthesis of brush border proteins associated with an enhanced glycoprotein content of the microvillus membrane. Subcellular fractionation studies demonstrated a large increase in the membrane-bound ribosomal RNA content of the enterocytes consistent with an enhanced synthesis of membrane proteins. These findings implicate a direct action of prednisolone on the enterocytes to increase their absorptive and digestive capacities by the induction of specific functional proteins.

These effects on the absorptive and digestive functions of the small intestine were sustained with long-term (28 days) prednisolone feeding. An equivalent long-term oral dose of betamethasone-17-valerate, a locally rather than a systemically active glucocorticoid, had a similar effect on the enterocytes. However, an inhibition of crypt cell turnover resulted in a marked hypoplasia and hence no net change in the functional capacity of the mucosa. These findings emphasise the separate and opposing actions of glucocorticoids on the adult mucosa, on the one hand to stimulate enterocyte function, but on the other to reduce the enterocyte population. The predominant activity appears to be a function of each individual steroid.

The predominant stimulatory action of prednisolone was further emphasised by investigating the effects of this glucocorticoid on the adapted ileum following jejunal resection. Indeed, short-term prednisolone enhanced the adaptive hyperplasia in the ileal remnant by increasing the functional capacity of the expanded population of enterocytes.

*R. M. Batt, Department of Veterinary Pathology, University of Liverpool, P.O. Box 147, Liverpool L69 3BX, U.K.*

## INTRODUCTION

Glucocorticoids have been used extensively for the management of many diseases including those of the gastrointestinal tract (1, 33, 37, 43, 51, 52), yet their effects on the small intestinal mucosa are not clearly defined. Indeed, an understanding of these effects and their molecular basis is fundamental to the interpretation of their value in intestinal disease and to the anticipation of their potential side effects on normal mucosa.

The following series of studies were therefore undertaken to determine the effects of pharmacological doses of oral glucocorticoid on the normal small intestine of the rat and to investigate the mechanism of action in detail.

## SHORT-TERM PREDNISOLONE

These studies were performed to explore the effects of a short-term dose of prednisolone on

Table I. Short-term study. Histological measurements and kinetic parameters in control and prednisolone-treated animals.

| | Jejunum | | Ileum | |
|---|---|---|---|---|
| | Control | Prednisolone | Control | Prednisolone |
| Villus height (μm) | 521 ± 7 | 519 ± 7 | 197 ± 4 | 214 ± 3 |
| | | $p < 0.05$ | | $p < 0.01$ |
| Crypt depth (μm) | 184 ± 7 | 144 ± 4 | 142 ± 4 | 145 ± 5 |
| | | $p < 0.001$ | | $p < 0.05$ |
| Epithelial cell density (no/200 μm length midvillus) | 30.2 ± 0.8 | 30.8 ± 0.5 | 37.1 ± 1.1 | 38.5 ± 1.1 |
| | | $p > 0.05$ | | $p > 0.05$ |
| Migration rate (μm/h) | 17 ± 0.6 | 15 ± 0.7 | 11 ± 0.6 | 14 ± 0.5 |
| | | $p > 0.05$ | | $p < 0.001$ |
| Villus transit time (h) | 36 ± 1.4 | 39 ± 1.9 | 26 ± 1.5 | 19 ± 0.8 |
| | | $p > 0.05$ | | $p < 0.001$ |

Data, from 6 animals in each group, are expressed as mean ± SEM

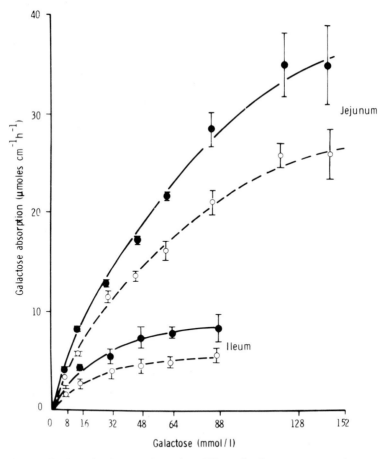

Fig. 1. Kinetics of galactose absorption. Effect of galactose concentration on absorption in the jejunum and ileum of control (○) and short-term prednisolone-treated (●) animals. Data, from at least five perfusions at each concentration, are expressed as mean ± SEM.

the small intestinal mucosa (6, 9, 46, 47). In each experiment prednisolone-21-phosphate (Merck, Sharp & Dohme Ltd., Hoddesdon, Herts, UK) was fed to adult male Wistar rats for 7 days at a dose of 0.75 mg/kg body weight/day.

*Intestinal morphology and cell kinetics*

This short-term administration of prednisolone produced only minor structural alterations in the jejunum and ileum (6) (Table I) findings in contrast to the marked functional and biochemical changes in the enterocytes described below. In the prednisolone-treated jejunum the kinetic parameters were also unaltered, however, in the

ileum the epithelial cell migration rate was enhanced and cell turnover time decreased (Table I).

*Intestinal function*

Intestinal function was assessed in vivo by determining the kinetics of D-galactose absorption with a recirculation-perfusion technique (6, 7). In both the jejunum and ileum of the prednisolone-treated animals absorption per centimetre of intestine was increased at each galactose concentration perfused (Fig. 1). Further analysis of these data demonstrated that this was due to a significant increase in maximum absorp-

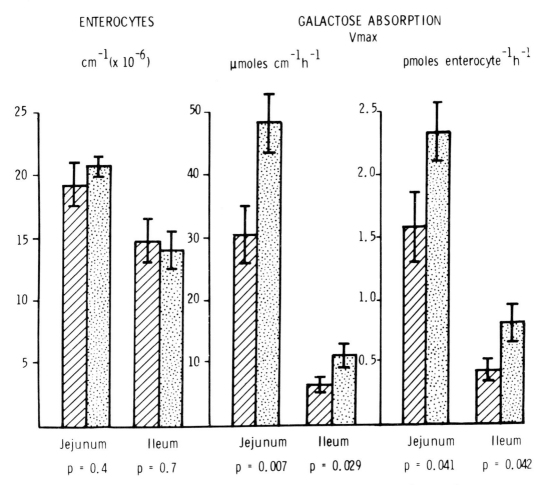

Fig. 2. Numbers of enterocytes/cm and $V_{max}$ of galactose absorption expressed per centimetre and per enterocyte in control (cross-hatched) and short-term prednisolone-treated animals (stippled). Data, from at least six rats in each group, are expressed as mean ± SEM.

tive capacity ($V_{max}$) without an alteration in the apparent affinity constant ($K_t$). Enterocytes were isolated and quantitated biochemically following a correction for yield (7). This procedure revealed no change in the number of enterocytes per centimetre in the steroid-treated group, in agreement with the morphological findings, and demonstrated that the increased $V_{max}$ per centimetre was due to enhanced absorptive capacity of the individual enterocytes (Fig. 2). Phlorrhizin, a competitive inhibitor of hexose absorption, almost completely inhibited galactose absorption in control and prednisolone-treated animals emphasising that the increase in the latter was due to carrier-mediated transport and not passive diffusion (6).

*Enzymology*

Enhancement of absorptive function in the prednisolone treated animals was paralleled by increased activities of brush border enzymes in both the jejunal and ileal enterocytes (6) (Fig. 3).

Activities of a basal-lateral membrane enzyme ($5^1$-nucleotidase) and of mitochondrial marker enzymes (cytochrome oxidase and malate dehydrogenase) were also elevated, however, there were no changes in the activities of lysosomal or peroxisomal marker enzymes in the enterocytes from the steroid-treated animals. The increase in the RNA content of prednisolone-treated enterocytes (Fig. 3) suggested that prednisolone action might be mediated by an enhanced rate of protein synthesis.

*Subcellular biochemical changes*

The data presented above suggested that short-term prednisolone has a direct effect on the enterocyte, particularly the brush border, to enhance the absorptive and digestive capacities of the small intestine. These effects were further investigated by use of analytical subcellular fractionation, a procedure which permitted a more detailed study of the biochemical changes in the enterocyte at a subcellular level (8, 9).

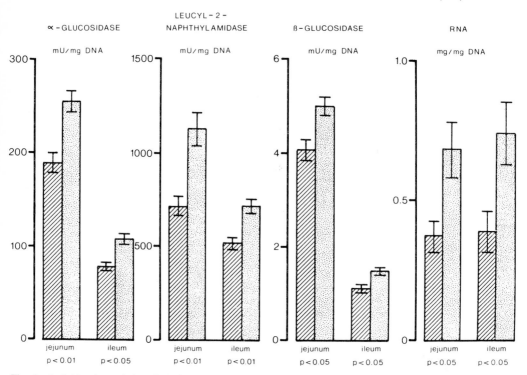

Fig. 3. Activities (m units/mg DNA) of brush border enzymes and RNA content (mg/mg DNA) in control (cross-hatched) and short-term prednisolone-treated (stippled) enterocytes. Data, from at least six rats in each group, are expressed as mean ± SEM.

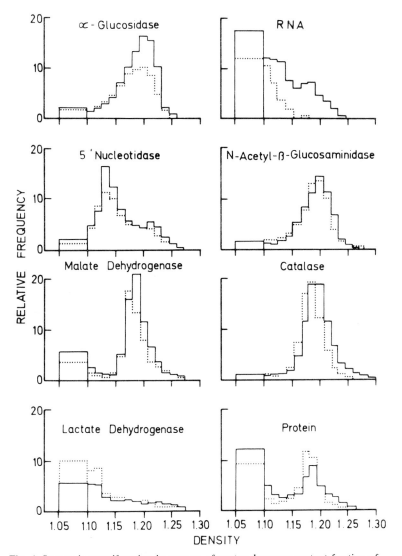

Fig. 4. Isopycnic centrifugation in sucrose of postnuclear supernatant fraction of jejunal enterocytes from control (. . . .) and short-term prednisolone-treated (———) animals. Graphs show the relative frequency-density distributions of six marker enzymes, RNA and protein. The areas of the distributions comparing the two groups are proportional to the relative specific activities per mg enterocyte DNA. Frequency is defined as that portion of the total recovered activity present in an individual fraction divided by the density span covered by that fraction. Relative frequency was derived by multiplying the frequency data for prednisolone-treated enterocytes by the relative specific activity of these compared with the control cells.

The relative activities and sucrose density gradient distributions of the principal marker enzymes, RNA and protein in extracts of jejunal enterocytes from control and prednisolone-treated animals are shown in Fig. 4. The main observations concerned the distributions of α-glucosidase and of RNA.

Soluble α-glucosidase activity was essentially unaltered in the prednisolone-treated cells, but there was a large increase in particulate brush

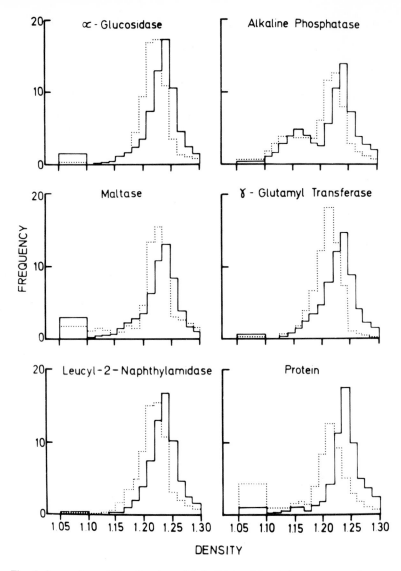

Fig. 5. Isopycnic centrifugation in sorbitol of jejunal brush border preparations from control (. . . . .) and short-term prednisolone-treated (———) animals. Graphs show the frequency density distributions of five marker enzymes and protein.

border enzyme activity and a shift in the distribution of this component towards the denser fractions. An increase in the density of the brush border following prednisolone administration was confirmed by density gradient centrifugation of isolated brush border preparations (Fig. 5). This finding was consistent with an increase in the glycoprotein content of the brush border membrane, a suggestion confirmed by the analysis of isolated microvillus membrane fractions (46).

Prednisolone also resulted in a striking alteration in the distribution of enterocyte RNA in the sucrose density gradients (Fig. 4). The increased RNA content was associated partly with the soluble fractions but predominantly with a distinct particulate component suggestive of a

Table II. RNA content of enterocytes from control and short-term prednisolone-treated rats

| Fraction | Control | Prednisolone | |
|---|---|---|---|
| Homogenate | 420 ± 45 | 556 ± 86 | p < 0.05 |
| Nuclear | 23 ± 8 (6) | 36 ± 11 (6) | p > 0.05 |
| Non-sedimentable fraction | 61 ± 2 (15) | 79 ± 11 (13) | p > 0.05 |
| Bound ribosomes | 135 ± 14 (33) | 239 ± 28 (43) | p < 0.01 |
| Free ribosomes | 181 ± 17 (37) | 145 ± 23 (26) | p > 0.05 |
| Ratio of bound to free ribosomes | 0.75 | 1.65 | |

Data, (µg RNA/mg enterocyte DNA) from 6 experiments are presented as mean ± SEM with the percentage recovered RNA in each fraction between parentheses.
Statistical analysis by paired t test.

proliferation of the rough endoplasmic reticulum. This was supported by differential centrifugation (11) which demonstrated a large increase specifically of bound ribosomal RNA associated with an increase in the ratio of bound to free ribosomes (Table II). Membrane proteins are synthesised on the rough endoplasmic reticulum (14) so that this finding and the increased glycoprotein content of the microvillus membrane are consistent with enhanced synthesis of specific brush border proteins in enterocytes from prednisolone-treated animals.

*Turnover of brush border proteins*

In order to determine whether prednisolone does enhance specific enzyme protein synthesis the turnover of brush border membrane proteins was investigated (47). Animals were injected with L-[$^{14}$C]tyrosine 16 hours and L-[$^{3}$H]tyrosine 6 hours before sacrifice. As a measure of turnover the $^{3}$H/$^{14}$C ratio was determined (16) in purified brush border membranes and also following the isolation of aminopeptidase using anti-aminopeptidase-protein A Sepharose. Prednisolone resulted in an increase in the $^{3}$H/$^{14}$C ratio of

the brush border preparations (Table III) associated predominantly with the high molecular weight protein subunits (47). In addition, an increase in the specific activity of aminopeptidase was accompanied by an elevation in the $^{3}$H/$^{14}$C ratio in the isolated enzyme (Table III). These findings indicate that prednisolone increases brush border aminopeptidase activity by enhancing steady-state enzyme synthesis and suggest that other microvillus membrane proteins may be similarly affected.

## LONG-TERM ADMINISTRATION—COMPARISON BETWEEN PREDNISOLONE AND BETAMETHASONE

In this study (44) the period of prednisolone feeding has been extended from 7 to 28 days to determine whether the short-term effects on the jejunal mucosa are maintained with continued administration. This longer period has also been chosen to compare prednisolone with betamethasone-17-valerate, as the latter is a topically rather than a systemically active glucocorticoid. In common with the short-term study prednisolone was fed

Table III. Brush border protein turnover and soluble tyrosine pools in enterocytes from control and short-term prednisolone-treated animals

| | Control | Prednisolone | |
|---|---|---|---|
| Brush border membrane ($^{3}$H/$^{14}$C ratio) | 1.30 ± 0.16 | 1.79 ± 0.21 | p < 0.01 |
| Aminopeptidase ($^{3}$H/$^{14}$C ratio) | 1.63 ± 0.13 | 2.42 ± 0.15 | p < 0.01 |
| Soluble [$^{14}$C] tyrosine specific activity (dpm/n mol) | 39.7 ± 4.3 | 41.2 ± 7.2 | |
| Aminopeptidase specific activity (mU/mg membrane protein) | 5600 ± 200 (19%) | 8300 ± 667 (22%) | p > 0.05 |

Data are expressed as mean ± SD with percentage recovered aminopeptidase activities between parentheses

Table IV. Long-term study. Histological measurements and kinetic parameters in control, prednisolone-treated and betamethasone-17-valerate treated animals

| | Control | Prednisolone | | Betamethasone-17-valerate |
|---|---|---|---|---|
| Villus height (µm) | $535 \pm 5$ | $492 \pm 9$ ($p < 0.05$) | $p < 0.01$ | $401 \pm 10$ ($p < 0.01$) |
| Crypt depth (µm) | $178 \pm 7$ | $165 \pm 4$ ($p > 0.05$) | $p > 0.05$ | $143 \pm 4$ ($p < 0.05$) |
| Epithelial cell density (no/200 µm length midvillus) | $30.4 \pm 0.7$ | $28.9 \pm 0.6$ ($p > 0.05$) | $p > 0.05$ | $31.5 \pm 0.4$ ($p > 0.05$) |
| Migration rate (µm/h) | $15 \pm 1$ | $16 \pm 1$ ($p > 0.05$) | $p < 0.05$ | $9 \pm 1$ ($p < 0.05$) |
| Villus transit time (h) | $35 \pm 1$ | $31 \pm 1$ ($p > 0.05$) | $p < 0.05$ | $44 \pm 2$ ($p < 0.05$) |

Data, from 8 rats in each group, are expressed as mean $\pm$ SEM

to rats at a dose of 0.75 mg/kg body weight/day. An equivalent dose of 0.06 mg/kg body weight/day of betamethasone-17-valerate (Glaxo, Greenford, UK) was chosen based on the anti-inflammatory properties of these two steroids and their effects on hepatic glycogen deposition.

*Intestinal morphology and cell kinetics*

In common with the 7 day study longer-term prednisolone administration had little effect on the structure of the jejunal mucosa, although the small decrease in villus height was significant (Table IV). Betamethasone-17-valerate, in contrast, produced a marked decrease in villus height and crypt depth compared to both the control and prednisolone-treated groups.

The kinetic parameters (Table IV) were unaffected by long-term prednisolone, however, betamethasone-17-valerate decreased epithelial cell migration rate and increased the villus transit time compared to the other two groups.

*Intestinal function*

Assessment of intestinal function in vivo (Fig. 6) demonstrated that prednisolone significantly increased the absorption of D-galactose per enterocyte and per centimetre of intestine, in agreement with the short-term study. Absorption per enterocyte was also increased by betamethasone-17-valerate, however, this steroid resulted in a reduction in the enterocyte population and hence no change in the absorption per centimetre compared to the control group.

*Enzymology*

The activities of brush border enzymes reflected the changes already described for absorptive function (Fig. 6). Prednisolone and betamethasone-17-valerate both enhanced these activities in jejunal enterocytes but only prednisolone resulted in increased brush border enzyme activities per centimetre of intestine. This pattern was also observed when the RNA content of the isolated epithelial cell preparations per mg DNA and per centimetre of intestine was quantitated (Fig. 6). The activity of $5^{1}$-nucleotidase (basal-lateral membrane) was similarly affected, but there were no significant changes in the activities of mitochondrial or lysosomal marker enzymes.

## ENHANCEMENT OF ILEAL ADAPTATION BY PREDNISOLONE

The short-term prednisolone studies demonstrated an increase in the digestive and absorptive capacities of the small intestine by an effect on the existing population of enterocytes. Following partial resection, in contrast, the dominant component of the adaptive response in the small intestinal remnant consists of a large increase in the number of absorptive epithelial cells (12, 19, 54). This study was designed to determine

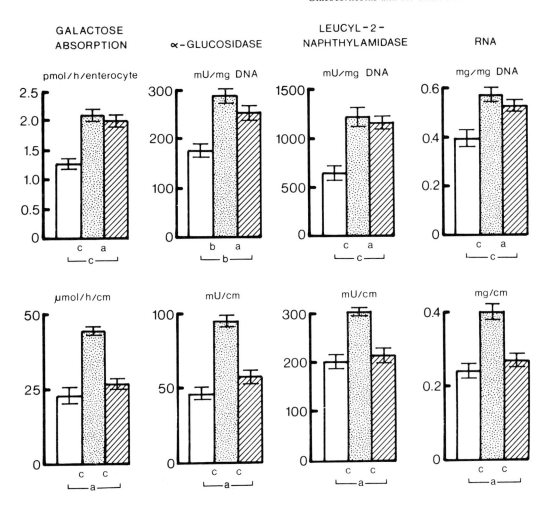

Fig. 6. Long-term study. Absorption of galactose, activities of brush border enzymes and enterocyte RNA content in control (unshaded), prednisolone-treated (stippled) and betamethasone-17-valerate-treated (cross-hatched) animals. Data, from 8 rats in each group, are expressed as mean ± SEM per enterocyte (or mg enterocyte DNA) and per cm of intestine. Galactose was perfused at a concentration of 64 m mol/l. The letters under the histograms denote statistical significance: a = not significant; b = $p < 0.05$; c = $p < 0.01$.

Table V. Histological measurements and kinetic parameters in control, resection alone and resection plus prednisolone-treated animals

| | | | | | |
|---|---|---|---|---|---|
| Villus height (μm) | 278 ± 12 | | 478 ± 12 | | 467 ± 6 |
| | | $p < 0.01$ | | $p > 0.05$ | |
| Crypt depth (μm) | 142 ± 4 | | 173 ± 3 | | 167 ± 5 |
| | | $p < 0.01$ | | $p > 0.05$ | |
| Epithelial cell density (no/200 μm length midvillus) | 36 ± 0.6 | | 38 ± 0.5 | | 38 ± 0.4 |
| | | $p > 0.05$ | | $p > 0.05$ | |
| Migration rate (μm/h) | 11 ± 0.4 | | 17 ± 0.2 | | 14 ± 0.4 |
| | | $p < 0.05$ | | $p < 0.05$ | |
| Villus transit time (h) | 23 ± 0.7 | | 29 ± 0.4 | | 31 ± 0.4 |
| | | $p < 0.05$ | | $p < 0.05$ | |

Data, from 8 animals in each group, are expressed as mean ± SEM

whether prednisolone could enhance this adaptive response in the ileal remnant following jejunal resection (45).

Proximal small intestine (50 cm) was removed from adult male Wistar rats and at 28 days after surgery the ileal remnant was compared to a similar segment from transection—reanastomosis controls. A third group comprising resected animals were also examined at this time but following the feeding of prednisolone in a daily dose of 0.75 mg/kg body weight for the last 7 days.

### Morphology and cell kinetics

Resection resulted in the anticipated increases in villus height and crypt depth, and these effects were not altered by the administration of prednisolone (Table V). Epithelial cell migration rate

and villus transit time were significantly increased in both resection groups compared to the controls (Table V). Prednisolone, however, slightly reduced migration rate so that the time for an epithelial cell to migrate the length of an adapted villus was marginally increased.

### Enzymology

Resection alone resulted in no changes in the activities of brush border enzymes in the individual enterocytes (mU/mg DNA) but increased the activities per centimetre of intestine (Fig. 7) emphasising that the adaptive response is primarily due to an increased enterocyte population. Prednisolone, however, considerably enhanced these enzyme activities in the enterocytes of the adapted ileum resulting in a further increase in

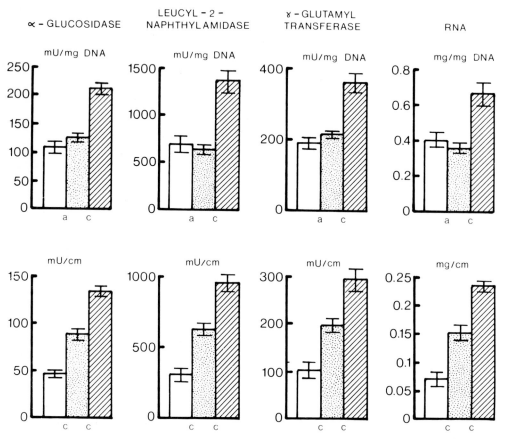

Fig. 7. Brush border enzyme activities and enterocyte RNA content in control (unshaded), resection-alone (stippled) and resection plus prednisolone-treated (cross-hatched) animals. Data, from eight rats in each group, are expressed as mean ± SEM per mg enterocyte DNA and per cm of intestine. Significance values as for Fig. 6.

brush border enzyme activities per centimetre. These findings in the two resection groups were paralleled by changes in the enterocyte RNA content (Fig. 7). In contrast to the effects on the brush border enzymes, prednisolone did not alter the activities of either mitochondrial or lysosomal marker enzymes in the resected animals.

## DISCUSSION

### Short-term prednisolone

Many studies have demonstrated the influence of corticosteroids on the structure and function of the normal intestinal tract of the rat (3, 5, 10, 13, 15, 18, 22, 26, 32, 40, 50, 53, 55). Particular attention has been focused on the immature animal in which glucocorticoids have been shown to induce the precocious development of adult brush border enzyme activities (18, 26) and to facilitate the induction of specific enzymes by dietary carbohydrate (32). In the adult rat the potent effects of mineralocorticoids and of glucocorticoids on the transport of fluid and electrolytes in the intestinal tract have been well documented (10, 13, 22, 40), however, the effects of glucocorticoids on the digestion and absorption of nutrients in the small intestine are less clearly defined. Indeed, interpretation of some apparently conflicting results has been hindered by fundamental differences in experimental design, particularly the dose, potency, half-life, route and period of administration of the individual steroid investigated (3, 5, 13, 50, 53, 55). The short-term studies described in this paper were undertaken in order to explore the effects of prednisolone on the normal small intestinal mucosa and to investigate the mechanism of action of glucocorticoids in detail.

Prednisolone, administered orally for 7 days, resulted in an enhancement in the absorptive and digestive capacities of both jejunum and ileum by an effect on the individual enterocytes without an alteration in the size of the cell population. There was little effect on mucosal structure, a finding confirmed by the biochemical calculation of the enterocyte population. Indeed, even a much higher oral dose (5 mg/kg body weight/day) given for 8 days has been found to result in only a slight villus atrophy. In contrast, more prominent morphological changes may result from the administration of long-acting glucocorticoids as they appear to have a more marked effect on DNA metabolism and can inhibit crypt cell proliferation (55). This is considered further when the long-term studies are discussed. Short-term prednisolone, however, resulted in no changes in the migration rate or cell turnover in the jejunum and both parameters were enhanced in the ileum. This emphasises that the increased absorptive and digestive capacities of the individual enterocytes are likely to be due to a direct action of prednisolone and not secondary to a reduced migration rate resulting in an older and hence more mature enterocyte population (24).

Other studies have shown an enhancement of hexose absorption and increased activities of brush border enzymes in the small intestine following the administration of glucocorticoids to the adult rat (3, 5, 13, 53). Conversely, decreased absorptive function and reduced brush border enzyme activities have been reported following adrenalectomy, although these changes may not reflect a primary effect of adrenal steroids on the intestine (2, 17, 34, 41). The present studies have demonstrated an enhancement of brush border function by prednisolone and suggested that these effects might be mediated by the control of protein synthesis.

Evidence for the mechanism of action of prednisolone was derived particularly from the protein turnover and subcellular fractionation studies. Prednisolone enhanced the maximum absorptive capacity of the enterocytes for galactose, implicating an increase in the number of galactose carriers, and increased the specific activities of brush border enzymes. An increase in enzyme activity may be due to activation of an existing enzyme, an increase in the rate of enzyme synthesis or a decrease in the rate of degradation (20, 25). The turnover studies, however, indicated increased synthesis of microvillus membrane proteins, a finding consistent with the enhanced glycoprotein content of this organelle. In agreement with these findings, the subcellular fractionation studies demonstrated a large increase in the membrane-bound ribosomal RNA content of the enterocyte, the rough endoplasmic reticulum being the site of synthesis of membrane proteins (14). Prednisolone therefore might act to enhance the number and to induce the attachment of protein-synthesising units to the endoplasmic reticulum, a mechanism postulated for growth and developmental hormones (48).

Further insight into these mechanisms may be gained from the investigations of hepatic enzyme induction by glucocorticoid (23, 36, 42). Indeed, detailed studies have demonstrated that corticosteroids increase the content of messenger RNA for specific proteins and hence induce RNA polymerase I (21, 27), the enzyme responsible for ribosomal RNA snythesis (31). This appears to be mediated by binding of the receptor-glucocorticoid complex to chromatin resulting in an increase in the numbers of initiation sites for RNA polymerase II and enhanced template activity (28, 29).

*Long-term administration—Comparison between prednisolone and betamethasone*

In this study, the consequences of sustained prednisolone feeding have been investigated and compared to the effects of a topically active glucocorticoid, betamethasone-17-valerate. In common with the short-term studies, long-term prednisolone increased the absorptive and digestive functions of the jejunal mucosa by an effect on the individual enterocytes. Betamethasone-17-valerate had a similar effect on the enterocytes, however, this effect was negated by a reduction in the enterocyte population resulting in no net change in the functional capacity of the mucosa.

These findings have clearly distinguished the stimulatory effect of glucocorticoids on protein synthesis, discussed above, from the potentially inhibitory action on crypt cell proliferation. In common with previous studies (3, 53) long-term prednisolone did result in villus atrophy, however, this effect was minor and was not accompanied by an alteration in cell turnover. Betamethasone-17-valerate, in contrast, had a profound inhibitory effect on epithelial cell turnover resulting in a marked hypoplasia of the jejunal mucosa. Although equivalent doses of these two steroids were fed, a high local concentration of betamethasone-17-valerate might explain these differences as it is a topically rather than a systemically active glucocorticoid (35, 38). Indeed, insufficient betamethasone-17-valerate was absorbed to cause adrenal atrophy although this was a consequence of the prednisolone administration (44). The differences might also reflect the longer biological half-life of betamethasone-17-valerate compared to prednisolone (4), as longer-acting glucocorticoids appear to have a more marked effect on DNA replication. Indeed, prenisolone tertiary butyl acetate, a long-acting depot preparation, has been shown to inhibit jejunal crypt cell proliferation in the adult rat (55) the increased proliferation reported previously (50) probably representing a rebound phenomenon (55). The mechanism of this inhibition in the small intestine has not been established but, in common with other tissues, a reduction in the activity of DNA polymerase might play a role (30, 49).

This study has revealed that glucocorticoids can have separate and opposing effects on the adult small intestinal mucosa, on the one hand to stimulate enterocyte function, but on the other to reduce the population of these cells by an inhibition of crypt cell proliferation. The consequences depend on which of these activities predominates and appear to be a function of each individual steroid.

*Enhancement of ileal adaptation by prednisolone*

This study explored the effects of short-term oral prednisolone on the adapted ileum following jejunal resection and emphasised the direct action of this steroid on the enterocytes. In agreement with previous studies, the adaptive response to resection was primarily due to an expansion of the enterocyte population (12, 19, 54). Prednisolone further enhanced this adaptive response by an increase in the functional capacities of the enterocytes and hence added a functional hypertrophy to an adaptive hyperplasia. In common with the short-term studies discussed above, prednisolone increased the epithelial cell RNA content, suggesting that the mechanisms of action on the normal and adapted mucosa are likely to be identical.

# CONCLUSIONS

The direct action of glucocorticoids to enhance the absorptive and digestive capacities of the enterocytes illustrates the flexibility of the adaptive potential of the small intestinal mucosa. Stimulatory effects mediated by the induction of specific proteins, however, may be opposed by an inhibitory action on crypt cell proliferation resulting in a reduction of the enterocyte population. These pharmacological effects probably represent an exaggeration of underlying physiological mechanisms initiated by binding to specific cytoplasmic receptors present in the epithelial cells (39). In intestinal disease, prednisolone might act not only as an immuno-suppressive and anti-inflammatory agent (43) but also to stimulate enterocyte function and hence assist repair of a damaged mucosa. For glucocorticoids such as betamethasone-17-valerate, however, these beneficial effects may be negated by the inhibition of cell proliferation, a property that could limit their therapeutic value in the small intestine.

# ACKNOWLEDGEMENTS

The authors thank Dr. T. J. Peters for constant encouragement and both the Medical Research Council and the Wellcome Trust for financial support during the course of these studies. We also thank Mrs. Pat Laws for secretarial assistance and Mrs. Paula Jenkins for the figures.

Data in Fig. 1, 2, 3, 4, 5, and Table I are reproduced from *Clinical Science and Molecular Medicine* (refs 6, 9), in Fig. 6 and Table IV from the American Journal of Physiology (ref 44) and in Fig. 7 and Table V from *Gut* (ref 45) with permission of the Editors.

# REFERENCES

1. Adlersberg D, Colcher H, Drachman SR. Gastroenterology 1951, 19, 674–697
2. Althausen TL, Anderson EM, Stockholm M. Proc Soc Exp Biol Med 1939, 40, 342–344
3. Ananna A, Eloy R, Bouchet P, Clendinnen G, Grenier JF. Lab Invest 1979, 41, 83–88
4. Axelrod L. Medicine (Baltimore) 1976, 55, 39–65
5. Banerjee S, Varma SD Proc Soc Exp Biol Med 1966, 123, 212–213
6. Batt RM, Peters TJ. Clin Sci Mol Med 1976, 50, 511–523
7. Batt RM, Peters TJ. Clin Sci Mol Med 1976, 50, 499–509
8. Batt RM, Peters TJ. Clin Sci Mol Med 1978, 55, 157–165
9. Batt RM, Wells G, Peters TJ. Clin Sci Mol Med 1978, 55, 435–443
10. Binder HJ. Gastroenterology 1978, 75, 212–217
11. Blobel G, Potter VR. J Mol Biol 1967, 26, 293–301
12. Booth CC, Evans KT, Menzies T, Street DF. Br J Surg 1959, 46, 403–410
13. Charney AN, Kinsey MD, Myers L, Giannella RA, Gots RE. J Clin Invest 1975, 56, 653–660
14. Dallner G, Siekevitz P, Palade GE. J Cell Biol 1966, 30, 73–96
15. Daniels VG, Hardy RN, Malinowska KW, Nathanielsz PW. J Physiol (Lond) 1973, 229, 681–695
16. Dehlinger PJ, Schimke RT. J Biol Chem 1971, 246, 2574–2583
17. Deren JJ, Broitman SA, Zamcheck N. J Clin Invest 1967, 46, 186–195
18. Doell RG, Kretchmer N. Science 1964, 143, 42–44
19. Dowling RH, Booth CC, Clin Sci 1967, 32, 139–149
20. Feigelson P, Greengard O. J Biol Chem 1962, 237, 3714–3717
21. Feigelson P, Kurtz DT. Adv Enzymol 1978, 47, 275–312
22. Field M. Gastroenterology 1978, 75, 317–319
23. Gelehrter TD. Metabolism 1973, 22, 85–100
24. Gleeson MH, Cullen J, Dowling RH. Clin Sci 1972, 43, 731–742
25. Greengard O, Feigelson P. J Biol Chem 1961, 236, 158–161
26. Herbst JJ, Koldovsky O. Biochem J 1972, 126, 471–476
27. Jacob ST, Sajdel EM, Munro HN. Eur J Biochem 1969, 7, 449–453
28. Johnson LK, Baxter JD. J Biol Chem 1978, 253, 1991–1997
29. Johnson LK, Lan NC, Baxter JD. J Biol Chem 1979, 254, 7785–7794
30. Kim YS, Jatoi I, Kim Y. Exp Mol Pathol 1979, 30, 255–263
31. Kulkarni SB, Netrawali MS, Pradhan DS, Sreenivasan A. Mol Cell Endocrinol 1976, 4, 195–203
32. Lebenthal E, Sunshine P, Kretchmer N. J Clin Invest 1972, 51, 1244–1250
33. Lepore MJ. Am J Med 1958, 25, 381–390
34. Levin RJ, Newey H, Smyth DH. J Physiol (Lond) 1965, 177, 58–73
35. Marks R, Williams K. In; Mechanisms of Topical Corticosteroid Activity 1976, Ed. LC Wilson, R Marks. Edinburgh, Churchill Livingstone, pp 39–46
36. Miner PB, Sutherland E, Simon FR. Gastroenterology 1980, 79, 212–221
37. Otaki AT, Daly JR, Morton-Gill A. Gut 1967, 8, 458–462
38. Philips GH. In: Mechanisms of Topical Corticosteroid Activity 1976, Ed. LC Wilson, R Marks. Edinburgh, Churchill Livingstone, pp 1–18

39. Pressley L, Funder JW. Endocrinology 1975, 97, 588–596
40. Rachmilewitz D, Fogel R, Karmeli F. Gut 1978, 19, 759–764
41. Rodgers JB, Riley EM, Drummey GD, Isselbacher KJ, Gastroenterology 1967, 53, 547–556
42. Rousseau GG, Amar-Costesec A, Verhaegen M, Granner DK. Proc Natl Acad Sci 1980, 77, 1005–1009
43. Scott J. Clin Gastroenterol 1981, 10, 627–652
44. Scott J, Batt RM, Maddison YE, Peters TJ. Am J Physiol 1981, 241, G 306–312
45. Scott J, Batt RM, Peters TJ. Gut 1979, 20, 858–864
46. Scott J, Hounsell E, Feizi T, Peters TJ. Cell Biol Int Rep 1980, 4, 814
47. Scott J, Peters TJ, Gastroenterology 1981, 80, 1279
48. Tata JR. Nature (Lond) 1968, 219, 331–337
49. Tesch DJ, Wilce PA, Ircs J Med Sci 1980, 8, 729–730
50. Tutton PJM. Virchows Archiv Cell Pathol B 1973, 13, 227–232
51. Wall AJ. Med Clin N Am 1973, 57, 1241–1252
52. Wall AJ, Douglas AP, Booth CC, Pearse AGE. Gut 1970, 11, 7–14
53. Wall AJ, Peters TJ. Gut 1971, 12, 445–448
54. Weser E, Hernandez MH. Gastroenterology 1971, 60, 69–75
55. Wright NA, Al-Dewachi HS, Appleton DR, Watson AJ. Virchows Archiv Cell Pathol B 1978, 28, 339–350

# Effect of Exogenous Gut Hormones on Gastrointestinal Mucosal Growth

L. R. JOHNSON
Department of Physiology, University of Texas Medical School,
Houston, Texas, U.S.A.

Numerous GI hormones and peptides, such as gastrin, CCK, secretin, glucagon, somatostatin and EGF, have been shown to stimulate at least part of the trophic response in GI tissues. Whether any of these (or a different one) accounts for gastrointestinal adaptation is unknown. Final proof will entail the demonstration that the endogenous serum levels of one of these increases during the adaptation period to amounts significant to cause the response.

*Department of Physiology, University of Texas Medical School, Houston, U.S.A.*

## INTRODUCTION

Two general types of stimulation result in growth of gastrointestinal (GI) mucosa. One is provided by non-GI hormones such as thyroxine and growth hormone. The other consists of the many factors brought into play by the ingestion and digestion of food. Alterations in this second group have been hypothesized by many investigators to be responsible for the adaptive responses of GI mucosa following partial intestinal resection or other procedures which result in adaptation of the gut. Three of these, local nutrition (the direct action of luminal nutrients stimulating the growth of the mucosa absorbing them), pancreatic and biliary secretions, and GI hormones are of particular interest and have been the subject of numerous investigations.

The local nutrition and secretion theories are gradient based. That is, the proximal bowel is normally exposed to the highest concentration of both nutrients and secretions, and the amounts of these and their effects would decrease distally. These concepts, therefore, could explain the presence of intestinal villus height and crypt depth gradients (1), the atrophy of proximal bowel removed from continuity as a Thiry-Vella loop (17), the hyperplasia of distal mucosa following resection of proximal bowel (22), and the observation that transposition of proximal and distal segments results in hyperplasia of the former distal segment and hypoplasia of the mucosa of the proximal segment now located distally (1, 6). These phenomena cannot be totally explained by a humoral mechanism. On the other hand, a trophic factor has not been isolated from bile or pancreatic juice, and there is no strong evidence that nutrients stimulate growth of the cells absorbing them.

There is growing evidence, however, that at least a portion of the adaptive response is humorally mediated (10). Numerous results including the demonstration of hyperplasia in by-passed intestinal loops after resection (7) and hyperplasia of the mucosa of both animals of a parabiotic pair following partial intestinal resection in one of them (23) must be explained by systemic factors.

Attention has naturally focused on GI hormones and peptides, some of which have known trophic effects (8), as possible mediators of these humoral responses. The purpose of this paper is to review the trophic effects of these substances and to indicate the criteria which must be satisfied before a response can be attributed to a particular hormone.

## TROPHIC EFFECTS OF EXOGENOUS HORMONES

GI hormones and peptides reported to have

Table I. Summary of trophic effects of GI peptides on GI tissues. +, stimulation; 0, no effect; blank spaces indicate tissues which have not been tested

| | Tissue | | | |
|---|---|---|---|---|
| Hormone or Peptide | Oxyntic Gland | Duodenum | Colon | Pancreas |
| Gastrin | + | + | + | + |
| CCK | 0 | 0 | 0 | + |
| Secretin | 0 | 0 | 0 | + |
| Glucagon | + | | + | |
| EGF | + | +,0 | 0 | |
| Somatostatin | + | | | |

trophic effects on either GI mucosa or the pancreas are shown in Table I. The growth stimulating properties of gastrin are well known and studies reported in 1969 involving this hormone led to the hypothesis that GI hormones regulated the growth of mucosal tissues as well as their secretions (11). Exogenous gastrin or pentagastrin stimulates the growth of mucosa of the oxyntic gland stomach, duodenum and colon and increases the DNA content of the pancreas (8, 16, 19, 20). Removal of endogenous gastrin by antrectomy results in hypoplasia of much of the GI mucosa and the pancreas. This loss of cells is prevented by treatment with exogenous gastrin (2). Exogenous gastrin in doses which do not increase serum levels of the hormone more than those which occur after the ingestion of a meal stimulate gastric mucosal DNA synthesis (21). These data justify the conclusion that the stimulation of mucosal growth is a physiological action of gastrin.

Cholecystokinin (CCK) stimulates the growth of the exocrine pancreas. In 1974 Mainz et al. (19) demonstrated that CCK led to increased pancreatic RNA, DNA, and protein content. CCK does not appear to have potent trophic effects on oxyntic gland or duodenal mucosa (14). Doses of exogenous CCK octapeptide which increased pancreatic DNA content significantly had no effect on either oxyntic gland or duodenal mucosal DNA in the same rats. Much higher doses of CCK caused a slight stimulation of DNA synthesis in duodenal mucosa but this effect was not physiological (14).

Secretin inhibits the trophic effect of gastrin and has little or no effect of its own on the growth of GI mucosa (13). In the pancreas exogenous secretin increases DNA synthesis and DNA content and potentiates the trophic action of CCK (3). The effects of exogenous CCK and secretin on pancreatic growth are probably physiological, for they can be mimicked by intraduodenal perfusion of physiological amounts of hydrogen ion and amino acids (12). These are the normal releasers of the endogenous hormones.

Two other members of the secretin family of peptides, glucagon and VIP, have been tested for trophic effects on GI mucosa. In both oxyntic gland and colonic mucosa glucagon increases DNA synthesis significantly (9). Optimal stimulation was caused by 50 μg/kg glucagon; doubling the dose caused no further stimulation. The effect of glucagon was equal to approximately 40% of the effect produced by pentagastrin in the same tissues. VIP behaves in a manner essentially identical to that of secretin. In other words it inhibits the effect of gastrin on mucosal growth and has no effect of its own (9).

Feldman et al. (5) have shown that EGF, epidermal growth factor, stimulates ornithine decarboxylase activity in the stomach and duodenum of 8-day old mice. Evidence exists relating polyamines to RNA synthesis and indicating that ornithine decarboxylase actually activates RNA polymerase I. Thus, the induction of ornithine decarboxylase has been used as an index of trophic activity. In adult rats EGF increased DNA synthesis and RNA and DNA content of oxyntic gland mucosa (15). The maximal effect was produced by 20 µg/kg EGF and was equal to the trophic response to pentagastrin. In the same study EGF had no effect on growth of duodenal or colonic mucosa (15).

Konturek et al. (18) have recently reported that somatostatin stimulates DNA synthesis of rat oxyntic gland mucosa. It was also able to decrease the severity of aspirin induced gastric ulcers in both rats and cats in doses which did not inhibit gastric acid secretion.

## PHYSIOLOGICAL SIGNIFICANCE OF THE EFFECT OF AN EXOGENOUS HORMONE

Many of the effects of exogenous GI hormones and peptides are not physiological. In fact given the proper dose gastrin and CCK alter secretion, motility and growth of almost all GI tissues. Determination of whether or not a particular peptide is a physiological regulator of growth is more difficult than assessing its significance on, for example, gastric secretion. Increases in the various components of the pleiotypic or trophic response take hours and days after hormone administration to become statistically significant. Growth is stimulated usually by the continuing presence of hormone rather than by short term release as normally occurs after a meal. In general, however, if the trophic effect of an exogenous hormone is reproduced by endogenous hormone, and if the trophic effect occurs in response to exogenous hormone which does not raise serum hormone levels over those produced by normal endogenous release, the effect is considered physiologically significant.

These criteria have been satisfied for the trophic effect of gastrin. Hypergastrinemia in cases of Zollinger-Ellison syndrome produce hyperplasia of oxyntic gland and duodenal mucosa (4). Removal of the source of gastrin following antrectomy results in the atrophy of many GI tissues (2). In dogs with gastric fistulas and denervated pouches the $D_{50}$ dose of porcine gastrin II (160 ng/kg-h) for the stimulation of acid secretion was infused continuously for 4 h (21). Using a biopsy instrument for repeated samples of pouch mucosa Ryan et al. (21) demonstrated that 16 h

after the start of infusion, DNA synthesis had increased 500% compared to animals receiving saline or histamine. Serum gastrin levels were not increased significantly over those resulting from the ingestion of a normal meal in the same animals.

## CONCLUDING REMARKS

Numerous GI peptides have been shown to exert trophic effects on GI tissues. In order to prove that one of these (or a different one) is responsible for a part of the adaptational response it will be necessary to show that levels of that peptide increase endogenously to levels sufficient to produce the effects caused by exogenous administration.

## ACKNOWLEDGEMENTS

The work reported in this paper was supported by NIH grant AM 18164.

## REFERENCES

1. Altman GV, Leblond CJ. Am J Anat 1970, 127, 15–36
2. Dembinski AB, Johnson LR. Endocrinology 1979, 105, 769–773
3. Dembinski AB, Johnson LR. Endocrinology 1980, 106, 323–328
4. Ellison EH, Wilson SD. pp 363–369 in Shnitka TK, Gilbert JAL, Harrison RC. (eds). Gastric Secretion, Pergamon Press, New York, 1967
5. Feldman EJ, Aures D, Grossman MI. Proc Soc Exp Biol MEd 1978, 159, 400–402
6. Gronqvist B, Engstrom B, Grimilias L. Acta Chir Scand 1975, 141, 208–217
7. Hanson WR, Rijke RPC, Plaisier HM. Cell Tiss Kinet 1977, 10, 543–555
8. Johnson LR. Ann Rev Physiol 1977, 39, 135–148
9. Johnson LR. Gastroenterology 1977, 72, 788–792
10. Johnson LR. World J Surg 1979, 3, 477–487
11. Johnson LR, Aures D, Yuen L. Am J Physiol 1969, 217–251–254.
12. Johnson LR, Dudrick SJ, Guthrie PD. Am J Physiol 1980, 239, G400–G405
13. Johnson LR, Guthrie PD. Gastroenterology 1974, 67, 601–606
14. Johnson LR, Guthrie PD. Gastroenterology 1976, 70, 59–65
15. Johnson LR, Guthrie PD. Am J Physiol 1980, 238, G45–G49
16. Johnson LR, Lichtenberger, LM, Copeland EM, Dudrick SJ, Castro GA. 1975, 68, 1184–1193
17. Keren DF, Elliott HL, Brown GD, Yardley JH. Gastroenterology 1975, 68, 83–93

18. Konturek SJ, Radecki T, Brzozowski T, Piastucki I, Dembinski A, Dembinska-Kieć A, Zmuda A, Gryglewski R, Gregory H. Gastroenterology 1981, 81, 438–443.

19. Mainz DL, Block O, and Webster PD. J Clin Invest 1974, 52, 2300–2304

20. Mak KM, and Chang WWL. Gastroenterology 1976, 71, 117–120

21. Ryan GP, Copeland EM, and Johnson LR, Am J Physiol 1978, 235, E32–E36

22. Weser E, Heller R, and Tawil T. Gastroenterology 1977, 73, 524–529

23. Williamson RCN, Buchholtz TW, and Malt RA. Gastroenterology 1978, 75, 249–254

# The Hormonal Pattern of Intestinal Adaptation

## A major role for Enteroglucagon

S. R. BLOOM & J. M. POLAK
Royal Postgraduate Medical School, Du Cane Road, London W12 0HS, UK

A number of human diseases with intestinal adaptation have been investigated, including acute infective diarrhoea, intestinal resection, jejuno-ileal bypass, coeliac disease, tropical sprue, chronic pancreatitis and cystic fibrosis. In all, the newly isolated hormone enteroglucagon appeared to be elevated in proportion to the degree of adaptation. In rats after gut resection and cold adaptation, enteroglucagon was also elevated and the degree of elevation correlated closely with the crypt cell production rate (CCPR). Chronic administration of somatostatin suppressed both enteroglucagon and CCPR, while bombesin stimulated both. A crude preparation of enteroglucagon was found to directly stimulate DNA synthesis in enterocyte cultures. It is thus concluded that, at present, the most likely candidate for the humoral component of intestinal adaptation is the hormonal peptide enteroglucagon.

*Dr. S. R. Bloom, Department of Medicine, Hammersmith Hospital, Du Cane Road, London W12 0HS, U.K.*

## INTRODUCTION

One of the major advances in gastroenterology has been the discovery that the gut is regulated by local and hormonal peptides (regulatory peptides). The history of their discovery parallels the development of biological knowledge over the last 60 years. The process is, however, not yet complete. Bayliss & Starling in 1902 (3) discovered that control of an intestinal function (neutralisation of acid in the duodenum by pancreatic bicarbonate juice) was mediated through a circulating hormone. Thus its physiological role was discovered first and there was never any doubt, therefore, about the function of the hormone secretin. Subsequently proposed hormonal peptides have come on the scene in various accidental ways and their functional significance is far less secure. For example, two new peptides have recently been isolated on the basis that they possessed C-terminal amides, a structural feature which is common in regulatory peptides (24). Preliminary evidence suggests that both these peptides (known as PHI and PYY from their terminal amino acids) are found in neuroendocrine tissues and their role as regulatory peptides is thus strongly suggested. There is almost no evidence, however, as to what that role might be. Thus currently we have a number of active peptides, some of which are easy to measure by radioimmunoassay and localise by immunocytochemistry, but whose physiological role is uncertain. To balance this there are a number of physiological actions which are clearly under hormonal control, but of which the hormones have not yet been identified. Is intestinal adaptation such a hormonally controlled process? At first sight the answer to the question is no, as adaptation appears to depend on luminal nutrition.

Thus a bypassed segment of the bowel atrophies, while a greater local nutriment load (due either to nutriment diversion to an area not normally receiving it or to a greater whole body food intake) causes hypertrophy. However this simple relationship (more nutriment equals more mucosal growth) is not an adequate explanation for all situations (for example considerable hypertrophy is seen above an area of resected bowel even when food intake is unchanged). Indeed an extreme alternative hypothesis is that the luminal nutriment is required only as a background enabling factor and mucosal growth is mainly under hormonal control. Such a theory could explain the observed facts quite adequately. The problem of deciding which theory is correct can be approached in two ways. First, the effect of exogenous hormone can be studied (see previous chapter by Johnson), and secondly the hormone milieu can be investigated in naturally-occurring or experimental situations where intestinal adaptation develops. This chapter follows the latter approach and attempts to demonstrate that one particular hormone, enteroglucagon, correlates very well with mucosal growth. Indeed this relationship is so close that enteroglucagon has been nicknamed growth hormone of the gut (7).

## HORMONES INVESTIGATED

The hormones measured in these studies included gastrin from G cells in the gastric antrum and upper small intestinal mucosa, secretin from S cells in the duodenum and jejunum, gastric inhibitory peptide (GIP) from K cells of the jejunal mucosa, motilin from the D1 cells of the jejunum and ileum, neurotensin from the NT cells of the ileum, enteroglucagon from the EG cells of the ileal and colonic mucosa and pancreatic polypeptide (PP) from PP cells of the pancreas. With the exception of secretin and PP, each of these hormonal peptides is normally produced and released into the circulation in multiple forms. Radioimmunoassay is a sufficiently sensitive technique to detect the low concentrations that are present in the circulation, but a number of technical problems prevent agreement between laboratories as to the correct absolute concentrations. This is because the particular antibodies being employed by different laboratories for each peptide differ in the part of the amino acid sequence they detect and may, for example, react to different degrees with different molecular forms of each peptide. Related problems affect tissue localisation by immunocytochemistry. Fortunately a better understanding of factors which interfere in antibody-antigen reactions and the employment of antibodies which react with a defined part of the hormone molecule (optimally the biologically active part of the sequence) have greatly improved the absolute value of these immunological detection techniques in recent times. Further their reliability in comparative situations is excellent so that the effect of disease or experimental procedure can be very accurately determined. The sequence of almost all the major porcine forms of the peptides has now been established with the recent publication of the sequence of enteroglucagon (also termed glucagon-like immunoreactivity of intestinal origin or GLI, more recently abbreviate to glicentin because of the supposed presence of 100 amino acids). This latter peptide was found to contain the entire amino acid sequence of pancreatic glucagon in its C-terminal sequence thus explaining the crossreactivity of enteroglucagon with pancreatic glucagon antibodies (25).

## PATHOLOGY

### Tumours

Diseases can be regarded as a series of natural experiments throwing light on the way physiological processes normally work. A singular example was the discovery of a tumour at the beginning of the last decade where the patient was found to have gross mucosal hypertrophy. Indeed the villi were so large that they were visibly enlarged to naked eye inspection (15). A tumour was found and after resection all the patient's abnormalities disappeared. The preoperative plasma contained massive quantities of enteroglucagon which was found to be produced by the tumour (6). When extracts of tumour material were injected into the mice it appeared to result in considerable hypertrophy of the intestinal mucosa, reproducing the clinical syndrome. The idea was thus born that enteroglucagon may have been the trophic factor responsible. There have been no subsequent reports of further non-pancreatic enteroglucagonomas. The discovery, however, that the difference between the alpha cell of the pancreas and the EG cell of the intestinal mucosa appeared to reside solely in the post-translational enzymic processing, suggested the possibility that pancreatic alpha cell tumours might also produce enteroglucagon if the hormone synthesis was sufficiently deranged. This has indeed been found to be the case and a small number of pancreatic glucagonomas have been found associated with intestinal villous hypertrophy on jejunal biopsy. No systematic documentation of this phenomenon and its association with large molecular weight glucagon production has yet been undertaken, however (13).

*Acute infection*

While performing experiments on glucagon metabolism in calves, we discovered that large amounts of crossreacting substance were sometimes present in the plasma. This material turned out to be enteroglucagon and it was found to be elevated only in those calves which had developed acute scour (diarrhoea). The levels returned to normal when the animals recovered. Subsequently we have found this phenomenon in a number of different animal species. It is particularly marked in gnotobiotic animals, when an enteropathic organism is introduced for the first time. The only other hormone to be consistently elevated in diarrhoea is motilin. This 22 amino acid polypeptide hormone has very potent effects on smooth muscle contractility and it seems more likely that it has a role in the abnormal intestinal motility seen in these circumstances. A four-fold increase of motilin and a three-fold increase in enteroglucagon was seen in a group of 12 previously healthy young adult patients who had developed acute infective diarrhoea (11). No other hormone was significantly changed and, following recovery, both motilin and enteroglucagon returned to normal. It is known that such infections produce damage to the mucosa and thus presumably an adaptive response occurs in the healing phase.

*Intestinal resection*

The most classical situation of intestinal adaptation follows intestinal resection. Although resections are sometimes performed in patients with healthy bowels, the most common setting for this procedure is in inflammatory bowel disease. This was the case in a series of 18 patients

we studied with partial small intestinal resection, who were looked at in contrast with 9 patients with partial resection of the large intestine and 11 sex and age matched healthy controls (9). Pancreatic polypeptide was the most elevated hormone in both intestinal resection groups but this may have been related more to the presence of inflammatory bowel disease as, in a separate study, inflammatory bowel disease by itself was also associated with raised levels of this hormone. Enteroglucagon was approximately two-fold elevated in the small intestinal resection group in the basal state and three-fold elevated at the peak concentration after a meal.

In contrast the large intestinal resection group showed basal plasma enteroglucagon concentrations that were approximately half those of the control group. When the distribution of enteroglucagon is examined in the human alimentary tract, the highest concentration is found in the distal ileum while in the upper small intestine the concentrations are vanishingly low. In the large bowel the average concentration ($35 \pm 10$ pmol/g) is approximately an eighth that of the ileum, but because of the greater weight of this region the total amount of enteroglucagon is considerably larger and is not dissimilar from the total in the small intestine (12). Thus the lower level of enteroglucagon after colonic resection was not unexpected. Whether the fall in plasma enteroglucagon concentration is associated with any reduction in mucosal growth, is at present unknown. Certainly after small intestinal resection increased mucosal growth is seen and, since no other measurable peptide is grossly changed in these circumstances (including motilin), if there is a circulating trophic factor enteroglucagon remains the candidate. Enteroglucagon is released by fat and carbohydrate, both in the small intestine and also in the large intestine (18) and thus malabsorption of food in the upper small intestine allows it to pass into the area of greater enteroglucagon cell density within the ileum or even, with more severe malabsorption, to spill over into the colon with the possibility of affecting a still larger number of enteroglucagon cells. Thus the distribution of this hormone would fit it for a role in intestinal malabsorption.

*Bypass operations*

Morbid obseity is a major problem of the civilised world and is extremely resistant to any form of simple treatment. Various surgical procedures have been tried to ameliorate this condition. The jejunoileal bypass procedure became particularly popular about 10 years ago. We were able to study a group of patients 12 months after a 7″ jejunum to a 7″ ileum anastomosis, bypassing the rest of the small intestine. A significant, though not massive, weight loss ensued and, at the time of investigation, the patients were $181 \pm 8\%$ of ideal body weight, compared with a control pre-operative group of $222 \pm 7\%$ of ideal body weight (n = 19). Hormones released from the part of the bowel that was bypassed (eg GIP, Fig. 1) were greatly reduced in the postprandial period, whereas hormones released in the part of the bowel beyond anastomosis (ie neurotensin and enteroglucagon, Fig. 2) were greatly increased (8). Unfortunately the operation has several problems, including a high initial mortality and

toxic effects from bacterial overgrowth in the blind loop. In addition, although initial weight loss can be quite spectacular, adaptation of the bowel remaining in continuity results in diminishing effectiveness over time. Thus a typical patient ceases to lose weight after about a year and approximately 5 years after the procedure may show a considerable regain of weight. If laparotomy is required for any reason, massive hypertrophy is noted of the segment of intestine still in continuity. It has also been noted that the bypassed bowel fails to atrophy in the expected fashion. Thus it has been postulated that there is a considerable trophic drive to the mucosa of the small intestine in these patients, some component of which may operate via the circulation. Again enteroglucagon would appear to be a good candidate as a massive 16-fold elevation in the postprandial concentrations is found. Interestingly an alternative procedure (bilio-pancreatic bypass) developed by Scopinaro and colleagues, also produces a massive elevation of enteroglu-

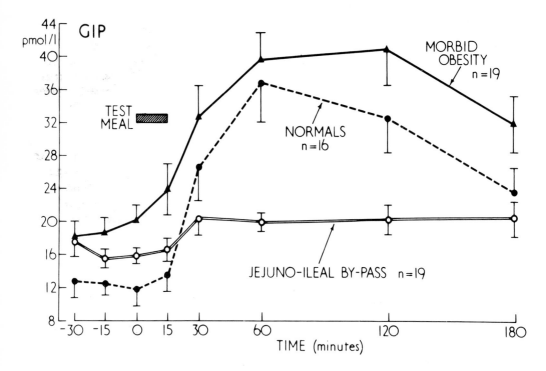

Fig. 1. Plasma GIP concentrations following a 530 calorie test breakfast in patients after jejuno-ileal bypass with matched (sex and age) groups of pre-operative obese subjects and normal weight controls.

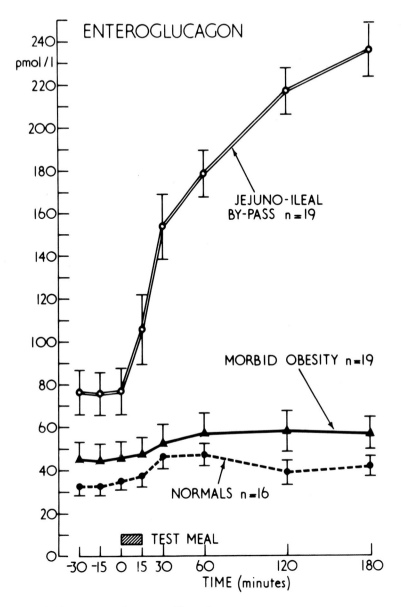

Fig. 2. Plasma enteroglucagon as Figure 1.

cagon (23) but in this case the design of the bypass is such as to prevent compensatory hyperabsorption in the relevant segment.

### The sprues

There are a number of conditions where the gross appearance of the small intestine suggests atrophy but where, in fact, rates of intestinal growth are maximal though they are unable to overcome the chronic destructive process. In these circumstances one would anticipate any hormonal mediator of intestinal adaptation would be present in very high concentrations. This has indeed been found to be the case. Thus in a group of 11 patients with active coeliac disease, studied in comparison with 13 patients now symptom-free

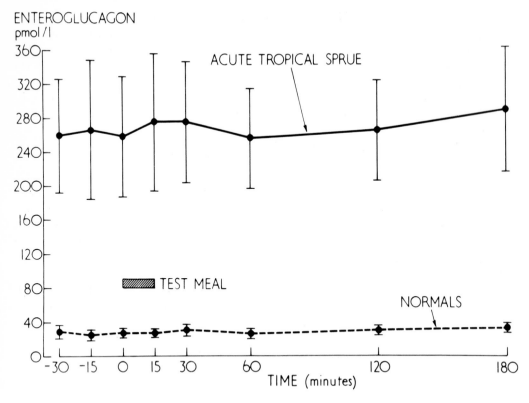

Fig. 3. Plasma enteroglucagon in a group of previously healthy young adults, who developed acute malabsorption following a period in the tropics, with a group of matched controls, following ingestion of a 530 calorie test breakfast.

on a gluten-free diet and 13 healthy controls, enteroglucagon was found to be extremely elevated (Fig. 3), more so than any other hormones (4). In this condition, as in every other one examined, gel permeation chromatography of the enteroglucagon in plasma demonstrates a single major peak with a Kav on G-50 sephadex of approximately 0.25. This is distinctly different from pancreatic glucagon and matches exactly the position in which the purified 69 amino acid porcine enteroglucagon (glicentin) is eluted from the same column. Several other minor peaks of immunoreactivity can be detected but do not alter significantly following stimuli and are not responsible for the elevated concentrations seen in disease states. Enteroglucagon levels were completely normal in those patients treated with a gluten-free diet, in contrast to the ten-fold elevation of enteroglucagon seen in patients with

active disease. A very small elevation (one and half-fold) of neurotensin was also noted in the latter but upper small intestinal hormones were distinctly depressed. Gastrin and pancreatic polypeptide were not significantly altered. A rather similar pattern of hormonal change was seen in another group of patients suffering from acute tropical malabsorption (tropical sprue). Eight young adults were studied who had been completely healthy until they visited the tropics, developed chronic diarrhoea, and returned with malabsorption and subtotal villous atrophy. A strikingly abnormal gut hormone profile was seen, where, again, the major abnormality was a gross elevation of enteroglucagon concentrations. The pattern was, however, different from that seen in coeliac disease in that the basal elevation was particularly marked with little further increase after a meal (5). In these subjects neurotensin was not abnormal but motilin was four-fold elevated, commensurate with their diarrhoea. Other hormones were not significantly different from the matched control group. The same patients have been re-studied 4 years later by which time they were completely symptom-free, residing in London, and at this time their gut hormone profile was completely normal. It was of interest that the degree of elevation of enteroglucagon correlated closely with breath hydrogen which reflects the degree of functional malabsoprtion of carbohydrate in the small intestine and its consequential metabolism by colonic bacteria. In patients with malabsorption due to pancreatic disease, the pancreatic hormone, PP, is considerably reduced and enteroglucagon is again elevated. In a group of 10 children with cystic fibrosis, GIP was significantly diminished and the pancreatic polypeptide response to a meal abolished. Enteroglucagon was four-fold elevated in the basal state but showed little response to a milk stimulus (1). Similarly in patients with steatorrhoea due to chronic pancreatitis, there was a distinct elevation of plasma enteroglucagon (10).

*The first meal*

At birth there is a complete and irreversible switch from parenteral to enteral feeding. In the following days very rapid gut adaptation occurs and the organ increases in size significantly. The mechanism controlling this adaptation is unknown. In the human infant it fails to occur if, for any reason, the parenteral feeding is artificially continued by the medical attendants. Indeed, it then becomes difficult to re-establish oral feeding and, as prolonged intravenous feeding is associated with a high incidence of infections, the failure of oral feeding can result in considerable morbidity.

Gastrointestinal hormones are known to be produced in the human foetal intestine from an early stage (14) and cord concentrations at birth are not dissimilar from those seen in the fasting adult. Dramatic elevations of almost all the hormones occur as soon as feeding is commenced and high plasma concentrations are achieved. Subsequently, the normal fasting and fed pattern

is developed and after a few weeks the average concentration returns towards that seen in the adult. These changes are completely absent in infants fed parenterally. A hormone showing one of the biggest rises is enteroglucagon but very significant elevations occur with gastrin and neurotensin (2, 19).

EXPERIMENTAL STUDIES

The finding in the studies mentioned above that enteroglucagon was always elevated when stimuli to intestinal growth were present, led us to concentrate on this peptide in particular. To date no experimental circumstance has been found to vitiate this connection and no other hormone demonstrates this relationship.

In a series of 3 different rat models of intestinal adaptation, measurements were made of small intestinal growth, fasting plasma and small intestinal tissue content of enteroglucagon. In 17 rats, 5 weeks after resection of the proximal two-thirds of the intestine, plasma and tissue enteroglucagon concentrations nearly doubled. In a group of 17 rats undergoing cold acclimation, plasma levels tripled and tissue levels doubled. In a third group investigated on the 12th day of lactation, while tissue enteroglucagon levels were more than double, plasma concentrations were not significantly different. Thus in these preliminary experiments there appeared evidence that enteroglucagon was elevated during 3 different sorts of mild stimulus to intestinal adaptation (17). In another series of rats, after varying degrees of intestinal resection, enteroglucagon concentrations were elevated in proportion to the amount of bowel resected (16). A more recent series of 48 rats were studied after either a 75% proximal small bowel resection or a jejunal transection (as control). The animals were divided into 3 groups, the first of which was allowed food ad libitum, the second was kept hypothermic (resulting in hyperphagia), while the third group were nourished intravenously. All animals were killed 12 days later and plasma enteroglucagon, gastrin and crypt cell production rate (CCPR, see Chapter by Wright) was used to evaluate cellular proliferation. A significant hyperplasia of the enteroglucagon-producing cells

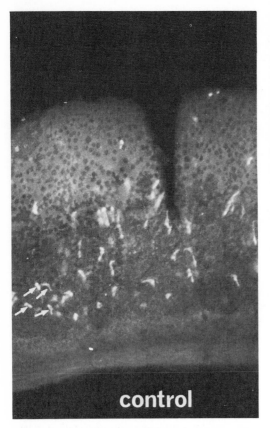
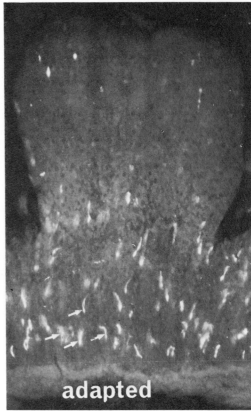

Fig. 4. Thin slices of ileal wall from a control rat (left) and a rat with hypertrophic intestinal adaptation (right, 40 days after 80% proximal small bowel resection) (immunofluorescence, X 116). Tissue samples were fixed in p-benzoquinone (0.4% in phosphate buffered saline – PBS – 0.01 mol/l, pH 7.2) for 1 hour, dehydrated, cleared in xylene, re-hydrated and divided into strips (0.5–1 mm wide). These were immunostained in toto for entero-glucagon cells, using N-terminal specific glucagon antibodies. After immunostaining thin tissue slices (1 villus wide) were obtained and single villi and crypts were microdissected for quantitative assessment of the enteroglu-cagon cell density (cells per crypt/villus). In the adapted ileum the mucosa shows striking hypertrophic changes. At this time-length after intestinal resection enteroglucagon cells (arrows) are clearly more numerous in the crypt region, as confirmed by preliminary quantitative studies.

was seen in the orally-fed resected or hyperphagic rats (Figs. 4 & 5). In each group resected rats had a significantly greater crypt cell production rate and higher enteroglucagon level compared to transected animals. Plasma gastrin, in contrast, did not show any significant change (Fig. 6) (22). In an attempt to establish the presence of a humoral mechanism, a further series of rats were studied with 75% proximal small bowel resection in which the resected bowel was refashioned to form a Thiry-Vella fistula. Half the group were fed by mouth, while the remainder were fed

isocalorically by an intravenous line. The animals were killed at 12 days and plasma gastrin, entero-glucagon and CCPR measured. Plasma entero-glucagon was much greater with oral feeding (566 ± 59 pmol/l) than with intravenous feeding (250 ± 42 pmol/l), though the gastrin levels did not differ. The CCPR/h was similarly much greater in the orally fed animals (48 ± 5) than in the intravenously fed animals (18 ± 3). The CCPR in the excluded fistula was very much lower but again was greater in the orally fed rats (24 ± 2) than in the intravenously fed animals

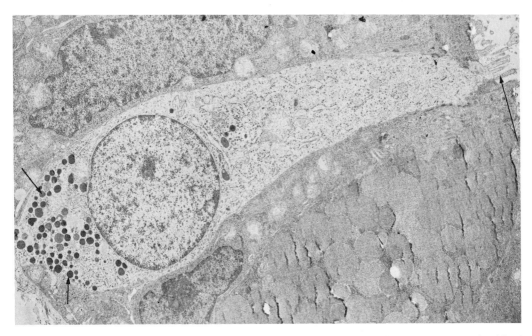

Fig. 5. Electron micrograph of an L-cell in the human ileum showing characteristic secretory granules (short arrows) containing enteroglucagon, microvilli can be observed (long arrow) X 7,040.

(16 ± 1.5). This study therefore suggested that there was indeed a humoral agent affecting the rate of enterocyte proliferation, but it also underlined the importance of the nutriment stream (20).

Two regulatory peptides have been found which influenced the rate of enteroglucagon release, somatostatin which inhibits it and bombesin which stimulates it. Using both a long-acting subcutaneous depot preparation and also the Alzet 7 day subcutaneous pump, the effect of these 2 agents on enteroglucagon concentrations and CCPR was investigated in a further group of rats. After administration of somatostatin, plasma enteroglucagon fell in rats, that had previously had a 75% small intestinal resection, from 667 ± 70 pmol/l to 73 ± 9 pmol/l and CCPR fell in parallel from 49 ± 5 to 15 ± 1. The effects of bombesin were slight in animals undergoing near maximal adaptation and were most clearly seen in rats that had not undergone intestinal resection, causing a rise in enteroglucagon concentrations from 99 ± 10 pmol/l to 218 ± 34 pmol/l. Again the

CCPR increased in parallel from 17 ± 1 to 25 ± 2 (21). This study therefore demonstrates that regulatory peptides can indeed influence intestinal adaptation though whether the effect is a direct one or an indirect one (e.g. via enteroglucagon) requires further experimentation.

## CONCLUSION

In surveying the hormonal pattern of intestinal adaptation, one hormonal peptide stands out above all others as correlating closely with the rate of enterocyte growth, namely enteroglucagon. This substance, which is produced by endocrine cells in the mucosa of the lower small intestine and colon has recently been isolated and sequenced. Preliminary studies, with a partly purified enteroglucagon preparation, show a stimulation of DNA synthesis in cultured jejunal mucosa (26). Further experiments of this nature can be expected and will hopefully demonstrate that this material is indeed trophic to the enterocyte. The degree to which this hormonal peptide

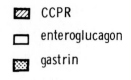

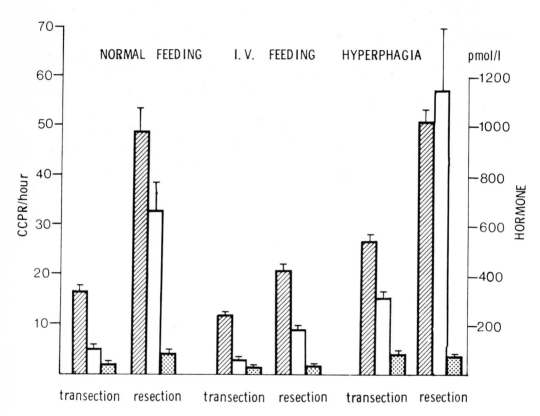

Fig. 6. Changes in crypt cell production rate in the terminal ileum and plasma gastrin and enteroglucagon in transected and resected rats fed orally, intravenously or in the cold (hyperphagia).

acts alone or in conjunction with other trophic influences, and the role of local nutrition, remain to be established.

## ACKNOWLEDGEMENTS

Support from the Stanley Thomas Johnson Foundation is gratefully acknowledged.

## REFERENCES

1. Adrian TE, McKiernan J, Johnstone DI, Hiller EJ, Vyas H, Sarson DL, Bloom SR. Gastroenterology 1980, 79, 460–465

2. Albuquerque RH, Owens CWI, Bloom SR. Experientia 1979, 35, 1496–1497
3. Bayliss WM, Starling EH. J Physiol (Lond) 1902, 28, 325–353
4. Besterman HS, Bloom SR, Sarson DL, Blackburn AM, Johnston DI, Patel HR, Stewart JS, Modigliani R, Guerin S, Mallinson CN. Lancet 1978, I, 785–788
5. Besterman HS, Cook GC, Sarson DL, Christofides ND, Bryant MG, Gregor M, Bloom SR. Brit Med J 1979, 1, 1252–1255
6. Bloom SR. Gut 1972, 13, 520–532
7. Bloom SR. In: Gray CH, James VHT, (eds) Hormones in Blood, 3rd edition, Academic Press, London 1979, 321–356
8. Bloom SR. In: Maxwell JD, Gazet J-C, Pilkington

TR (eds). Surgical Management of Obesity, Academic Press, London 1980, 115–123

9. Bloom SR, Besterman HS, Adrian TE, Christifides ND, Sarson DL, Mallinson CN, Pero A, Modigliani R. Gastroenterology 1979, 76, 1101.

10. Bloom SR, Besterman HS, Adrian TE, Christofides ND, Sarson DL, Mallinson CN, Pera A, South M, Modigliani R, Guerin S. Gastroenterology 1978, 74, 1012

11. Bloom SR, Besterman HS, Welsby PD, Christofides ND, Sarson DL. Gastroenterology 1979, 76, 1102

12. Bloom SR, Polak JM. In: Bloom SR (ed). Gut Hormones, Churchill Livingstone, Edinburgh 1978, 3–18

13. Bloom SR, Polak JM. In: Abe K (ed). Clinics in Endocrinology & Metabolism, Saunders Ltd, London 9 1980, 285–298

14. Buchan AMJ, Bryant MG, Polak JM, Gregor M, Ghatei MA, Bloom SR. In: Bloom SR, Polak JM (eds). Gut Hormones, 2nd Edition, Churchill Livingstone, Edinburgh 1981, 119–124

15. Gleeson MH, Bloom SR, Polak JM, Henry K, Dowling RM. Gut 1971, 12, 733–782

16. Gregor M, Bryant MG, Buchan AMJ, Bloom SR, Polak JM. Gut 1980, 21, A907

17. Jacobs LR, Bloom SR, Dowling RH. Life Sci 1981, 29, 2003–2007

18. Jian R, Besterman HS, Sarson DL, Aymes C, Hostein J, Bloom SR, Rambaud JC. Dig Dis Sci 1981, 26, 195–201

19. Lucas A, Bloom SR, Aynsley-Green A. Arch Dis Child 1980, 55 678–682

20. Sagor GR, Ghatei MA, Al Mukhtar MYT, Wright NA, Bloom SR. Submitted

21. Sagor GR, Ghatei MS, O'Shaughnessy DJ, AL Mukhtar MYT, Wright NA, Bloom SR. 1982 Submitted

22. Sagor GR, Al Muktar MYT, Ghatei MA, Wright NA, Bloom SR. Br J Surg 1982, 69, 14–18

23. Scopinaro N, Sarson DL, Civalleri D, Gianetta E, Bonalumi U, Friedman D, Bloom SR. Ital J Gastroenterol 1980, 12, 93–96

24. Tatemoto K, Mutt V. Nature 1980, 285, 417–418

25. Thim L, Moody AJ. Reg Pep 1981, 2, 139–150

26. Uttenthal LO, Batt RM, Carter MW, Bloom SR. Reg Pep 1982, 3, 84

# Non-Hormonal Regulation of Intestinal Adaptation

E. WESER, A. VANDEVENTER & T. TAWIL

Medical Service, Audie L. Murphy Veterans Administration Hospital and
The University of Texas Health Science Center at San Antonio, Texas, USA

Infusion of simple sugars and some amino acids into the lumen of the small bowel stimulates local mucosal growth where these substrates come into direct contact with the mucosa. This stimulation does not require active absorption or mucosal metabolism of the substrate and in the case of glucose can be inhibited by phlorizin. Infusion of sugars and some amino acids into ileal lumen results in mucosal growth of proximal bowel distant from the site of infusion. Diverting pancreatico-biliary secretions from proximal to distal small bowel lumen markedly stimulates growth in distal small bowel, while the absence of these secretions from the duodenojejunum paradoxically results in growth of the mucosa at this site. Such regional differences in adaptation suggest that regulation of mucosal growth is different in proximal and distal small bowel.

*E. Weser, M.D., Medical Service, Audie L. Murphy Veterans Administration Hospital and The University of Texas Health Center at San Antonio, Texas, U.S.A.*

## I. INTRODUCTION

Multiple mechanisms may jointly interact to regulate growth of small bowel mucosa. Under physiologic conditions, exposure of the small intestinal mucosa to intraluminal nutrients is necessary for maintenance of normal mucosal growth or adaptive hyperplasia after extensive small bowel resection (7, 4–11, 15, 17, 18, 20, 26). Nutrient contact with the mucosa, absorption, or intramucosal metabolism may stimulate mucosal growth either directly or via release of pancreatico-biliary secretions. These secretions have been shown to increase villus height and mucosal mass in both normal and intestinally resected animals (1, 2, 14, 21, 30, 35, 37, 38). Even the type of oral or enteral nutrition may influence small bowel adaptation. Recent studies have indicated that isocaloric amounts of defined formula diets do not maintain small bowel mucosal mass as well as macromolecular diets (6, 23, 40). Small quantities of long chain triglycerides (20% of total calories) however, seem to produce growth effects equal to complete macromolecular nutrients (22). In recent years therefore, investigation has focused on the specific effects of single nutrients or pancreatico-biliary secretions on mucosal growth hoping to clarify some non-hormonal mechanisms of regulation.

## II. EXPERIMENTAL STUDIES

### Enteric Infusion of Specific Sugars

Glucose infused into the gastrointestinal tract has been shown to stimulate small bowel mucosal growth and maintain the proximal-distal gradient of mucosal mass (6, 26). In order to determine whether mucosal metabolism of glucose or its active transport was necessary for its growth effects on mucosa, several types of sugars were infused either into the stomach or mid-gut and compared with glucose. Male Sprague-Dawley rats (240 g) were maintained on total parenteral nutrition (TPN) (29) and infused continuously via a gastric catheter with glucose (20% in normal saline), galactose (20%), 3-O-methyl glucose (10%), or normal saline for 7 days. At the end of this period the entire small bowel was divided into 8 equal segments and mucosal mass measured. As shown in Fig. 1, gastric infusion of glucose, galactose, and 3-O-methyl glucose increased mucosal weight in all segments compared with saline controls. The significant and peak increases were located in the proximal gut segments for glucose and galactose, establishing the usual proximal-distal gradient of mucosal mass. However, the growth changes with 3-O-methyl glucose (at 50% the weight concentration of other sugars) were found in mid- and distal gut

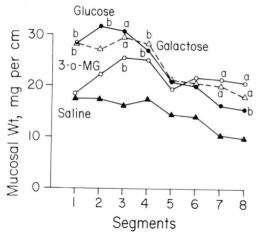

Fig. 1. Stimulation of mucosal growth by gastric infusion of actively absorbed sugars in TPN rats. Glucose 20% (●), n = 5; Galactose 20% (△), n = 6; 3-O-methyl glucose 10% (○), n = 4; Saline 0.9% (▲), n = 5. Values represent Means. Significance (analysis of variance): a = p < 0.01; b = p < 0.05. Adapted from Weser, E., Tawil, T., and Fletcher, J. T. Stimulation of small bowel mucosal growth by gastric infusion of different sugars in rats maintained on total parenteral nutrition. In Intestinal Adaptation 2. Proceedings of an International Conference, Titisee/Black Forest, West Germany, 1981, MTP Press, Lancaster, England (In Press).

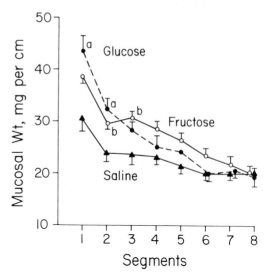

Fig. 2. Stimulation of mucosal growth by gastric infusion of fructose in TPN rats. Fructose 15% (○), n = 6; Glucose 15% (●), n = 5; Saline 0.9% (▼), n = 7. Values represent Mean ± SEM. Significance (analysis of variance): a = p < 0.01; b = p < 0.05. Adapted from Weser, E., Tawil, T., and Fletcher, J.F. Stimulation of small bowel mucosal growth by gastric infusion of different sugars in rats maintained on total parenteral nutrition. In Intestinal Adaptation 2. Proceedings of an International Conference, Titisee/Black Forest, West Germany, 1981, MTP Press, Lancaster, England (In Press).

segments. While this sugar is actively transported (albeit at a slower rate than glucose), it is not metabolized. Similarly, galactose is not metabolized by the intestinal mucosa (5, 39). Therefore, it is unlikely that direct mucosal metabolism of actively absorbed sugars explains the effects on mucosal growth. The reduced rate of 3-O-methyl glucose absorption may result in greater amounts of this sugar reaching the lumen of mid- and distal gut, accounting for its more distal growth effects.

Similar experiments with gastric infusion of mannose and mannitol surprisingly revealed these carbohydrates also stimulated mucosal growth throughout the length of the small bowel with a peak effect in the proximal bowel segment (35). These sugars are limited but to some extent absorbed by non-active transport, suggesting that active absorption is not a requirement for stimulating mucosal growth. As shown in Fig. 2, gastric fructose infusion was similar to glucose in maintaining the proximal-distal gradient of mucosal mass compared with saline infusion.

When phlorizin was added to the gastric glucose infusion solution mucosal mass increased in mid-gut segments compared to glucose infusion without phlorizin (Fig. 3). There was no such effect on mucosa when phlorizin was added to the control saline infusion solution (Fig. 3) or fructose or mannose solutions (not shown in figure). Thus phlorizin was specific in shifting the glucose-induced gradient of mucosal growth caudally. Phlorizin may have partially decreased glucose uptake in proximal gut segments, exposing the lumen of more distal segments to the unabsorbed glucose.

In other experiments, TPN rats were infused continuously via a catheter placed in mid-small intestine with solutions of glucose (15%), fructose (15%), mannose (7.5%), or mannitol (7.5%) for a period of 7 days. As shown in Fig 4, mid-gut infusion of glucose and fructose significantly increased mucosal mass (as indicated by mucosal

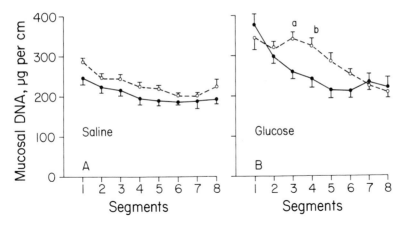

Fig. 3. Stimulation of mucosal growth by gastric infusion of mannose and mannitol in TPN rats. Mannose 7.5% (●), n = 5; Mannitol 7.5% (○), n = 4; Saline 0.9% (▼), n = 7. Values represent Mean ± SEM. Significance (analysis of variance); a = p < 0.01; b = p < 0.05. Adapted from Weser, E., Tawil, T., and Fletcher, J.F. Stimulation of small bowel mucosal growth by gastric infusion of different sugars in rats maintained on total parenteral nutrition. In Intestinal Adaptation 2. Proceedings of an International Conference, Titisee/Black Forest, West Germany, 1981, MTP Press, Lancaster, England (In Press).

DNA) downstream from the site of infusion, with a peak effect in segment 5. It should also be noted that both glucose and fructose mid-gut infusions also caused significant increases in mucosal mass in proximal small bowel segments, maximal in segment 1, even though this location was far removed from the infusion site. It is likely that this proximal response was mediated via some

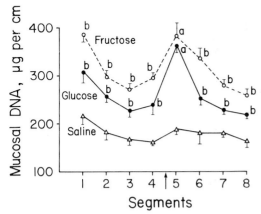

Fig. 4. Stimulation of mucosal growth by mid-gut infusion of glucose and fructose in TPN rats. Glucose 15% (●), n = 5; Fructose 15% (○), n = 6; Saline 0.9% (△), n = 7. Values represent Mean ± SEM. Arrow indicates site of infusion. Significance (analysis of variance): a = p < 0.01; b = p < 0.05.

humoral or neurovascular mechanism since retrograde flow of the sugar is improbable and would not account for the distribution of segmental growth effects.

When phlorizin was added to the glucose and fructose solutions, only with glucose did it cause a shift caudally in the local glucose-stimulated growth of mucosa, peaking in segment 6 (Fig. 5). This shift probably resulted from some unabsorbed glucose in the lumen reaching more distal segments where exposure to greater amounts of glucose caused increased mucosal growth.

Mid-gut infusions of both mannose and mannitol also caused a diffuse increase in mucosal mass throughout the small intestine compared to saline infusion. No striking peak effect was noted around or downstream from the mid-gut infusion site.

These studies indicate that metabolized and non-metabolized intraluminal sugars absorbed by active or non-active transport, stimulate local and remote mucosal growth in the small intestine. While sugar contact with the mucosa, entry into the mucosal cell, and release of trophic mucosal agents may all be factors in the observed mucosal growth, it is not possible to exclude the effects of chronic hyperosmolar stress. Previous studies

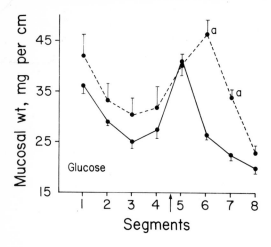

Fig. 5. Effect of phlorizin on mucosal growth stimulated by mid-gut infusion of glucose in TPN rats. Glucose 15% (●--●), n = 5; Glucose 15% + phlorizin (200 mg/ml) (●—●), n = 5; Values represent Mean ± SEM. Arrow indicates site of infusion. Significance (Student's t test): a = p < 0.001.

with hyperosmolar solutions have all been acute and indicate that these solutions cause loss of gut epithelium (16, 29).

### Enteral Infusion of Specific Amino Acids

Since a mixture of 5% amino acids infused into the stomach or mid-small intestine caused local mucosal growth in rats otherwise maintained on TPN (26), the effect of enteral infusion of single class-specific amino acids on mucosal growth was studied (27). In TPN rats 5% glycine, valine, or histidine was continuously infused intragastrically or into the mid-gut lumen for a period of 7 days and growth effects compared with normal saline or a 5% mixture of amino acids (FreAmine®II). As shown in Fig. 6, intragastric infusions of both valine and particularly histidine stimulated mucosal growth in proximal bowel segments compared to saline. Glycine did not stimulate growth and was no different than saline. The growth

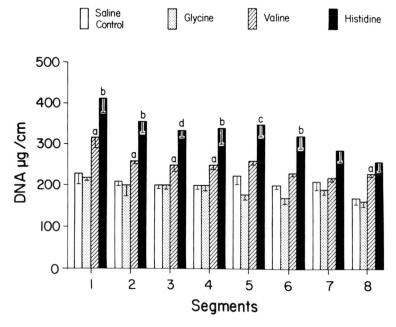

Fig. 6. Effect of gastric infusion of 5% single amino acids on small bowel mucosal growth in TPN rats compared to saline. Bars represent Mean ± SEM. Segment 1, duodenum; segment 8, terminal ileum. Significance: a, p < 0.05; b, p < 0.01; c, p < 0.05; d, p < 0.001. n = 5 rats for each group. Adapted from Spector, M.H., Traylor, J., Young, E.A., and Weser, E. Stimulation of mucosal growth by gastric and ileal infusion of single amino acids in parenterally nourished rats. Digestion 21:33–40, 1981.

effects produced by histidine infusion were equal to those produced by the 5% mixture of amino acids (not shown).

After infusion of each amino acid into mid-small intestine, all three were associated with significant mucosal growth compared to saline (Fig. 7) and comparable or greater growth in the mucosa of distal segments when compared with mixed amino acids (not shown). Furthermore, mid-gut infusion of valine and histidine stimulated significant increases in mucosal mass in the remote segments 1 and 2 compared with both saline and the amino acid mixture. Glycine had not such distant proximal effects.

These studies demonstrate that regional differences exist in the mucosal growth response to single amino acid infusions. Whereas intragastric glycine infusion did not maintain proximal mucosal mass and resulted in atrophy with loss of the proximal-distal mucosal gradient, its infusion into mid-gut stimulated ileal mucosal growth comparable or better than a mixture of amino acids. The remote stimulation of mucosal growth in proximal intestine by mid-gut infusion of valine

and histidine (but not glycine) is probably similar to the observations noted with mid-gut sugar infusions and mediated via humoral or neuro-vascular mechanisms. All three amino acids studied are transported actively against a concentration gradient but by different carrier mechanisms.

To determine if an absorbable, but non-metabolized amino acid would stimulate mucosal growth in TPN maintained rats, 5% alpha amino isobutyric acid (AIB) was infused into the stomach or mid-gut for 7 days. As indicated in Fig. 8, there was no difference in mucosal weight of any segment between AIB and saline controls after gastric infusion. AIB infusion did not prevent atrophy of the proximal segments in the TPN maintained rats and was similar in this regard to glycine infusion. After mid-gut infusion however, AIB caused an increase in mucosal weight in segments downstream from the infusion site compared with saline (Fig. 9), and again was similar to glycine infusion at this site. No remote stimulation of mucosal growth in proximal segments was noted with AIB infusion.

Since both AIB and glycine stimulated local

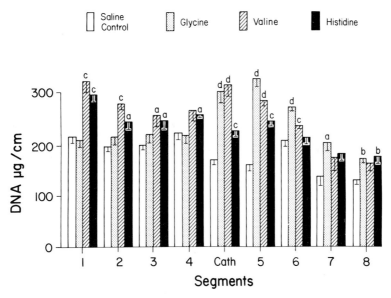

Fig. 7. Effect of mid-gut infusion of 5% single amino acids on small bowel mucosal growth in TPN rats compared to saline. Cath = catheter segment. Bars, segments, and p values as in Figure 6. Adapted from Spector, M.H., Traylor, J., Young, E.A., and Weser, E. Stimulation of mucosal growth by gastric and ileal infusion of single amino acids in parenterally nourished rats. Digestion 21:33–40, 1981.

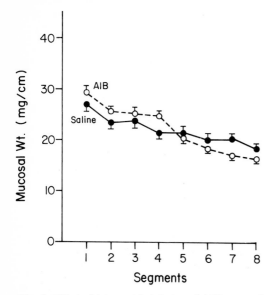

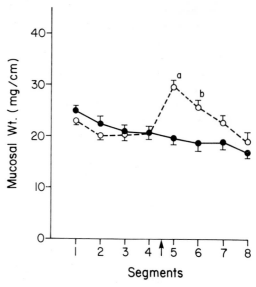

Fig. 8. Effect of intragastric infusion of AIB on small bowel mucosa compared to saline in TPN rats. AIB 5% (○), n = 6; Saline 0.9% (●), n = 5. Values represent Mean ± SEM. No significant difference between AIB and saline.

Fig. 9. Stimulation of mucosal growth by mid-gut infusion of AIB compared to saline in TPN rats. AIB 5% (○), n = 6; Saline 0.9% (●), n = 5. Values represent Mean ± SEM. Arrow indicates site of infusion. Significance (Student's t test); a, p < 0.01; b, p < 0.02.

growth only after mid-gut infusion, the absorption of these two amino acids from different regions of the small intestine was measured to determine if absorption correlated with their effects on mucosal growth. Rats were maintained on either TPN or isocaloric intragastric infusion of the TPN solution for 5 days. A 10 cm segment of proximal, middle, or distal small bowel was cannulated in-vivo and perfused for 2 hours with a 200 μM solution of AIB or glycine containing 0.2% polyethylene glycol. Absorption of AIB or glycine was calculated for each of the three gut segments. As indicated in Table I, there were no significant differences in absorption between proximal, middle, or distal bowel segment for either AIB or glycine in rats maintained on TPN. In rats fed intragastrically, absorption of AIB and glycine was least in distal gut segments, without significant differences between proximal and middle gut segments.

These results of the experiments suggest that the regional growth effects caused by mid-gut infusion of AIB or glycine are not related to greater local absorption or metabolism of the amino acid and again, imply different mechanisms

exist for regulating proximal and distal small bowel mucosal growth.

*Influence of bile and pancreatic secretions on small bowel mucosa*

Nutrients in the lumen of the small bowel stimulate the flow of pancreatico-biliary secretions into the proximal intestine. This enteric-pancreatico-biliary response is mainly mediated via the release of enteric secretogogues into the circulation such as cholecystokinin and secretin, as well as others

Table I. In-vivo intestinal absorption of AIB or glycine (200 μM) in TPN or gastric-fed rats

|  | μmoles/cm/10 min | | |
|---|---|---|---|
|  | Proximal | Middle | Distal |
| TPN Rats |  |  |  |
| AIB (4)* | 1.0 ± 0.4† | 0.8 ± o.4 | 0.7 ± 0.2 |
| Glycine (6) | 1.4 ± 0.4 | 1.7 ± 0.3 | 1.3 ± 0.3 |
| Gastric-Fed Rats |  |  |  |
| AIB (4) | 1.4 ± 0.2 | 1.4 ± 0.3 | 0.7 ± 0.2‡ |
| Glycine (5) | 2.2 ± 0.4 | 1.8 ± 0.4 | 1.5 ± 0.3 |

* Number in parentheses equals number of animals
† Mean ± SEM
‡ p < 0.02 compared with proximal segment

with less clear secretory function. The original studies of Altmann (1) transplating the duodenal papilla (containing the biliary and pancreatic ducts) into the ileum of rats fed chow diets demonstrated that villus size doubled in the ileal segment nearest to the transplanted duodenal papilla. This effect of relocating the duodenal papilla into the ileum was noted even in a "blind" or isolated loop of ileum not in continuity with the nutrient stream suggesting that pancreatico-biliary secretions stimulated by ingested nutrients were responsible for the increase in villus size. Similar studies transplating only the bile duct into the ileum revealed much less of an increase in villus size (1, 2) suggesting that pancreatic secretions or the combination of pancreatic secretions and bile were the potent factor(s) for villus growth. More recent studies in rats have confirmed that pancreatico-biliary diversion into the ileum produces ileal mucosal hyperplasia in rats orally fed chow and defined formula diets as well (21, 36–38). Male Sprague-Dawley rats were divided into four experimental groups: sham operation for duodenal papilla transplant, duodenal papilla transplant into the ileum, sham operation for bile duct transplant, and transplantation of bile duct into the ileum. After 28 days comparable segments of the small bowel were examined for mucosal mass (two jejunal segments, and four ileal segments). As shown in Fig. 10, transplating the duodenal papilla into the ileum resulted in significant mucosal growth in ileal segments adjacent to the site of transplant compared with the sham controls. Also note there was significant growth of mucosa in the most proximal jejunal segment remote from the site of transplant. Transplantation of the bile duct into the ileum also resulted in significant mucosal growth in ileal segments adjacent to the site of bile entry (Fig. 11) but not as great as combined pancreatico-biliary diversion. No change in mucosa was noted in the remote proximal jejunal segment.

These results indicate that pancreatico-biliary diversion not only stimulates adaptive mucosal hyperplasia in the pancreatico-biliary secretion enriched ileum, but also in the jejunum deprived of these secretions. It has been shown that the

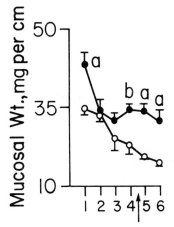

Fig. 10. Effect of duodenal papilla transplant into ileum on small bowel mucosa. Each value represents Mean ± SEM of five rats. Duodenal papilla transplant (●); Sham (○). Arrow indicates site of transplant. Significance: a, p < 0.01; b, p < 0.05. Adapted from Weser, E., Drummond, A., and Tawil, T. Effect of diverting bile and pancreatic secretions into the ileum on small bowel mucosa in rats fed a liquid formula diet. Journal of Parenteral and Enteral Nutrition. 1981. (In Press).

absence of these secretions from the jejunum can prevent the hypoplasia typically seen in rats maintained on TPN (21). Other authors have reported no change in jejunal mucosa after diverting

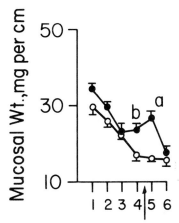

Fig. 11, Effect of bile duct transplant into ileum on small bowel mucosa. Each value represents Mean ± SEM of five rats. Bile duct transplant, (●); Sham (○). Arrow indicates site of transplant. Significance: a, p < 0.001; b, p < 0.02. Adapted from Weser, E., Drummond, A., and Tawil, T. Effect of diverting bile and pancreatic secretions into the ileum on small bowel mucosa in rats fed a liquid formula diet. Journal of Parenteral and Enteral Nutrition, 1981, (In Press).

pancreatico-biliary secretions into remnant ileum following proximal bowel resection (14), even though ileal hyperplasia was enhanced by pancreatico-biliary diversion. In these studies, neither bile alone nor pancreatic secretion alone influenced ileal adaptation, only the combination enhanced mucosal growth. Absence of bile from the duodenum (and presence of pancreatic juice) caused hypoplasia of the duodenojejunal mucosa. Despite these somewhat different observations, all results indicate that duodenojejunal mucosa has greater mass when combined pancreatico-biliary secretions are diverted from proximal intestine into ileum compared to bile diversion alone. These findings suggest that bile and pancreatic secretions have different influences on mucosal growth in jejunum and ileum. It is possible that secretions from the stomach or duodenum selectively contribute to proximal mucosal growth (3).

It is not yet clear by what mechanisms pancreatico-biliary diversion into ileum may stimulate local ileal mucosal growth. A direct nutritive stimulating effect of these secretions on ileal mucosa is possible. Infusion of hog pancreatic extract or commercial pancreatin into ileum for 5–12 days caused greater ileal mucosal hyperplasia than infusion of an amino acid mixture (2), suggesting that nutritive amino acids derived from pancreatic extracts only partially contributed to the mucosal growth. Pancreatic secretions may have specific trophic factors leading to mucosal growth. Other studies on bile have suggested that its absence from the small bowel lumen may decrease cell renewal in the ileum, but not affect proximal jejunum (12, 24). Infusion of fresh hog bile into ileum however was not observed to cause mucosal hyperplasia (2). Other studies have reported that bile acids in the intestinal lumen stimulate epithelia cell generation time (13, 24). Further studies of chronic pancreatico-biliary diversion on cell replication, epithelial turnover, and mucosal metabolism in different regions of small intestine may better define the role of these secretions in mucosal growth regulation.

*Neurovascular Regulation of Adaptation*

There still is little information on whether altered blood flow to a bowel segment plays a primary role in adaptive hyperplasia. After mid-gut resection, circulation to the ileum increases after 2 days, but returns to normal after 2 months (31). Adrenergic denervation of remnant small bowel was reported to cause a transient decrease in blood flow (32). Although epinephrine inhibits mucosal mitosis, beta-adrenergic blockade can reverse this effect (34). Cellular proliferation has been inhibited by sympathectomy (8, 34), and cholinergic drugs may stimulate epithelial cell division (33). Abdominal vagotomy has produced intestinal hypoplasia with subsequent stimulation of cell turnover (4, 19, 25). These observations suggest that vascular and neural responses of the intestinal tract are related, but their role in relation to other factors involved in intestinal adaptation is unclear.

## III. CONCLUDING REMARKS

Non-hormonal regulation of intestinal adaptation is well supported by experimental evidence. It seems clear that simple sugars and some amino acids present in the lumen of the small intestine stimulate mucosal growth locally where they come in direct contact with the mucosa. It has been suggested that this stimulation does not require active absorption or metabolism of the substrate by the mucosa. In the case of sugars, if absorption is impeded locally, the distribution of sugar-stimulated mucosal growth can be shifted downstream in the small intestine. When sugars and some amino acids come in contact with distal small bowel mucosa, they cause remote mucosal growth in the proximal intestine by mechanisms which may be mediated via humoral substances. Whether pancreatico-biliary secretions or other secreted substances are important in this phenomenon awaits further study.

It is also clear that diverting combined pancreatico-biliary secretions into distal small bowel produces local mucosal growth in the distal intestine. This may be particularly important in ileal adaptation after jejunal resection. Absence of these secretions from the duodeno-jejunum may also influence growth in this region, although the magnitude of this phenomenon is still not clear. The regional differences in adaptation to pancreatico-biliary secretions, as well as to local infusion of some amino acids suggest that regulation of mucosal growth is different between proximal and distal small bowel. The relative effects of non-hormonal, hormonal, and neuro-vascular stimuli to overall intestinal adaptation under various conditions (TPN, bowel resection, bowel bypass, and pancreatico-biliary fistulae) remain to be determined.

## ACKNOWLEDGEMENTS

This work was supported in part by the Research Service of the Veterans Administration and the Morrison Trust of San Antonio (K GAHI 30 024 480). The authors wish to express their appreciation to Jill Traylor and Karen Falksen for the technical assistance, and to Wanda Shaw for typing the manuscript.

## REFERENCES

1. Altmann GC. Am J Anat 1971, 132, 167–178
2. Altmann GC. pp 75–86 in Dowling RH, Riecken EO. (ed). Intestinal Adaptation. Schattauer Verlag, Stuttgart and New York, 1974
3. Altmann GC, Leblond CP. Am J Anat 1970, 127, 15–30
4. Ballinger WF II, Iida J, Aponte GE, Wirts W, Goldstein F. Surg Gynecol Obstet 1964, 118, 1305–1311
5. Barry RJC, Eggenton J, Smyth DH. J Physiol 1969, 204, 299–310
6. Buts J, Morin CL, Ling V. Clin Invest Med. 1979, 2, 59–66
7. Dowling RH, Feldman EJ, McNaughton J, Peters TJ. Digestion 1974, 10, 216–217
8. Dupont JR, Biggers DC, Sprinz H. Arch Pathol 1965, 80, 357–362
9. Eastwood GL. Surgery 1977, 82, 613–620
10. Feldman EJ, Dowling RH, McNaughton J, Peters TJ. Gastroenterology 1976, 70, 712–719
11. Fenyo G, Hallberg D, Soda M, Roos KA. Scand J Gastroenterol 1976, 11, 635–640
12. Fry RJM, Kisieleski WE, Kraft B, Staffeldt E, Sullivan MF. pp 142–147 in Sullivan, MF (ed). Gastrointestinal Radiation Injury Excerpta Medica, Amsterdam, 1968
13. Fry RJM, Staffeldt E. Nature 1964, 203, 1396–1398.
14. Gelinas MD, Morin CL. Can J Physiol Pharmacol 1980, 58, 1117–1123
15. Johnson LR, Copeland EM, Dudrick SJ, Lichtenberger LM, Castro GA. Gastroenterology 1975, 68, 1177–1183
16. Kameda H, Abei T, Nasrallah S, Iber F. Am J Physiol 1968, 214, 1090–1095
17. Levine GM, Deren JJ, Steiger E, Zinno R. Gastroenterology 1974, 67, 975–982
18. Levine GM, Deren JJ, Yezdimir E. Am J Dig Dis 1976, 21, 441–445
19. Liavag I, Vaage S. Scand J Gastroent. 1972, 7, 23–27
20. Menge H, Werner H, Lorenz-Meyer, Riecken EO. Gut 1975, 16, 462–467
21. Miazza BM, Levan H, Vaja S, Dowling RH. in Intestinal Adaptation 2. MTP Press, Lancaster, England, 1982, In Press
22. Morin CL, Grey VL. in Intestinal Adaptation 2. MTP Press, Lancaster, England, 1982, In Press
23. Morin CL, Ling V, Bourassa D. Dig Dis Sci 1980, 25, 123–128
24. Roy CC, Laurendeau G, Doyon G, Chartrand L, Rivest MR. Proc Soc Exp Biol Med 1975, 149, 1000–1004
25. Silen W, Peloso O, Jaffe RF. Surgery 1966, 60, 127–135
26. Spector MH, Levine GM, Deren JJ. Gastroenterology 1977, 72, 706–710
27. Spector MH, Traylor J, Young EA, Weser E. Digestion 1981, 21, 33–40
28. Steiger E, Vars HM, Dudrick SJ. Arch Surg 1972, 104, 330–332
29. Teichberg S, Lifshitz F, Pergolizzi R, Wapiur RA Pediat Res 1978, 12, 720–725
30. Terpstra OT, Peterson-Dahl E, Shellito PC, Malt, RA. Arch Surg 1981, 116, 800–802
31. Touloukiain RJ, Spencer RP. Ann Surg 1972, 175, 320–325
32. Touloukiain RJ, Aghajanian GK, Rothe RH. Ann Surg 1972, 176, 633–637
33. Tutton PJM. Med Biol 1977, 55, 201–208
34. Tutton PJM, Heline RD. Cell Tissue Kinet 1974, 7, 125–136
35. Weser E, Tawil T, Fletcher JT. in Intestinal Adaptation 2. MTP Press, Lancaster, England, 1982, In Press
36. Weser E, Drummond A, Tawil T. J Paren Ent Nutr 1982, In Press
37. Weser E, Heller R, Tawil T. Gastroenterology 1977, 73, 524–529
38. Williamson RC, Bauer FLR, Ross JS, Watkins JB, Malt RA. Gastroenterology 1979, 70, 1386–1392
39. Wilson TH, Landau BR. Am J Physiol 1960, 198, 99–102
40. Young EA, Cioletti LA, Winborn WB, Traylor JB, Weser E. Am J Clin Nutr 1980, 33, 2106–2118

# Adaptive Cell-proliferative Changes in the Small-intestinal Mucosa in Coeliac Disease

A. J. WATSON[1], D. R. APPLETON[2] & N. A. WRIGHT[3]
Departments of Pathology[1] and Medical Statistics[2], University of Newcastle upon Tyne
and Department of Histopathology[3], Royal Postgraduate Medical School, London, England.

Cell proliferation in the small-intestinal crypts of rodents has been intensively investigated and lends itself to the deployment of techniques which are inapplicable in man. In particular there are ethical and economic objections to methods involving the use of tritiated thymidine in vivo for specific labelling of DNA, while the validity of in vitro studies using organ culture is uncertain. It is possible, nevertheless to construct a profile of the size and cytokinetic status of the mucosal crypts by analysis of serial sections prepared from well orientated routine diagnostic biopsy specimens. Such studies can provide a measure of mean total crypt-cell population, and by studying the distribution of mitoses in the crypts relative measurements can be obtained of proliferation and maturation compartment sizes, and of crypt cell production rate (CCPR). These parameters have been compared in 62 patients with 'flat' avillous coeliac mucosae and in 85 patients with normal villous mucosae. A heterogeneous group of 47 patients with lesser degrees of abnormality (convoluted mucosae) were similarly studied. In addition, estimates of cell cycle times were obtained in a small group of patients with normal, convoluted and 'flat' mucosae by taking biopsies before and after the administration of the metaphase-arresting agent vincristine. 'Flat' coeliac mucosae show a threefold increase in the size of the proliferation compartment compared with normal and the cell cycle time is approximately halved leading to a net sixfold increase in CCPR. This is the basis of the change in mucosal morphology and presumably represents a compensatory reaction to the gluten-induced increase in loss of enterocytes from the mucosal surface. Convoluted mucosae occupy an intermediate position in terms of the parameters studied and should be regarded as stages in a continuum of adaptive change.

*Dr. A. J. Watson, University Department of Pathology, Royal Victoria Infirmary, Newcastle upon Tyne, NE1 4LP, U.K.*

## INTRODUCTION

Coeliac disease was first recognised as a clinical entity defined in terms of its symptoms and signs, with emphasis on evidence of malabsorption and in particular of steatorrhoea. In common with many other syndromes its characterisation as a specific nosological entity could be achieved only when a specific aetiological agent was identified (19). It is now well established that the condition of overt coeliac disease occurs in susceptible individuals whose diet includes products prepared from the grain of wheat, rye, barley and oats. The starch fraction of the flour from these grains is innocuous, but the heterogeneous alcohol-soluble component (gliadin) of the protein fraction (gluten) was soon shown to be capable of inducing the condition (20) and this harmful property was still present in a water-soluble peptide fraction produced by peptic-tryptic digestion of wheat gliadin (26). However, it has not yet proved possible to identify the responsible factor precisely, at molecular level, despite intensive investigation. The first reliable demonstration of the morphological changes in the small-intestinal mucosa in untreated coeliac disease was based on the examination of specimens obtained fortuitously at laparotomy (39). Subsequently the development of peroral suction-biopsy techniques (18, 25, 44, 50) allowed the characteristic histopathological features to be fully documented (1, 21, 47, 60) together with the sequence of changes by which normal morphology is restored during successful treatment, and the mode of reversion when treatment is discontinued (49). Additional important information has also been derived from the application of techniques such as stereomicroscopic examination with the dissecting microscope (27, 45) and the more sophisticated scanning electron microscope (3, 35, 36). The nature of the cellular and subcellular changes affecting the enterocytes, i.e. the monolayer of closely packed columnar epithelial cells which normally cover the villi, and whose residual population of shortened, pseudostratified cells cover the surface of the avillous coeliac mucosa, have been intensively studied by enzyme histochemistry (43, 54), by transmission electron microscopy (48, 51) and by analytical subcellular fractionation techniques (41).

The first hypothesis propounded to explain the pathogenesis of coeliac disease in terms of gluten sensitivity stipulated the constitutional absence of some specific enzyme, possibly a peptidase, normally present within the surface epithelium. Short-term organ-culture studies appeared to indicate that gluten or gliadin digests had no direct deleterious effect on treated coeliac mucosa in vitro (22, 29). Recently, however, it has been reported that gluten-sensitivity can be demonstrated during organ culture not only in untreated, but also in treated coeliac mucosa by actual quantitative assessment of changes in enterocyte height (28). Peters, Jones & Wells (41) found a persistent defect in brush-border enzyme activities in morphologically normal coeliac mucosa after prolonged gluten withdrawal; this defective activity was particularly marked for beta-glucosidase. The concept of a primary enzyme deficiency cannot yet be regarded as entirely abandoned.

The weight of current opinion tends to favour the major alternative explanation which postulates that the harmful effects of gluten are mediated by immunological mechanisms (38). Of course these two hypotheses are not necessarily mutually exclusive, and if there is an inherited abnormality in the coeliac enterocyte it may be concerned with surface receptors (38) rather than enzymes. Although the role of these mechanisms is not fully understood, and it is probable that local humoral activity is not central to the pathogenesis (37) there are indications that local cell-mediated immune reactions to gluten may be involved (8, 23, 24, 32). Marsh's report (37) that a high mitotic index in the population of intra-epithelial lymphocytes in untreated coeliac disease is specifically indicative of a state of gluten-sensitive enteropathy is of great theoretical interest and is likely to be of practical importance.

The difficulties in achieving an acceptable definition of coeliac disease have been pithily expressed by Creamer (16), but we suggest for most practical purposes that it be regarded as a malabsorptive condition resulting from a probably permanent state of intolerance to dietary gluten associated with a flat avillous duodeno-jejunal mucosa on stereomicroscopy, usually with a mosaic pattern, and with characteristic histological changes, in particular, total villous atrophy, crypt hyperplasia and a marked infiltration of the lamina propria by plasma cells and macrophages. Strict adherence to a gluten-free diet is followed in some 85% of cases by clinical and morphological improvement, but there is a liability to relapse following reintroduction of gluten. If the finding of mitoses amongst intraepithelial lymphocytes is as diagnostically discriminatory as Marsh (37) asserts, this will help to overcome the difficulty presented by the occasional finding of a 'flat' pseudocoeliac mucosa in a variety of unrelated conditions; it will also obviate the need for second and third biopsies to check response to treatment and reversion of the improvement on gluten challenge.

It is the purpose of this paper to present an integrated account of the proliferative status of the crypt-cell population in the 'flat' avillous small-intestinal mucosa of untreated coeliac disease and to attempt to correlate this with the altered morphology of the crypts and villi. A comparison will be drawn with the findings in a series of morphologically normal mucosae and it will also be established that mucosae with intermediate morphological abnormalities probably represent stages in a continuum of increasingly pronounced cytokinetic adjustments. This present account incorporates results published elsewhere (58, 60, 61, 64, 65, 66, 67, 68). Despite the necessary limitations related to ethical and technical considerations we believed that it was necessary to carry out a direct study of human material; this has been conducted mainly by analysis of routine diagnostic biopsies with the exception of a few instances in which a stathmokinetic technique was applied in a small group of fully informed volunteers.

## MATERIALS AND METHODS

### Patients

In most instances a single biopsy sample of proximal small-intestinal mucosa was obtained by the peroral route, primarily for diagnostic purposes, usually to confirm or to exclude a provisional diagnosis of coeliac disease. Other mucosal biopsies were obtained from patients, with psoriasis (52) or other dermatoses, in whom the presence of dermatogenic enteropathy was being investigated (33). During the course of such studies the association between dermatitis herpetiformis (DH) and coeliac disease was discovered (34, 53, 59); in this association the coeliac condition is usually clinically latent.

A total of 62 patients had a 'flat' coeliac-type mucosa; this group comprised 13 adults and 29 children with untreated coeliac disease and 20 adults with dermatitis herpetiformis. Morphologically normal biopsy specimens were obtained

from 85 patients (75 adults and 10 children) and these mucosal samples constituted our control series. A further series of 47 biopsy specimens, designated 'convoluted' mucosae for reference purposes, showed an intermediate range of abnormalities (Table I). The patients from whom these mucosal samples were obtained constituted a heterogeneous group in term of clinical diagnosis, but it is noteworthy that 15 had DH and 2 were first degree relatives of DH patients. Six were coeliac patients in various stages of remission or relapse, and 4 were suffering from giardiasis.

### Methods

Peroral biopsy specimens were taken under radiological control from the vicinity of the duodeno-jejunal junction using a modified Crosby suction-biopsy capsule. The capsule was immediately withdrawn and the specimen retrieved without delay; it was then orientated under a dissecting microscope and gently spread, mucosal surface upwards, on to a thin piece of glass. Primary fixation was 10% neutral buffered formol saline and detailed stereomicroscopic examination was postponed for at least 24 hours, when obscuring mucus and debris could be removed by gentle brushing without risk of damage. In order to improve the quality of fixation and to give better nuclear staining, the specimen

Table I. Synopsis of changes which characterise convoluted mucosae assigned to each of three arbitrarily defined groups.

| Group | Stereomicroscopy | Histology |
|-------|------------------|-----------|
| 1 | Not more than a few convolutions, distributed amongst leaves and ridges, and occupying less than 10% of mucosal surface | No notable abnormality |
| 2 | From 10 to 70% of mucosal surface occupied by convolutions | Some shortening of villi evident on inspection; little or no apparent lengthening of crypts; surface epithelium normal; density of inflammatory cell infiltration normal or just perceptibly increased |
| 3 | Mucosal surface completely or predominantly (over 70%) convoluted | Short stubby villi; crypts obviously lengthened; surface epithelium abnormal; obvious increase in density of inflammatory cell infiltration |

was post-fixed in a 5% solution of mercuric chloride in formol saline; it was then processed for embedding in vertical orientation in paraffin wax. Approximately 200 serial sections, cut at a thickness of 3 μm and stained by Harris's haematoxylin, were used for the purpose of crypt analysis (see below). For immediate diagnostic assessment several sections were stained by haematoxylin and eosin and by the periodic-acid Schiff method after amylase digestion; 'flat' coeliac mucosae were also routinely stained by the haematoxylin-van Gieson and by the picro-Mallory methods to detect collagenisation of the lamina propria.

## Morphological classification

The biopsy specimens were assigned to one of three main categories on the basis of their morphological appearances as seen by stereomicroscopic examination under the dissecting microscope and by conventional light microscopy of histological sections. Although the use of stereomicroscopy has been decried (31, 40, 46) it

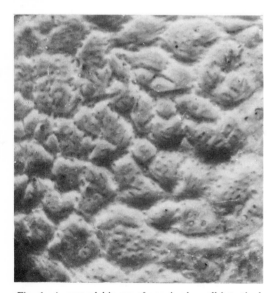

Fig. 1. A peroral biopsy of proximal small-intestinal mucosa from a patient with untreated coeliac disease. The 'flat' avillous mucosal surface shows a characteristic mosaic pattern. Some of the hyperplastic crypts open directly on to the surface, but it is more usual for several crypts to open into short communal vestibules whose orifices are dispersed over the surface. (× 12) (From Watson et al., 58).

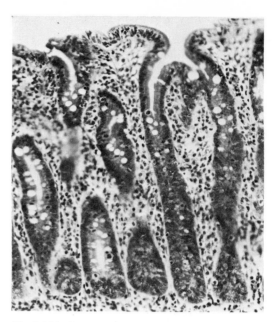

Fig. 2. This shows the characteristic histological findings in an untreated coeliac mucosa. There is total villous atrophy whereas the crypts are hyperplastic; two crypts are seen opening into a shared vestibule; dividing crypt cells are plentiful and occur to a high level in the crypts, the lamina propria shows a heavy infiltration of chronic inflammatory cells; there are numerous lymphocytes in the surface epithelium which also shows nuclear pseudostratification. (Haematoxylin and eosin × 150) (From Watson et al., 58).

remains a valuable adjunct to histological examination and should not be neglected.

*'Flat', avillous, coeliac-type mucosae.* A characteristic stereomicroscopic appearance is seen (Fig. 1) of which the most significant feature is the complete absence of any projecting structures which could conceivably merit the term villi. The adjective 'flat' is somewhat inappropriate, but is in general use and its connotation is unambiguous. The corresponding histological features are equally characteristic (Fig. 2).

*Normal mucosae.* These specimens showed a normal villous appearance on stereomicroscopy and conformed to the conventional appearance of normality on histological examination. In adults especially it is relatively unusual to find mucosa from the region sampled showing exclusively a population of tall finger-shaped villi; narrow or broad leaf-shaped forms were accepted as normal, and the presence of curved or angular leaves, of joined leaves, of straight or sinuous ridges amonst the more regular leafy villi did not exclude specimens from this category. But specimens showing convolutions were invariably excluded.

*Convoluted mucosae.* Specimens in this category are most easily and reliably identified when the various forms of villous structure described above have been wholly replaced by a complex of intertwining flexuous ridged formations (Fig. 3) reminiscent of the cerebral convolutions; the height of the convolutions often appears comparable to that of normal villi. For our purposes we have included all mucosae with convolutions in this category irrespective of the prevalence of these forms and it is clear, therefore, that this is a heterogeneous group. It is heterogeneous also in respect of the histological appearances which range from normality through varying degrees of villous atrophy, crypt hyperplasia, with inflammatory and other changes eventually approaching in severity those of untreated coeliac disease. Indeed, markedly atrophic forms of convolutions are occasionally seen which are more appropriately regarded as variants of 'flat' mucosae. Consequently we have divided the convoluted mucosae into three subgroups on the basis of increasing severity of morphological abnormality according to arbitrary criteria (Table I). In those instances where there was disparity between the extent of the convoluted state and the degree of accompanying histological abnormality, the specimen was assigned to its subgroup on the basis of the more marked alteration.

### Methods of analysis

In all of the morphological categories the aim was to analyse thirty separate crypts, each of which had been sectioned in its longitudinal axis so as to include the base, middle and mouth in the plane of the histological section. Crypt length was measured in terms of cell units by enumerating the 'left-hand' column of cells from the bottom to the mouth of the crypt as seen in section. In villous mucosae the mouth corresponds approximately to the plane of the crypt villous junction, whereas in avillous coeliac mucosae the mouth is represented by the apparent

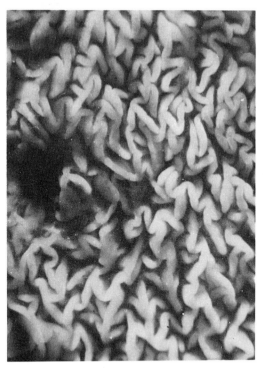

Fig. 3. A peroral biopsy of proximal small-intestinal mucosa as viewed through one eyepiece of a dissecting microscope; after fixation the epithelium is no longer transparent. Villi have been replaced by so-called convolutions and this specimen would be assigned to group 3. ($\times$ 12) (From Watson, Wright & Appleton, 58).

junction of the crypt with the surface epithelium (Fig. 2). Within the crypt column the positions of all cells with mitotic nuclei were recorded and, by pooling the data for all crypts examined in any group of mucosae, the distribution of the mitotic index ($I_m$) values at each cell position, in a crypt with a length equal to the mean for the appropriate group, was determined (9, 63).

A useful description of the extent of cell proliferation up the length of the crypt is the so-called cut-off position (10, 11, 55) at which cells in effect receive a signal to complete the present cycle, but not to enter a further cycle. We have described elsewhere (2) how this can be found from the results of stathmokinetic experiments provided an estimate of the cell cycle time is available. As this requires determination of the frequency of labelled mitoses (FLM) following injections of tritiated thymidine we have been unable to ascertain the cut-off position in our human material. Instead, we have derived from the mitotic index distribution curves, estimates of the cell position at which $I_m$ falls to 50% of its maximum value (13); we term this the half-maximum position (HMP). In the hypothetical situation in which all cells below this position were proliferating with a cell cycle time of equal duration then the cut-off position would be half this distance from the bottom of the crypt.

### Stathmokinetic study

Five patients participated in this study having given their informed consent after receiving a full explanation of the procedure involved. The project was also approved by the Ethical Committee of the Newcastle University Hospital Group. Two procedures were used to permit measurement of the crypt-cell birth rate ($k_B$) after inducing stathmokinesis by rapid intravenous infusion of vincristine sulphate in a dosage of 0.045 mg per kg body weight.

Three patients underwent a two-biopsy procedure. On day 1 a peroral biopsy of proximal small-intestinal mucosa was taken from the region of the duodeno-jejunal junction at 13:30h, using a modified Crosby capsule whose position was monitored radiologically. On day 2 a second biopsy was obtained from the same position at the same time of day, exactly 2.5h after the vincristine infusion. The birth rate for the whole crypt was estimated from the equation

$$k_B = \frac{I_m\,(day\,2) - I_m\,(day\,1)}{2.5}$$

and a value for the crypt-cell production rate (CCPR) was obtained from the sum of the birth rates at each cell position in a single crypt column multiplied by the total number of columns in the crypt i.e. the column count.

*Patient AA* was a man aged 61 with a history of rosacea and varicose ulcers of the legs. Both biopsy specimens showed finger-shaped and narrow leaf-shaped villi and appeared histologically normal.

*Patient BB* was a man aged 25 suffering from dermatitis herpetiformis; he presented no clinical or biochemical evidence of malabsorption. Both

biopsy specimens showed a completely convoluted surface associated with histological changes of group 3 severity.

*Patient CC* was a man aged 37 with a history of DH for ten or more years, who had recently developed a megaloblastic anaemia due to folic acid deficiency: his skin condition was controlled by Dapsone and he was taking a normal diet. His biopsy specimens both showed a 'flat' avillous appearance with histological changes indistinguishable from those of untreated coeliac disease.

Another two patients were studied by a multiple biopsy procedure using a Quinton multiple biopsy machine. The biopsy capsule was passed to the region of the duodeno-jejunal junction as before and a sample of mucosa retrieved; after intravenous infusion of vincristine further specimens of mucosa were retrieved at approximately 15 minute intervals over a period of about 2 h in one instance and 2.5 h in the other. The cell birth rate for the whole crypt was estimated from the slope of a straight line fitted to the mitotic accumulation data; as before the CCPR was obtained from consideration of the cumulative birth rates at each cell position.

*Patient DD* was a man aged 61 who was being investigated to ascertain the cause of his chronic diarrhoea. Eleven biopsies, obtained over a period of 150 minutes, were considered to be morphologically normal.

*Patient EE* was a woman aged 55 in whom a provisional clinical diagnosis of coeliac disease had been made. Nine biopsies, obtained over 105 minutes, showed a 'flat' avillous appearance and characteristic histological changes of untreated coeliac disease.

The handling, fixation, processing and sectioning of all these specimens was exactly as described above for single biopsies; crypt analysis was also essentially similar but even more meticulous in that at least 3000 crypt-cell nuclei were counted for each biopsy specimen.

## RESULTS

### Morphometric variables

The mean values for crypt length and column count in the eight groups of patients studied are

Table II. Cell population data for crypts in different clinical/morphological groups. ACD = adult coeliac disease; CCD = childhood coeliac disease; DH = dermatitis herpetiformis. All figures are for cells

| Mucosa | Patients | Crypt length | Column count | Total cells | Proliferation zone | Maturation zone |
|--------|----------|--------------|--------------|-------------|-------------------|-----------------|
| Normal | Adults (75) | 32 | 25 | 800 | 550 | 250 |
|        | Children (10) | 34 | 25 | 850 | 600 | 250 |
| Convoluted: |  |  |  |  |  |  |
| group 1 (15) |  | 37 | 26 | 950 | 750 | 200 |
| group 2 (18) |  | 39 | 27 | 1050 | 750 | 300 |
| group 3 (14) |  | 49 | 31 | 1550 | 1150 | 350 |
| 'Flat' avillous | ACD (13) | 74 | 41 | 3050 | 1700 | 1350 |
|        | CCD (29) | 75 | 35 | 2650 | 1550 | 1100 |
|        | DH (20) | 76 | 36 | 2700 | 1650 | 1050 |

shown in Table II together with estimates of the total crypt-cell population obtained from the product of these two measurements. The most marked contrast in the values both for crypt length and column count is between the normal controls and the groups with flat mucosae; all of the latter have crypt length values which are more than double those of the controls, and all include crypts more than 100 cells long. Column counts are greatly increased in the coeliac-type groups, but especially in adult coeliacs. The estimates of total crypt-cell population show a threefold or greater increase compared with controls.

All three groups with convoluted mucosae have an increased mean crypt length, though the increase is greatest in group 3 as might be anticipated from the definition of these groups (Table I). In group 3 the column count is also clearly increased and consequently the total crypt-cell population is double that of the controls.

The location of the half maximum position (HMP) can be identified from the mitotic index distributions (Fig. 4) and we refer to the total population of cells below this position as occupying the 'proliferation zone' although it is possible that some of the cells in this zone are not in cycle. The zone above the HMP is termed the 'maturation zone'. The sizes of these populations in the different groups are shown in Table II. In the convoluted mucosae the proliferation zone increases in size in absolute terms and also appears to be slightly increased as a proportion of the whole population. The flat mucosae show an even greater increase in the proliferation zone

Table III. Observed number of mitoses per crypt column and estimated crypt cell production rate (CCPR) in the different clinical/morphological groups. Abbreviations as in Table II

| Mucosa | Patients | Mitoses per column | CCPR (cells/crypt/h) |
|--------|----------|--------------------|----------------------|
| Normal | Adults (75) | 1.0 | 17 |
|        | Children (10) | 1.2 | 21 |
| Convoluted: |  |  |  |
| group 1 (15) |  | 1.3 | 23 |
| group 2 (18) |  | 1.5 | 28 |
| group 3 (14) |  | 2.7 | 59 |
| 'Flat' avillous | ACD (13) | 3.9 | 110 |
|        | CCD (29) | 3.4 | 84 |
|        | DH (20) | 4.1 | 105 |

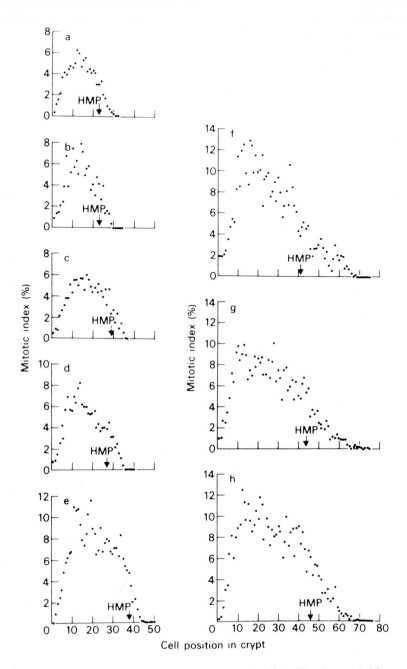

Fig. 4. Mitotic index distributions in (a) adult controls, (b) childhood controls (c) group-1 convoluted, (d) group-2 convoluted, (e) group-3 convoluted, (f) adult coeliac disease, (g) childhood coeliac disease and (h) dermatitis herpetiformis. Mitotic indices (%) are indicated on the vertical axes and cell position in the crypt on the horizontal axes. Half-maximum positions (HMP) are shown. (From Watson et al., 58).

Table IV. Data relating to three patients studied by the two-biopsy stathmokinetic technique. The mitotic index has been corrected for the size of the proliferation zone; $k_B$ = birth rate at top of crypt; CCPR = crypt cell production rate

| Patient | Category | Crypt cell population | Corrected mitotic index (%) | | Birth rate ($k_B$) (cells/1000 cells/h) | CCPR (cells/crypt)h) |
|---|---|---|---|---|---|---|
| | | | Day 1 | Day 2 | | |
| AA | Adult control | 700 | 1.7 | 5.4 | 15 | 11 |
| BB | Group 3 convoluted | 1450 | 3.2 | 9.6 | 26 | 38 |
| CC | Dermatitis herpetiformis | 2050 | 3.6 | 10.4 | 27 | 55 |

in terms of cell numbers, but the size of the increase is exceeded in the maturation zone which has some five times more cells than in the controls.

Provided certain assumptions are made it is possible to estimate the crypt-cell production rates from the $I_m$ data. Table III shows the mean numbers of mitoses observed per crypt column; if the duration of mitosis is taken as 1 h, then these are also the numbers of cells produced by a column every hour and multiplication by the column counts will give values for the CCPR. Because mitotic nuclei are found nearer the central axis of the crypt than intermitotic nuclei Tannock (56) pointed out that they tend to be over-represented in longitudianl sections and that this leads to an overestimate of the mitotic index. It is necessary to apply a correction factor which can be derived from the ratio of the mean radial displacement of mitotic nuclei from the central axis, to the corresponding mean distance for intermitotic nuclei. We derived a correction factor of 0.7, applicable both to normal and to abnormal mucosae, by appropriate measurements in histological cross-sections of the mucosal samples of

patients taking part in the stathmokinetic studies. The estimates of CCPR entered in Table III have been reduced by this factor; it can readily be seen that any inaccuracies in the estimate of mitotic duration or failure to apply Tannock's correction factor will be reflected in a similar loss of accuracy in estimating CCPR.

*Stathmokinetic observations*

The mitotic indices, corrected by multiplying by 0.7 as explained above, for the patients subjected to the two-biopsy procedure are shown in Table IV along with the cell birth rates and the CCPRs derived from them.

The results of the multiple biopsy stathmokinetic technique on the two patients DD and EE are illustrated in Figure 5 and Table V shows the calculated birth rates together with estimates of CCPR obtained from the population sizes for the appropriate groups as given in Table II.

The estimates of CCPR in the five stathmokinetic investigations all show the same general pattern of variation between the different morphological types of mucosa as do the estimates

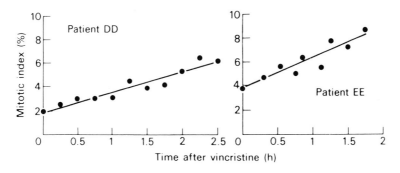

Fig. 5. Stathmokinetic data from patients DD and EE. (From Watson et al., 58).

Table V. Data relating to two patients studied by the multiple biopsy stathmokinetic technique. Crypt cell production rate is estimated from cell populations of corresponding categories in Table II

| Patient | Category | Birth rate (cells/1000 cells/h) | CCPR (cells/crypt/h) |
|---------|----------|--------------------------------|----------------------|
| DD | Adult control | 17 | 14 |
| EE | Adult coeliac | 25 | 76 |

in Table III although the stathmokinetic results are all slightly lower than would be expected. Amongst the reasons which might account for this are failure of vincristine to arrest all cells in metaphase, degeneration of arrested metaphases, and normal variability within or between individuals. On the other hand it is likely that the values found by simple enumeration of mitoses are too high because the mitotic duration has been underestimated.

## DISCUSSION

### Normal versus coeliac crypts

*Morphometric parameters.* Simple inspection of well orientated histological sections suffices to show that coeliac crypts are longer than normal crypts, but is less apparent that they are also increased in girth. If we compare the arithmetic means of the measurements for the two control groups and for the three coeliac groups respectively then we find that the mean crypt length is increased by a factor of 2.3 from 33 cells in the controls to 75 cells in the coeliacs. Similarly the mean column count is increased by a factor of 1.5 from 25 cells to 37 cells. The product of these two parameters gives a reliable estimate of the total crypt cell population (62) (Table II), and if the mean values are compared we see that the total cell population in coeliac crypts is 3.4 times greater than in control crypts. The proliferation zone and the maturation zone both show an absolute increase in cell numbers, but the increase in size of the maturation zone is disproportionately greater than the increase in size of the whole crypt.

*Proliferative parameters.* Despite the total atrophy and disappearance of villi from the proximal small-intestinal mucosa in untreated coeliac disease it is quite inappropriate to refer to the general state of the mucsoa as one of atrophy; indeed the crypts are both hyperplastic and hyperproliferative. The assumption that this state constitutes a response to an abnormally high rate of cell loss, from the surface of the mucosa into the lumen of the the bowel, was confirmed and quantified by Creamer and his colleagues (17, 42). They assessed the rate of cell loss by measuring the DNA content of the washings from perfused segments of small bowel and concluded that patients with untreated coeliac disease showed a six-fold increase over the normal rate of cell loss. Ordinarily the 'flat' coeliac mucosa must achieve a new state of equilibrium to compensate for this change by a corresponding increase in the rate of cell production from the crypts. From the data in Table III it is evident that the CCPR from coeliac crypts is 5.2 times greater than from normal crypts. If the comparison is restricted to adult controls and adult coeliacs the increase in CCPR is 6.5 times, an estimate which matches closely the estimated increase in the rate of cell loss. These comparisons are valid only if we assume that there is no significant increase in the number of crypts per unit length of small bowel in coeliacs as compared with normals.

The increase in CCPR can be partly accounted for by the near trebling of cell number in the proliferation zone of the crypt, and for the rest by an appproximately 50 per cent reduction in cell cycle time, always assuming that the duration of mitosis remains virtually constant. The results from the stathmokinetic studies are similar though lower (Tables IV and V) and possible explanations for this slight discrepancy have already been mentioned.

## Significance of a convoluted mucosa

The duodeno-jejunal mucosa can assume a 'flat' avillous appearance, with crypts opening directly or through shared vestibular chambers on to the surfaces of a mosaic of low plateaux, in conditions other than coeliac disease (30). Nevertheless, these changes are so characteristic as to be virtually diagnostic of untreated coeliac disease in appropriate clinical circumstances. On the other hand a convoluted appearance is often of unknown significance as an isolated finding even when all other aspects of the case have been taken into account (60, 61, 64). In the context of coeliac disease a convoluted appearance represents an intermediate stage in the recovery or in the development of a 'flat' mucosa. The distal limit of a 'flat' coeliac mucosa may be separated from unaltered villous mucosa by an intermediate convoluted zone. Islands of convoluted mucosa may be found in an otherwise 'flat' coeliac mucosa by multiple sampling. Convolutions may be a feature of various other disorders and the prevalence in apparently healthy subjects differs between different population groups (4, 33, 64).

Our studies of the morphometric and proliferative parameters show that group-3 convoluted mucosae are in a hyperproliferative state intermediate between normal and 'flat' mucosae whereas groups 1 and 2 differ little from normal controls. Our data are consistent with the hypothesis that group-3 convoluted mucosae represent a morphological adaptation to a moderately reduced population of villous enterocytes consequent upon increased cell loss and balanced by an appropriate increase in cell production. If the rate of cell loss should increase further, then preservation of surface integrity would entail loss of convolutions leading to total villous atrophy and further stepping-up of cell production, perhaps to near maximum rates.

## Nature of adaptive responses

In the light of present knowledge we can reasonably discard certain suggestions some of which are now of little more than historical interest. These include mitotic arrest as a cause of the increased mitotic index in coeliac crypts (45); though experimental models based on this con-

cept show villous atrophy they differ from coeliac disease in that this change is accompanied by crypt atrophy (12). The concept of enteroblastic hypoplasia (15) is not in keeping with the characteristically increased mitotic index in flat coeliac mucosae; the patient shown by in vivo tritiated-thymidine studies to have a reduced output of cells from the crypt must be regarded as atypical (14). In theory, maturation arrest or delay might account for a reduction in CCPR, but this explanation can be accommodated only if we also postulate loss or death of cells in the maturation zone; there is no morphological evidence for this occurrence (48). Furthermore, studies of coeliac mucosae maintained in organ culture have convincingly shown an increased labelling index compared to normal when tritiated-thymidine was added to the culture medium, and an increase in the rate of migration from the crypts (57). In terms of an analogy with the haemopoeitic system (5, 6, 7) our studies support the concept of an enteroblastic hyperplasia in the coeliac mucosa comparable to the erythroblastic hyperplasia which occurs in haemolytic anaemia. In the small-intestinal mucosa this response is mediated by a threefold increase in the population of proliferating crypt cells, an increase which entails considerable enlargement of the length and girth of the crypts to accommodate these and the enlarged population of maturing cells. Also contributing to the roughly sixfold increase in the rate of output of cells from the crypts is a reduction in cell cycle time to about half its normal value. Whether these compensatory changes occur synchronously, or to some greater or lesser extent sequentially, and if the latter in what order of sequence, cannot be ascertained from our observations or from those of any currently available, acceptable techniques.

## ACKNOWLEDGEMENTS

The work reported in this paper was supported by a grant from the North of England Council of the Cancer Research Campaign. Figs. 1 to 5 are reproduced in whole or in part from the publication cited as reference (58), and Tables I to V have been adapted from the same source, with the permission of the publishers Pitman Medical. The authors are grateful to Miss E. Wark for secretarial assistance.

## REFERENCES

1. Anderson CM. Arch Dis Child 1960, 35, 419–427
2. Appleton DR, Sunter JP, Watson AJ. Cell Tissue Kinet (In Press)
3. Asquith P, Johnson AG, Cooke WT. Am J Dig Dis 1970, 15, 511–521
4. Baker SJ. Pathol Microbiol (Basel) 1973, 39, 222–237
5. Booth CC. Postgrad Med J 1968, 44, 12–16
6. Booth CC. Br Med J 1970, 3, 725–731
7. Booth CC. Br Med J 1970, 4, 14–17
8. Bullen AW, Losowsky MS. Gut 1978, 19, 126–131
9. Cairnie AB, Bentley RE. Exp Cell Res 1967, 46, 428–440
10. Cairnie AB, Lamerton LF, Steel GG. Exp Cell Res 1965, 39, 528–538
11. Cairnie AB, Lamerton LF, Steel GG. Exp Cell Res 1965, 39, 539–553
12. Clark PA, Harland WA. Br J Exp Path 1963, 44, 520–523
13. Cleaver JE. Thymidine Metabolism and Cell Kinetics. North Holland Publishing Co., Amsterdam, 1967
14. Creamer B. Gut 1962, 3, 295–300
15. Creamer B. Br Med Bull 1967, 23, 226–230
16. Creamer B. pp 91–114 in Creamer B. (ed.), The Small Intestine, William Heinemann Medical Books, London, 1974
17. Creamer B, Croft DN. pp 21–25 in Booth CC, Dowling RH, (eds.), Coeliac Disease, Churchill-Livingstone, 1970
18. Crosby WH, Kugler HW. Am J Dig Dis 1957, 2, 236–241
19. Dicke WK. Coeliakie, een onderzoek naar de nadelige invloed van sommige graansorten op de lijder aan coeliakie 1950, Thesis, Utrecht University. Cited in Lancet 1952, 1, 857–858
20. Dicke WK, Weijers HA, Van de Kamer JH. Acta Paediat 1953, 42, 34–42
21. Doniach I, Shiner M. Gastroenterology 1957, 33, 71–86
22. Falchuk ZM, Gebhard R, Sessons C, Strober W. J Clin Invest 1974, 53, 487–500
23. Ferguson A, Jarrett E. Gut 1975, 16, 114–117
24. Ferguson A, McClure J, MacDonald T, Holden R. Lancet 1975, 1, 895–897
25. Flick AL, Quinton WE, Rubin CE. Gastroenterology 1960 38, 964
26. Frazer AC, Fletcher RF, Shaw B, Ross CAC, Sammons HG, Schneider R. Lancet 1959, 2, 252–255
27. Holmes R, Hourihane DO'B, Booth CC. Lancet 1961, 1, 81–83
28. Howdle PD, Corazza GR, Bullen AW, Losowsky MS. Gastroenterology 1981, 80, 442–450
29. Jos J, Lenoir G, de Ritis G, Rey J. p 91 in Hekkens W, Pena AS. (eds.), Coeliac Disease, Stenfert-Kroese, Leiden, 1974
30. Katz AJ, Grand RJ. Gastroenterology 1973, 76, 375–377
31. Lee FD, Toner PG. Biopsy Pathology of the Small Intestine. Chapman and Hall, London 1980
32. MacDonald TT, Ferguson A. Gut 1976, 17, 81–91
33. Marks JM, Shuster S. Gut 1970, 11, 281–291
34. Marks J, Shuster S, Watson AJ. Lancet 1966, 2, 1280–1282
35. Marsh MN, Brown AC, Swift JA. pp 26–44 in Booth CC, Dowling RH. (eds.), Coeliac Disease, Churchill-Livingstone, London, 1970
36. Marsh MN. pp 81–135 in Badenoch J. Brooke BN. (eds.), Recent Advances in Gastroenterology (2nd ed.), Churchill-Livingstone, London 1972
37. Marsh MN. Scand J Gastroenterol 1981, 16 (70), 87–106
38. Marsh MN. Clin Sci 1981, 61, 497–503
39. Paulley JW. Br Med J 1954, 2, 1318–1321
40. Perera DR, Weinstein WM, Rubin CE. Human Pathol 1975, 6, 157–217
41. Peters TJ, Jones PE, Wells G. Clin Sci Molec Med 1978, 55, 285–292
42. Pink IJ, Croft DN, Creamer B. Gut 1970, 11, 217–222
43. Riecken EO. pp 20–41 in Card WI, Creamer B. (eds.), Modern Trends in Gastroenterology – 4, Butterworths, London, 1970
44. Royer M, Croxatto O, Biempica L, Balcazar Morrison AJ, Prensa Med Argent 1955, 42, 2515–2519
45. Rubin CE, Brandborg LL, Phelps PC, Taylor HC. Gastroenterology 1960, 38, 28–49
46. Rubin CE, Eidelman S, Weinstein WM. Gastroenterology 1970, 58, 409–413
47. Rubin W. Am J Clin Nutr 1971, 24, 91–111
48. Rubin W, Ross LL, Sleisenger MH, Weser E. Lab Invest 1966, 15, 1720–1747
49. Schenk EA, & Samloff IM. Am J Path 1968, 52, 579–593
50. Shiner M. Lancet 1956, 1, 85
51. Shiner M. pp 33–53 in Cooke WT, Asquith P. (eds.), Coeliac Disease. Clinics in Gastroenterology, Saunders, London, 1974
52. Shuster S, Watson AJ, Marks JM. Br Med J 1967, 3, 458–460
53. Shuster S, Watson AJ, Marks J. Lancet 1968, 1, 1101–1106
54. Spiro HM, Filipe MI, Stewart JS, Pearse AGE. Gut 1964, 5, 145–154
55. Steel GG. Growth Kinetics of Tumours. Clarendon Press, Oxford, 1977
56. Tannock IF. Exper Cell Res 1967, 47, 345–356
57. Trier JS, Browning TH. New Engl J Med 1970, 283, 1245–1250
58. Watson AJ, Wright NA, Appleton DR. pp 350–363 in Appleton DR, Sunter JP, Watson AJ. (eds.), Cell Proliferation in the Gastrointestinal Tract, Pitman Medical, Tunbridge Wells, 1980
59. Watson AJ, Shuster S, Marks JM. pp 798–800 in Gregor O, Riedl O. (eds.), Modern Gastroenterology, FK Schattauer Verlag, Stuttgart & New York, 1969
60. Watson AJ, Wright NA. pp 11–31, in Cooke WT, Asquith P. (eds.), Coeliac Disease. Clinics in Gastroenterology, Saunders, London, 1974

61. Watson AJ, Wright NA. pp 151–154 in Hekkens WTJM, Pena AS. (eds.), Coeliac Disease, Stenfert-Kroese, Leiden, 1974
62. Wimber DR, Lamerton LF. Rad Res 1963, 18, 137–146
63. Wright NA, Al-Dewachi HS, Appleton DR, Watson AJ. Cell Tissue Kinet 1975, 8, 361–368
64. Wright NA, Appleton DR, Marks J, Watson AJ. J Clin Path 1979, 32, 462–470
65. Wright NA, Watson AJ, pp 141–150 in Hekkens WTJM, Pena AS. (eds.), Coeliac Disease, Stenfert-Kroese, Leiden, 1974.
66. Wright N, Watson A, Morley A, Appleton D, Marks J, Douglas A. Gut 1973, 14, 603–606
67. Wright N, Watson A, Morley A, Appleton D, Marks J, Douglas A. Gut 1973, 14, 701–710
68. Wright A, Watson A, Morley A, Appleton D, Marks J, Douglas A. Virchows Archiv Pathol Anat 1975, 364, 311–323

# Jejuno-ileal Bypass: Clinical and Experimental Aspects

J. D. MAXWELL & R. C. McGOURAN
Department of Medicine, St. George's Hospital Medical School
London, SW17 0RE, U.K.

Small intestinal bypass was introduced over 25 years ago as a radical treatment for gross obesity, designed to cause weight loss by surgically induced malabsorption. The prototype operation, jejuno-colic bypass, was soon abandoned because of its unacceptably high mortality and metabolic complications, particularly liver disease. Jejuno-ileal bypass was subsequently shown to be a more satisfactory operation, resulting in substantial weight loss (around 35% initial weight) which was usually permanent. However weight reduction was achieved at the cost of a mortality between 4 to 8%, and a formidable number of surgical and medical complications. Many of these were understandable sequelae of the shortened small bowel, but others including the most serious complication, liver disease, were initially unexplained. Patients are at greatest risk during the early catabolic period after surgery, but nutritional and metabolic problems may emerge years after weight stabilisation.

Animal studies have indicated that the long bypassed segment of gut, initially considered inert, makes an important contribution to both the beneficial and unwanted effects of the operation. Jejuno-ileal bypass results in significantly greater weight loss and mortality than equivalent resection, and liver dysfunction is seen only after bypass. These differences in adaptive response appear to be due to the abnormal bacterial flora (principally anaerobes and colonic type organisms) which develops in the bypassed gut. Enhanced weight loss (due to diminished food intake), increased mortality and hepatic dysfunction occur whether or not bacteria in the excluded loop have direct access to functioning bowel. Bacterial toxins may be responsible, but the nutritional disorder accompanying bypass seems to play a permissive role in the development of liver disease.

As both the major advantage of small intestinal bypass, spectacular and sustained weight loss, and the increased risk of death and liver failure after this procedure seem to depend on bacterial overgrowth in the bypassed gut, prospects for improving the safety of this operation while retaining its efficacy seem limited. Thus newer gastric bypass procedures, which achieve similar weight loss without metabolic complications, are likely to replace small intestinal bypass. However although this pioneering surgical experiment is unlikely to make a permanent therapeutic contribution, it has taught us much about intestinal adaptation, and the role of intestinal bacteria in the regulation of food intake, and their potential for causing nutritional disturbance and hepatic dysfunction. These lessons may be relevant to other forms of malnutrition accompanied by intestinal bacterial overgrowth and liver disease.

*J. D. Maxwell, Dept. of Medicine, St. George's Hospital Medical School, London, SW17 0RE, U.K.*

Intestinal bypass for obesity was pioneered over 25 years ago, and it has been estimated that over 100,000 such operations have now been performed in the USA alone. This 'artificial disease' is of interest to gastroenterologists not only from a practical clinical viewpoint, but because of the insights into intestinal adaptation it has provided.

The historical background to the introduction of intestinal bypass for obesity and its clinical effects, both beneficial and adverse, will be described, before summarising some of the more important adaptive changes which follow the operation. Significant differences in response to small intestinal bypass and equivalent resection which have emerged from animal studies, can be ascribed to differences in host adaptation to these two similar procedures. These in turn provide a rational basis for our present understanding of the mechanisms involved in weight loss after bypass surgery, and in the pathogenesis of its most important complication, liver disease.

## HISTORICAL BACKGROUND

Although it is not known for certain who performed the first intestinal operation for the treatment of gross obesity, in 1954 Kremen and colleagues in a paper devoted to animal studies evaluating the nutritional importance of the proximal and distal small intestine, briefly reported the use of ileal bypass to treat a patient with extreme obesity (39). However the first in depth clinical study of intestinal bypass surgery was begun by Payne, De Wind and Commons in 1956 at the Hospital of the Good Samaritan, Los Angeles (59). Their interest was stimulated by a patient who had progressive weight loss after extensive small intestinal resection, with anastomosis of her remaining proximal jejunum to transverse colon. It was decided to carry out a similar operation (jejuno-colic anastomosis) to achieve weight loss in morbidly obese patients with the specific intent of re-establishing normal gastrointestinal continuity when patients reached ideal body weight. However elective jejuno-colic anastomosis proved to have serious side effects and an unacceptable mortality. The operation—described as 'a metabolic disaster'—was soon abandoned (42, 59). Moreover it was discovered that when patients had intestinal continuity restored, they quickly returned to their original hyperobese state.

Subsequently Payne experimented with the effects of jejuno-ileal bypass, anastomosing varying lengths of jejunum and ileum, and in 1965 decided that it was most appropriate to leave approximately 10% of small intestine in continuity, with 35 cm (14 inches) of proximal jejunum anastomosed end to side to 10 cm (4 inches) of distal ileum (22, 58). This has remained the standard operation, although various modifications have been introduced in attempts to increase the efficacy of the procedure (70) or to reduce complications (31). Small intestinal bypass was the first effective treatment for gross obesity, but is no longer the only form of radical surgery available. It is now being replaced by gastric bypass procedures which are as effective, but with minimal metabolic and electrolyte complications (1, 13, 46, 64).

## CLINICAL EFFECTS OF JEJUNO-ILEAL BYPASS

The benefits of jejuno-ileal bypass in obesity can be summarised as follows:

### Weight loss

Intestinal bypass surgery was the first form of treatment shown to produce substantial weight loss in the majority of patients with gross obesity. Moreover unlike that resulting from dieting, weight loss after surgery is usually permanent, although some weight regain has been noted after long term follow up (32, 61).

Variations of the original operation have been tried but have not produced significant differences in weight loss. Modifications include alteration in the ratio of jejunum to ileum (which may affect the risk of gallstone formation (19), and various operations designed to prevent reflux of food up the bypassed segment. However clinical and experimental studies have shown that reflux is of no practical significance (27, 43). In any event it is now accepted that malabsorption accounts for only a small proportion of weight loss after intestinal bypass. There is no clear relationship between the length of bowel left in continuity, and ensuing weight loss. Although there appears to be greater weight loss with shorter bypass, this may be fortuitous as weight loss correlates well with initial weight, and shorter shunts have usually been chosen for heavier patients (61). On the other hand animal studies indicate that the extent of weight loss is affected by the length of excluded gut remaining. In groups of rats with the same (10%) length of small intestine in continuity, weight loss was greater in animals with a long, than in those with a short or medium bypassed segment (76). The pattern of weight loss after intestinal bypass is very reproducible with an initial rapid weight reduction during the first three to four weeks followed by more gradual weight loss and eventual stabilisation around a year following surgery. Total weight loss correlates well with initial weight, and usually amounts to about 30–35% of preoperative weight (22, 61). Thereafter the new weight is usually maintained, although small increases have been observed after long term follow up (32).

*Psychosocial function*

Various studies have shown improved psychological adjustment after intestinal bypass, with enhanced self esteem following weight reduction (18, 72).

*Reduction in risk factors*

Improvement in adverse risk factors associated with obesity is a third benefit of intestinal bypass surgery. These include decrease in blood pressure, improved pulmonary function, improved glucose tolerance, and decrease in serum lipids (8, 11).

These benefits of intestinal bypass for obesity are obtained at the cost of an overall mortality of between 4 and 8% (11, 22, 32, 47, 48) and numerous complications (2, 3, 11, 15, 22, 48). These include not only problems associated with surgery in high risk patients, but a growing list of nutritional and metabolic disorders. Patients are most at risk of serious complications during the early catabolic period of weight loss after surgery. However it is now apparent that serious medical complications may first develop many years after surgery and weight stabilisation (32). These considerations underline the need for careful long term follow up.

*Operative complications*

In addition to operative mortality, there are many other surgical risks including pulmonary embolism, wound infection and breakdown, anastomotic leaks, gastrointestinal haemorrhage, renal failure and pancreatitis (11, 15). Over 50% of patients in the St. George's Hospital series developed significant problems in the perioperative period, and many subsequently required readmission for the management of bypass related complications (15, 22).

*Medical complications*

A large number of metabolic and nutritional disturbances are now recognised after intestinal bypass. Although patients are most at risk from life threatening medical complications—particularly liver disease—during the first 6 to 12 months after surgery, it is now appreciated that serious problems may develop many years after weight stabilisation (3, 32).

Many medical complications (such as diarrhoea, steatorrhoea, electrolyte disturbance, various nutritional disorders including deficiency of fat and water soluble vitamins, cholesterol gallstone formation, and hyperoxaluria with nephrolithiasis) are understandable consequences of adaptation to the short length of functioning small bowel after bypass (3, 8, 11, 15, 22). Other, initially unexplained, complications are now considered to result from the abnormal intestinal flora which follows the altered anatomy produced by this operation. These include polyarthritis, vasculitis and inflammatory skin disorders (77), as well as abdominal bloating and intestinal pseudo-obstruction. The most serious of these, post-bypass liver disease, will be discussed in more detail later. Before reviewing the experimental evidence which has led to our current understanding of the mechanism of weight loss after intestinal bypass, and of the pathogenesis of its most important complication, it is helpful to consider some of the adaptive changes occurring after jejuno-ileal bypass, and summarise important differences between the response to jejuno-ileal bypass, and to equivalent resection.

ADAPTATION    AFTER    JEJUNO-ILEAL BYPASS

Changes can be considered under the following headings:

*Small intestinal morphology and function*

Jejuno-ileal bypass causes similar structural changes in the small bowel left in functioning continuity, to those seen after resection (38, 78). However animal studies indicate that intestinal adaptation after bypass is significantly less pronounced than after resection, as gauged by measurements of intestinal length and weight, and mucosal weight, protein and DNA content (75, 78). Studies in man at reoperation after jejuno-ileal bypass, or using peroral mucosal biopsies, have also shown hypertrophy of the intestine in continuity (24, 38). Elongation of the jejunal and ileal segments in continuity occurs, together with increase in villous height. This adaptive response (as is the case after resection) is due to hyperplasia rather than to hypertrophy because the total number of normal sized cells increases (26, 78).

In view of these gross morphological changes and eventual weight stabilisation after bypass, functional adaptation of the remaining small intestine in continuity might be expected. Increased absorption of glucose per unit length of intestine six months after jejuno-ileal bypass for obesity has been reported (38). Both luminal factors as well as hormonal changes noted after bypass (see below) appear to be important for the development of these adaptive responses (78), but the impaired response compared to resection is poorly understood. Moreover the significance of these adaptive changes in determining eventual weight stabilisation after bypass is uncertain. Increases in segmental function are modest and take place on a quite different time-scale from weight changes. Furthermore the degree of malabsorption after jejuno-ileal bypass has been shown to be unrelated to the rate of weight loss (61, 62).

### Intestinal hormones

Gut hormones have a characteristic anatomical distribution through the gastrointestinal tract, and changes noted after jejuno-ileal bypass indicate a reduction of hormone release from areas of bypassed small bowel, with a concomitant increase from gut proximal to the bypass (stomach), and from intestine beyond the bypassed segment (6, 78). Thus postprandial gut hormone profiles following intestinal bypass for obesity have shown a very marked rise in enteroglucagon (6 to 16x) compared to age and sex matched controls, a considerable increase in neurotensin (8x), and small increases in gastrin release. Postprandial insulin release is diminished

(with a reduction in insulin secretion stimulated by oral glucose—the enteroinsular axis), and glucose dependent insulinotropic peptide (GIP) is also reduced. For details see chapter by Bloom and Polak (this issue).

These hormonal changes are similar to those seen after intestinal resection in man. The increased gastrin secretion may contribute to hyperplasia of small bowel in continuity after bypass, as this hormone is trophic to the alimentary mucosa. There is also circumstantial evidence for enteroglucagon being an additional trophic factor in local mucosal hypertrophy. In addition enteroglucagon and neurotensin both appear to have an inhibitory effect on gastrointestinal motility and gastric emptying. Thus the increased secretion of these hormones after bypass may contribute to the delayed intestinal transit observed in the short segment remaining in continuity after this operation. These hormonally mediated changes in intestinal motility and hypertrophy both appear to be advantageous adaptive responses in so far as they counteract surgically induced malabsorption (6, 78).

### Bile acid synthesis and enterohepatic circulation

Small bowel bile acid concentrations and lipolysis decrease after jejuno-ileal bypass, probably due to post-operative bile acid malabsorption resulting in reduced entero-hepatic circulation. However impaired fat digestion after intestinal bypass does not influence fat absorption in the duodenum or upper jejunum, suggesting that the steatorrhoea after bypass is mainly caused by reduction of absorptive intestinal surface (73).

Clinical studies have also shown that ileal bypass results in marked increase in cholesterol turnover and neutral sterol and bile acid excretion in hyperlipidaemic patients (51) (and partial ileal bypass is utilised in the treatment of hypercholesterolaemia). In rats jejuno-ileal bypass is reported to increase hepatic synthesis of cholesterol, and it is suggested that the enhanced synthesis of this bile acid precursor is related to interruption of the enterohepatic circulation of bile acids and consequent bile salt depletion (30).

After bypass in man bile becomes lithogenic, and there is an increased risk of cholesterol gallstones (19, 21). It seems likely that both bile acid depletion and the adaptive increase in hepatic cholesterol synthesis and excretion contribute to the substantially increased risk of gallstone formation observed after bypass surgery.

*Intestinal bacterial flora*

The small bowel does not normally harbour anaerobes or coliforms in significant numbers. However after jejuno-ileal bypass the development of an abnormal colonic type flora in the bypassed segment and functioning small bowel in continuity, with significant overgrowth of aerobic and anaerobic organisms has been well documented both in experimental animals and in clinical studies.

In unstarved rats the small bowel flora consists mainly of lactobacilli, but bacterial counts reduce markedly after 24 hours starvation (57). Small intestinal resection with end to end anastomosis causes a moderate increase in total bacterial counts throughout the small intestine, with relative reduction in lactobacilli and increase in colonic organisms (coliforms, bacteroides and clostridia). Jejuno-ileal bypass results in marked qualitative and quantitative changes in the bacterial flora distal to the anastomosis, and in the bypassed segment (57). It is concluded that bacterial overgrowth in the functioning small intestine results not only from contamination by the bypassed segment (acting as a bacterial reservoir) but that the anastomosis itself contribute to the development of a pathological intestinal flora, possibly by disturbing peristalsis. The delayed transit through the shortened functioning small bowel after resection or bypass (previously noted as an adaptive response) may also contribute to the altered bacterial flora after these operations. Other animal studies in rats (25, 45) and dogs (35) have shown similar abnormalities in the bacterial flora after jejuno-ileal bypass.

In man most studies on normal fasting individuals have shown only a sparse bacterial population in the small intestine, with a high proportion of aspirates from the upper jejunum being sterile. However several clinical reports have clearly established significant bacterial overgrowth in the long excluded segment of jejuno-ileum composed largely of anaerobic organisms and colonic flora (12, 17). A similar flora is present in the small intestine remaining in continuity (17, 20, 63).

## COMPARISON OF THE EFFECTS OF JEJUNO-ILEAL BYPASS AND RESECTION

When small intestinal bypass was introduced to treat patients with massive obesity the intention was to simulate an extensive intestinal resection, but to retain the long excluded segment in case there was need to restore intestinal anatomy at a future date. It was assumed that the bypassed segment of jejuno-ileum was inert, but subsequent experience has shown this not to be the case.

The major achievement of animal models of small intestinal bypass has been to demonstrate the important contribution of the bypassed segment of gut to both the beneficial and unwanted effects of the operation. Comparisons of bypass and equivalent small intestinal resection are not feasible in man because so few patients undergo massive resection, and in those who do the exact length and condition of the remaining small bowel is often unknown. Both the dog and the rat have been shown to be suitable animal models, provided an adequate bypass operation is performed. In the rat bypass of 90% of the small bowel between the pylorus and caecum (37, 45, 69) (an operation similar in extent to the standard procedure in man) and in the dog an 80% bypass, have been shown to reproduce many of the features of the human operation (7, 14, 35). Although genetically obese animals might seem most appropriate, they are expensive and fragile, and have been shown to respond to intestinal bypass in the same manner as their lean counterparts (29).

Four animal studies involving a comparison of small intestinal bypass and equivalent resection are summarised in Table I. They show that these similar operations differ in three major respects—extent of weight loss, propensity to liver dysfunction, and risk of postoperative mortality. Bondar and Pisesky (7) concerned at the high morbidity and frequency of metabolic disturbances after intestinal bypass for obesity, first

Table I. Four animal studies comparing small intestinal bypass with equivalent resection, demonstrating altered adaptive response due to the bypassed segment

|  |  | Number | Deaths | Liver damage | Weight loss |
|---|---|---|---|---|---|
| Bondar & Pisesky (7) |  |  |  |  |  |
| Dogs | 80% resection | 2 | 0/2 | No | + |
|  | 80% bypass | 12 | 10/12 | Yes | + + |
| Burney et al. (14) |  |  |  |  |  |
| Dogs | 90% resection | 6 | 1/5 | No | + |
|  | 90% bypass | 12 | 3/12 | Yes | + + |
| Hyland et al. (37) |  |  |  |  |  |
| Rats | 90% resection | 70 | ? | No | + |
|  | 90% bypass | 70 | ? | Yes | + + |
| McGouran et al. (45) |  |  |  |  |  |
| Rats | 90% resection | 42 | 0/30 | No | + |
|  | 90% bypass | 59 | 14/51 | Yes | + + |

used an animal model to compare the effects of bypass with equivalent small intestinal resection, and suggested that the increased weight loss, liver dysfunction and mortality after bypass all depended on retention of the long bypassed segment of gut. In their study two types of intestinal bypass—jejuno-ileal and jejuno-colic—were compared. The latter was found to have a more catastrophic effect, in accordance with clinical experience (42, 59).

Although numbers studied in earlier reports were small and conclusions tentative, recent studies have confirmed significant differences between bypass and resection, and have helped to clarify

the mechanisms involved. Interestingly these adverse effects of jejuno-ileal bypass occur whether or not the bypassed segment is left in contact with the functioning short small bowel (Fig. 1) (25, 43, 44).

The differences in adaptation between intestinal bypass and resection revealed by these animal studies have allowed a better understanding of the beneficial and adverse effects of jejuno-ileal bypass surgery in man. The remainder of this review will be devoted to a more detailed analysis of the mechanism of weight loss after jejuno-ileal bypass (the major justification for bypass surgery) and of the pathogenesis of

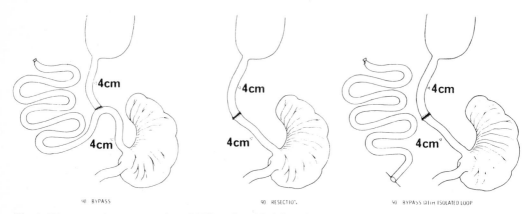

Fig. 1. Diagrammatic representation of 90% end to side jejuno-ileal bypass and equivalent resection in the rat. In additional experiments the long bypassed loop was isolated and exteriorised as an ileostomy. Enhanced weight loss and adverse effects on liver function occur whether or not the excluded segment has direct access to functioning bowel.
(From McGouran and Maxwell, 1980 (44))

post-operative liver disease (the most serious complication of this operation).

## MECHANISM OF WEIGHT LOSS AFTER INTESTINAL BYPASS

### Malabsorption

The initial rationale for intestinal bypass in obesity was that this operation would simulate the effects of extensive resection and produce a controlled malabsorption, which would eventually lessen as a result of intestinal adaptation (59). Malabsorption does indeed occur after surgical bypass, but is now known not to be the major factor in postoperative weight loss. Moreover the role of intestinal adaptation in the modulation of weight changes after bypass has been questioned, as the adaptive changes in intestinal structure and function after intestinal bypass are modest and take place on a quite different time scale from the weight changes (61). Pilkington investigated the role of malabsorption in producing weight loss by studying patients on identical dietary intakes before and at intervals up to 24 months after jejuno-ileal bypass (62). Faeces were collected and their energy content measured. Despite great differences in the rate of weight loss at various time intervals after surgery, malabsorption as measured by total faecal caloric loss did not change significantly during the 2 years. Four months after surgery faecal calorie loss amounted to 15% of the energy intake and could only account for one quarter of the large amount of weight lost at that time. The observation that there was little change in the extent of malabsorption two years after bypass also indicated that adaptive mucosal hypertrophy in the segment of jejuno-ileum left in continuity could not adequately account for reduction in the rate of weight loss and eventual stabilisation.

### Decreased food intake

Patients notice difficulty in eating after jejuno-ileal bypass, and measurements of food intake indicate that this decreases substantially during the first 6 months after surgery. Over the ensuing months food intake then gradually increases, but does not return to preoperative

levels (10, 28, 61). Controlled ad libitum feeding experiments before and after bypass surgery have shown a significant correlation between weight loss and the decrease in caloric intake after jejuno-ileal bypass. In addition bypass also modifies taste preferences for sweet solutions (10). These studies indicate that the reduction in food intake which follows intestinal bypass accounts for the major portion of weight lost, and that this results not only from decrease in size of individual meals, but from realignment of eating patterns. Animal studies confirm these findings (45, 69).

Several possible explanations have been offered for the diminished food intake after bypass. The signal(s) for a reduction in food intake might be triggered in the gastrointestinal tract (e.g. by mechanical distension) or relate to post-ingestional changes (such as alteration in circulating concentrations of nutrients or gut hormones). For example it has been speculated that the slow transit through the bowel leads to distension which may be responsible for satiety, as experimental studies have demonstrated that mechanical gut distension can affect food intake (66). Alternatively it has been proposed that hormonal changes observed after bypass might be responsible for altered eating patterns (6). However perhaps the most persuasive evidence comes from animal studies which implicate bacterial overgrowth in the excluded segment of small bowel as a major factor responsible for diminished food intake after bypass (44, 45).

Animal studies have clearly shown that weight loss is greater after small bowel bypass than equivalent resection, implicating the excluded segment in this effect (7, 14, 37, 44) (Fig. 2). Moreover as discussed earlier, there is ample evidence from clinical and animal studies that intestinal bypass alters the bacterial flora of both the excluded and functioning segments of small bowel. In studies designed to investigate the relative roles of nutrition (food intake, malabsorption) and bacteria on weight loss after bypass it was shown that rats with a 90% small bowel bypass (similar in design and extent to the standard human operation for obesity) lost approximately 30% of their starting weight, (equivalent to weight loss following bypass in obese patients) and double the weight

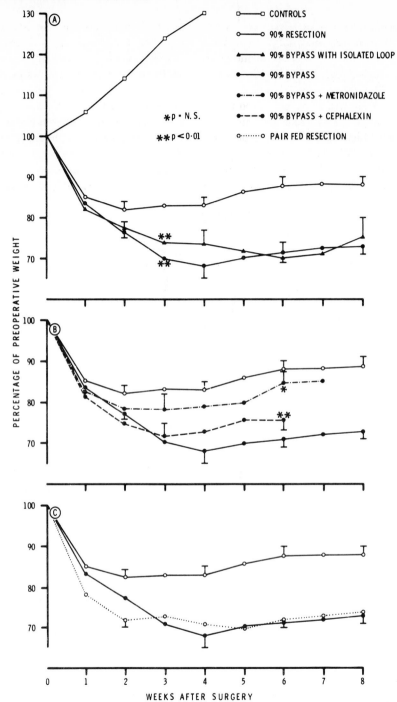

Fig. 2. A) Changes in body weight after sham operation, 90% small bowel resection and bypass in rats. I indicates mean ± SEM. Significance values relate to a comparison with 90% resection. B) Changes in body weight after 90% resection and bypass, and in bypassed rats treated with Metronidazole or Cephalexin. C) Body weight after 90% resection and bypass. The weight curve for a resected rat pair fed with a bypassed animal is also shown.
(From McGouran et al., 1982 (45))

loss in resected rats. This difference could not be explained by increased malabsorption, as faecal and caloric excretion were virtually identical after both procedures (Fig. 3). Pair feeding studies indicated that the increased weight loss by bypass rats could be explained by reduced food intake. Moreover treatment with a selective antianaerobic drug (metronidazole), but not a broad spectrum antiaerobic antibiotic (cephalexin) markedly reduced the degree of weight loss in bypass rats, so that six weeks after surgery these animals were not significantly different in weight from resected rats (44, 45) (Fig. 2). Thus these experimental studies demonstrate that only approximately half of the weight loss that follows bypass is due to shortening of the small bowel. The remainder is a consequence of retention of the bypassed loop. It appears that anaerobic organisms which are not normally present in the small bowel, but are found in large numbers after intestinal bypass, somehow reduce food intake and consequently increase weight loss. As these organisms are pres-

FAECAL LIPID AND CALORIE EXCRETION

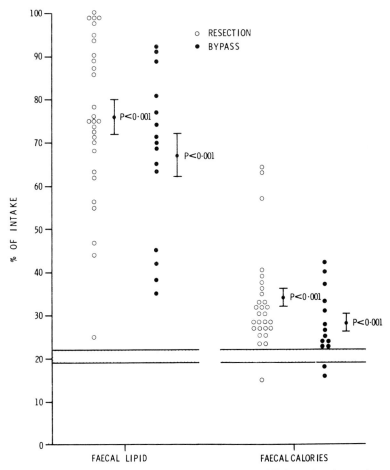

Fig. 3. Faecal lipid and total calorie excretion after 90% bypass and resection, expressed as a percentage of intake. **I** indicates mean ± SEM. Shaded area denotes mean ± SEM for sham operated controls. Significance values relate to a comparison with controls.
(From McGouran et al., 1982 (45))

ent in functioning small bowel after both bypass and resection, it is likely that the increased weight loss which follows bypass is due to the high concentration of anaerobes in the long excluded segment.

## LIVER DISEASE AFTER INTESTINAL BYPASS

Jejuno-colic anastomosis, the prototype intestinal bypass operation for obesity, was abandoned after it became apparent that it had an unacceptably high morbidity and mortality. The frequency of liver dysfunction and electrolyte disturbances earned the operation its unenviable reputation as a "metabolic disaster" (42, 47, 59). Subsequently experience with jejuno-ileal anastomosis has shown it to be a more satisfactory operation, but liver dysfunction, although infrequent remains its most serious complication (7, 22, 47, 48).

*Prevalence of post-bypass liver disease*

Analysis of published series allows a reasonably accurate estimate of the mortality associated with jejuno-ileal bypass, but it is more difficult to be sure of the proportion of deaths attributable to, or associated with, liver disease. The extent of clinically significant liver dysfunction after bypass is even more difficult to ascertain, as criteria vary and many published reports do not address themselves to these issues. With these reservations, data from a number of well documented reports (2, 4, 9, 22, 33, 48) from Europe and the USA including at least 50 patients are summarised in

Table II. This shows the overall mortality of jejuno-ileal bypass together with deaths associated with liver failure, and numbers of patients with clinically significant liver involvement. From these reports it appears that clinically significant liver disturbance occurs in between 3 to 10% of patients with jejuno-ileal bypass. Although the overall mortality is very much lower than seen after jejuno-colic anastomosis, deaths associated with liver disease continue to make a substantial contribution—between 25% and 75%—to total deaths.

*Liver changes before and after jejuno-ileal bypass*

*Obesity.* Histological abnormalities are found in the majority of obese subjects. Between 60 and 90% of morbidly obese patients have some degree of hepatic steatosis prior to surgery (47, 54). Much of this hepatic fat probably represents a local organ manifestation of a generalised increase in lipid stores, but it should be remembered that in a proportion of obese individuals alcohol provides a significant contribution to total calories, and to hepatic steatosis. Other abnormalities occasionally reported in preoperative biopsies include focal necrosis and inflammation, periportal fibrosis and even cirrhosis (47, 54). All these changes can be produced by alcohol excess, and such reports emphasise the importance of preoperative assessment of liver morphology.

*Post-bypass.* When weight loss is achieved by dieting hepatic histology improves, and there is reduction in steatosis (23). This is in striking contrast to weight reduction achieved after

Table II. Some reports on overall mortality rate, clinically significant liver dysfunction, and deaths associated with liver failure after jejuno-ileal bypass

| Author | Cases | Overall mortality | Liver dysfunction | Deaths associated with liver failure |
|---|---|---|---|---|
| DeWind & Payne (1976)   (22) | 230 | 19 (8%) | 14 (6%) | 10 (4%) |
| Bray et al. (1976)   (9) | 989 | 47 (4%) | not stated | 11 (1%) |
| Maxwell et al. (1977)   (48) | 120 | 5 (4%) | 3 (3%) | 3 (3%) |
| Halverson et al. (1978)   (33) | 101 | 5 (5%) | 6 (6%) | 3 (3%) |
| Andersen et al. (1980)   (2) | 2450 | 123/2450 (5%) | 83/1917 (4.3%) | not stated |

jejuno-ileal bypass, which is followed by worsening steatosis, often accompanied by hepatitic changes and fibrosis. Peters and his colleagues first drew attention to the remarkable similarity between post-jejuno-ileal bypass hepatic disease and alcoholic liver disease (60). The triad of steatosis, hepato-cellular necrosis and fibrosis seen in both disorders may persist or progress in apparently healthy patients five or more years after bypass (34).

*Fatty change.* A striking increase in hepatic fat occurs during the early postoperative catabolic phase of weight loss. Fat accumulation is maximal around six months postoperatively, subsiding to preoperative values about two to three years after surgery (68). The demonstration of a relationship between the extent of weight loss at intervals after bypass and the degree of fatty change in the liver (Fig. 4) (68) suggests a relationship between postoperative hepatic steatosis, and the rate of mobilisation of fat from peripheral stores to fulfil calorie requirements.

Most reports on fatty liver in obese subjects

before and after intestinal bypass have used histological assessment which provided only a very approximate guide to total hepatic fat. Chemical estimates show a net fat accumulation of at least three times preoperative values 13 months after bypass. This is largely due to increase in hepatic triglycerides, with little change in cholesterol or phospholipid concentration (36), but other studies have shown increased cholesterol turnover in liver (51).

Although extensive fatty metamorphosis is the most obvious change in the liver after bypass, fat accumulation per se is generally of little clinical significance. Greater importance should be attached to the other morphological changes, which although less striking, are more important determinants of hepatic dysfunction (34, 47, 60).

*Hepatocellular necrosis.* Hepatitic changes after bypass (patchy hepatocellular necrosis and polymorphonuclear inflammatory infiltrates) are well recognised (23, 34, 47). These changes are most prominent during the early postoperative period, but can be detected in asymptomatic individuals

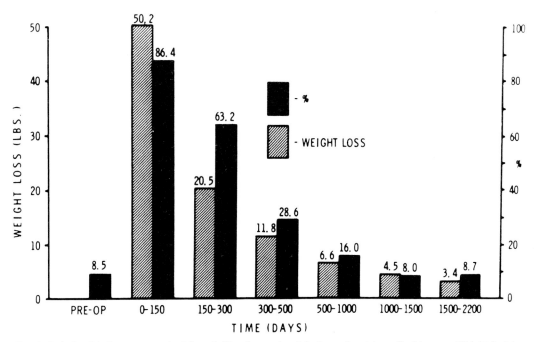

Fig. 4. Relationship between marked fatty infiltration and weight loss after jejuno-ileal bypass. Weight lost in each period is expressed as a percentage of total weight lost (shaded columns), and related to percentage of patients with marked hepatic steatosis (solid black columns) in each period.
(From Salmon and Reedyk, 1975 (68))

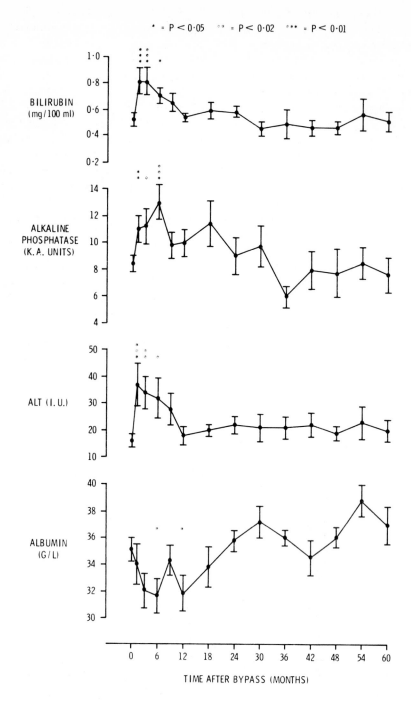

Fig. 5. Mean ± SEM plasma concentration of bilirubin, alkaline phosphatase, alanine aminotransferase (ALT), and albumin in 35 healthy patients followed up to 60 months after jejuno-ileal bypass. Asterisks denote significant change from preoperative values.

(From Maxwell et al., 1977 (48))

some years after surgery, well after weight stabilisation (32). They are reflected in routine liver function tests by elevation of hepatocellular enzymes, accompanied by small but significant changes in plasma bilirubin, alkaline phosphatase and albumin (Fig. 5). These biochemical changes are apparent during the early postoperative period, and revert to normal after a new stable weight is achieved (48). However unlike fat accumulation, biochemical disturbances after bypass do not seem to be related to the extent of weight loss, nor are they due to alcohol, halothane or hepatitis B infection (12, 48). It is of interest that the median time after bypass for the appearance of clinical liver dysfunction—3 months—is precisely the time when the most significant biochemical changes are noted in asymptomatic patients following surgery (12, 47, 48). Thus the development of jaundice and liver failure after intestinal bypass seems to represent the tip of an iceberg of widespread asymptomatic liver disturbance, rather than a rare idiosyncratic response.

*Hepatic fibrosis/cirrhosis.* Although minor degrees of fibrosis (and cirrhosis) may be present in obese individuals before surgery (47, 54) there is good evidence that these changes may develop *de novo*, or progress, after intestinal bypass (4, 5, 12, 33, 34, 47, 68). Only routine preoperative biopsy will detect these changes, but such studies are not invariably performed, and many published reports do not state whether or not all patients had this evaluation. Furthermore some cases of postbypass cirrhosis may be due largely or entirely to alcohol abuse (4, 68). Nevertheless it is well established that cirrhosis may be a genuine complication of the bypass procedure itself, with over 9% of patients developing this complication on long term follow up (34). Interestingly, increased activity of proline hydroxylase, the rate limiting enzyme in collagen synthesis, has been demonstrated in liver biopsies from patients after bypass who develop hepatocellular necrosis and fibrosis, but not in biopsies showing only fatty change (49).

The recognition that standard liver function tests may be entirely normal despite the presence of cirrhosis has emphasised the need for routine preoperative and regular follow up liver biopsies in all patients. Since adopting this procedure the detection rate for cirrhosis following jejuno-ileal bypass has doubled (5).

*Hepatic granulomas.* In a small proportion of liver biopsies after intestinal bypass non-caseating granulomas have been noted, unrelated to tuberculosis, sarcoid or liver failure. Although of no clinical significance, this interesting observation might assist in the understanding of post-bypass hepatic disease (9, 33) as granulomas may result from immune complex deposition (74).

## Pathogenesis of liver changes after bypass

The acceptability of intestinal bypass would undoubtedly be greatly increased if it were possible to diminish the metabolic hazards while retaining the efficacy of this operation. The cause of the adverse liver changes has been the subject of much investigation and controversy, but a better understanding has emerged from the study of animal models.

Clinical evidence indicates that whatever the explanation for post-bypass hepatic dysfunction, it is not due to halothane toxicity, alcohol (although this may have an additive effect) or hepatitis B infection (12, 48). The principal hypotheses propose that nutritional deficiency and/or intestinal bacterial overgrowth are responsible (Table III).

In evaluating the various hypotheses it is important to remember the similarity between post-bypass and alcoholic liver disease. Any acceptable explanation should account not only for the extensive fatty change after bypass, but also for the development of hepatocellular necrosis and fibrosis.

### Nutritional deficiency

The similarity to the hepatic changes seen in kwashiorkor prompted the suggestion that *protein malnutrition* might account for liver disease after bypass. This was supported by the observation that in the early catabolic period after bypass (when fatty change was marked, and liver function tests most deranged) plasma amino-acid profiles were typical of protein-calorie malnutrition (52). After weight stabilisation, the concentra-

Table III. Nutritional and bacterial hypotheses regarding the pathogenesis of liver dysfunction after jejuno-ileal bypass

| NUTRITIONAL DEFICIENCY? | and/or | BACTERIAL INVOLVEMENT? |
|---|---|---|
| —Protein/amino-acids<br>—Essential fatty acids<br>—Lipotropes<br>—Vitamins<br>—Minerals | | —Hepatotoxins produced by<br>  bacterial metabolism<br>  (deconjugated bile acids)<br>  (alcohol)<br>—Bacterial inactivation lipotropes<br>  (choline → trimethylamine)<br>—Direct hepatotoxicity<br>  (hepatic infection)<br>  (immune complexes)<br>  (endotoxins) |

tions of amino-acids returned to normal, and amino-acid tolerance tests improved, suggesting improved absorption. During the early catabolic phase when mobilisation of fat stores leads to increased hepatic triglyceride accumulation, lipid secretion by the liver is diminished, possibly because of its inability to synthesise or secrete lipoprotein carrier at a pace commensurate with triglyceride. Whether the availability of protein is rate limiting under these circumstances is not known. However protein deficiency, even of extreme degree, does not by itself cause hepatocellular necrosis, inflammation or fibrosis (49)—the most significant changes following bypass.

Other nutritional factors implicated include deficiency of *essential fatty acids*, and *lipotropes*. It has been speculated that essential fatty acid deficiency (as a result of the short gut and steatorrhoea) might cause disruption of lysosomal membranes and consequent hepatocellular damage (47). However there is no evidence from clinical studies to support this suggestion. Although intestinal adaptation is morphologically less pronounced after bypass than comparable resection, and it has been inferred from this that some (unspecified) nutritional defect might account for bypass liver disease (75), animals with experimental resection or bypass show no difference in malabsorption of fat or total calories (44, 45). As resected animals do not develop liver dysfunction (7, 14, 37, 44) selective nutritional

deficiency after bypass seems unlikely. Moreover there is no good evidence in man to support the suggestion that liver changes after bypass may be related to or aggravated by deficiency of vitamins, minerals or choline. Choline deficiency in rats may result in liver damage (an effect which appears to require participation of intestinal bacteria (56, 67)) but man's daily requirement is unknown, and primates are far less susceptible to protein and lipotrope deficiency than rodents. Intestinal bacterial overgrowth after bypass could theoretically produce deficiency by converting choline to inactive trimethylamines. If this does occur, it should properly be classified as a bacterial, rather than nutritional, effect. Some evidence from experimental animal studies has been presented to support the nutritional hypothesis. In dogs progression to liver damage and death was inevitable after 80% bypass, but this could be prevented by daily instillation of 15 g predigested gelatin, or 15–30 cc medium chain triglyceride (MCT) into the proximal end of an exteriorised bypassed loop. However 2 g sulphathalidine or 5 g methylcellulose had no such protective effect (41). It was concluded that the gelatin and MCT prevented liver damage by providing additional nutrition, but other interpretations are possible. The instilled nutrients might have encouraged the development of a normal flora, or may have exerted a cleansing effect on the bypassed loop. Thus in summary, while protein deficiency may contribute to hepatic steatosis, there is no good evidence that nutritional deficiency can account for the whole spectrum of hepatic changes seen after intestinal bypass.

*Intestinal bacteria*

The most persuasive evidence implicating bacteria in post-bypass hepatic dysfunction comes from experimental animal studies (Fig. 6). These demonstrate that liver dysfunction follows experimental jejuno-ileal bypass, but is not seen after equivalent intestinal resection (7, 14, 25, 37, 44). Further evidence for the role of intestinal bacterial overgrowth in the production of liver dysfunction after bypass has come from animal studies comparing control and antibiotic treated groups. Hepatic dysfunction after bypass in dogs could be prevented by doxycycline, a tetracycline like antibiotic with broad activity against gram +ve and gram −ve aerobes and anaerobes (35). In rats cephalexin (a cephalosporin with a

wide range of activity against gram +ve and gram −ve aerobes, but negligible activity against anaerobes) abolished the expected rise in plasma AST and ALT during the first 6 weeks after surgery, but subsequently the protective effect was lost, possibly due to emergence of resistant strains (44). In contrast metronidazole (activity against anaerobes but without effect on aerobes) had not protective effect on liver function, although influencing weight and survival (44, 45).

It is not clear whether bacteria exert their deleterious effects on the liver directly, or indirectly.

*Indirect hepatotoxic effect of bacteria.* It has been suggested that intestinal bacterial overgrowth, with abnormal intestinal metabolism by bacteria of ingested nutrients and bile acids could contribute to hepatic disease after bypass surgery via the production of endogenous hepatotoxins (63).

Enhanced bacterial deconjugation of bile salts

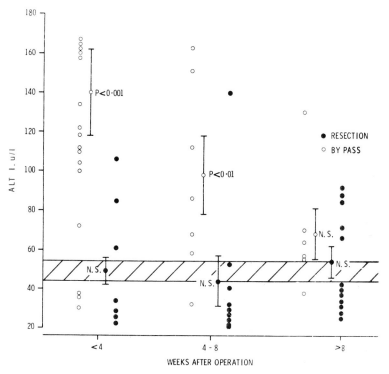

Fig. 6. Effect of 90% jejuno-ileal bypass (○) and resection (●) on plasma alanine amino-transferase (ALT) for three time periods after surgery. Shaded area denotes mean ± SEM for sham operated controls. Plasma ALT was unaffected by resection, but significantly elevated after bypass.
(From McGouran and Maxwell, 1980 (44))

and high plasma levels of potentially hepatotoxic secondary *bile acids* have been demonstrated after jejuno-ileal bypass (71). However it is unlikely that these are responsible for the development of liver disease, as this is not seen after equivalent bile salt malabsorption in patients undergoing ileal resection. Furthermore patients with the bilio-intestinal type of bypass (where the apex of the excluded jejuno-ileal segment is anastomosed to the gallbladder, allowing enhanced bacterial deconjugation and subsequent absorption of bile acids from the long excluded segment) do not appear to have an increased risk of liver dysfunction (47).

Intestinal bacterial fermentation of ingested carbohydrate to *alcohol* would provide a satisfactory explanation both for the occurrence of liver disease after bypass, and its similarity to alcoholic liver disease. Alcohol has been detected after bypass in venous samples from man and the dog (50) but levels were very low, and insufficient to implicate this as a hepatotoxin. Additionally it has been suggested that dietary choline could be converted to the lipotrophically inactive form—trimethylamine—by the increased numbers of intestinal bacteria present after bypass (47). Although such deficiency may cause experimental liver damage in rodents (an effect enhanced by intestinal bacteria) (56, 67) man's daily requirement for choline is unknown, and there is little evidence that deficiency of choline or other nutrients, vitamins or minerals ever cause clinically significant liver damage.

An ingenious experimental modification of the standard jejuno-ileal operation has also cast doubt on the relevance of intestinal bacterial metabolism (either by producing hepatotoxic products from bile sats or ingested food, or by inactivating dietary lipotropes) in the pathogenesis of post-bypass liver disease. In these studies the long excluded segment of jejuno-ileum was separated from the short section of functioning small bowel, and exteriorised (Fig. 1). Thus there was no longer any connection between the heavily colonised excluded loop, and ingested food or endogenous bile secretions. Nevertheless adverse effects on the liver were identical to those seen after standard jejuno-ileal bypass (25, 44).

*Direct hepatotoxic effect of bacteria* thus seems the most likely explanation for post-bypass liver dysfunction, but this conclusion is tentative and reached only after exclusion of possible indirect bacterial mechanisms discussed above.

There is no evidence to implicate bacterial colonisation of the liver after bypass. Although portal pyaemia is not infrequent, liver disease due to direct bacterial involvement is rate (55), and has not been reported after intestinal bypass. Circulating immune complexes have been implicated in skin and joint disease after bypass surgery (77) and it is possible that immunological sequelae to intestinal bacterial overgrowth may also be involved in disturbances of liver structure and function. Granulomas, which are occasionally found in the liver after bypass, can be produced by immune complexes (74). However bacterial endotoxins absorbed via the portal vein to the liver also seem likely candidates, and certainly are capable of causing hepatocellular damage, cholestasis and inhibiting liver phagocytes (Kupffer cells) (55, 56).

Thus in summary current evidence suggests that liver dysfunction after intestinal bypass is due to some enterohepatic factor related to bacterial overgrowth in the long excluded segment. Nevertheless associated nutritional deficiency may have an important permissive effect, as indicated by the need for an extensive bypass before liver disturbance occurs (14), and from previous studies showing that protein deficiency enhances the effects of various hepatotoxins (16, 40). Unfortunately it is not possible to predict patients at greatest risk of liver disease after jejuno-ileal bypass (47, 53). The management of this, and other complications of the operation, and indications for reanastomosis are reviewed elsewhere (5, 47).

## COSTS v BENEFITS AND THE FUTURE OF INTESTINAL BYPASS

It is now estimated that over 100,000 patients have undergone intestinal bypass surgery, but as the number has increased, the enthusiasm of doctors, if not of patients, for this procedure as a treatment for obesity has declined (2, 8, 11, 65).

Regardless of its spectacular effect on body weight jejuno-ileal bypass remains a major physical intervention, with a mortality far exceeding all other forms of treatment for obesity and a formidable list of complications. Such radical treatment for gross obesity should only be carried out by multidisciplinary teams able to evaluate prospective patients carefully before surgery, and committed to carrying out meticulous follow-up. In this way potentially life threatening complications can be recognised and treated in time, or if deterioration continues, reanastomosis performed (5). Although the majority of serious complications occur in the first year after surgery at the time of rapid weight loss, it is now recognised that significant nutritional and metabolic complications may emerge years after weight stabilisation, and life-long supervision seems mandatory (32).

Whether the reduction in weight and adverse risk factors achieved after jejuno-ileal bypass results in a significant gain in quantity or quality of life has not been established, but may be answered in due course by controlled studies such as the Danish Obesity Project (65). However it seems likely that intestinal bypass is in the process of being abandoned in favour of gastric bypass or partitioning procedures, which are almost as effective in achieving weight loss, but with minimal electrolyte or metabolic complications (1, 13, 46, 64). Partial ileal bypass however may retain a role in the treatment of severe hypercholesterolaemia.

Although intestinal bypass now seems unlikely to make a lasting therapeutic contribution, it was a bold surgical experiment, and the first effective treatment to be offered to thousands of grossly obese patients. A better understanding of adaptive changes occurring after jejuno-ileal bypass proved the initial rationale for the operation to have been incorrect, and clarified a number of unexpected complications. Paradoxically both the efficacy of small intestinal bypass in reducing food intake and body weight, and the increased risk of death and major metabolic complications after this procedure seem to depend on changes in small intestinal bacterial flora. Thus the prospects for improving the safety of this operation, while retaining its efficacy, seem limited. Inevitably newer operations with a similar potential for reducing food intake, but without the metabolic risks, will take its place. However, therapeutic considerations apart, intestinal bypass has proved a fascinating experimental model. This unique "artificial disease" has taught us much about intestinal adaptation, and the relationship between intestinal bacteria, food intake, nutritional status, and liver disease. These lessons may be relevant to an understanding of other, even more prevalent, nutritional disorders.

## ACKNOWLEDGEMENTS

We are indebted to Professor T.R.E. Pilkington for advice and encouragment, and to the St. George's Hospital Research Fund for financial support. Thanks are due to Liza Ang for technical assistance, and to Marion Amos for expert secretarial help.

Figures 1 and 6 are reproduced by kind permission of Academic Press, publishers of "Surgical Management of Obesity", Figures 2 and 3 by permission of the editor of International Journal of Obesity, Figure 4 by permission of the editor of Surgery, Gynecology & Obstetrics, and Figure 5 by permission of the editor of the British Medical Journal.

## REFERENCES

1. Alden JF. Arch Surg 1977, 112, 799–806
2. Andersen T, Juhl E, Quaade F. Am J Clin Nutr 1980, 33, 440–445
3. Anon. Nutr Rev 1980, 38, 238–240
4. Baddeley RM. Br J Surg 1976, 63, 801–806
5. Baddeley RM. pp 293–303 in Maxwell JD, Gazet J-C, Pilkington TRE. (eds.) Surgical Management of Obesity, Academic Press, London, 1980
6. Bloom SR. pp 115–123 in Maxwell JD, Gazet J-C, Pilkington TRE. (eds.) Surgical Management of Obesity, Academic Press, London, 1980
7. Bondar GF, Pisesky W. Arch Surg 1966, 94, 707–716
8. Bray GA. pp. 67–75 in Maxwell JD, Gazet J-C, Pilkington TRE. (eds.) Surgical Management of Obesity, Academic Press, London, 1980
9. Bray GA, Barry RE, Benfield JR, Castelnuovo-Tedesco P, Drenick EJ, Passaro E. Ann Intern Med 1976, 85, 97–109
10. Bray GA, Barry RE, Benfield J, Castelnuovo-Tedesco P, Rodin J. Am J Clin Nutr 1976, 29, 779–783
11. Bray GA, Greenway FL, Barry RE, Benfield JR,

Fiser RL, Dahms WT, Atkinson RL, Schwarz AA. Int J Obesity 1977, 1, 331–367

12. Brown RG, O'Leary JP, Woodward ER. Am J Surg 1974, 127, 53–58

13. Buckwalter JA. Am Surg 1980, 46, 377–381

14. Burney DP, Burnham SJ, Hough AJ, Scott HW. Am Surg 1977, 43, 778–786

15. Butler CM. pp. 209–219 in Maxwell JD, Gazet J-C, Pilkington TRE. (eds.) Surgical Management of Obesity, Academic Press, London 1980

16. Carey JB, Wilson ID, Zaki FG. Medicine (Balt) 1966, 45, 461–470

17. Corrodi P, Wideman PA, Sutter VL, Drenick EJ, Passaro E, Finegold S. J Infect Dis 1978, 137, 1–6

18. Crisp AH, Kalucy RS, Pilkington TRE. Am J Clin Nutr 1977, 30, 109–120

19. Dano P. pp. 137–146 in Maxwell JD, Gazet J-C, Pilkington TRE. (eds.) Surgical Management of Obesity, Academic Press, London 1980

20. Dano P, Lenz K, Justesen T. Scand J Gastroent 1974, 9, 767–774

21. Delaney AG, Duerson MC, O'Leary JP. Int J Obesity 1980, 4, 243–248

22. DeWind LT, Payne JH. JAMA 1976, 236, 2298–2301

23. Drenick EJ, Simmons F, Murphy JF. N Engl J Med 1970, 282, 829–834

24. Dudrick SJ, Daly JM, Castro G, Akhtar M. Ann Surg 1977, 185, 642–648

25. Edmiston CE, Hulsey TK, Scott HW, Hoyumpa AM, Wilson FA. J Infect Dis 1979, 140, 358–369

26. Fenyo G, Backman L, Hallberg D. Acta Chir Scand 1976, 142, 154–159

27. Gaspar MR, Movius HJ, Rosental JJ, Anderson D. Ann Surg 1976, 184, 507–515

28. Gazet J-C, Pilkington TRE, Kalucy RS, Crisp AH, Day S. Br Med J 1974, 4, 311–314

29. Grosfeld JL, Cooney DR, Csicsko JF, Madura JA. Surgery 1976, 80, 201–207

30 Grosfeld JL, Harris RA, Csicsko JF, Cooney DR, Madura JA. Surgery 1977, 81, 701–707

31. Hallberg D, Holmgren U. Acta Chir Scand 1979, 145, 405–408

32. Halverson JD, Scheff RJ, Gentry K, Alpers DH. Am J Surg 1980, 140, 347–350

33. Halverson JD, Wise L, Wazna MF, Ballinger WF. Am J Med 1978, 64, 461–475

34. Hocking MP, Duerson MC, Alexander RW, Woodward ER. Am J Surg 1981, 141, 159–163

35. Hollenbeck JI, O'Leary JP, Maher JW, Woodward ER. Rev Surg 1975, 32, 149–152

36. Holzback RT, Wieland RG, Lieber CS, De Carli LM, Koepke KR, Green S. N Engl J Med 1974, 290, 296–299

37. Hyland G, Stein T, Wise L. Surgery 1977, 81, 578–582

38. Iverson BM, Schjønsby H, Skagen DW, Solhaug JH. Eur J Clin Invest 1976, 6, 355–360.

39. Kremen AJ, Linner JH, Nelson CH. Ann Surg 1954, 140, 439–447

40. Lieber CS. Lipids 1974, 9, 103–107

41. McClelland RN, De Shazo CV, Heimbach DM, Eigenbrodt EH, Dowdy ABC. Surg Forum 1970, 21, 368–370

42. McGill DB, Humpherys SR, Baggenstoss AH, Dickson ER. Gastroenterology 1972, 63, 872–875

43. McGouran RC, Ang L, Maxwell JD. Int J Obesity 1982. In press

44. McGouran RC, Maxwell JD. pp. 159–169 in Maxwell JD, Gazet J-C, Pilkington TRE. (eds.) Surgical Management of Obesity, Academic Press, London 1980

45. McGouran RC, Rutter KP, Ang L, Goldie A, Maxwell JD. Int J Obesity 1982, 6, 197–204

46. Mason EE. pp. 29–39 in Maxwell JD, Gazet J-C, Pilkington TRE. (eds.) Surgical Management of Obesity, Academic Press, London 1980

47. Maxwell JD. pp. 235–255 in Maxwell JD, Gazet J-C, Pilkington TRE. (eds.) Surgical Management of Obesity, Academic Press, London 1980

48. Maxwell JD, Sanderson I, Butler WH, Gazet J-C, Pilkington TRE. Br Med J 1977, 2, 726–729

49. Mezey E, Imbembo AL. Surgery 1978, 83, 345–353

50. Mezey E, Imbembo AL, Potter JJ. Am J Clin Nutr 1975, 28, 1277–1283

51. Moore RB, Frantz ID, Buchwald H. Surgery 1969, 65, 98–108

52. Moxley RT, Pozefsky T, Lockwood DH. N Engl J med 1974, 290, 921–926

53. Nasrallah SM, Wills CE, Galambos JT. Ann Surg 1980, 192, 726–729

54. Nasrallah SM, Wills CE, Galambos JT. Dig Dis Sci 1981, 26, 325–327

55. Nolan JP. N Engl J Med 1978, 299, 1069–1071

56. Nolan JP, Ali MV. Proc Soc Exp Biol Med 1968, 129, 29–31

57. Nygaard K. Acta Chir Scand 1967, 133, 569–583

58. Payne JH, DeWind LT. Am J Surg 1969, 118, 141–147

59. Payne JH, De Wind LT, Commons RR. Am J Surg 1963, 106, 273–289

60. Peters RL, Gay T, Reynolds TB. Am J Clin Pathol 1975, 63, 318–331

61. Pilkington TRE. pp. 171–179 in Maxwell JD, Gazet J-C, Pilkington TRE. (eds.) Surgical Management of Obesity, Academic Press, London 1980

62. Pilkington TRE, Gazet J-C, Ang L, Kalucy RS, Crisp AH, Day S. Brit Med J 1976, 1, 1504–1505

63. Powell-Jackson PR, Maudgal DP, Sharp D, Goldie A, Maxwell JD. Br J Surg 1979, 66, 772–775

64. Printen KJ, Mason EE. Arch Surg 1973, 106, 428–431

65. Quaade F. pp. 317–331 in Maxwell JD, Gazet J-C, Pilkington TRE. (eds.) Surgical Management of Obesity, Academic Press, London 1980

66. Quaade F, Juhl E, Feldt-Rasmussen K, Baden H. Scand J Gastroent 1971, 6, 537–541

67. Rutenberg A, Sonnenblick E, Koven I, Apraham-ian HA, Reiner L, Fine J. J Exptl Med 1957, 106, 1–13

68. Salmon PA, Reedyk L. Surg Gynecol Obstet 1975, 141, 75–84

69. Sclafani A, Koopmans HS, Vasselli JR, Reichman M. Am J Physiol 1978, 234, 389–398

70. Scott HW, Dean R, Shull HJ, Abram HS, Webb W, Younger RK, Brill AB. Ann Surg 1973, 177, 723–735

71. Sherr HP, Nair PP, White JJ. Am J Clin Nutr 1974, 27, 1369–1379
72. Solow C, Silberfarb PM, Swift K. N Engl J Med 1974, 290, 300–304
73. Sorensen TIA, Krag E. Scand J Gastroent 1976, 11, 491–495
74. Spector WG, Heesom N. J Pathol 1969, 98, 31–39
75. Vanderhoof JA, Tuma DJ, Antonson DL, Sorrell MF. Dig Dis Sci 1981, 26, 328–333
76. Viddal KO, Nygaard K. Scand J Gastroent 1978, 13, 891–894
77. Wands JR, LaMont JT, Mann E, Isselbacher KJ. N Engl J Med 1976, 294, 121–124
78. Williamson RCN. N Engl J Med 1978, 298, 1393–1402 and 1444–1450

# Adaptation of the Small Intestine—Does It Occur in Man?

C. A. HUGHES* and D. A. DUCKER†
*Institute of Child Health, Francis Road, Edgbaston, Birmingham B16 8ET
†Department of Child Health, St. George's Hospital, Tooting, London

After resection and usually after shunt operations for obesity, the small bowel in-situ or in-continuity develops mucosal hyperplasia and enhanced absorption per unit length of intestine in animals and man, although the studies in man are limited. The opposite occurs in the small bowel deprived of food either by bypass or total parenteral nutrition (TPN). The changes which occur in the bypassed bowel are not consistent and cannot be explained by the luminal nutrition theory alone. The effect of TPN on jejunal function has been assessed in preterm infants using the one hour blood xylose test and potential difference changes after the infusion of glucose. The results of these tests suggest that the absorptive surface area is diminished during TPN, increases following enteral feeding, and is not related to post-natal age. Function at a cellular level probably remains constant. The mechanism of adaptation is poorly defined in man, but animal studies suggest that in addition to luminal nutrition, other factors such as hormones, and pancreatico-biliary secretions, are important but that there is a fine balance of agonists and antagonists.

*C. A. Hughes, Institute of Child Health, Francis Road, Edgbaston, Birmingham*

## INTRODUCTION

Experiments in animals have shown that morphological and functional changes occur in the small bowel in response to surgical procedures especially extensive resection of the gut (12, 13, 15, 48) and have added greatly to an understanding of the pathophysiology of the short bowel. Studies that have been performed in man (11, 38, 47) are limited, but the results of these studies correlate well with the results of animal experiments which demonstrate that adaptive growth occurs in the intestine remaining in-situ after resection.

Jejuno-ileal bypass, performed for obesity or hyperlipidaemia, although an imperfect model of short bowel syndrome, has enabled jejunal and ileal structure and function following massive resection to be studied further in man. The bypassed loop of bowel has allowed studies to be performed on small bowel which has been deprived of luminal nutrition and pancreatico-biliary secretions, both of which have been shown to be trophic to the intestine (10, 50).

The importance of luminal nutrition in maintaining normal gut structure and function has also been emphasised by experiments using parenterally fed animals (27, 28, 30). To determine whether gut changes similar to those seen in animals not fed orally were also seen in humans, babies born preterm who required feeding by total parenteral nutrition (TPN) were studied before and after commencing enteral feeds. The studies included: one hour blood xylose levels after the intraduodenal instillation of xylose, and potential difference changes following the infusion of differing concentrations of glucose.

The structure and function of the small intestine after adaptation following deprivation of luminal nutrition have been documented in man to a greater or lesser degree. However, the physiology or mechanisms of the adaptive response have been derived mostly from animal experiments.

## PHENOMENA OF ADAPTATION IN MAN

### Short bowel after resection

Clinically, it has been observed that the following factors determine the progress of the patient after a massive intestinal resection: the extent and location of the resected bowel; preservation of the ileo-caecal valve; the functional capacity of the remaining small bowel, stomach, colon, liver and pancreas, and the degree to which the remaining intestine adapts.

The adaptive response in man is apparent by the reduction in stool output and improvement in steatorrhoea which occurs after a period of time varying from weeks to months (52). The adaptation of the shortened bowel in-situ is demonstrated clinically by several stages (36). *Stage 1* is characterised by an initial period of profuse watery stools during which time the patient needs nutritional support which is given parenterally. The diarrhoea decreases as the patient enters *stage II* and is then able to tolerate the introduction of, and gradual increase in, oral intake of nutrients and energy. This stage may last for weeks or even a year or more and may require great patience in management. *Stage III* is the point at which maximum adaptation is reached and many patients are able to regain a normal home existence, tolerating sufficient energy and nutrients taken orally to maintain body weight and function. In infants and children, the ability of the intestine remaining in-situ after a massive resection to undergo adaptation with improve-

ment in function is demonstrated by the commencement of body growth and its gradual increase in velocity. Fig. 1 is an example of the daily weight chart of an infant who had a massive small bowel resection. Initially enteral food was not tolerated; this period of intolerance was followed by a gradual increase in tolerance to food given enterally and finally by the gut undergoing adaptation sufficiently to absorb enough energy, not only to maintain weight, but, also to grow satisfactorily. This is obviously an indirect index of the adaptive response of the gastro-intestinal tract to resection. Clinically, adaptation of the intestine to resection in man is a slow process and takes weeks to months to reach the stage of maximum adaptation. The process in animals appears to be much faster. The adaptive response to resection has been studied in much greater detail in animals than man and there are several recent reviews on the subject (10, 49, 50). The compensatory growth of the small intestine in-situ in man and animals involves all layers of the bowel, and includes dilatation and lengthening of the intestinal remnant, and an increase in villus height and crypt depth due to hyperplasia rather than hypertrophy (9, 12, 13, 35, 47) although one report has

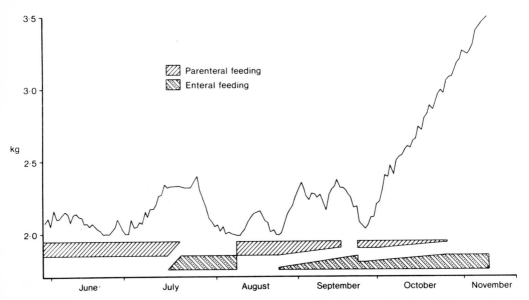

Fig. 1. Weight chart of infant K.E. who required a massive small intestinal resection for multiple atresias and demonstrates that the remaining small bowel adapts sufficiently to absorb energy and nutrients to support body growth.

described smaller enterocytes in the adapted bowel of rats (48). Measurements of the length and cellularity of the villi may under-estimate changes in mucosal surface area (37). This may be one explanation as to why the morphological findings in man are less striking than in animals.

Hyperplasia assessed by villous height measurements and enterocyte counts occurs in man following resection of small bowel of length greater than 50–80% (35). Children, who follow-ing a resection, have intestine remaining in-situ of length 25–120 cm have been shown to have a villus height which is 26 per cent greater than non-resected control children, although the results were not significantly different (38).

Results of absorption studies correlate with the indirect clinical evidence of improvement in symptoms and tolerance to food and show an increased absorption per unit length of intestine. Dowling & Booth (11) reported functional com-pensation by the jejunum in-situ of adult humans following gut resection. In these patients there was a modest increase in glucose absorption which, although modest, was greatest in those patients with the largest amount of intestine

resected. It is probable that the ileum shows a greater compensatory increase in function than the jejunum. In addition to glucose, enhanced intestinal absorption of water and electrolytes has been shown after small bowel resection in man (47).

In infants, the increase in glucose absorption by the intestine in-situ following resection is much greater than in adults. In a recent study of 5 children who had small bowel resections during the neonatal period, Schmitz et al. (38) demon-strated a marked increase in glucose absorption by these children compared with three normal control children, this became more marked as the quantity infused increased (Fig. 2).

One of the criticisms of using glucose to study intestinal function, is that it is, theoretically, metabolised by the enterocytes and therefore an increased luminal disappearance could be due to metabolism by an increased mucosal mass. How-ever, the results of the perfusions are in keeping with the clinical observations.

Sucrose hydrolysis and the activities of brush border hydrolases were also studied in the chil-dren with short bowel (38). Sucrose hydrolysis

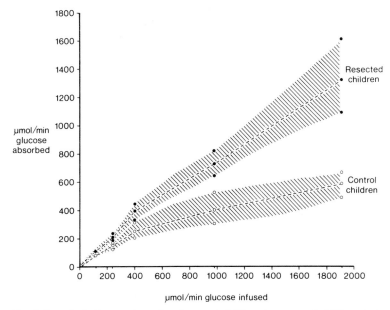

Fig. 2. Intestinal glucose absorption in resected (5) and non-resected (3) control infants. The mean results and range are given. (Data drawn from Schmitz et al. (38).)

correlated well with the glucose absorption studies and showed an increase of 66% in hydrolysis by the children with short bowel compared to the control children. However, there was no difference between the brush border enzyme activities of the bowel of children who had a resection or the control children. These studies correlate well with animal studies which demonstrate an increased absorption or function per unit length of intestine but which is unchanged or possibly decreased when expressed per cell (13).

In addition to an increase in glucose absorption, the absorption of vitamin $B_{12}$ has been shown to be increased after proximal small bowel resection in man probably due to local changes in the ileum (32) with an increase in the number of receptor sites.

It appears that providing the ileo-caecal valve is intact, 15 cm of jejunum and/or ileum is necessary to allow sufficient absorption of energy and nutrients to support life and growth in infants (51) although long term survival has been reported following the loss of the entire jejunum, ileum and ascending colon in man (29). However, the intestine in-situ is extremely difficult to measure and precise measurements have not been obtained.

The response of the intestine in-situ to resection is one of hypertrophy and adaptive growth with improvement in segmental function.

## JEJUNO-ILEAL BYPASS FOR OBESITY

### Bowel in-continuity

The adaptive response in man has been studied to a greater extent in patients with jejuno-ileal bypass. Morphological comparisons have been made between mucosal biopsies obtained at the initial bypass operation and those obtained at re-operation (2, 5, 17, 40, 45) or by peroral biopsies performed on the bowel in-continuity before and at intervals after the operation (6, 23, 41). The excluded segment of bowel has been studied either at re-operation or by taking biopsies using a flexible sigmoidoscope passed along the colon into the distal end of the bypassed loop of bowel (41).

The bowel in-continuity has been shown to

elongate and dilate (17, 23, 41). The jejunum gradually increases in length over a period of 18 months post-operatively, but is more pronounced and rapid in the ileal segment (41). In general, the mucosa has been found to hypertrophy (2, 5, 17, 23, 40, 41) with the villus height increasing in the jejunal remnant by 33 to 55 per cent after six months to one year and in the ileal remnant by 66 to 73 per cent (17, 41). Ninety per cent of the ultimate villus height is probably not reached until at least one year after the construction of the bypass (19). However, in some patients, it has not been possible to show an increase in surface or volume of the villi after surgery (4, 6, 45). Only the jejunum was studied in these patients and it is possible that adaptive hyperplasia occurred in the ileum in-continuity particularly as the weight stabilised after the initial loss following the surgical procedure.

Studies of enzyme activities in the remaining functional jejunum have yielded contradictory results, for example, the disaccharidase activities have been reported to be unchanged (1, 5, 6), increased (2, 42) or decreased (4, 39). Enzyme specific activities may, however, be raised in the functioning ileum in-continuity (1, 2). The interval between the operation and time of study is important, for example, lactase activity was found to be decreased during the first month post-operatively, but to have increased after six months (1, 24). In addition, the specific activities of the enzymes depend upon the protein content of the cell which may depend upon the state of the patient's nutrition at the time of the study. These studies are difficult to interpret and relate only to function at a cellular level, they tell us nothing of segmental activity in the adapted bowel. Studies of segmental absorption in some of those patients who showed no evidence of hyperplasia in the jejunum in-continuity following bypass construction show decreased leucine absorption and unchanged absorption of glycyl leucine (4), decreased (4) or unchanged (18) glucose absorption and an unchanged maltose hydrolysis rate (18), but the studies were performed 6–7 months after bypass surgery, before the maximum adaptive changes have occurred (19).

On the whole, the changes seen in the bowel in-continuity following bypass operations are similar to those observed following massive resection. In other words, the remaining functional bowel shows adaptive growth. There is indirect evidence from the clinical progress, but little direct evidence from studies of enzyme activities and direct intestinal absorption of increased function. The changes are related to the time interval following the initial operation.

The reverse change to that seen in the bowel in-continuity occurs in the bypassed loops. Although studied more fully in animals (13, 20), in general, a similar mucosal response has been seen in the limited studies performed in man.

The results of animal experiments suggest that the mucosa would become hypoplastic (13, 20). This has been observed in human bypassed jejunum (2, 5, 17) and bypassed ileum (41), although this has not been a universal finding for either bypassed jejunum (23, 40, 45) or ileum (5). There are several reasons why the bypassed loop may not show signs of atrophy. The mucosal biopsies may have been taken near to an anastomosis which may have affected the morphology, since studies in rats have shown that the area around an anastomosis becomes hyperplastic (34). Hypoplastic or atrophic changes may have been prevented by the reflux of colonic contents, which includes nutrients, minerals and bacteria, into the bypassed intestine. In addition, atrophic changes in the ileal mucosa are less obvious than in the jejunum since the mucosal thickness of the ileum in its normal environment is considerably less than that of the jejunum. The specific activities of disaccharidases does not appear to be affected by bypass (5) however the specific activities of alkaline phosphatase and thymidine kinase are decreased in the bypassed loops (42).

### Ileal conduits

This surgical manipulation isolates the ileum from gastro-intestinal secretions and nutrients, but it is exposed to fluid which contains nitrogen and minerals. The morphological changes are those of a patchy progressive villous atrophy (7, 21) which may be minimal (8). In these studies

the cell cycle time using tritiated thymidine labelling has been shown to be thirty six hours (8).

### The effect of total parenteral nutrition on the gut

Animal studies have shown that hypoplasia of the small bowel occurs during total parenteral nutrition (TPN) (27, 28, 30) and that the changes are more marked in the jejunum. In rats, hypoplasia, shown by decreased mucosal thickness and diminished wet weight, protein and DNA per unit length of bowel, occurs within three days of commencing TPN (Fig. 3). At the same time, a decrease in absorption per unit length is seen but the disaccharidase specific activities remain unchanged. Thus in animals, luminal nutrition or enteral food is necessary for the maintenance of normal gut structure and function. This has important implications. If the same phenomenon applies to man, it is essential that the gastro-intestinal tract should be deprived of food as little as possible.

### Adaption to extra-uterine life and the effect of food on the gut

To see what effect feeding babies by TPN had on their gut function, xylose absorption and

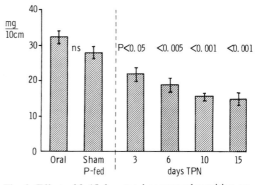

Fig. 3. Effect of 3–15 days total parenteral nutrition on mucosal protein/unit length of jejunum compared with those in conventionally housed orally fed control rats and in a second group of orally fed controls which had intravenous catheters and harnesses and were housed in metabolic cages (sham p-fed controls). Results are mean ± S.E.M. for five to seven rats in each group. The P values refer to the significance of differences between total parenteral nutrition groups and the sham parenterally fed control group of rats. N.S., not significant.

potential difference changes after the infusion of glucose were studied in two groups of preterm neonates, i.e. neonates born before 37 weeks gestation but with a birthweight appropriate for their age.

## PATIENTS STUDIED

Two groups of preterm neonates were studied: A) 5–7 neonates who had been fed by TPN from within the first few days of life because of respiratory problems. The period of TPN varied from 2–26 days. Enteral feeds were not given before or during TPN.
B) 4 preterm neonates fed enterally from birth with breast milk or a modified cows milk formula.

### 1. One hour blood xylose

All patients were given 0.5 g xylose/kg body weight as a 10 per cent solution by transpyloric infusion over five minutes. Group A were studied at the end of the period of TPN, immediately prior to commencing enteral feeds and thereafter

at intervals up to 16 days afterwards as shown in Fig. 4.

Group B were studied within the first week of birth and thereafter at intervals to age 16 days (16 days of enteral feeding). Xylose was assayed as reported previously (14).

### 2. Changes in transmural potential difference (PD) after glucose infusion

Neonates on TPN were studied immediately prior to commencing enteral feeds and the control preterm neonates (Group B) within the first three days of life. Studies were repeated after one week of further enteral feeding.

The technique used has been described previously (33).

Briefly, solutions containing 10 mM, 20 mM, 40 mM D-glucose in 134 mM sodium chloride, made iso-osmolar with mannitol, were infused at 0.05 l/h in an ascending order. Baseline recordings were made by infusing a solution without glucose. Changes in PD were recorded using paired silver–silver chloride electrodes connected to a

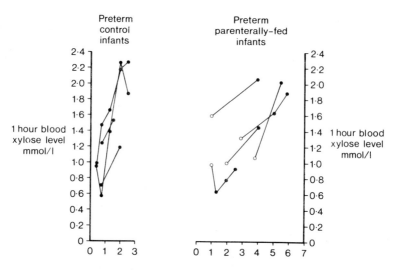

Fig. 4. Results of 1 hour blood D (+) xylose level in individual preterm infants fed enterally or by TPN. The enterally fed control group were studied within three–five days of birth and at intervals to 16 days. The TPN group were studied before, and at intervals to 16 days after commencing enteral nutrition.

Table I. PD$_{max}$ for glucose absorption in preterm infants fed normally and by TPN. Results are means ± S.E.M.

| Preterm infants fed normally | | Preterm infants fed by TPN | |
| --- | --- | --- | --- |
| Within 3 days of birth | After one week of enteral feeding | Before enteral feeding | After one week of enteral feeding |
| 10.9 ± 2.6 mV | 10.4 ± 1.12 mV | 10.9 ± 1.25 mV | 10.13 ± 1.3 mV |

battery powered voltmeter and via an isolation current to a chart recorder. PD max was calculated using Eisenthal–Cornish–Bowden plots.

## RESULTS

The results for the one hour blood xylose levels are shown in Fig. 4 and for the PD$_{max}$ after glucose infusion in Table I.

The one hour blood xylose level increased in both groups of infants after commencing enteral feeding and was not influenced by the post-natal or conceptional age.

The PD$_{max}$ for glucose absorption (Table I) was not affected by enteral feeding or the post-natal or conceptional age.

## COMMENT

The one hour blood xylose was used as a test of xylose absorption and the main reason for selecting its use in the above study was to detect induced changes in the structure of the mucosa. Our previous study (14) showed that the one hour blood xylose level was probably related to the amounts of the pentose reaching the absorption sites when the sugar was infused distal to the pylorus. It appears therefore that the absorption site for xylose increases with enteral feeding. The PD$_{max}$ however, remains unchanged and, on the face of it, appears to contradict the results for xylose absorption. However, the electrode is 'looking at' a very small area and absorption assessed by PD changes may well reflect absorption at a cellular level and not segmental absorption. This pattern of results, with changes in function or absorption segmentally but not at a cellular level has been seen in other models of intestinal adaptation where mostly it has been concluded that

adaptive changes are predominantly due to hypo- or hyperplasia.

Morphological and functional changes in the infant gut are influenced by factors involved in development and maturation but it is not known whether these factors are the same as those which influence the adaptive response of the adult intestine to food intake or surgical procedures.

## MECHANISM OF ADAPTATION IN MAN

So far, the phenomena of intestinal adaptation have been described. The mechanism of these changes has not really been investigated in man, indeed such experiments would be difficult to perform, and therefore it has been necessary to extrapolate from animal experiments, which have included complex surgical manipulations. It is not known whether factors which maintain normal gut structure and function are responsible for the adaptive response. It appears that several factors are involved and there is an interrelationship between these factors.

### Luminal nutrition

This appears to be one of the most important factors in the adaptive response of the intestine following resection in animal experiments (10, 12). The intestine of dogs does not adapt following resection in animals fed exclusively by the parenteral route and from these experiments it has been concluded that luminal nutrition or exogenous food is necessary for the adaptive response of hyperplasia to occur (16). There is little information on the effect of food or luminal nutrition on the shortened bowel following resection in man. In the studies on preterm infants, it appears that food must be given enterally for an increase in gut absorption to occur. Gastrointestinal absorption increases in enterally or normally fed babies with the increase in post-natal age. This does not necessarily apply to the adult patient who has undergone an intestinal resection.

Luminal nutrition is not the only factor which influences gut structure and function. Villous hypertrophy has been demonstrated in the segment of intestine distal to an atresia (44, 46) and therefore this area has not been exposed to food unless a fistula around the atretic segment existed. It is possible that local causes, such as those producing hyperplasia around an anastomosis (34), or denervation producing an increase in local perfusion (46) or the placenta supplying 'hyperalimentation' were responsible for the changes. These factors could have 'over ridden' the effect of absent luminal nutrients.

Patients who have undergone bypass surgery are the group of patients which have been studied most. However, it would be expected that the bypassed loop of bowel, deprived of luminal nutrition would atrophy, but this has not been the universal finding. It is due to the fact that the loop is not completely isolated and drains into the bowel but the reason for this observation is not clear. In some instances, the findings may have been due to the sampling site chosen but this does not explain the results in every case. This also suggests that factors other than luminal nutrition are important in maintaining gut structure, e.g. hormones.

### Hormones

Experiments in rats have shown that oral feeding compared with TPN partially prevents the mucosal atrophy which occurs in isolated intestine even when the bypassed intestine was not exposed to luminal nutrition (15). This argues strongly for a circulatory hormone being the factor responsible for partially maintaining gut structure.

The hormone(s) which produce a trophic effect on the gut are not known. Gastrin has been investigated as a candidate trophic hormone. In animals it has been shown to be trophic to the very proximal small bowel (28) but not in man. In man, circulating gastrin levels, although raised in some patients following resection have not been found to be raised in others and there are a few inconsistencies (50). Enteroglucagon is likely to be a trophic hormone (10, 50) but confirmation of its trophicity will have to wait until sufficient quantities can be obtained for infusion studies.

There is very little knowledge of the effect of hormones in maintaining normal gut structure and function. During TPN, given that the human gut behaves in a similar manner to that of experimental animals, it could be expected that trophic hormone levels would be low and/or hormone(s) with an anti-trophic effect would be high. Studies in human adults on TPN have recently shown that the fasting and post prandial gut endocrine reponse is well maintained (22). However, patients on TPN would not experience the post prandial release which may be important in maintaining gut structure and function. Until we have more knowledge of the effect of excluding luminal nutrition from patients by feeding them with TPN, it is impossible to assess the relationship between gut hormones and gut structure and function.

We know that intestinal function inproves in the post-natal period when the infant receives luminal nutrition. Studies have also shown that, after birth, there is a marked elevation in basal plasma gut hormone concentrations and that these changes are progressive (3, 31). It is probable that enteral feeding is the trigger for the hormonal surges. The role played by these hormones in the post-natal adaptive response of the intestine to enteral feeding is not known.

### Pancreatico-biliary secretions

Pancreatico-biliary secretions have been shown to be trophic to the intestine in animals (10, 50) and the daily stimulation of pancreatico-biliary secretions by CCK and secretin during TPN prevents the hypoplasia of the intestinal mucosa usually seen in animals fed in this way (26). Their role as a trophic factor in man has not been determined.

Whether pancreatic adaptation to resection, bypass or absent luminal nutrition occurs in man is not known. Pancreatic hyperplasia has been shown to occur in rats after massive intestinal resection (25) but whether this was associated with increased pancreatic secretion is not known.

If pancreatic hyperplasia and increased secretion occurs in man, it is one mechanism whereby the reduced total enzyme activities in the intestine could be compensated for, and one reason for the improvement in steatorrhoea weeks to months after the operation.

## OTHER FACTORS

Other factors which may influence the structure and function of the intestine are neurovascular and bacterial but the role played by them in adaptation in man is undefined, even more so than the roles of hormones.

## CONCLUSION

Compensatory hypertrophy occurs following resection of the gastro-intestinal tract probably as a result of interrelated luminal and systemic factors, which may include both agonists and antagonists. Whether, the same factors are involved in the maintenance of normal gut structure and function and whether the hypoplasia which results from absent or diminished luminal nutrition is due to an alteration in the integrated system, is undetermined.

## ACKNOWLEDGEMENTS

We thank Professor A. S. McNeish and Mr. G. Aucott, Department of Medical Physics, Leicester Royal Infirmary and Institute of Child Health for their help and Mrs. J. Fleming for typing the manuscript.

## REFERENCES

1. Asp NG, Gudmand-Høyer E, Andersen B. Scand J Gastroenterol 1979,14,469–473
2. Asp NG, Gudmand-Høyer E, Andersen B, Berg NO. Gut 1979, 20, 553–558
3. Aynsley-Green A, Bloom SR, Williamson DH, Turner RC. Arch Dis Child 1977, 52, 291–295
4. Barry RE, Barisch J, Bray GA, Sperling MA, Morin RJ, Benfield J. Amer J Clin Nutr 1977, 30, 32–42
5. Daly GM, Castro GA, Akhtar M, Dudrick SJ. Gastroenterology 1977, 72, 1042 & Ann Surg 1977, 185, 642–648
6. Dano P, Nielson OV, Petri M, Jorgensen B. Scand J Gastroenterol 1976, 11, 129–134
7. Deschner EE, Goldstein MJ, Melamed MR, Sherlock P. Gastroenterology 1973, 64, 920–925
8. Deschner EE, Goldstein MJ, Melamed MR, Sherlock P. Gastroenterology 1976, 71, 832–834
9. Dowling RH. MD Thesis, Belfast 1968
10. Dowling RH. pp. 251–261 in Peters DK (ed) 12 Symposium in Advanced Medicine, 1976 Pitman Medical, London
11. Dowling RH, Booth CC. Lancet 1966, 11, 146–147
12. Dowling RH, Booth CC. Clin Sci 1967, 32, 139–149
13. Dowling RH, Gleeson MH. Digestion 1973, 8, 176–190
14. Ducker DA, Hughes CA, Warren I, McNeish AS. Gut 1980, 21, 133–136
15. Dworkin LD, Levine GM, Farber NJ, Spector MH. Gastroenterology 1976, 71, 626–630
16. Feldman EJ, Dowling RH, MacNaughton J, Peters TJ. Gastroenterology 1976, 70, 712–719
17. Fenyo G, Backman L, Hallberg D. Acta Chir Scand 1976, 142, 154–159
18. Fogel MR, Ravitch MM, Adibi SA. Gastroenterology 1976, 71, 729–733
19. Friedman HI, Chandler JG, Peck CC, Nemeth TJ, Odum SK. Surg Gynecol Obstet 1978, 146, 757–767
20. Gleeson MH, Cullen J, Dowling RH. Clin Sci 1972, 43, 731–742
21. Goldstein MJ, Melamed MR, Grabstald H, Sherlock P. Gastroenterology 1967, 52, 859–864
22. Greenberg GR, Wolman SL, Christofides ND, Bloom SR, Jeejeebhoy KN. Gastroenterology 1981, 80, 988–993
23. Grenier JF, Eloy MR, Jaeck D, Dauchel J. Chirurgie 1974, 100, 59–65
24. Gudmand-Høyer E, Asp NG, Skovbjerg H, Andersen B. Scand J Gastroenterol 1978, 13, 641–647
25. Haegel P, Stock C, Marescaux J, Petit B, Grenier JF. Gut 1981, 22, 207–212
26. Hughes CA, Bates T, Dowling RH. Gastroenterology 1978, 75, 34–41
27. Hughes CA, Dowling RH. Clin Sci 1980, 59, 317–327
28. Johnson LR, Copeland EM, Dudrick SJ, Lichtenberger GM, Castro GA. Gastroenterology 1975, 68, 1177–1183
29. Kinney JM, Goldwyn RM, Barr JS. JAMA 1962, 179, 529–532
30. Levine GM, Deren JJ, Steiger E, Zinno R. Gastroenterology 1974, 67, 975–982
31. Lucas A, Adrian TE, Christofides ND, Bloom SR, Aynsley-Green A. Arch Dis Child 1980, 55, 673–677
32. Mackinnon AM, Short MD, Elias E, Dowling RH. Dig Dis 1975, 20, 835–839
33. McNeish AS, Ducker DA, Warren IF, Davies DP, Harran MJ, Hughes CA. pp. 267–276 in Ciba Foundation Symposium 20 (new series) Development of Mammalian Absorptive Processes. Excerpta Medica Amsterdam, 1979
34. Nygaard K. Acta Chir Scand 1966, 132, 731–742
35. Porus RL. Gastroenterology 1965, 48, 753–757
36. Pullan JM. Proc Roy Soc Med 1959, 52, 31–37

37. Robinson JWL, Menge H, Schroeder P, Riecken EO, Van Melle G. Eur J Clin Inv 1980, 10, 393–399

38. Schmitz J, Rey F, Bresson JL, Ricour C, Rey J. Arch Fr Pediatr 1980, 37, 491–495

39. Skovbjerg H, Gudmand-Høyer E, Noren O, Sjostrom H. Gut 1980, 21, 662–668

40. Solhaug JH. Scand J Gastroenterol 1976, 11, 155–160

41. Solhaug JH, Tvetes S. Scand J Gastroenterol 1978, 13, 401–408

42. Stein TA, Wise L. Am J Clin Nut 1978, 31, 1143–1148

43. Tilson MD. Arch Surg 1972, 104, 69–72

44. Tilson MD. Am J Surg 1972, 123, 733–734

45. Tompkins RK, Waisman J, Watt CMH, Corlin R, Keith R. Gastroenterology 1977, 73, 1406

46. Touloukian RM, Wright HK. J Pediatr Surg 1973, 779–784

47. Weinstein LD, Shoemaker CP, Hersh T, Wright HK. Arch Surg 1969, 99, 560–562

48. Weser E, Hernandez MH. Gastroenterology 1971, 60, 69–75

49. Williamson RCN. N Eng J Med 1978, 298, 1393–1402

50. Williamson RCN. N Eng J Med 1978, 298, 1444–1450

51. Wilmore DW. J Pediatr 1972, 80, 88–95

52. Winawer SJ, Broitman SA, Wolochaw DA, Osborne MP, Zamcheck N. N Eng J Med 1966, 274, 72–78

# Subject Index

# Date Due